Radiation Carcinogenesis and DNA Alterations

NATO ASI Series

Advanced Science Institutes Series

A series presenting the results of activities sponsored by the NATO Science Committee, which aims at the dissemination of advanced scientific and technological knowledge, with a view to strengthening links between scientific communities.

The series is published by an international board of publishers in conjunction with the NATO Scientific Affairs Division

A	**Life Sciences**	Plenum Publishing Corporation
B	**Physics**	New York and London
C	**Mathematical and Physical Sciences**	D. Reidel Publishing Company Dordrecht, Boston, and Lancaster
D	**Behavioral and Social Sciences**	Martinus Nijhoff Publishers
E	**Engineering and Materials Sciences**	The Hague, Boston, Dordrecht, and Lancaster
F	**Computer and Systems Sciences**	Springer-Verlag
G	**Ecological Sciences**	Berlin, Heidelberg, New York, London,
H	**Cell Biology**	Paris, and Tokyo

Series A: Life Sciences

Radiation Carcinogenesis and DNA Alterations

Edited by

F. J. Burns and

A. C. Upton

New York University Medical Center
New York, New York

and

G. Silini

U.N. Scientific Committee on the Effects of Atomic Radiation
Vienna, Austria

Plenum Press
New York and London
Published in cooperation with NATO Scientific Affairs Division

Proceedings of a NATO Advanced Study Institute on
Radiation Carcinogenesis and DNA Alterations,
held October 7–20, 1984,
in Corfu, Greece

Library of Congress Cataloging in Publication Data

NATO Advanced Study Institute on Radiation Carcinogenesis and DNA Alterations (1984: Kerkyra, Corfu)
    Radiation carcinogenesis and DNA alterations.

    (NATO ASI series. Series A, Life sciences; v. 124)
    "Proceedings of a NATO Advanced Study Institute on Radiation Carcinogen-
esis and DNA Alterations, held October 7–20, 1984, in Corfu, Greece"—T.p. verso.
    Includes bibliographies and index.
    1. Tumors, Radiation-induced—Genetic aspects—Congresses. 2. Deoxyribo-
nucleic acids—Effect of radiation on—Congresses. 3. Mutation (Biology)—Con-
gresses. 4. Human chromosome abnormalities—Congresses. I. Burns, F. J.
(Fredric J.) II. Upton, Arthur C., 1923–   . III. Silini, G. IV. Title. V. Series.
[DNLM: 1. DNA—radiation effects—congresses. 2. Neoplasms, Radiation-
Induced—congresses. QZ 200 N287r 1984]
RC268.55.N37   1984   616.99′4′071   87-2224
ISBN 0-306-42495-9

© 1986 Plenum Press, New York
A Division of Plenum Publishing Corporation
233 Spring Street, New York, N.Y. 10013

Printed in the United States of America

PREFACE

This volume is based on the proceedings of an Advanced Study Institute (ASI) sponsored by the North Atlantic Treaty Organization (NATO) held October 1984 in Corfu, Greece. The meeting received financial support from the United States Department of Energy and the United States National Cancer Institute.

A plethora of recent developments in the molecular biology of DNA are leading to new ideas concerning how DNA alterations might be involved in the mechanism of radiation carcinogenesis. Evidence is accumulating that genetic sequences, known as oncogenes, are involved in the translation of DNA molecular alterations into phenotypic changes associated with malignant cells.

For example, a chromosome break often occurs at or near the location of a specific oncogene in Burkitt's lymphoma. Such breaks could represent initial lesions in a translocation process that activates the oncogene by inserting it at a new location, eg., near an active promoter. Since breakage of the DNA is one of the principal ways that ionizing radiation affects mammalian cells, these new molecular ideas suggest ways that radiation-induced DNA breaks might be involved as initial events in carcinogenesis.

While the possible involvement of oncogenes in radiation carcinogenesis is an exciting new development, a direct sequential connection between early molecular changes in DNA and later tumor development has yet to be established. Accordingly, there is a tremendous need for experimental studies of how DNA alterations might convert normal cells to cancer cells.

One purpose of the Corfu meeting was to bring together people working on the molecular biology of radiation-induced DNA damage with others interested in the mechanisms of radiation carcinogenesis. Participants at the meeting, as well as the designated faculty, were encouraged to make informal presentations of their work, and many of these are included in the current volume. The book is organized into general subject areas, each containing a number of chapters. Within each subject area, review chapters are located at the beginning, and the research-type contributions are located closer to the end.

Pleasant memories of the meeting itself still linger, including recollections of the excitement of productive discussions among people with diverse interests and backgrounds. We hope that some of the excitement has been captured in the contents of the current volume. The editors warmly thank all contributors who so willingly shared their knowledge and ideas. We also thank Mary Bader for typing the manuscript in its entirety and Michael Snow for expertly applying the finishing touches.

Fredric J. Burns
Arthur C. Upton
Giovanni Silini

September 1986

CONTENTS

CARCINOGENESIS IN HUMANS AND ANIMALS

TRANSFORMATION IN VITRO

ULTRAVIOLET RADIATION

DNA STRAND BREAKS AND CHROMOSOME ALTERATIONS

NON-STOCHASTIC AND CELL CYCLE EFFECTS

MODELS OF RADIATION CARCINOGENESIS

FOLLOW-UP STUDIES OF PATIENTS TREATED BY X-RAY EPILATION FOR TINEA CAPITIS

R. E. Albert*, R. E. Shore*, N. Harley* and A. Omran**

*Department of Environmental Medicine
Institute of Environmental Medicine
New York University Medical Center
550 First Avenue
New York, N.Y. 10016
**School of Public Health
University of North Carolina
Chapel Hill, North Carolina 27514

INTRODUCTION

Tinea capitis is one of the most common fungal diseases of children. It has been a major public health problem in many countries and is especially prevalent in low socioeconomic groups (1). In the United States, tinea capitis was relatively uncommon until a major epidemic occurred throughout the country during World War II (2). Treatment for ringworm of the scalp by X-ray epilation was introduced by Sabouraud in 1904 and standardized by Kienbock in 1907 (3) and Adamson in 1910 (4). The purpose of the epilation was to permit effective fungal decontamination of the scalp. Before the Adamson-Kienbock X-ray procedure was introduced, epilation was done manually. Exposure of the scalp produced complete epilation in approximately two to three weeks which lasted one to two months (5). X-ray epilation proved to be much superior to the alternative forms of topical therapy and was widely used until the introduction of griseofulvin in 1958. No accurate figures exist for the total number of children treated by X-ray epilation during the one-half century of its use. On a worldwide basis, it is possible that as many as 200,000 children have received this form of irradiation (1).

In spite of the large population and the substantial radiation exposures of scalp, bone marrow, brain, and other head structures associated with X-ray epilation, until recently only a few follow-up studies have been made to characterize the nature and magnitude of delayed radiation damage; such studies have been concerned almost entirely with the effects on the scalp. Amongst the early studies a one-year follow-up by Beare (6) and a 5-year follow-up by Thorne (7) reported no evidence of scalp damage. Studies involving longer post-treatment periods by Berlin (8) and Symann (9) did show a low incidence of hair damage and Symann's study raised the possibility of mental retardation in the irradiated cases.

A follow-up study of irradiated and nonirradiated tinea capitis cases treated at the Skin and Cancer Unit of the New York University (NYU) Hospital between 1940 and 1959 was initiated in 1962. The purpose of the study was to determine whether X-ray epilation produced chronic radiation injury and to relate the nature and magnitude of any observed effects to the radiation dose received by the various structures of the head.

DOSIMETRY (10, 11, 12)

The X-ray treatment was given using the standard Adamson-Kienbock procedure (4), in which an exposure of 300-380 R of 180 KeV, unfiltered X-rays was given to five overlapping fields on the scalp so as to cause complete temporary epilation. The treatment protocol was highly standardized, with all five exposure being administered in a uniform order within the space of 10-20 minutes. Nearly all treatments at NYU were given by one technician, who was highly skilled and methodical in her procedures. The child was prone for all treatments and rotated as necessary for different exposure fields. Correct placement of the X-ray port was achieved with the aid of a "tinea treatment cap" fashioned from steel bands, each field being joined together. Three different sized caps were used to accommodate different head sizes. The position for each field was then marked on the child's shaved head before treatment. Sandbags were placed around the head to help minimize the child's potential for movement during the exposure. Head surfaces other than the scalp were protected by lead shielding. Lead foil 0.36 mm thick was taped over the ears and eyes. A large sheet of the same foil was cut to shape around the edge of the hairline to protect all except the scalp from the direct X-ray beam in the anterior and lateral positions. For the vertical and posterior irradiation positions the lead foil was not present, but a lead impregnated rubber apron was placed over the lower neck and shoulders for all five positions.

X-ray equipment operating between 60 and 100 kvp was used for this treatment. In order to achieve high output, which was very important since short treatment times were essential, and also a rapid fall-off in depth dose only the inherent filtration of the X-ray tube was employed. Treatment distances varied between 20 and 30 cm mainly in order to retain high output. Inasmuch as epilation had to be complete for successful results, the X-ray field sizes were sufficiently large so that there was considerable overlapping of adjacent treatment fields. All of these factors combine to make the radiation dosimetry of the tinea capitis treatment quite complicated.

The head phantom used in the estimation for the doses to the head structures consisted of the skull of a 7-year-old child covered with a tissue-equivalent wax to simulate the head and neck. The top section of the skull was removable and a simulated brain filled the entire skull volume. The simulated brain was constructed of masonite and tissue-equivalent wax. The average doses to the head structures are shown in Table 1. The effects of the lead shield placed below the hair line and the unbalanced vertical field produced a dosage gradient from about 75 rad at the base of the brain to 165 rad at the apical region. The average dose recorded by the 15 dosimeters for the standard five field treatment, 370 R exposure per field, was 140 rad. The scalp doses were measured at 30 locations. The regional distribution of the scalp dose is shown together with the skin tumor locations in Figure 1.

Table 1. Dose to the organs of the head and neck during a typical
          tinea capitis treatment

Organ	Average Dose at 25 cm TSD (rad)	Average Dose at 20 cm TSD (rad)
Scalp	220-540	
Brain	140	
Eye	16±2	
Internal Ear	71	
Cranial Marrow	385	
Pituitary	49±6	49±2
Thyroid	6±2	3±0.2
Thyroid Maximum Credible*	9	
Skin (eyelid)	16±2	
Skin (nose)	11±2	
Skin (mid-neck region)	9±2	
Parotid Gland	39±9	

*Dose determine assuming leaded rubber apron slipped from neck when
 under the lead foil.

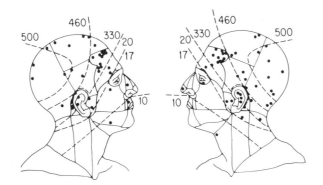

Fig. 1.   X-ray dose in rads for tinea treatment and
          location of basal cell lesions.

CHARACTERISTICS OF THE TINEA CAPITIS POPULATION AVAILABLE FOR STUDY
(13)

     The recovery of irradiated case charts from the clinic files was
greatly facilitated by a registry that had been maintained in the X-ray
Department of the Skin and Cancer Unit of the New York University Hospital.
Charts of nonirradiated tinea capitis cases were winnowed from the clinic
files. The population available for study therefore included virtually all
the tinea capitis cases seen at the NYU Skin and Cancer Unit between 1940
and 1959. No cases prior to 1940 were available because the charts had
been discarded, while X-ray treatment was not used beyond 1959 because of

Table 2. Clinic population

	Irradiated	Nonirradiated
White	1832	1358
Male	1548	1047
Female	284	311
Black	572	436
Male	522	362
Female	50	74
Total Male	2070	1409
Total Female	334	385
Total Cases	2404	1794
% Male	86	79
% White	76	76
% Black	24	24

the introduction of griseofulvin. Of the 4,198 tinea capitis cases treated during the 1940-59 time interval at the NYU Hospital Skin and Cancer Unit, 2,404 cases received X-ray epilation and 1,794 were treated by other methods.

Table 2 shows the tinea capitis case census at the Skin and Cancer Unit during the target years stratified according to treatment, race, and sex. The peak load of tinea capitis cases occurred near the end of World War II: 48% of irradiated cases and 53% of the nonirradiated cases were treated within the four-year period, 1943 through 1947. The use of X-ray epilation over the 19-year period was fairly constant. An average of 57% of the tinea capitis cases were irradiated, with extremes of 49% (during 1943 to 1945) and 74% from 1954 to 1955. The sex distribution of cases remained relatively constant over the years with a marked predominance of males, averaging 86% in the irradiated and 79% in the control groups. There was also a marked predominance of whites, averaging about 75% for both the irradiated and control groups. From 1952 onward, however, there was a progressive increase in the proportion of blacks in the irradiated and control groups, reaching 55% to 60% in 1958. This shift was undoubtedly due to the change in the ethnic character of the local population.

The subjects were from one to 19 years of age at the time of their tinea treatment, with 98% of the irradiated group and 92% of controls in the age range 3-13 years. (Those under the age of three were less likely to be treated with X-rays.) The mean age ($\pm$ standard deviation) at treatment was 7.9 ± 2.5 years in the irradiated group and 7.5 ± 3.1 years in the control group.

The socioeconomic status of a random sample of 1,359 irradiated and 1,021 control cases was compared on the basis of the family income reported on the clinic admission cards at the time of treatment. The reported incomes, normalized to the 1957-1959 consumer price index for the New York City area, were equally low at approximately $3,200.

Table 3. Distribution of cases according to treatment group, race, and sex

	Irradiated No.	Irradiated %	Nonirradiated No.	Nonirradiated %
White				
Male	1326	64.9	824	58.3
Female	226	11.1	241	17.1
Black				
Male	451	22.1	287	20.3
Female	40	2.0	61	4.3
Total				
Male	1777	87.0	1111	78.6
Female	266	13.0	302	21.4
Total				
White	1552	76.0	1065	75.4
Black	491	24.0	384	27.2
Total Cases	2043	100.0	1413	100.0

MAIL SURVEYS OF THE POPULATIONS (13, 14, 15, 16)

The irradiated and control groups have been followed up with three rounds of mailed questionnaires during 1962-66, 1968-73, and 1975-79 to ascertain their health status, as well as to provide further information on sociodemographic characteristics.

The location methods included: (a) certified mailings to the address shown in the patient's clinic chart; (b) the use of telephone directories (both name and address) for locating the patient, his relatives, or neighbors; (c) the use of school records for information about change of family residence; (d) the use of private and governmental agency records, e.g., Social Service Exchange, State Motor Vehicle Bureaus; and (e) neighborhood inquiries by field workers.

In the first survey 85% of the irradiated cases and 79% of the nonirradiated cases were located. There was no difference between the irradiated and nonirradiated groups with respect to the type of case-finding method which was successful. The frequency distributions of race and sex in the located and nonlocated irradiated and control cases were almost identical. The distribution of cases according to treatment group, race, and sex is shown in Table 3. Both the irradiated and control cases averaged 23 years of age at contact.

Table 4 shows that the located and nonlocated irradiated and control groups were comparable with respect to fungus infection diagnoses with almost all of the irradiated cases (96.4%) having had M. audouini infections due to the predominance of these infections in the clinic population as a whole and the infrequent use of X-ray epilation in the patients with M. lanosum infection.

Health Questionnaires

Questionnaires were sent by mail with a letter indicating that the purpose of the study was to determine the late health effects of ringworm of the scalp. The relevance of the study to possible radiation injury was

Table 4. Percentage of cases with the indicated fungus diagnosis
          according to treatment group

Fungus	Irradiated	Nonirradiated
Audouini	96.4	69.0
Lanosum	2.0	23.8
Other	1.4	7.0

not mentioned. The questionnaire solicited information on birth date,
occupation, height, weight, and martial status. A series of illnesses was
listed in the questionnaire and the patient was instructed to check "yes,"
"no," or "don't know" after each item. The list included illnesses
unrelated to possible radiation sequelae in order to mask the purpose of
the study. Another check list was included for previous medical and
surgical treatments as well as radium or X-ray therapy.

The patients were asked to provide the name of the hospital and
physician involved in the treatment of each illness. The physicians and
hospitals were contacted to obtain confirmatory diagnoses and medical
records. Attempts were made to obtain the death certificates for deceased
cases.

In the first survey patients were asked about their treatment for
scalp ringworm. Only a small proportion of the patients (6.5% and 10.0% of
the irradiated and control cases, respectively), denied that they had
attended the NYU Skin and Cancer Unit for treatment of ringworm of the
scalp. However, 33% of the irradiated patients indicated they had not
received X-ray therapy at the Skin and Cancer Unit, and 23% of the
nonirradiated patients said that they had been given X-ray treatment.
Thus, the majority of irradiated patients or their parents were aware of
having received X-ray epilation, but some of the nonirradiated patients
also thought they had been irradiated.

The percent of irradiated and control subjects who either completed a
questionnaire or were known dead were 85 and 79 respectively in the first
survey, with almost all of the remainder being unlocatable. The
corresponding percents were 89 and 90 in the second survey, and 89 and 83
in the third survey. (The discrepancy in the last rates occurred largely
by error; after study termination it was discovered that a batch of 4% of
the control subjects had inadvertently been filed away without having had
adequate location efforts.)

The treatment, sociodemographic, and life-style characteristics of the
irradiated and controls groups in the third survey, which were typical of
those on the earlier surveys as well, are shown in Table 5. The mean age
at latest follow-up was about 33 years for both groups, and the mean
follow-up interval was 25-26 years. Thus, the length of follow-up and ages
were very similar for these groups. The two treatment groups were
comparable in race, with both being about 25% black, but there were
proportionately fewer females in the irradiated group (13%) than in the
control group (21%).

Table 5. Characteristics of the irradiated and control groups

	Irradiated	Control
Age at Tinea Treatment ($\bar{X}$, yr.)*	7.9±2.5	7.5±3.1
At at Last Follow-up ($\bar{X}$, yr.)	33.6±7.1	32.7±7.9
Interval between Treatment and Follow-up ($\bar{X}$, yr.)	25.7±6.5	25.2±7.0
Ringworm Genus: Audouini (%)	95.9	69.2
Sex: Female (%)	12.9	21.3
Race: Black (%)	24.5	25.7
Ethnicity: Irish (%)	17.4	15.7
Italian (%)	18.4	19.2
Jewish (%)	10.5	10.7
Birthplace: Ouside of New York Metropolitan Area (%)	22.0	13.2
Married (%)	68.9	65.9
Education ($\bar{X}$, yr.)	13.6±2.8	13.3±2.8
Occupational Status: Managerial, Professional, Technical (%)	33.6	28.1
Occupational Status: Laborer, Unskilled Service (%)	14.9	15.7
Bureau of Census Socioeconomic Index ($\bar{X}$)**	6.5±1.7	6.3±1.7
Average Length of Time Jobs Held ($\bar{X}$, yr.)	7.1±8.3	6.9±8.1
Smoke (%)	56.0	56.9
Alcohol Use: Moderate to Heavy (%)	23.6	23.2
Drug Use: Regular (Past or Present (%)	5.3	5.2
Name of Subject	226	1387

*Mean ±S.D. is given when X is indicated.
**Based on education and occupation

The educational, occupational, and socioeconomic indices showed that the groups were similar, but the irradiated group had a slightly higher socioeconomic status. Marital status was comparable in the two groups. The personal habits--smoking, drinking and drug use--were almost identical in the irradiated and control groups. There were 48,193 person-years at risk in the irradiated group and 29,252 person-years in the control group. However, at latest follow-up the irradiated group was still young; there were few person-years at risk over the age of 40.

Illness Reported by Patients

In the first survey, no significant differences in the responses of the irradiated and control cases were observed in 15 of the 18 reported-illness categories. Significantly higher responses were obtained in the following categories: neuropsychiatric, scalp and hair, and cysts. The prevalence of reported neuropsychiatric disorders was 9.5% in the irradiated group compared to 5.3% in the controls. Cysts of various types and locations were reported by 9.3% of the irradiated cases compared to 6.4% in the controls. The incidence was especially high for cysts (and tumors) of the scalp. Baldness and hair thinning were reported by 12.3% of the irradiated group and 5.7% of the nonirradiated group. The contrasts between the two groups on the second survey were similar to those found on the first questionnaire survey, but with the addition of trends in elevated rates of thyroid tumors, central nervous system (CNS) tumours and skin cancer, which will be discussed below.

In the remainder of the paper, we will present and discuss the findings concerning the principal categories of disease which were elevated in the irradiated group, along with the clinical evaluation programs which were conducted to learn more about possible late radiation sequeallae.

Psychiatric Disorders

In the first survey, the incidence of medically verified psychiatric disorders of all types was 2.5 times higher in the irradiated cases compared to the controls (3.2% and 1.3%, respectively). This difference was statistically significant p <0.01).

Further cases of psychiatric disorders were accumulated during the second survey. Analyses of the cumulative diagnosed psychiatric disorders were conducted, controlling for race, sex, socioeconomic status, age at tinea treatment, and interval from treatment to diagnosis. There was a 30% excess of psychiatric disorders in the irradiated group overall. To further explore the validity of this result, the consistency of the relative risk (RR) within subgroups was examined. This revealed a distinct difference between blacks and whites. Adjusted RR among whites was 1.40 but among blacks was only 1.07 for treated psychiatric disorders. Among whites the irradiated group had consistently higher rates for each category of psychiatric disorder--psychoses, neuroses, and personality disorders. A life-table analysis showed that, among the white sample, an increase in psychiatric disorders in the irradiated groups developed over the 30 year span, but among blacks, the irradiated and control groups did not differ in any consistent way.

Several indirect indicators of emotional disorders were also examined in the second survey. Possible psychosomatic illnesses were evaluated. The groups did not differ in the incidence of peptic ulcer, hypertension or asthma (verification of allergies and headaches proved to be too unreliable for use). Neither did they differ in the prevalence of reported criminal infractions, drug abuse, or alcoholism. The groups were comparable in military status. Of the males with draft classifications, 16% in both groups were classified 1Y or 4F. In both groups, dishonorable or bad conduct discharges were found in 2.7% of those with military service. Thus, the two groups did not differ in the prevalence of indirect markers of emotional disorders.

In the third survey further psychiatric diagnoses were obtained, for a total of 186 treated cases in the irradiated group and 79 among controls, of whom 64 and 30, respectively, were hospitalized. Based on a life-table tabulation, the cumulative incidence of treated psychiatric disorders by 35 years post-irradiation was 10.6% ± 0.8 percent and 7.4 ± 0.8 percent among controls. The relative risk was 1.44 (90% confidence limits of 1.14-1.82, p <0.01), with race, sex, socioeconomic status, and interval since irradiation controlled. Thus, there was a continuing, though small, excess of treated psychiatric disorders in the irradiated group. The difference in rates of hospitalized psychiatric disorders was not significant, probably owing to the smaller numbers of cases.

Clinical Psychiatric and Psychometric Evaluation (17)

The findings of apparent differences between the groups in frequency of psychiatric disorders led to the development of a clinical protocol to examine differences in psychiatric function in more detail.

A psychiatric and psychrometric evaluation was performed on 109 irradiated cases and 68 controls. Each individual was tested with the Minnesota Multiphasic Personality Inventory (MMPI) and interviewed by one psychiatrist using a standardized semi-structured format. All the subjects were male; 25 irradiated and 24 control cases were black and the remainder white.

The mean intervals between tinea treatment and clinical evaluation for the white, male irradiated and control groups were 19 and 21 years, respectively, while the intervals for the respective black groups were 16 and 17 years. The groups were compared for age, education, occupation, marital status, and religion. Among blacks the irradiated and control groups did not differ, but among whites the irradiated cases were younger (30% vs. 58% over the age of 30), more often single (51% vs. 31%), and better educated (45% vs. 29% with some college education) than the control group.

Analyses which controlled for educational level and family psychiatric disorders showed that, among whites, the irradiated group manifested more psychiatric symptoms and more deviant MMPI profiles. They were also (blindly) judged more maladjusted from their MMPI profiles, and more frequently had a history of treated psychiatric disorders; however, the psychiatrist's overall rating of current psychiatric status showed only a borderline difference between the two groups. There were no significant differences between irradiated and control blacks.

CLINICAL EXAMINATIONS (1965-1967) (18)

Because of concern over possible damage to the scalp and other organs of the head, as suggested by the first questionnaire survey, a medical examination program was conducted.

The purpose of these examinations was to determine whether there was any objective evidence of chronic radiation injury in the irradiated tinea capitis cases, e.g., alopecia of the scalp, lenticular opacities of the eye, neurological and auditory disturbances, and hematological abnormalities.

In addition to the specialized clinical examinations of the scalp, eye, and ear, general physical examinations were done to detect abnormalities which might otherwise be overlooked. Measurements were obtained of height, weight, blood pressure, and visual acuity. Specimens were taken for hematologic and hair studies.

The population that attended the clinic included 319 irradiated cases and 2 control groups totaling 285 cases. One control group consisted of

127 nonirradiated tinea capitis cases in the study, and the second control group consisted of 158 volunteers from neighborhood boys and girls clubs who had no history of either tinea capitis or X-ray therapy.

Most of the cases in the irradiated and tinea-control groups were male (86% to 89%), and about 85% were whites. The nontinea controls were also predominately male (70%) and almost all whites. The median age at the time of clinical examination of the irradiated tinea capitis patients were 17.0 years, which was similar to that for the control groups.

Examination of the Scalp and Hair

Generalized Alopecia   Three patterns of hair loss were observed in these cases: (a) normal male baldness, (b) generalized diminution (alopecia) of the hair population, and (c) focal alopecia consisting of single or multiple discrete patches of hair loss usually only a few centimeters in diameter. The outstanding clinical finding was a generalized alopeica which occurred in about one fifth of the irradiated patients. This abnormality was observed with remarkable consistency throughout the clinical study and was limited almost entirely to the irradiated patients. The incidence of this generalized alopecia tended to be higher in whites, particularly white females, where the hair loss was usually cosmetically disfiguring. In men, this type of hair loss was readily differentiated from the patterned hair loss of male baldness. The irradiated patients with and without generalized alopeica did not differ with respect to the age at the time of X-ray epilation or the post-irradiation elapsed time, or the type of fungus which caused the tinea capitis infection.

Baldness   As expected, the incidence of both mild and severe baldness increased with age in the irradiated and control groups, with blacks having a lower incidence of baldness than whites. In the 10- to 20-year age group, there were only a few cases of mild baldness in either the irradiated or control groups. In the 20- to 34-year age range, there was no substantial difference between the irradiated and tinea-control groups in the incidence of severe baldness; and the incidence of mild baldness was actually higher in the controls.

Hair Color and Texture   Graying was not produced by X-ray epilation in the examined patients under 20 years of age. There was a slightly higher incidence of patients with gray hair in the irradiated group between the ages of 20 and 34, but the significant of this difference is doubtful.

The irradiated and control cases had the same distribution of hair color. Within the irradiated group, there was a significantly higher incidence of generalized alopecia in the males with straight hair.

Scalp Hair Counts   A quantitative assessment of radiation damage to the scalp hair was obtained by measurement of the average number of hairs per square centimeter of scalp and their average diameter. Hair counts were done on a total of 205 patients. The data, sorted according to treatment group, race or sex, and baldness were pooled to yield average values for the number of hairs per 0.28 cm^2 sample site and the average diameter of the sample hairs.

The individuals with generalized alopecia had a reduction in both the total number and average diameter of the sampled hair. The combined effect served to exaggerate the loss of larger hairs. The more severe cases of baldness had fewer hairs but without a reduction in the average diameter.

Hair pulled out by the roots from the occiput in clumps of about 40 to 80 hairs from 151 cases were classified by microscophic examination according to their morphologic appearance as anagen (growing), catagen (intermediate), telogen (resting), and dystropic (abnormal). The cases were stratified according to treatment group, race, and sex, baldness and generalized alopecia, and the data for each of these categories were pooled.

There were no consistent differences between the irradiated and control cases with respect to the anagen-telogen ratios or the proportion of the dystrophic hair, regardless of generalized alopecia. However, a pronounced decline in the anagen-telogen ratios with increasing severity of baldness was observed.

Examination of the Ear

The ear examination consisted of an otoscopic inspection of ear canals and drums and an audiometric evaluation of hearing loss. The examination was done in the same mammer for all cases: hearing was tested at six frequencies (256, 512, 1024, 2048, 4096 cycles per second) in 5 db decrements starting from an audible intensity. A total of 452 individuals were examined, 85% of whom were males; and of those, 70% were white.

Structural ear damage, demonstrated by otoscopic examination, was observed in very few patients with no appreciable differences between the irradiated and control cases. The audiograms were classified as abnormal when the hearing loss was at least 15 db below the arbitrary standard for normal hearing at any frequency. The controls had a relatively high incidence of abnormal audiograms, and the incidence of abnormal audiograms was consistently higher in the older age groups. The irradiated patients did not have a higher incidence of abnormal audiograms than the control patients.

Examination of the Eye

Eye examinations were done on 306 irradiated and 247 control patients. There were no differences in the visual acuity of the irradiated and control cases. Few gross abnormalities of the eye were noted. The slit-lamp examinations were done with a biomicroscope. The abnormalities that were noted included abnormal degrees of luminescence caused by backscatter of light within the lens and minute opacities scattered throughout the lens or located preferentially in specific regions, i.e., subcapsular, sutural, etc. The observed abnormalities were graded as mild or moderate. There were no severe and very few moderately severe abnormalities. There was a very pronounced increase in the incidence of abnormal luminescence in the older-age category. The incidence of lens opacities was not age dependent. There were no significant differences between the irradiated and control groups with respect to the incidence of abnormal luminescence of lens opacities which did not involve the posterior cortex. There was a small but significantly higher incidence of lens opacities involving the posterior subcortical region in the irradiated cases; the severity of these posterior lens opacities was very mild.

Leukemia and Cancer

There were no differences between the irradiated and control groups in the incidence of tumors in areas other than the head and neck. In the irradiated group, the cancers, excluding head/neck/hematopoietic, were: 1 breast, 1 lung, 1 stomach, 1 rectum, and 1 testicular, for a prevalence of 22×10^{-4}. In the control group, the cancers were: 1 breast, 2 lung, 1 colon, 3 testicular, 1 kidney, 1 bladder, and 1 fibrosarcoma of the hand, for a prevalence of 72×10^{-4}.

Table 6. Summary tabulation of tumors of the head and neck, cumulative for all three surveys

Tumors	Irradiated No.	Irradiated Prevalence[a]	Control No.	Control Prevalence[a]
Neurogenic				
Brain	6	27	0	—
Acoustic Neuroma	2	9	0	—
Neck: Schwannoma or Neurilemoma	2	9	0	—
Total	10	45	0	—
Parotid[b]	4	18	1	7
Skin-Epithelial				
Basal Cell	41	184	3	22
Cylindroma	4	18	0	—
Other[c]	3	13	2	14
Total	48	216	5	36
Bone-Skull and Jaw[d]	4	18	0	—
Mouth-Larynx				
Papilloma	7	31	2	14
Thyroid				
Adenoma	8	36	0	—
Hemopoietic/ Lymphopoietic				
Leukemia	4	18	1	7
Hodgkin's Disease	5	22	2	14
Other Lymphoma[e]	2	9	0	—

[a] Cumulative prevalence per 10,000 subjects, not corrected for length of follow-up.
[b] Includes an acinous cell carcinoma of the parotid in the irradiated group.
[c] Excludes nevi and other minor types of benign skin tumors. Includes a trichoepithelioma, a clear cell hidradenoma (myoepithelioma) and a pigmented eccrine poroma in the irradiated group; a calcifying epithelioma and a benign acanthoma in the control group.
[d] Includes a fibrosarcoma of the mandible.
[e] Includes a lymphosarcoma of a submandibular node.

There were four patients with leukemia in the irradiated group, all of whom died, and one leukemia in the control group. The cases of leukemia in the irradiated group all occurred within 20 years of irradiation and the types were consistent with a radiation etiology: two cases of acute lymphocytic, one case of acute myeloblastic, and one case of chronic myelogenous leukemia. One patient in the control group had chronic lymphocytic leukemia occurring 25 years after tinea treatment.

Data in Table 6 show in irradiated cases a higher incidence of head and neck tumors, including: brain, salivary glands, skin, bone, and thyroid. The hematopoietic and lymphopoietic tumors are included in this tabulation because such tissues were present in the head and neck at the time of X-ray epilation. The malignant tumors of the head and neck in the irradiated group included: an acinous cell carcinoma of the parotid gland, a fibrosarcoma of the mandible, a lymphosarcoma of a submandibular node, 3 malignant brain tumors (a glioma, an astrocytoma and a hemangioblastoma), and 41 cases of basal cell carcinoma of the skin. The tumors of the thyroid, CNS, and skin, in particular, merit further analysis and discussion.

THYROID TUMORS

A total of 8 thyroid tumors were surgically removed in the irradiated group vs. none among the controls. All of these were pathologically diagnosed as benign adenomas (Table 7). Six of the eight thyroid tumors were diagnosed as follicular in cell type, one was mixed papillary-follicular, and the other was unspecified as to type. One of these cases also had multiple parathyroid adenomas.

For years 5+ post-irradiation, the thyroid incidence was 8/48,123 PY = $16.6/10^5$. Since published data on the age-specific incidence of benign thyroid tumors are not available from large populations, the spontaneous incidence was estimated by combining the present control group data and the control data from Hempelmann's study (19). This yielded a rate of $5.1/10^5$ PY. The excess in the irradiated group was therefore about $11.5/10^5$ PY, and the relative risk was 3.25. If the thyroid dose is assumed to be 6 rads, then the overall risk estimate would be about $19/10^6$ PY-rad (p = 0.004 by an exact Poisson test), with a 95% lower confidence limit of $3.6/10^6$ PY-rad.

The temporal course of the thyroid tumor response was of interest. The intervals between irradiation and thyroid tumor diagnosis are shown in Table 7. The mean latency (adjusting for censored data) was 30.6 years with 90% confidence limits of 27 to 34 years. A life-table analysis yielded a cumulative incidence estimate of 7.6 per thousand irradiated persons by 35 years post-irradiation (90% confidence limits of 3.8 to 15.4 per thousand). Whether the excess thyroid tumor incidence diminishes after a period of time, i.e., has a wavelike temporal pattern, can be crudely addressed. The thyroid tumor incidences in the irradiated group for years 5-14, 15-24, and 25-35 post-irradiation were 9, 16, and $37/10^5$ PY. If one subtracts out rates, comparable by sex distribution and age, derived from the combined thymus and tinea control series, the net rates (i.e., excesses) are 7, 15, and $22/10^5$ PY, respectively. Thus, there is no indication that the benign thyroid tumor effect is diminishing with longer follow-up time.

The data were examined for several host susceptibility factors which might modify the magnitude of radiation-induced thyroid tumorigenesis. A log-linear analysis of thyroid tumors in the irradiated group was performed by: sex, race, age at irradiation (1-7 vs. 8+ yr.) and interval since irradiation (using coarse groupings of 5-14, 15-24, and 25-35 years because of the sparse data). The analysis showed a significant effect for sex (p = 0.0001), such that the risk was higher among females. Although only 13% of the irradiated group were females, five of the eight thyroid tumors occurred among them. The effects of race, age at irradiation and interval since irradiation were not significant. An examination of interactions revealed a weak interaction between sex and age at irradiation, but this was not readily interpretable.

Table 7. Thyroid tumors in the irradiated group

Race-Sex	Interval Since X-ray (yr.)	Age at Diagnosis	Pathologic Diagnosis
WM	6	17	Adenoma, degenerating foetal (follicular)
WF	9	14	Adenoma, papillary-follicular
WM	19	28	Adenoma
WF	21	26	Adenoma, follicular
WM	22	32	Adenoma, microfollicular (+ parathyroid adenomas)
WF	32	36	Adenoma, follicular
WF	34	39	Adenoma, follicular
WF	34	41	Adenoma, follicular

No thyroid cancers were observed in this study. This raises the question of the magnitude of thyroid carcinogenesis at low radiation doses. To determine the number of thyroid cancers expected under the linear dose-response hypothesis, the expected spontaneous thyroid cancer frequency (based on sex and age specific rates from the Connecticut Tumor Registry) and the expected radiation-induced frequency (based on sex-specific estimates from Hempelmann's study) were summed, yielding an expectation of 1.5 thyroid cancers. Observing zero is statistically compatible ($p = 0.22$) with this expectation.

CENTRAL NERVOUS SYSTEM TUMORS

A list of the eight intracranial neoplasms in the irradiated group is shown in Table 8. No central nervous system (CNS) tumors were observed in the control group. Of the eight tumors, the glioma, the hemangioblastoma, and one of the astrocytomas were malignant. The other astrocytoma was diagnosed as benign. Only the glioma case has died.

One peculiarity of these tumors was that all eight occurred on the left side of the brain, whereas spontaneous brain tumors occur with equal frequency on the right and left sides (20). Thus, this distribution is nominally a significant deviation from expectation ($p = 0.004$).

As with thyroid tumors the minimum latent period was taken to be five years, since in both this study and the study by Modan (21) brain tumors occurred before 10 years post-irradiation. For years 5+ post-irradiation, the CNS tumor incidence was $8/48,115$ PY $= 16.6/10^5$ PY. Based on age-specific rates derived from the Connecticut Tumor Registry (20) for combined malignant and benign brain tumors, about 1.4 brain tumors would have been expected. The ratio of observed to expected gives a relative risk of 5.7 ($p = 0.0001$ by the exact Poisson test) with 90% confidence limits of 2.8 to 10.3. About 0.9 CNS tumors were expected in the control group, which is compatible with the zero observed ($p = 0.40$).

The dose to the brain ranged from about 70 rads at the base to 175 at the top, with an average of about 140 rads. The excess of 6.6 (= 8-1.4)

Table 8. CNS tumors in the irradiated tinea group

Sex Race	Age at Tinea (yrs)	Interval: X-Ray to Diagnosis (yrs)	Tumor Type	Location
WM	7	5	Glioma	L. Frontal Lobe
WM	4	6	Astrocytoma	L. Optic Chiasm
WM	8	26	Astrocytoma	L. Cerebellum
WF	9	26	Hemangio-blastoma	L. Cerebellum
WM	6	21	Meningioma	L. Convexity
NM	6	17	Meningioma	L. Temporal Lobe
WM	10	26	Neuroma	L. Acoustic Nerve
WM	4	17	Neuroma	L. Acoustic Nerve

was $13.7/10^5$ PY, which translates into an excess of about $1.0/10^6$ PY-rad. A more refined analysis controlling for sex, age at irradiation and interval since irradiation (as for thyroid tumors above), gave a significant Mantel-Haenszel summary chi-square, with a 95% lower confidence limit on the relative risk of 1.2.

The temporal distribution of the CNS tumors is shown in Table 8. A life-table analysis showed a cumulative incidence by 35 years post-irradiation of 4.8 per thousand persons (90% confidence limits of 2.7 to 8.7). For the grouping of 5-14, 15-24, and 25-35 years post-irradiation, the CNS tumor rates were respectively 9, 16, and $38/10^5$ PY. From these rates one might conclude that the tumor yield is increasing with time out to at least 35 years post-irradiation. However, the lack of CNS tumors after 26 years raises the question of whether the CNS tumor excess may instead be diminishing at longer intervals in a wave-like fashion. Further years of observation will be required to settle this, since the number of PY in the longest intervals is currently too small to draw any conclusion. Supportive of the "wave" interpretation is the fact that mean latency for the CNS tumors was only 19.6 years (90% confidence limits of 15 to 24), which was much shorter than the mean latency for thyroid tumors.

Log-linear analyses of the CNS tumor data for the irradiated group by sex, race, age at irradiation and interval since irradiation (with subgroups defined as the for the thyroid tumor analyses) did not reveal any significant host-susceptibility factors.

SKIN CANCER

The dose to the scalp from the tinea treatment ranged from about 270 rads to 540 rads, depending on scalp location because of the overlapping fields. The margins of the scalp also received about 270 rads, but the rest of the face and neck received 10-50 rads. The results of the dosimetric study and the locations of skin cancers are shown in Figure 1.

In the three surveys of these study groups, a total of 31 cases of skin cancer of the head and neck have been found in the irradiated group and 3 in the control group. In addition to the 31 found on survey in the irradiated group, 10 more cases were found in a dermatological clinic evaluation program of 203 irradiated subjects (vs. zero among 90 control subjects). Thus, a total of 41 irradiated subjects is known to have had skin cancer. For the purpose of calculating incidence rates only the 31 found on survey can properly be used, but in examining the risk factors for skin cancer all 41 will be used where possible.

Ionizing radiation is known to produce squamous cell carcinomas and basal cell carcinomas of the skin. In this study all 41 irradiated cases had basal cell carcinomas (including one person with both a basal cell and a squamous cell carcinoma). Multiple basal cell lesions--found both synchronously and sequentially--were common among the irradiated cases. There were a total of 80 skin cancer lesions among the 41 cases.

Even though 25% of the irradiated group was black, all 41 skin cancer cases were in whites. An analysis of the 31 found on survey in the irradiated group showed a highly significant difference by race. Based on the PY 15 or more years post-irradiation, the numbers were 31/21646 vs. 0/4596 (p = 0.003 by the Fisher exact test, with a 95% lower confidence limit of RR of 2.1).

One way of assessing the radiation-skin cancer effect is to compare the observed number of skin cancers among irradiated whites with an expected number derived form general-population rates. Because most cancer registries do not have adequate reporting of non-melanoma skin cancers, expected values were generated from the special skin cancer incidence survey of caucasians which was performed in Iowa and parts of Minnesota, California and Texas (22). Since the Texas rates were aberrant from the others, probably due to the extremely high levels of sun radiation in that area, only the other three locations were used to obtain average rates for sex- and age-specific groups, with the reported more recent increases in basal cell carcinoma rates also factored in (23, 24, 16). Because our interest was in skin cancers of the head and neck only, the rates needed to be adjusted to exclude skin cancers at other body sites. Based on a large series of basal cell carcinomas, Kopf has reported that 85% of them occur on the head and neck (25). The population rates were therefore multiplied by 0.85 to obtain appropriate expected values.

The expected number of head and neck skin cancers among irradiated whites proved to be 7.4. Comparing this to the 31 observed skin cances gave a highly significant (p < 0.0001) relative risk of 4.2 (90% confidence limits of 3.0 to 5.7). If one assumes a minimal latent period of 15 years (which is discussed further below) and an average skin dose of about 450 rads, then the absolute risk of skin cancers is about $2.4/10^6$ PY-rad (90% confidence limits of 1.5 to 3.4). The expected value in the control group was 4.4, which did not differ significantly (p = 0.72) from the three observed skin cancers.

A Mantel-Haenszel analysis among whites, adjusting for age at treatment, sex and interval since irradiation, also yielded a highly significant different (p = 0.007) between the irradiated and control group and a relative risk of 6.1 (90% confidence limits of 2.1 to 20.8).

Temporal Pattern and Risk Models for Skin Cancer

The temporal pattern of the radiation-induction of skin cancer was striking. No excess was observed before 20 years post-irradiation, but thereafter the excess risk became pronounced (Figure 2). The cumulative

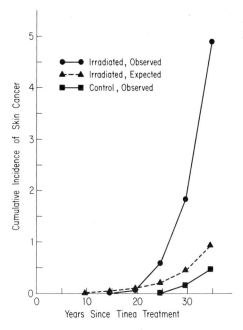

Fig. 2.   Temporal skin cancer response.

incidence of skin cancer in the irradiated group by 35 years post-irradiation was 49 per thousand persons (90% confidence limits of 30 to 79). The median latency for the skin cancers, adjusting for censored data was 32.3 years (90% confidence limits of 31 to 34). When the "spontaneous" incidence curve for the control group was subtracted out, the residual, "radiation-induced" curve had a median of 33 years. The risk appeared to be increasing with time, as shown in Table 9. The excess rates increased over time from zero to about $400/10^5$ PY, respectively.

This result raises the issue of whether the radiation induction of skin cancer over time better fits the absolute risk or relative risk model of radiation effects. The absolute risk model predicts that the magnitude

Table 9.   Skin cancers among irradiated white subjects by interval since irradiation

Interval (years)	Person years	Observed Cancers*	Expected Cancers	Excess Cancers (Rate/10^5 PY)
1-14	23,309	0	0.26	-
15-19	7,939	1	0.98	0.3
20-24	6,797	7	1.64	78.9
25-29	4,801	12	2.38	200.4
30-35	2,109	11	2.15	419.6

*Cases entered only once. Those with multiple skin cancers were entered according to date of first cancer.

Table 10. Complexion and sun-exposure factors vs. skin cancer among white irradiated subjects

	Skin Cancer (%)	No Skin Cancer (%)	Odds Ratio
Complexion: Fair	60.0	43.4	1.96
Blue Eyes	51.4	27.2	2.83
Freckles: Moderate to Many	22.9	11.8	2.22
Hair: Blonde, Red	14.3	10.5	1.42
Sunburn Easily	77.1	66.6	1.69
Tan Little	37.1	10.5	2.29
Ethnicity: Irish	33.3	22.3	1.74
Sun Exposure: 15 hr/wk	30.3	23.4	1.42
Sun Exposure: hr/wk (X)	12.8	11.5	----
Sunbathe: "Yes"	34.3	44.5	0.65
Outdoor Activities: "Yes"	74.3	73.5	1.04

of radiogenic risk is independent of the size of the spontaneous risk for some outcome. The relative risk model, on the other hand, hypothesizes that the radiogenic risk is proportional to the spontaneous risk. Trend statistics suggested that radiogenic skin cancer risk fits a relative risk model better than an absolute risk model.

Modifying Factors for Skin Cancer Risk

Factors which could be examined were based on responses to questions concerning complexion and sunlight exposure. The distributions of these factors among skin cancer cases and the remainder of the white irradiated group who completed these questions is shown in Table 10. A stepwise multiple regression analysis of skin cancer vs. these variables was first performed to select the most important variables, which proved to be: eye color, freckles, and ease of tanning. Since no variables were retained which reflected the amount of sunlight exposure, the number of hours per week spent outdoors was also added for the main analysis.

The main analysis of these factors vs. skin cancer was performed using a log-linear model of PY, including a factor of interval since tinea treatment. Each factor was examined controlling for all other factors. The significance of each factor was: interval ($p = 0.0001$), sun exposure ($p = 0.08$), freckles ($p = 0.02$), tanning ability ($p = 0.008$), and blue eyes ($p = 0.01$). Thus, the amount of sun exposure was not significant, but the three complexion variables were. No interactions among these factors were significant. The conclusion from the analysis is that several variables having to do with lightness of complexion and skin reactions to sunlight exposure are modifiers of radiogenic skin cancer risk. Variation among individuals in amount of sunlight exposure appears to be only a marginal modifier of radiogenic skin cancer risk in this study (but another interpretation is that the questions on sunlight exposure may have been inadequate to provide reliable and accurate discrimination among persons).

However, Figure 1 suggests that UV exposure is an important co-factor for radiogenic skin cancers in another way. A total of 23 skin cancers occurred near the margins of the scalp (excluding the ears which had special shielding) where there was a substantial radiation dose on the order of 270 rads, but no hair-shielding of the UV exposure. The skin surface area of these margins is about 140 cm^2. Similarly, there were 13 skin cancer lesions on areas of the face which received   50 rads. By contrast, only 35 skin cancers occurred on the hairy scalp, which received an average dose of about 440 rads and has a surface area of about 570 cm^2. A calculation on the basis of dose and skin area indicates that UV exposure has increased the X-ray carcinogenic effect on the face, relative to that on the UV-protected scalp, by approximately a factor of 4.5.

It is of interest to determine whether those who developed skin cancers on the scalp may have had radiation-induced alopecia or early baldness, so that the scalp would have had more UV exposure than normal. Table 11 presents the available data on this point, as well as on complexion factors. This table compares irradiated subjects who had skin cancers on the scalp (with or without additional skin cancers on the face) with those who had skin cancers only on the face and with other irradiated and control subjects. The scalp cancer group had an (insignificantly) lower prevalence of baldness, both self-reported and as judged in our dermatologic clinic program, than the non-tumor irradiated group. The self-reported and dermatologist-judged prevalence of generalized hair thinning was somewhat, but not significantly, greater in the scalp cancer group. However, the objective hair count from the dermatologic evaluation showed less (p = 0.05) hair thinning in the scalp cancer group than in the non-tumor group. Hence, there was no evidence that the subjects with skin cancers of the scalp had more UV exposure to the scalp than others did.

One interesting sidelight of Table 11 is that the scalp tumor group was intermediate between the non-tumor group and the facial skin cancer group for the complexion factors. Put in other words, the complexion variables seem to matter the most for skin cancers on areas with major UV exposure. This is as one would expect, since skin pigmentation is thought to confer susceptibility/resistance primarily to the effects of UV irradiation.

RADIATION EFFECTS VS. OTHER TREATMENTS

To verify that variations in the other tinea treatments received by the subjects do not account for the tumors, a tabulation of the frequency and types of local medications was made. Checks were made of (a) if the subjects who had developed thyroid tumors, brain tumors or skin cancers had any unusual patterns of tinea treatment with local medications, as compared with a random sample of irradiated subjects (n = 50), and (b) if the local medications used in the irradiated group differed substantially from those used in a random sample of the control group (n = 52).

Tabulations of medications revealed that the following were commonly used on both the irradiated and control groups (in descending order of frequency; percent use in the combined irradiated samples given in parentheses): ammoniated mercury ointment (82%), salicyclic acid (19%), benzoic acid (13%), iodine compounds (13%), and sulfur compounds (12%). In the irradiated sample, 32% were given local medications prior to irradiation, and 94% received them after irradiation.

Table 11. Hair and complexion variables by skin cancer status

	Skin-Cancer Face*	Skin-Cancer Scalp*	Other Irrad.	Controls
Reported Baldness (%)	11.1	4.5	9.3	4.6
Hair Thinning (%)	33.3	31.8	25.9	14.0
Bald Clinic (%)	33.8	18.1	25.4	20.9
Hair Thinning–Clinic (%)	70.0	73.3	58.5	65.9
Hair Count–Clinic**	36±16.9	48.2±15.3	42.0±11.1	46.0±11.6
Wear a Hat in the Sun (%)	37.5	58.8	27.0	24.0
Fair Complexion (%)	64.7	55.6	38.8	37.3
Blue Eyes (%)	64.7	38.9	22.3	20.0
Blond/Red Hair (%)	17.6	11.1	8.6	6.9

* "Skin-cancer face" includes those with skin cancer(s) only on the face or neck
   (n=18). "Skin-cancer scalp" includes all cases with skin cancer on the hairy
   scalp, with or without skin cancers on the face or neck (n=22).
**Hair count given as Mean ± S.D. hairs per cm^2. Items noted as "clinic" are obser-
   vations based on those attending the dermatological clinic program.

Comparisons of subjects with thyroid tumors, CNS tumors or skin
cancers respectively with the random sample of irradiated subjects revealed
no significant differences in receiving treatment before or after
irradiation, or in the frequency of treatment with any of the specific
medications listed above. Thus, there was no evidence that the tumor cases
had any unusual treatment.

A comparison of the random samples of irradiated and control subjects
revealed only one nominally significant difference: the irradiated group
was more likely to have received treatment with ammoniated mercury ointment
than the control group (82 vs. 60%, respectively; p = 0.02). Even though
this difference was statistically significant, the high frequency of use of
ammoniated mercury among the controls, as well as cases, makes it seem
unlikely that the modest inter-group differences in its use could account
for the high relative risks observed in the irradiated group for the
several tumor sites. The fact that the frequency of application of
ammoniated mercury did not differ between the random irradiated sample and
anyof the three tumor-site groups, also favors an interpretation that the
compound was not tumorigenic; the percents with ammoniated mercury
applications in the groups with CNS, thyroid, and skin tumors were 54, 83
and 88%, respectively, as compared with 82% in the random irradiated sample.
Thus, one is left with the inference that x-irradiation is the only likely
candidate for the tumorigenic agent.

DISCUSSION

From an epidemiological standpoint, the tinea capitis study population
is exceptionally good: the cases and controls are closely matched for age,
sex, and race; the radiation treatments were administered by a single
technician with a frequently calibrated X-ray machine; a high proportion of
cases were located and followed. The study population is mostly white,
male, irradiated at about 7 years of age and followed to date for an

average of 25 years. The major findings are an excess of cancers of the scalp, brain, thyroid, bone marrow (leukemia) and mental disorders. Pronounced hair thinning was observed in 20% of the cases, and minor ocular lens opacities and hearing loss was also noted. As of 25 years post-irradiation, there has been no radiation associated excess mortality.

A parallel study is being carried out in Israel with a larger population followed by means of a national cancer registry (21, 26, 27). A similar pattern of tumors of the brain, thyroid, and leukemia has been seen. Skin tumors were not evaluated.

Mental disorders were evaluated as part of the follow-up surveys. There was a generalized excess of mental disorders in whites only, beginning after 9 years post-irradiation, which was confirmed by hospital and physician records as well as by direct psychiatric and psychologic examination in a subset of cases. In the Israeli irradiation population there has been an indication of electroencephalographic changes in the irradiated group and some suggestion of poorer mental function among them, as compared with their control groups (28, 29).

The contrast in psychiatric disorders between the irradiated and control groups has diminished: in the first survey, 3.2% of the irradiated group had verifiable past or current psychiatric illness compared with 1.3% of the controls. The irradiated cases thus had two and a half times more psychiatric illness than the controls. The additional follow-up time has increased the total frequency in the irradiated and control groups to 8.1% and 6.4%, respectively. The absolute difference is about the same as before, but the relative difference is small, although statistically significant for treated psychiatric disorders in white cases (p = .04). The populations themselves revealed no antecedent differences that might explain the difference in the rates of psychiatric disorders, as, for example, socioeconomic status or familial mental illness.

Although the thyroid gland has long been known to be radiosensitive, data were not available to permit assessment of effects of exposures to levels below about 20 rads until recently (21, 27). An extension of the previously reported dosimetry in this study (11) showed that the thyroid received about 6 ± 2 rads, which is in agreement with an estimate by Werner et al. of 6.5 rads (30). The lack of thyroid cancers was notable in this study, since Modan's larger tinea radiation study (27) found an appreciable excess of thyroid cancers. Nevertheless, the present finding is statistically compatible with the expected magnitude of the excess found in most other thyroid irradiation studies. The principal reasons for the lack of an excess are the relatively small number of person-rads in this study and, secondarily, the small fraction of irradiated females (since females have been shown to have 2-4 times more radiation-induction of thyroid cancer than males).

The temporal course of the thyroid tumors was of interest because of the apparently conflicting findings in the literature. Until recently, the Japanese A-bomb data suggested that thyroid cancers appear as a "wave" which has largely subsided by 25 years post-irradiation (31); however, the most recent data indicate that the risk is continuing out to 40 or more years among those irradiated in the first 2-3 decades of life, but it appears to have diminished or stopped in those with irradiation at older ages (32). The large Michael Reese Hospital series showed a temporal curve (for combined thyroid carcinomas and adenomas) which was tapering off after 30 years but had not yet fallen to baseline level by 40 years post-irradiation (33). The Rochester thymus radiation series gave no evidence of a tapering-off for either thyroid carcinomas or adenomas out to 40 years post-irradiation (34). The temporal results in the present study appear compatible with the Rochester study, although the numbers were too small to provide strong support for any particular temporal pattern.

The results indicating that females have more radiation-induction of thyroid tumors than males is consistent with the other major studies. The Israeli tinea radiation study (27) found evidence that irradiation at an earlier age (ages 0-5) induced a greater risk of thyroid cancer than irradiation at older ages. A similar effect was not found in the present study, although the null results might be attributable to the small number of thyroid tumors in this study.

Neural tissue has traditionally been thought to be radioresistant, but at least four prospective studies, including this one, have now found excess brain tumors following postnatal irradiation (26, 35, 36). However, only Modan's study and the present one have brain dosimetries to permit quantitative estimates of risk. The agreement between these two studies is relatively good--about 0.6 in Modan's study and $1.0/10^6$ PY-rad in the present study.

The distribution of histological types of CNS tumors in this study is similar to the distribution found in large series of spontaneous CNS tumors. Based on an average from several series (37) about 40% are gliomas (including astrocytomas), 17% are meningiomas, 6% are neuromas, and 1% are hemangioblastomas. The present study found 3 gliomas-astrocytmas, 2 meningiomas, 2 neuromas and 1 hemangioblastoma. The similarity of histologic types in this study to the background distribution is in contrast to what has been found after exposure to certain chemicals. For example, the brain tumors found after vinyl chloride exposure were all glibolastoma multiforme (glioma) type (38).

No explanation has been found for the finding that all eight of the CNS tumors were on the left side, although several hypotheses were explored. The radiation dose at the left and right hemispheres was equivalent. The distribution of left and right handedness among these cases was about as one would expect from the general population. An hypothesis that lesions in the left hemisphere might lead to earlier and more likely detection because of the unique symptoms produced by lesions on the left side also could not account for this difference: in only one case was there a "left sided" symptom (viz. impaired speech) which led to medical attention and diagnosis. The larger Israel tinea irradiation study did not find a preponderance of brain tumors on the left side (39).

One possibly relevant fact was that all of our cases were irradiated first over the left lateral aspect of the head; the side with the CNS tumors. Perhaps the first radiation exposure produced ischemia of the brain by vascular spasm which made the subsequent head exposures less tumorigenic. In the Israeli irradiations, each of the five fields was treated on successive days which would probably permit recovery from any such vascular effect if, in fact, it did occur.

The excess of skin cancers was striking in this study. The risk per rad is greater in the present study than in any other. The skin of the face is the most frequent site of basal cell carcinomas due to ultraviolet radiation (25). Since the face received appreciable doses in this study, but not in most other comparison studies, a synergism between ultraviolet (UV) and ionizing radiation may account for the large effect here. On the other hand, the relatively young age at irradiation may also be an important factor; juvenile irradiation may confer more skin cancer risk than adult irradiation. At present, there is no way of deciding between these possible explanations. However, there is evidence in this study that factors related to susceptibility to UV radiation play an important role.

The lack of skin cancers among blacks is one line of evidence, and the finding that fair complexion factors increase the risk from ionizing radiation is another. There was also more UV exposure among skin cancer cases than among other subjects, but this was not as strong a factor as the complexion diathesis.

The data from animal studies of radiation-induced skin cancer have generally suggested a dose-squared relationship, which implies there will be little skin cancer risk at lower doses. Similarly, it has frequently been posited that in humans there was little skin cancer risk below 1000 rads. The present study shows that this conception is probably incorrect, at least for a site such as the face where there is also appreciable UV insolation. In particular, a clear excess risk was seen in facial areas which received only 10-50 rads.

REFERENCES

1. A. C. Cipollaro, A. Kallos, and J. P. Rupper, Jr., Measurement of gonadal radiation during treatment for tinea capitis, New York J. Med. 59:3033-3040 (1959).

2. G. M. Lewis, et al., Measures to prevent and control an epidemic of ringworm of scalp, New York J. Med. 44:1327-1333 (1944).

3. R. Kienbock, Uber radiotherapie der haarerkrankungen, Arch. Derm. Syph. Wien. 83:77-1111 (1907).

4. H. G. Adamson, A simplified method of x-ray application for the cure of ringworm of the scalp; Kienbock's method, Lancet 1:1378-1380 (1909).

5. F. C. Combes and H. T. Behrman, Technique and problems of roentgen epilations, Arch. Derm. 57:74-89 (Jan. 1948).

6. J. M. Beare and E. A. Chesseman, Tinea capitis, Brit. J. Derm. 63:165-186 (1951).

7. M. A. Thorne and R. V. Grange, A survey of tinea capitis five years after treatment by x-ray epilation, Postgrad. Med. J. 30:423-424 (1954).

8. C. Berlin and C. Meyrovitz, The management of tinea capitis: report on 1877 treated cases, Brit. J. Derm. 67:397-401 (1955).

9. T. Symann, Untersuchungen zur frage der spawirkungen der epilationsbestgrahlungen in Bezug auf die geistige entwicklung des des kindes, Strahlentherapie 55:248-261 (1936).

10. R. Schulz and R. Albert, Dose to organs of the head from the x-ray treatment of tinea capitis, Arch. Environ. Health 17:935-950 (1963).

11. N. Harley, R. Albert, R. Shore, and B. Pasternack, Follow-up study of patients treated by x-ray epilation for tinea capitis. Estimation of the dose to the thyroid and pituitary glands and other structures of the head and neck, Phys. Med. Biol. 21:631-642 (1976).

12. N. H. Harley, A. Kolber, R. Shore, et al., The skin dose and response for the head and neck in patients irradiated with x-ray for tinea capitis: implications for environmental radioactivity, in: "Epidemiology Applied to Health Physics," (Proceedings of the Health Physics Society meeting, Jan. 9-13, 1983), Health Physics Society, Albuquerque (1983), pp. 125-142.

13. R. E. Albert and A. Omran, Follow-up study of patients treated by x-ray epilation for tinea capitis: I. Population characteristics, posttreatment illnesses, and mortality experience, Arch. Environ. Health 17:899-918 (1968).

14. R. Shore, R. Albert, and B. Pasternack, Follow-up study of patients treated by x-ray epilation for tinea capitis, Arch. Environ. Health 31:21-28 (1976).

15. R. Shore, A follow-up study of children given x-ray treatment for ringworm of the scalp (tinea capitis), Dissertation, Columbia University, New York (1982), pp. 168.

16. R. E. Shore, R. Albert, M. Reed, et al., Skin cancer incidence among children irradiated for ringworm of the scalp, Radiat. Res. 100:192-204 (1984).

17. A. R. Omran, R. E. Shore, R. A. Markoff, et al., Follow-up study of patients treated by x-ray epilation for tinea capitis: psychiatric and psychometric evaluation, Am. J. Public Health 68:561-567 (1978).

18. R. Albert, A. Omran, E. Brauer, et al., Follow-up study of patients treated by x-ray epilation for tinea capitis. II. Results of clinical and laboratory examinations, Arch. Environ. Health 17:919-934 (1968).

19. L. Hempelmann, W. Hall, M. Phillips, et al., Neoplasms in persons treated with x-rays in infancy: fourth survey in 20 years, J. Natl. Cancer Inst. 55:519-530 (1975).

20. B. Schoenberg, B. Christine, and J. Whisnant, The descriptive epidemiology of primary intracranial neoplasms: the Connecticut experience, Am. J. Epidemiol. 104:499-510 (1976).

21. B. Modan, D. Baidatz, H. Mart, et al., Radiation-induced head and neck tumours, Lancet 1:277-279 (1974).

22. J. Scotto, A. Kopf, and F. Urbach, Non-melanoma skin cancer among caucasians in four areas of the United States, Cancer 34:1333-1338 (1974).

23. T. Fears and J. Scotto, Changes in skin cancer morbidity between 1971-72 and 1977-78, J. Natl. Cancer Inst. 69:365-370 (1982).

24. J. Scotto, T. Fears, and J. Fraumeni, "Incidence of Nonmelanoma Skin Cancer in the United States," Pub. No. 83-2433, National Cancer Institute, Washington, D.C. (1983).

25. A. Kopf, Computer analysis of 3531 basal-cell carcinomas of the skin, J. Dermatol. 6:267-281 (1979).

26. E. Ron and B. Modan, Benign and malignant thyroid neoplasms after childhood irradiation for tinea capitis, J. Natl. Cancer Inst. 65:7-11 (1980).

27. E. Ron and B. Modan, Thyroid and other neoplasms following childhood scalp irradiation, in: "Radiation Carcinogenesis: Epidemiology and Biological Significance, Vol. 26," J. D. Boice, Jr. and J. F. Fraumeni, Jr., eds., Raven Press, New York (1984), pp. 139-151.

28. I. Yaar, E. Ron, B. Modan, et al., Long-lasting cerebral functional changes following moderate dose x-radiation treatment to the scalp in childhood: an electroencephalographic power spectral study, J. Neurol. Neurosurg. Psychiat. 45:166-169 (1982).

29. E. Ron, B. Modan, S. Floro, et al., Mental function following scalp irradiation during childhood, Am. J. Epidemiol. 116:149-160 (1982).

30. A. Werner, B. Modan, and D. Davidoff, Doses to brain, skull and thyroid, following x-ray therapy for tinea captis, Phys. Med. Biol. 13:247-258 (1968).

31. G. Beebe, H. Kato, and C. Land, "Mortality Experience of Atomic Bomb Survivors, 1950-74, Life Span Study, Report 8," Radiation Effects Research Foundation, Hiroshima (1977), (Technical Report: RERF TR 1-77).

32. R. Prentice, H. Kato, K. Yoshimote, et al., Radiation exposure and thyroid cancer incidence among Hiroshima and Nagasaki residents, Natl. Cancer Inst. Monogr. 62:207-212 (1982).

33. A. Schneider, M. Favus, M. Stachura, et al., Incidence prevalence and characteristics of radiation-induced thyroid tumors, Am. J. Med. 64:243-252 (1978).

34. R. Shore, E. Woodward, B. Pasternack, et al., Radiation and host factors in human thyroid tumors following thymus irradiation, Health Phys. 38:451-465 (1980).

35. G. Matanoski, R. Seltser, P. Sartwell, et al., The current mortality rates of radiologists and other physician specialists: specific causes of death, Am. J. Epidemiol. 101:199-210 (1975).

36. M. Colman, M. Kirsch, and M. Creditor, Tumours associated with medical x-ray therapy exposure in childhood, in: "Late Biological Effects of Ionizing Radiation, Vol. 1," Intl. Atomic Energy Agency, Vienna (1978), pp. 167-179.

37. H. L. Zimmerman, Introduction to tumors of the central nervous system, in: "Pathology of the Nervous System, Vol. 2," J. Minckler, ed., McGraw-Hill, New York (1971), pp. 1947-1951.

38. R. Waxweiler, W. Stringer, J. Wagoner, et al., Neoplastic risk among workers exposed to vinyl chloride, Ann. N.Y. Acad. Sci. 271:40-48 (1976).

39. E. Ron, Personal communication (1983).

TUMOUR INDUCTION IN EXPERIMENTAL ANIMALS AFTER NEUTRON AND X-IRRADIATION

J. J. Broerse

Radiobiological Institute TNO
Rijswijk, The Netherlands

ABSTRACT

Cancer induction is generally considered to be the most important
somatic effect of low dose ionizing radiation. It is therefore of great
concern to obtain information on the dose-response relationships for
carcinogenesis and to assess the quantitative cancer risk of exposure to
radiations of different quality.

Tissues in the human with a high sensitivity for cancer induction
include the bone marrow, the lung, the thyroid and the breast in women. If
the revised dosimetry estimates for the Japanese survivors of the atomic
bomb explosions are correct, there is no useful data base left to derive
RBE values for human carcinogenesis. As a consequence, it will be
necessary to rely on results obtained in biological systems, including
experimental animals, for these estimates.

The following aspects of experimental studies on radiation carcinogenesis are of relevance:

1. Assessment of the nature of dose-response relationships.

2. Determination of the relative biological effectiveness of
    radiations of different quality.

3. Effects of fractionation or protraction of the dose on tumour
    development.

For the analysis of tumour data in animals, specific approaches, such
as nonparametric actuarial methods and proportional hazard functions, have
to be applied. The dose response curves for radiation induced cancer in
different tissues vary in shape. This is exemplified by studies on myeloid
leukemia in mice and mammary neoplasms in different rat strains. The
results on radiation carcinogenesis in animal models clearly indicate that
the highest RBE values are observed for neutrons with energies between 0.5
and 1 MeV.

The diversity of dose-response relationships point to different
mechanisms involved in the induction of different tumours in various
species and even in different strains of the same species.

INTRODUCTION

The biological effects of ionizing radiation include cell
inactivation, chromosome aberrations, induction of mutations and malignant
transformation. The latter effect, cancer induction, is generally
considered to be the most important somatic risk of irradiation at low
doses. For this endpoint, there is a noticeable lack of quantitative
information in contrast to the vast amount of data obtained on cell
survival and chromosome aberrations. For radiation protection, it is of
great concern to assess the quantitative risk of exposure to radiations of
different quality which is correlated with the actual dose-response
relationships for carcinogenesis. The process of carcinogenesis is an
intriguing biological phenomenon. After irradiation some changes in the
genetic material of one or more cells are initiated. The lesions can be
dormant for some time, however, finally the damage expresses itself and
will result in the manifestation of a tumour after a latency period which
can easily be in excess of 10 to 15 years in humans. When a tumour with a
volume of 1 cm^3 is observed, a number of 30 volume doubling times has
elapsed. The processes of initiation, promotion and proliferation of the
malignant cells can be influenced by immunological, endocrinological and
dietary factors.

Tumour induction in man and larger experimental animals has clearly
been demonstrated after irradiation with doses in excess of 1 Gy (1).
Total body irradiations of monkeys (2) and dogs (3) with high doses of
neutrons (up to 3 Gy), and X-rays (up to 7 Gy) have resulted in a large
number of neoplasms, underlining the risk of some medical procedures.

For radiation protection applications, however, one is concerned about
the effects of low doses of ionizing radiation. Neoplasms induced by
ionizing radiation are indistinguishable from those occurring spontaneously
and any carcinogenic effect has to be inferred from relatively small
increases above the natural incidence by means of statistical approaches.
In the present review, results on neutron carcinogenesis in experimental
systems are discussed. The present day recommendations for radiological
protection including the quality factor as a function of neutron energy and
risk factors for tissues with high susceptibility for tumour induction are
summarized. Due to the reappraisal of the dosimetry of the Japanese
survivors of the atomic bomb explosions, there is no longer evidence
available on the effectiveness of fast neutrons for carcinogenesis in man.
In consequence, a number of investigators have tried to formulate models of
radiation carcinogenesis with the aim of obtaining reliable extrapolations
for radiation risks and RBE values to the range of low doses. Studies on
tumour induction in experimental animals and on in vitro carcinogenesis
will be discussed in connection with the following aspects: (1)
interpretation of tumour incidence data; (2) assessment of the shapes of
dose-response relationships, (3) determination of the relative biological
effectiveness (RBE) of radiations of different quality and (4) effects of
fractionation or protraction of the dose on tumour initiation and
development. The data on neutron carcinogenesis in experimental animals
are sometimes contradictory and it will be concluded that, at the present
time, a number of questions still remain.

PRESENT DAY RECOMMENDATIONS

Regarding stochastic effects, such as carcinogenesis, the ICRP (4) has
recommended a linear relationship without threshold between dose and the
probability of an effect within the range of exposure conditions usually
encountered in radiation work. Further, it has been stated (4) that the
use of linear extrapolations from the frequency of effects observed at high

doses, may suffice to assess an upper limit of risk with which the benefit of a particular practice or the hazard of an alternative practice, e.g., one not involving radiation exposure, may be compared. The assumption of linearity may lead to an overestimation of the radiation risk factors which in turn could result in a choice of alternatives that are more hazardous than practices involving radiation exposures. For neutron beams, the ICRP (5) has recommended effective quality factors as a function of neutron energy. These factors were calculated by dividing the maximum dose equivalent by the absorbed doses at the depth where the maximum dose equivalent occurs.

Siebert et al. (6) derived mean quality factors for neutrons in tissue directly from initial recoil energy spectra. They reported a maximum quality factor of 14 for neutron energies around 0.5 MeV. The dependence of the quality factor on neutron energy is in accordance with studies on RBE for a large number of biological endpoints (7).

Cancer may be induced by radiation in nearly all tissues of the human body. However, it has been shown, that tissues and organs can vary considerably in their sensitivity to the induction of cancer by radiation. A tabulation of the sensitivity of various tissues to the oncogenic effect of radiation can be found elsewhere (8). The tissues in the human with the highest sensitivity for cancer induction are summarized in Table 1 together with the risk factors which have been recommended by the ICRP (4).

As stated before, these risk factor are based on a linear dose-effect relationship. However, experimental studies have shown that other types of dose-response functions can be applied to the observed data. A number of attempts have been made to explain these dose-response relationships by introducing specific models of radiation carcinogenesis.

HUMAN DATA ON NEUTRON CARCINOGENESIS

During the past years, considerable efforts have been made to reassess the absorbed doses received by the survivors of the atomic bomb explosions at Hiroshima and Nagasaki (9-13). The most important conclusion of these calculations is that the contribution from neutrons at Hiroshima is considerably lower than that estimated by the 1965 tentative dose calculations, T65D. Dobson and Straume (14) combined the new radiation dose estimates for Hiroshima and Nagasaki with epidemiological data from the A-bomb survivors and also examined the data for compatibility with

Table 1. Sensitivity of various tissues to onocogenic influence of radiation according to BEIR(S) and ICRP(4)

site or type of cancer	spontaneous incidence of cancer	relative sensitivity to radiation induction of cancer	mortality risk factor per sievert
female breast	very high	high	$2.5 \ 10^{-3}$
lung (bronchus)	very high	moderate	$2 \ \ 10^{-3}$
alimentary tract	high	moderate to low	10^{-3}
leukaemia	moderate	very high	$2 \ \ 10^{-3}$
thyroid	low	very high, especially females	$5 \ \ 10^{-3}$

other human and experimental radiobiological results. The results of their
analysis are shown in Figure 1. RBE values obtained from the Japanese
studies for breast cancer and acute leukaemia are close to unity and do not
change with neutron dose. The data for chronic granulocytic leukaemia and
total malignancies would still follow a similar trend as calculated by
Rossi and Mays (15) for induction of all types of leukemias in the A-bomb
survivors. However, in a discussion of this analysis (16), it was stated
that the neutron doses are simply too low to derive any conclusion. Dobson
and Straume (17) have recently pointed out, that the apparent
radiobiological discrepancies between the A-bomb results and other
radiobiological data would be reconciled if the neutron component in
Hiroshima was a factor of five higher (or alternatively about a 50% greater
device yield) at Hiroshima than recently estimated. Although there may be
some additional adjustments in the Japanese dose estimates, it seems very
unlikely that these results will provide meaningful human data on the RBE
for tumour induction. Other sources of human population exposed to
neutrons are also as yet unlikely to produce useful information on the RBE.
In consequence at the present time one has to rely on studies in animals
and other biological systems with regard to estimates of RBE of neutrons
especially in the low dose range.

MODELS OF RADIATION CARCINOGENESIS

The adoption of a linear model for risk estimation has not received
unanimous approval of the scientific community. The so-called BEIR
controversy centered around arguments in favour of a linear-quadratic
versus a purely linear dose-response relationship (18-20). Linear-

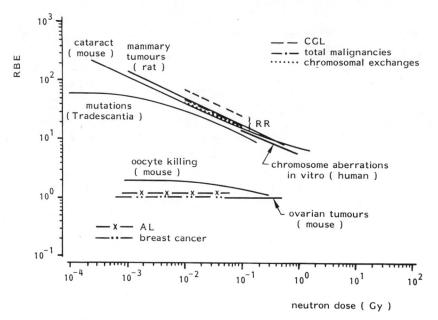

Fig. 1.   RBE values for acute leukaemia (AL), breast cancer,
          chromosomal exchanges, chronic granulocytic leukaemia
          (CGL), and total malignancies for the A-bomb survivors
          derived on the basis of the radiobiologically
          reconciled (RR) dose estimates in comparison with
          experimental results obtained with 0.4 MeV neutrons
          (Dobson and Straume (14)).

quadratic relationships have been suggested by different authors introducing various mechanisms. Leenhouts and Chadwick (21) argue that such a relationship can be understood on the basis of double strand breaks in the DNA which will lead to a mutation of the cell to a pre-malignant state. Kellerer and Rossi (22) postulated in their theory of dual radiation action that the induction of two non-specified sublesions is necessary for the production of the effect. They consider energy depositions by individual charged particles in critical structures with dimensions in the order of 1 µm. On the basis of their microdosimetric considerations, the probability of the effect will depend on the first and second power of the absorbed dose:

$$E = a_1D + a_2D^2$$

In addition, Rossi and colleagues (23, 24) conclude that also for carcinogenesis the RBE of high-LET radiation should vary as an inverse function of the square root of its dose. This relation is valid when the magnitude of the high-LET dose is sufficiently low to act by single, dose rate independent, events whereas the effect of low-LET radiation is principally due to the action of multiple events.

The relevance of the theory of dual radiation action to interpret dose-response relationships for human cancer is under debate (19). Barendsen (25) and Goodhead and coworkers (26) have provided theoretical and experimental arguments that mechanisms of radiation action should be based on interaction of lesions within nanometer sites, and on dose dependent repair processes. Tumour induction involves a number of sequential steps including physico-chemical lesions, cell death, cellular repair and possibly mutations (27). If the primary mechanisms underlying the induction of cellular and molecular damage are similar for various cellular responses, the dose-effect relationships should have some characteristics in common. The effectiveness of single events can be expressed in terms of a cross section or interaction volume and corresponds to the value of a_1 in the dose-effect relationships. A comparison of the effectiveness of different radiations for a number of biological endpoints by Barendsen (28) showed that a_1 values for morphological transformation are a factor of 50 to 1000 smaller than for reproductive death and chromosome aberrations. Results on mutations show even lower a_1 values, by factors 10^4 to 10^5 than for cell death. A compilation of cross sections for cell inactivation, transformations and mutations induced by radiations of different linear energy transfer (LET) by Goodhead (27) leads to the same conclusion (see Figure 2).

The large ratio between the frequency of transformations and specific mutations suggests that a mechanism of a more general nature than de-repression or activation of a specific oncogene would be involved in the malignant transformation. Barendsen (28) has therefore postulated that the primary chromosomal changes induced by radiation do not affect transformation genes or oncogenes directly but that the primary changes occur at other sites or in other genes which are present at multiple sites on all chromosomes.

In their theory of the gene transfer-misrepair mechanism of radiation carcinogenesis, Van Bekkum and Bentvelzen (29) propose interaction between DNA fragments containing oncogenes coming from a destroyed cell (the donor cell) and a cell which is capable of incorporating such fragments into its own genome. The probability of transformation is dependent on the number of DNA fragments reaching a certain proportion of recipient cells engaged in scheduled DNA synthesis. This theory would result in a multi-phase dose-response curve for low LET radiation with a threshold at about 0.01 Gy.

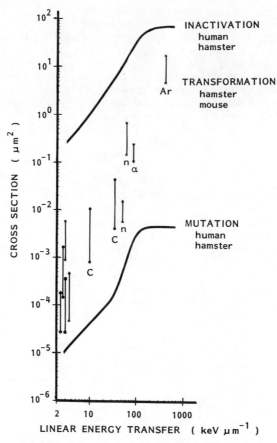

Fig. 2. Cross sections for cell inactivation, transformations and mutations induced in mammalian cells
by radiation of different LET (Goodhead (27)).

According to Baum (30), clones with large number of cells at risk have
a relatively high probability of response (transformation of at least one
cell) leading to a steep dose response curve. Depletion of the number of
untransformed cells with increasing dose would leave primarily
untransformed smaller clones with smaller probability of response per unit
dose. The response function is related to the mean number of charged
particle traversals per cell and the effectiveness of the secondaries.
This clonal theory of radiation carcinogenesis is applied to explain a
linear dose-response for x-irradiations and a power function of the dose,
with an exponent less than one for neutron exposure, as observed in mammary
tumour induction in American Sprague-Dawley rats (31-33).

On the basis of their microdosimetric considerations, Rossi and
coworkers (34) have postulated that cancer induction must be due to a
collective response of several cells. Although their theory is not
generally accepted, other authors came to comparable conclusions. In his
studies on the induction of myeloid leukaemia in mice, Mole (35) has
observed a purely quadratic dose-response relationship for low-LET
radiation (see Figure 3). This would rule out explanations of the kind
that microdosimetry provides for cell mutation and inactivation. Mole (35)
suggests that the induction of malignant disease by ionizing radiation
requires an action of radiation on two immediately adjacent cells
(diplosyncytic mechanism). It should be stressed, however, that any one

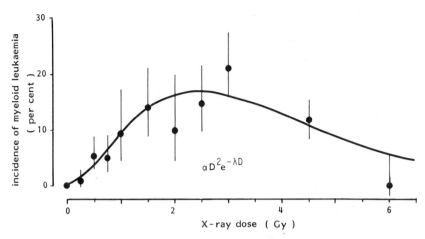

Fig. 3. Dose-response for nduced myeloid leukaemia in male CBA/H mice after exposure to 250 kVp X-rays (Mole (35)).

model will not be universally applicable to all radiation-induced types of cancer.

INTERPRETATION OF TUMOUR INCIDENCE DATA

The simplest approach in the analysis of tumour induction studies in animals is to score the proportion of animals that develop a tumour or the mean number of tumours per animal, observed after a given dose. However, this use of so-called uncensored data, may lead to erroneous interpretation of results. During the observation time, the group of animals at risk may be reduced due to intercurrent death, or other losses of animals from the experiment due to unknown reasons. Appropriate corrections for competing risks can be made by using life table analysis methods as formulated by Kaplan and Meier (36). The resulting quantities such as the integral tumour rate (37) or the cumulative prevalence and actuarial incidence (38) provide meaningful expressions of the response. The probability curves, produced by the life table analysis, inevitably show discontinuities in the course of time. The stochastic effect of carcinogenesis, however, can be described by hazard functions which result in curves with a common shape. In this type of analysis, the time elapsing from when an animal enters the experiment until a specified type of mammary tumour becomes palpable, is taken as the endpoint. In these studies one deals with incomplete observations or so-called right-censored data (39, 40). This expresses the fact that one knows either the actual time that a tumour is observed in an animal or that the animal has not developed such a tumour up to its time of disappearance from the experiment. Methods of analysis that accommodate censoring are generally called failure time distributions. Let T be a random variable, representing the onset time of a tumour, hereafter referred to as a failure. Particularly useful for the description of the probability distribution of T are the survivor function, the probability density function and the hazard function (40).

The survivor function or cumulative distribution function, S, is defined as the probability that T is at least as great as a value t, which means:

$$S(t) = Prob.(T \geq t).$$

The probability density function f of T is defined as:

$$f(t) = \lim_{\Delta t \downarrow 0} \frac{\text{Prob.}(t \leq T < t + \Delta t)}{\Delta t} = -\frac{dS(t)}{dt}.$$

The hazard function, h, specifies the instantaneous rate of failure at T = t, conditional upon survival to time t and is defined as:

$$h(t) = \lim_{\Delta t \downarrow 0} \frac{\text{Prob.}(t \leq T < t + \Delta t \mid T \geq t)}{\Delta t} = \frac{f(t)}{S(t)}$$

This quantity refers to the animals which are still at risk (i.e., without a failure). It is easy to see that h(t) specifies the cumulative distribution function of T since by integrating the above equation and using the fact that S(0) = 1, the following relation can be derived:

$$S(t) = e^{-\int_0^t h(u)\,du} = e^{-H(t)},$$

in which H(t) is the cumulative hazard function or more concisely the hazard. The hazard depends not only explicitly on the time, but also on a number of co-variates or variables such as the rat strain, hormonal status, irradiation schedule, etc. The proportion of animals surviving without evidence of tumour up to time t can be analyzed with a continuous parametric failure time model. The three parameter Weibull distribution, a generalization of the exponential distribution, can be used to describe failure rates of complex systems. This model allows for a power dependency of the hazard function with time, usually written as:

$$h(t) = \beta/\alpha \left(\frac{t-\gamma}{\alpha}\right)^{\beta-1},$$

where:

α = the time scale parameter which indicates the time at which the survivor function is equal to 37% ($\gamma = 0$)

β = the shape parameter, which is a measure of the time dependence and

γ = the location parameter, which is a finite time prior to which no failure will occur. The experimental results obtained at TNO show that the location parameter can vary between 0 and 6 months. In the present analysis, γ is taken to be zero.

The Weibull hazard can be written as follows:

$$H(t;D) = (t-\gamma)^{\beta} \left\{1/\alpha(D)\right\}^{\beta},$$

where only the time scale parameter is dependent on the absorbed dose. Thus, concurrently, a weighted least squares fit of the Weibull distribution parameters can be derived from the Kaplan-Meier estimate for the cohorts of interest. In such a procedure, the value of the time scale parameter depends on the different absorbed doses (with no constraints) while the shape parameter has the same value for all cohorts. This procedure is presently applied at TNO, as shown in Figure 4, to calculate the proportion of WAG/Rij rats surviving without known mammary fibroadenomas after X-irradiation.

The relative excess hazard can be defined independently of the time function and describes the net effect in the hazard of an irradiated cohort relative to the hazard of the control cohort. The relative excess hazard is then equal to:

$$\eta(D) = \frac{H(t;D) - H(t;0)}{H(t;0)} = \left\{ \alpha(0)/\alpha(D) \right\}^{\beta} - 1.$$

It becomes rather complicated to prove the carcinogenic action of ionizing radiation when only a few tumours have been observed even at high dose values. This has been the case for the induction of mammary carcinomas in the Sprague-Dawley rats studied at TNO (see Figure 5). Under these circumstances, the tumour incidence data can be analyzed employing contingency tables with a computer programme developed by Peto et al. (41). The number of animals dying with a specific tumour is compared with the number that would have been expected, taking into account the group size, and intercurrent mortality which does not have as the underlying cause, tumours of the type of interest. On the basis of this

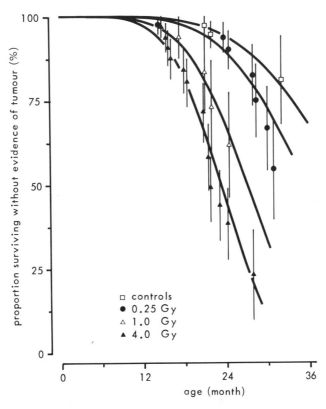

Fig. 4.   Probability of surviving without evidence of
           fibroadenomas in WAG/Rij rats after X-irradiation.

35

approach, the carcinogenic effect of a specific agent would only be clearly demonstrated when the ratio of observed and expected events is in excess of 1 (42).

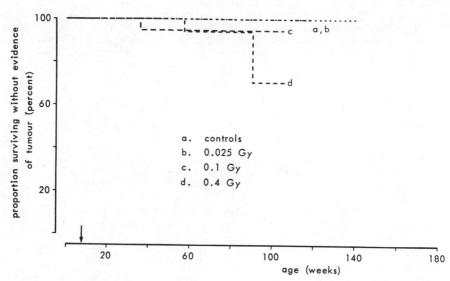

Fig. 5.   Probability of surviving without evidence of mammary carcinomas in TNO Sprague-Dawley rats after irradiation with 0.5 MeV neutrons. The arrow indicates the time of irradiation.

NATURE OF DOSE-RESPONSE RELATIONSHIPS

Dose-effect curves for tumour induction after neutron irradiation have been reported for a number of tissues. In this review attention will be given to induction of mammary neoplasms, myeloid leukaemia and lung tumours.

Initially, studies on radiation-induced mammary neoplasms concentrated on the use of the Sprague-Dawley rat as employed by Shellabarger and colleagues (31) and Vogel (32). The first group derived dose-response relations on the basis of the excess number of neoplasms per animal at a specified time. Shellabarger et al. (37) admit that the disadvantage of this procedure is that the choice of the reference time is arbitrary and that not all of the experimental data are utilized. Alternative approaches are the scoring of the forward shift in time of occurrence of the tumours, or the determination of the loss of tumour-free life-span. Regardless of the procedures applied, the resulting dose-response relationship (43) for induction of fibroadenomas in the Sprague-Dawley rats for neutrons generally corresponds to a dose exponent of approximately 0.5 (see Figure 6). The data for X-rays appear to be consistent with a dose exponent of 1. The number of radiation induced adenocarcinomas in the studies of Shellabarger et al. was too small to permit definitive statements on the dose-response relationships.

It may be questioned to what extent data on induction of benign tumours will be of relevance for risk assessment in man. At TNO a number of successive programs on mammary tumourigenesis in three rat strains, notably Sprague-Dawley, WAG/Rij and Brown Norway rats have been initiated for single and fractionated irradiations with X-rays and monoenergetic

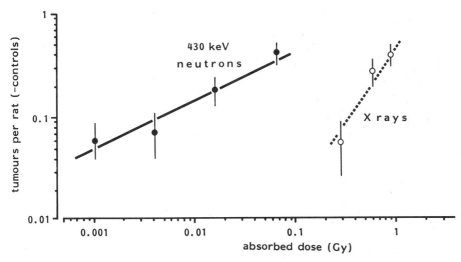

Fig. 6. Incidence of mammary neoplasms in American Sprague-Dawley rats as a function of absorbed dose of 250 kVp X-rays and 430 keV neutrons (Rossi (43)).

neutrons of three energies (see Table 2). These studies have shown that only in WAG/Rij rats an appreciable number of carcinomas was induced by irradiation (44). Earlier analyses of the TNO results (45) were based on the excess actuarial incidence at an age of 22 months or on the forward shift in time. For the incidence of fibroadenomas in the WAG/Rij rats, the exponent of the dose effect curve for excess actuarial incidence after irradiation with 0.5 MeV neutrons was also lower than 1. However, the addition of new data and the analysis of the data by the hazard functions has resulted in a linear dose-response curves for fibroadenomas in Sprague/Dawley rats and for fibroadenomas (Figure 7) and carcinomas (Figure

Table 2. Summary of studies on mammary carcinogenesis in the female rat

	STUDY NO.					
	I	II	III	IV	V	VI
Rat strains	WAG,BN,SD	WAG	WAG	WAG,SD	BN,SD	WAG,BN
Type and Dose of Irradiation (rad)	X:10-400 N: 2-150	X:200-400 N: 20-30	X:20-200 N:20 γ:200	X:200-400 N: 50-100	X:1-50	X: 2-400 N:0.5- 40 ß: 2-400
Total body (TBI) or Local (L) Irrad.	TBI	TBI	TBI	TBI	TBI	L
No. of fractions (Fraction intervals, days)	1 –	1,5 (14,30)	1,10,50 (1,30)	1,10 (7)	1,5 (30)	1,10 (30)
Hormonal status (normal,OVH,E_2)	normal OVH E_2	normal	normal E_2	normal E_2 (E_2 – 1,3 or 6 mo after irrad.)	normal	normal
Age at irrad. (mo)	2	2	2	2	2,6	2
No. of rats in study	5000	240	960	1000	1800	2280

8) in the WAG/Rij rats for the two irradiation conditions notably X-rays and 0.5 MeV neutrons.

It has been established that American Sprague-Dawley rats show a larger and more rapid mammary neoplastic response than do the TNO Sprague-Dawley rats studied in the Netherlands. As indicated in Figure 9, similar differences were observed after DMBA administration indicating that there are inherent differences between the two lines of rats (46). Genetic differences between the two lines were confirmed by establishing dissimilarities in the expression of erythrocyte antigens. Vogel and Turner (47) studied mammary tumour development in five different strains of female rats during the first year after irradiation with fission neutrons. A genetic factor in rat mammary tumourigenesis is also evident from this study with the highest susceptibility for tumour induction in Sprague-Dawley rats.

Upton and coworkers (48, 49) investigated the induction of myeloid leukaemia in RF mice after exposure to X- and gamma rays and neutrons at different dose rates. Although the number of experimental data in the low dose region is limited, Barendsen (50) derived linear and quadratic terms for the malignant transformation process and the induction of cell reproductive death:

$$I (D) = (a_1 D + a_2 D^2) \; e^{-(b_1 D + b_2 D_2)}$$

The competition between tumour induction and inactivation of cells has also been observed by Mole and colleagues (35, 51) for induction of myeloid leukaemia in male CBA mice. The initial part of the dose-response curve for low LET radiation had to be fitted with a quadratic dose term without a statistically significant linear dose component (see Figure 3). For irradiation with fission neutrons the initial part of the response curve followed a linear relation with the dose.

The induction of lung adenocarcinomas in mice after irradiation with fission neutrons or gamma radiation has been studied by Ullrich and colleagues (52, 53). The dose-response curve for gamma irradiation could be fitted with a linear quadratic relation. However, the dose-response curve after fission neutron irradiation shows a convex upward shape which is described by Ullrich with a square root dose dependence. It seems speculative to ascribe the downward bending of the curve to inactivation of the alveolar cells after fission neutron irradiation. Studies on life time shortening in mice performed by Thomson et al. (54) after irradiation with fission neutrons have shown linear dose-effect relationships for photons and a convex upward shape for neutrons.

RELATIVE BIOLOGICAL EFFECTIVENESS OF FAST NEUTRONS

For radiation protection applications, the main emphasis is on the assessment of the RBE at low dose levels, e.g., at a neutron dose of 1 cGy. It is sometimes rather difficult to distinguish the carcinogenic effect for these low dose irradiations from background incidence. Specific models have been postulated for the extrapolation to the low dose regions, e.g., the dependence of RBE on the inverse square root of the neutron dose. When the estimates are based on different assumptions the same set of experimental data can result in widely differing RBE values. In reporting his own data on lung adenocarcinomas, Ullrich (53) derived an RBE of 18.5 on the basis of the linear slope constants for the neutron and gamma ray dose response curves, whereas Fry (55) quoted an RBE of 60 on the same

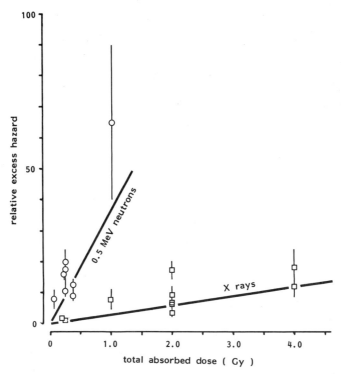

Fig. 7.   Relative excess hazard as a function of total
            absorbed dose for fibroadenomas induced in WAG/Rij
            rats irradiated with X-rays and 0.5 MeV neutrons.

criteria. When Ullrich applied the inverse square root dose dependence he
derived an RBE of 71 for a neutron dose of 1 cGy, however, Rossi (24)
obtained an RBE of 133 at the same dose level. That different RBE values
were derived from the same experiment implies that considerable caution
should be exercised in the interpretation of such data. In addition, it
has to be realized that high RBE values for neutron carcinogenesis will be
mainly due to the low effectiveness of small doses of low-LET radiation.

    The above mentioned insufficiencies should be realized when RBE values
are quoted for carcinogenesis in different tissues. Malignant
transformation has been studied in vitro employing short-term cultures of
Syrian hamster embryo cells (56). The RBE values of 430 keV monoenergetic
neutrons as a function of the dose for both transformation and cell
survival are shown in Figure 10. The vertical bars in the figure indicate
RBE values for in vitro malignant transformation that can be excluded with
80% confidence. Borek and Hall (56) conclude from their study that the RBE
changes with dose for both cell killing and in vitro transformation and
that the RBE values are similar over the limited dose range in which both
endpoints have been scored. However, their data do not indicate a clear
increase in RBE with decreasing dose for malignant transformation.

    The studies on mammary neoplasms in Sprague-Dawley rats performed by
Shellabarger et al. (37) have indicated proportionality of RBE to the
inverse square root of the neutron dose (see Figure 1). Only a minor
fraction of all mammary tumours observed in this study were
adenocarcinomas. However, the authors claim that the RBE-dose dependence
for fibroadenomas alone and the combined group of fibroadenomas and
adenocarcinomas is consistent also for the more limited data pertaining to

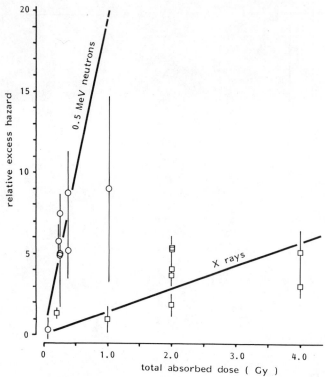

Fig. 8.　Relative excess hazard as a function of total
absorbed dose for carcinomas induced in WAG/Rij
rats irradiated with X-rays and 0.5 MeV neutrons.

adenocarcinomas.　The Brookhaven group has extended their studies to
another rat strain, notably ACI rats, in which they investigated (57) the
effect of exposure to low- and high-LET radiation and the administration of
diethylstilbestrol (DES).　The synthetic estrogen DES induced an
appreciable increase in adenocarcinomas, a finding similar to observations
at TNO (44) where the natural hormone estradiol-17β has been employed.　The
mammary carcinogenic response of non-DES-treated ACI rats to radiation,
appeared to be relatively small, thus requiring relatively high doses of X-
rays and neutrons to produce incidence values large enough to be analyzed
statistically.　The dose dependence of the RBE of 430 keV neutrons for
induction of mammary neoplasms in ACI and American Sprague-Dawley rats is
shown in Figure 11.　For the ACI rats treated with DES, the RBE values are
larger than those for Sprague-Dawley rats at comparable neutron doses.

The most recent analysis of the results on mammary tumourigenesis in
three rat strains performed at TNO, have resulted in linear dose-response
curves for both X-rays and 0.5 MeV neutrons.　This implies constant values
for the RBE, independent of the neutron dose.　It cannot be excluded that
the diversity of dose-response relationships for radiation carcinogenesis
may be due to the genetic characteristics and environmental status (e.g.,
hormonal levels) of the cells at risk.

A summary of RBE values for neutrons with energies between 0.5 and 1
MeV is given in Table 3.　The RBE values for induction of myeloid leukaemia
are based on the data of Upton et al. (49) and Mole (35, 51).　For the
latter set of data, the RBE was calculated as the square root of the ratio
a_1 for neutrons to a_2 for photons.　Because of the absence of a linear

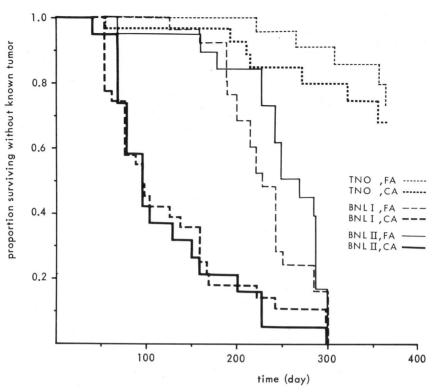

Fig. 9. Actuarial incidence of mammary carcinomas (CA) and
fibroadenomas (FA) after DMBA administration in
Sprague-Dawley rats from TNO, Rijswijk and BNL,
Brookhaven National Laboratory (Van Zwieten et
al. (46)).

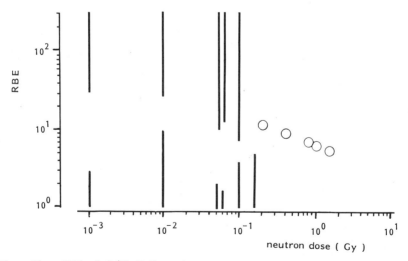

Fig. 10. RBE of 0.43 MeV neutrons for hamster embryo cells as a
function of neutron dose. The vertical bars
corresponding to oncogenic transformation indicate RBE
values excluded with 80% confidence. The open symbols
represent cell survival (Borek and Hall (56)).

coefficient in the dose-response curve observed by Mole for induction of
myeloid leukaemia after x-irradiations, it could be argued that these data
do not allow the calculation of genuine RBE values.

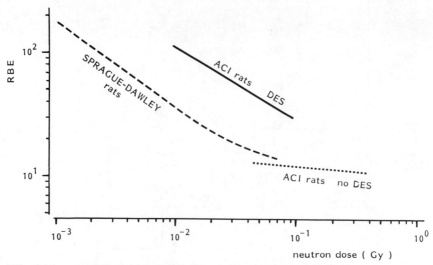

Fig. 11.   RBE of 0.43 MeV neutrons for induction of mammary
neoplasms in Sprague-Dawley rats and ACI rats (with and
without DES treatment) as a function of neutron dose
(Shellabarger et al. (57)).

     In a recent study by Covelli et al. (58), life shortening and tumour
induction in mice were investigated after exposure to fission neutrons and
X-rays. RBE values for different endpoints were found to be in the range
of 3 to 18. However, these results do not allow to quote an RBE at a
neutron dose of 1 cGy.

EFFECTS OF FRACTIONATION OR PROTRACTION OF THE DOSE

     When the radiation dose is administered in a number of fractions or at
a reduced dose rate, the biological response is different from that
obtained after single acute doses. For cell survival the modifying
processes include repair of sublethal damage, repopulation and re-
distribution over the cell cycle. For tumour induction the nature of
modifying mechanisms is not yet well understood, and it is rather difficult
to interpret all experimental results obtained after fractionated or
protracted exposures.

     Elkind and colleagues (59) studied the transformation of 10T1/2 cells
(fibroblast-like cells derived from a mouse embryo) after irradiation with
gamma rays and fission neutrons at different dose rates. The reduction in
dose rate resulted in a decreased transformation frequency for the gamma
irradiation and an enhancement for the fission neutrons. These authors
postulated different mechanisms for the transformation damage: after high-
LET irradiation, cells would experience a repair process the net effect of
which is error-prone, whereas following low-LET irradiation, the net effect
of repair is error-free. These results could indicate that the dose-effect
curve would have a negative curvature (convex upward) for neutrons and a
positive curvature (concave upward) for photons as postulated by Rossi and
Hall (34). However, it should be mentioned that there are appreciable

Table 3. Relative biological effectiveness at a dose of 1 cGy of neutrons with energies 0.43-1 MeV for different endpoints

	RBE at 1 cGy
Lung adenocarcinoma in mice, a_1 neutrons/a_1 photons	18.5
Ullrich, 1982 $\quad D_N^{-1/2}$	71
Malignant transformation in hamster embryo cells Borek and Hall (1984)	10-25
Myeloid leukemia in mice, daily chronic irradiation Upton et al. (1970)	16
Myeloid leukemia in mice, acute irradiation square root of a_1 neutrons/a_2 photons, Mole (1984)	13
Fibroadenomas in Sprague-Dawley rats, $D_N^{-1/2}$ Shellabarger et al. (1980)	50
Adenocarcinomas in ACI rats treated with DES, $D_N^{-1/2}$ Shellabarger et al. (1982)	100
Adenocarcinomas in WAG/Rij rats, TNO	15
Fibroadenomas in WAG/Rij rats, TNO	13
Fibroadenomas in Sprague Dawley rats, TNO	7

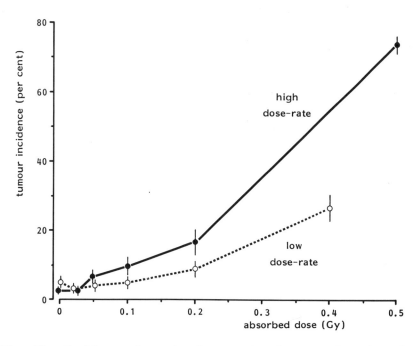

Fig. 12. Incidence of ovarian tumours in mice as a function of absorbed dose after high- or low-dose rate irradiations with fission spectrum neutrons (Ullrich (61)).

differences of opinion regarding the methodology and significance of transformation assays. For X-irradiations at relatively high doses in excess of 0.5 Gy, fractionation leads to a sparing effect for transformation, but between 0.1 and 0.5 Gy fractionation enhances the transformation incidence (56). The plating procedures and serum condition can effect the expression of malignant transformation.

Reviewing the present status of radiation transformation in vitro, Little (60) recalled that the ultimate yield of transformed foci per dish may be independent of the number of cells initially at risk. Caution should be employed in extrapolating results of in vitro transformation studies to predict the effects of radiation on cancer induction in humans.

Experimental studies on in vivo carcinogenesis suggest that effects of fractionation and protraction are different for the various tumour types presumably because of the different mechanisms of tumorigenesis that may be involved. For the induction of ovarian tumours in mice, Ullrich (61) observed that fission neutron irradiation was less effective when delivered at low dose rates in comparison with high dose rates (see Figure 12). However, the mammary carcinogenic effect of neutrons was enhanced at low dose rates, a finding similar to that of Vogel and Dickson (33). Studies performed at TNO on the induction of mammary carcinomas in WAG/Rij rats after single and fractionated irradiations with X-rays and 0.5 MeV neutrons indicate that for equal total absorbed dose the tumours appeared at approximately the same age (see Figure 13). This result might be due to a higher susceptibility for tumour induction at an older age. Another explanation for this phenomenon could be that fractionated irradiation has a higher efficiency for neutrons as well as for photons, for induction of mammary cancer. In this connection it should be noticed that the experimental studies on mammary carcinogenesis were generally based on total body irradiation of the animals. The induction of mammary cancer can easily be modified by hormonal factors, and it might well be that specific endocrinological conditions, necessary for tumour induction, are influenced to a lesser extent by fractionated or protracted exposures.

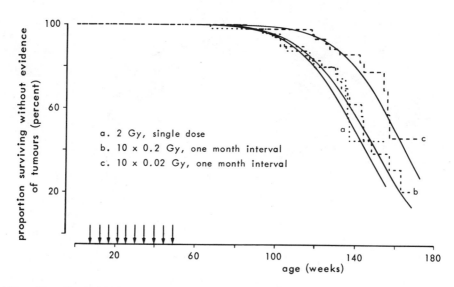

Fig. 13. Probability of surviving without evidence of mammary carcinomas in WAG/Rij rats after single-dose and fractionated irradiation with X-rays. The arrows indicate the times of irradiation.

CONCLUSIONS

The studies on neutron carcinogenesis in rodents do not provide risk factors applicable for man. The dose-effect relationships for photons clearly indicate linear and linear-quadratic relationships which provide a sound basis for linear extrapolations for risks of low-LET radiation. For exposure to fast neutrons, different investigators have reported responses proportional to the dose or to the square root of the dose. This aspect needs further experimental investigation. The experimental data on the relative biological effectiveness of fast neutrons for carcinogenesis suggest that the present values for the quality factor might be increased. The dependence of the RBE on the inverse square root of the neutron dose is not generally applicable. At low doses the RBE will be determined by the linear slope constants of the neutron and gamma-ray dose-response curves. In consequence, an increase of the quality factor by a factor of 2 to 3 seems more realistic than a tenfold rise. Such an adjustment of the quality factor will generally be accepted to provide an adequate margin of safety (62, 63). Neutrons of relatively low energy have been observed outside the shielding of nuclear installations. It will be important to register the doses received by radiation workers who may possibly be exposed to neutrons fields. Cancer patients treated with external beams of fast neutrons might also constitute an important group for human epidemiological studies in the future.

In addition to the probable consequences for radiation protection, it was expected that the experimental studies on neutron carcinogenesis could contribute to our understanding of fundamental mechanisms. Reviewing the currently available results, it is impossible to formulate general statements on carcinogenic action of low- versus high-LET radiation. The diversity of dose-response relationships suggest that different mechanisms may be involved in the induction of different tumours in various species and even in different strains of the same species. It is therefore of great importance to design new approaches to investigate the process of carcinogenesis at the cellular and subcellular level.

ACKNOWLEDGEMENTS

The experimental studies at TNO have been supported by the Commission of the European Communities, the U.S. National Cancer Institute, the Dutch Praeventiefonds and the Koningin Wilhelmina Fonds. The efficient cooperation with Dr. L. A. Hennen on the statistical analysis of the tumour incidence data, and with Dr. M. J. van Zwieten on the histological scoring of tumours in rat and monkeys is gratefully acknowledged. The contributions and constructive support of Dr. G. W. Barendsen, Dr. D. W. van Bekkum, Dr. C. F. Hollander and Dr. R. H. Mole have been of great assistance in the preparation of this review.

REFERENCES

1. United Nations Scientific Committee on the Effects of Atomic Radiation, "Sources and Effects of Ionizing Radiation," United Nations, New York (1977).

2. J. J. Broerse, C. F. Hollander, and M. J. van Zwieten, Tumour induction in Rhesus monkeys after total body irradiation with X-rays and fission neutrons, Int. J. Radiat. Biol. 40:671-676 (1981).

3. H. J. Deeg, R. Prentice, T. E. Fritz, G. E. Sale, L. S. Lombard, E. D. Thomas, and R. Storb, Increased incidence of malignant tumours in dogs after total body irradiation and marrow transplantation, _Int. J. Radiat. Oncol. Biol. Phys._ 9:1505-1511 (1983).

4. ICRP Publication 26, "Recommendations of the International Commission on Radiological Protection," Pergamon Press (1977).

5. ICRP Publications 15 and 21, "Protection against Ionizing Radiation from External Sources and Data for Protection against Ionizing Radiation from External Sources. Recommendations of the International Commission on Radiological Protection," Pergamon Press (1976).

6. B. R. L. Siebert, R. S. Caswell, and J. J. Coyne, Calculations of quality factors for fast neutrons in materials composed of H, C, N and O, _in:_ "Proc. Eighth Symposium on Microdosimetry," EUR 8395, J. Booz, and H. G. Ebert, eds., Commission of the European Communities, Luxemburg, (1983), pp. 1131-1140.

7. ICRU Report 26, "Neutron Dosimetry for Biology and Medicine," International Commission on Radiation Units and Measurements, ICRU, Washington (1977).

8. Committee on the Biological Effects of Ionizing Radiations, "The Effects on Populations of Exposure to Low Levels of Ionizing Radiation," National Academy Press, Washington (1980).

9. W. E. Loewe, and E. Mendelsohn, Revised dose estimates at Hiroshima and Nagasaki, _Health Phys._ 41:663-666 (1981).

10. G. D. Kerr, Review of dosimetry for the atomic bomb survivors, _in:_ Proc. Fourth Symposium on Neutron Dosimetry, Vol. 1," EUR 7448, G. Burger, and H. G. Ebert, eds., Commission of the European Communities (1983), pp. 501-513.

11. "Reassessment of Atomic Bomb Radiation Dosimetry in Hiroshima and Nagasaki," Proc. Workshop held at Nagasaki, D. J. Thompson, ed., (1983).

12. "Reassessment of Atomic Bomb Radiation Dosimetry in Hiroshima and Nagasaki, with Special Reference to Shielding and Organ Doses," Proc. Workshop held at Hiroshima (1983).

13. W. K. Sinclair, Revisions in the dosimetry of atomic bomb survivors, _in:_ "Proc. Seventh International Congress of Radiation Research," J. J. Broerse, G. W. Barendsen, H. B. Kal, and A. J. van der Kogel, eds., Martinus Nijhoff (1983), pp. 63-73.

14. R. Lowrey Dobson, and T. Straume, Cancer risks and neutron RBE's from Hiroshima and Nagasaki, _In:_ "Neutron Carcinogenesis," EUR 8084, J. J. Broerse, and G. B. Gerber, eds., Commission of the European Communities (1982), pp. 279-300.

15. H. H. Rossi, and C. W. Mays, Leukemia risk from neutrons, _Health Phys._ 34:353-360 (1978).

16. G. W. Barendsen, Summary of round table discussion on neutron carcinogenesis and implication for radiation protection, in: "Neutron Carcinogenesis," EUR 8084, J. J. Broerse and G. B. Gerber, eds., Commission of the European Communities (1982), pp. 445-453.

17. R. Lawrey Dobson, and T. Straume, Hiroshima and Nagasaki: expanded radiobiological analysis and dose reconciliation, in: "Proc. Seventh International Congress of Radiation Research," J. J. Broerse, G. W. Barendsen, H. B. Kal, and A. J. van der Kogel, eds., Martinus Nijhoff (1983), pp. C8-05.

18. J. I. Fabrikant, The BEIR III controversy, Radiat. Res. 84:361-368 (1980).

19. E. P. Radford, Human health effects of low doses of ionizing radiation: the BEIR III controversy, Radiat. Res. 84:369-394 (1980).

20. H. H. Rossi, Comments on the somatic effects section of the BEIR III report, Radiat. Res. 84:395-406 (1980).

21. H. P. Leenhouts, and K. H. Chadwick, Association between stochastic and non-stochastic effects and cellular damage, in: "Biological Effects of Low-level Radiation," IAEA, Vienna (1983), pp. 129-138.

22. A. M. Kellerer, and H. H. Rossi, The theory of dual radiation action, Current Topics Radiat. Res. 8:85-158 (1972).

23. H. H. Rossi, E. J. Hall, and M. Zaider, The role of neutrons in cell transformation research, in: "Neutron Carcinogenesis," EUR 8084, J. J. Broerse, and G. B. Gerber, eds., Commission of the European Communities (1982), pp. 371-380.

24. H. H. Rossi, Microdosimetry and carcinogenesis, in: "Proc. Eighth Symposium on Microdosimetry," J. Booz, and H. G. Ebert, eds., Commission of the European Communities (1983), pp. 539-549.

25. G. W. Barendsen, Influence of radiation quality on the effectiveness of small doses for induction of reproductive death and chromosome aberrations in mammalian cells, Int. J. Radiat. Biol. 36:49-63 (1979).

26. D. T. Goodhead, J. Thacker, and R. Cox, The conflict between the biological effects of ultrasoft X-rays and microdosimetric measurements and application, in: "Proc. Sixth Symposium on Microdosimetry," Vol. II, J. Booz and H. G. Ebert, eds., Commission of the European Communities (1978), pp. 829-843.

27. D. T. Goodhead, Deductions from cellular studies of inactivation, mutagenesis, and transformation, in: "Radiation Carcinogenesis: Epidemiology and Biological Significance," J. D. Boice, Jr., and F. Fraumeni, Jr., eds., Raven Press, New York (1984), pp. 369-385.

28. G. W. Barendsen, Effects of radiation on the reproductive capacity and proliferation of cells in relation to carcinogenesis, in: "Radiation Carcinogenesis" A. C. Upton, R. E. Albert, F. J. Burns and R. E. Shore, eds., Elsevier, New York (1986) pp. 85-105.

29. D. W. van Bekkum, and P. Bentvelzen, The concept of gene transfer-misrepair mechanism of radiation carcinogenesis may challenge the linear extrapolation model of risk estimation for low radiation doses, Health Phys. 43:231-237 (1982).

30. J. W. Baum, Clonal theory of radiation carcinogenesis, in: "Proc. Eighth Symposium on Microdosimetry," J. Booz, and H. G. Ebert, eds., Commission of the European Communities (1983), pp. 575-584.

31. C. J. Shellabarger, R. D. Brown, A. R. Rao, J. P. Shanley, V. P. Bond, A. M. Kellerer, H. H. Rossi, L. J. Goodman and R. E. Mills, Rat mammary carcinogenesis following neutron or X-radiation, in: "Proc. Symposium Biological Effects of Neutron Irradiation," IAEA, Vienna (1974), pp. 391-401.

32. H. H. Vogel, Jr., High let irradiation of Sprague-Dawley female rats and mammary neoplasm induction, in: "Proc. Symposium Late Biological Effects of Ionizing Radiation," Vol. II, IAEA, Vienna (1978), pp. 147-164.

33. H. H. Vogel, Jr., and H. W. Dickson, Mammary neoplasia in Sprague-Dawley rats following acute and protracted irradiation, in: "Neutron Carcinogenesis," EUR 8084, J. J. Broerse and G. B. Gerber, eds., Commission of the European Communities (1982), pp. 135-154.

34. H. H. Rossi, and E. J. Hall, The multicellular nature of radiation carcinogenesis, in: Radiation Carcinogenesis: Epidemiology and Biological Significance," J. D. Boice, Jr., and J. F. Fraumeni, Jr., eds., Raven Press, New York (1984), pp. 359-367.

35. R. H. Mole, Dose-response relationships, in: "Radiation Carcinogenesis: Epidemiology and Biological Significance," J. D. Boice, Jr., and J. F. Fraumeni, Jr., eds., Raven Press, New York (1984), pp. 403-420.

36. E. L. Kaplan and P. Meier, Nonparametric estimation from incomplete observations, J. Amer. Stat. Assoc. 53:457-481 (1958).

37. C. J. Shellabarger, D. Chmelevsky, and A. M. Kellerer, Induction of mammary neoplasms in the Sprague-Dawley rat by 430-keV neutrons and X-rays, JNCI 64:821-833 (1980).

38. J. J. Broerse, S. Knaan, D. W. van Bekkum, C. F. Hollander, A. L. Nooteboom, and M. J. van Zwieten, Mammary carcinogenesis in rats after X- and neutron irradiation and hormone administration, in: "Proc. Symposium Late Biological Effects of Ionizing Radiation," Vol. II, IAEA, Vienna (1978), pp. 13-27.

39. A. M. Kellerer, and D. Chmelevsky, Analysis of tumour rates and incidences--a survey of concepts and methods, in: "Neutron Carcinogenesis," EUR 8084, J. J. Broerse, and G. B. Gerber, eds., Commission of the European Communities (1982), pp. 209-231.

40. J. D. Kalbfleisch and R. L. Prentice, "The Statistical Analysis of Failure Time Data," John Wiley and Sons, New York (1980).

41. R. Peto, M. C. Pike, N. E. Day, R. G. Gray, P. N. Lee, S. Parish, J. Peto, S. Richards, and J. Wahrendorf, Guidelines for simple, sensitive significance tests for carcinogenic effects in long-term animal experiments, in: "IARC Monographs on the Evaluation of the Carcinogenic Risk of Chemicals to Humans, Suppl. 2, Long-Term and Short-Term Screening Assays for Carcinogens: A Critical Appraisal," IARC, Lyon (1980), pp. 311-423.

42. J. J. Broerse, L. A. Hennen, M. J. van Zwieten, and C. F. Hollander, Mammary carcinogenesis in different rat strains after single and fractionated irradiations, in: "Neutron Carcinogenesis," EUR 8084, J. J. Broerse, and G. B. Gerber, eds., Commission of the European Communities (1982), pp. 155-168.

43. H. H. Rossi, The role of the theory of dual radiation action in radiation protection, in: "Advances in Radiation Protection and Dosimetry in Medicine," R. H. Thomas, and V. Perez-Mendez, eds., Plenum Press, New York (1980), pp. 131-141.

44. M. J. van Zwieten, The rat as animal model in breast cancer research, Martinus Nijhoff (1984).

45. J. J. Broerse, L. A. Hennen, M. J. van Zwieten, and C. F. Hollander, Dose-effect relations for mammary carcinogenesis in different rat strains after irradiation with X-rays and monoenergetic neutrons, in: "Proc. Symposium Biological Effects of Low-Level Radiation," IAEA, Vienna (1983), pp. 507-519.

46. M. J. van Zwieten, C. J. Shellabarger, C. F. Hollander, D. V. Cramer, J. P. Stone, S. R. Holtzman, and J. J. Broerse, Differences in DMBA-induced mammary neoplastic responses in two lines of Sprague-Dawley rats, Eur. J. Cancer Clin. Oncol. 20:1199-1204 (1984).

47. H. H. Vogel, Jr., and J. E. Turner, Genetic component in rat mammary carcinogenesis, Radiat. Res. 89:264-273 (1982).

48. A. C. Upton, F. F. Wolff, J. Furth, and A. W. Kimball, A comparison of the induction of myeloid and lymphoid leukemias in X-ratiated RF mice, Cancer Res. 18:842-848 (1958).

49. A. C. Upton, M. L. Randolph, and J. W. Conklin, Late effects of fast neutrons and gamma-rays in mice as influenced by the dose rate of irradiation: induction of neoplasia, Radiat. Res. 41:467-491 (1970).

50. G. W. Barendsen, Fundamental aspects of cancer induction in relation to the effectiveness of small doses of radiation, in: "Proc. Symposium Late Biological Effects of Ionizing Radiation," Vol. II, IAEA, Vienna (1978), pp. 263-275.

51. Mole, R. H., and J. A. G. Davids, Induction of myeloid leukaemia and other tumours in mice by irradiation with fission neutrons, in: "Neutron Carcinogenesis," EUR 8084, J. J. Broerse, and G. B. Gerber, eds., Commission of the European Communities (1982), pp. 31-39.

52. R. L. Ullrich, M. C. Jernigan, and L. M. Adams, Induction of lung tumors in RFM mice after localized exposures to X-rays or neutrons, Radiat. Res. 80:464-473 (1979).

53. R. L. Ullrich, Lung tumour induction in mice: neutron RBE at low doses, in: "Neutron Carcinogenesis," EUR 8084, J. J. Broerse, and G. B. Gerber, eds., Commission of the European Communities (1982), pp. 43-55.

54. J. F. Thomson, L. S. Lombard, D. Grahn, F. S. Williamson, and T. E. Fritz, RBE of fission neutrons for life shortening and tumourigenesis, in: "Neutron Carcinogenesis," EUR 8084, J. J. Broerse, and G. B. Gerber, eds., Commission of the European Communities (1982), pp. 75-93.

55. F. J. M. Fry, Experimental radiation carcinogenesis: what have we learned?, Radiat. Res. 87:224-239 (1981).

56. C. Borek, and E. J. Hall, Induction and modulation of radiogenic transformation in mammalian cells, in: "Radiation carcinogenesis: Epidemiology and Biological Significance," J. D. Boice, Jr., and J. F. Fraumeni, Jr., eds., Raven Press, New York (1984), pp. 291-302.

57. C. J. Shellabarger, D. Chmelevsky, A. M. Kellerer, and J. P. Stone, Induction of mammary neoplasms in the ACI rat by 430-keV neutrons, X-rays, and diethylstilbestrol, JNCI 69:1135-1146 (1982).

58. V. Covelli, V. diMajo, B. Bassani, S. Rebessi, M. Coppola, and G. Silini, Influence of age on life shortening and tumour induction after X-ray and neutron irradiation, Radiat. Res., 100, 348-364 (1984).

59. M. M. Elkind, A. Han, and C. K. Hill, Error-free and error-prone repair in radiation-induced neoplastic cell transformation, in: "Radiation Carcinogenesis: Epidemiology and Biological Significance," J. D. Boice Jr., and J. F. Fraumeni, Jr., eds., Raven Press, New York (1984), pp. 303-318.

60. J. B. Little, Radiation transformation in vitro/review, in: "Proc. Seventh International Congress of Radiation Research," J. J. Broerse, G. W. Barendsen, H. B. Kal, and A. J. van der Kogel, eds., Martinus Nijhoff (1983), pp. 377-384.

61. R. L. Ullrich, Tumor induction in BALB/c mice after fractionated or protracted exposures to fission-spectrum neutrons, Radiat. Res. 97:587-597 (1984).

62. NCRP Statement on Dose Limit for Neutrons (1980).

63. J. B. Storer, and T. J. Mitchell, Limiting values for the RBE of fission neutrons at low doses for life shortening in mice, Radiat. Res. 97:396-406 (1984).

DOSE-RESPONSE FOR RADIATION-INDUCED CANCER IN RAT SKIN

F. J. Burns and R. E. Albert

Institute of Environmental Medicine
New York University Medical Center
550 First Avenue
New York, N.Y. 10016

INTRODUCTION

Skin has been extensively utilized to study the carcinogenic effects of environmental and industrial agents (1). Compared to internal organs, skin is relatively easy to manipulate, and tumors are detectible at earlier times. The skin contains a comparatively large variety of cell types many of which are susceptible to the action of carcinogens. For example, rat skin exposed to radiation develops a variety of tumor types including, squamous carcinomas, basal cell carcinomas, sarcomas, and sebaceous cell tumors, each of which presumably arises from different cell populations in the skin. Rat skin is sensitive to a number of environmentally-important carcinogens, including radiation, where perhaps the most extensive comparison of animal results with human epidemiological data are available (2, 3). Rat and mouse skin have proved to be sensitive and reproducible systems for studying the dose-response and time-response characteristics of radiation carcinogenesis and for investigating the mechanism relating to how the absorption of the radiation by the cells leads to cancer (4). The following chapter will describe and summarize these studies many of which have been carried out at the Institute of Environmental Medicine at New York University.

The Time-Response Function

Upon exposure of the skin of rats to single doses of ionizing radiation, epithelial tumors begin to appear about 10 weeks after irradiation and continue to appear at an accelerating rate thereafter. The reproducibility and consistency of this time pattern is remarkable and is the basis for constructing dose response functions. A time-independent dose-response function requires that tumor yield be described by a separable function. Separability means that the function is a product of a function only of time with a function only of dose (5). This important concept can be expressed as follows:

$$Y(D,t) = f(D) \cdot g(t) \tag{1}$$

where $Y(D,t)$ is the yield in tumors per animal as a function of dose, D, and time, t. The function $f(D)$ depends on dose only and the $g(t)$ depends on time only.

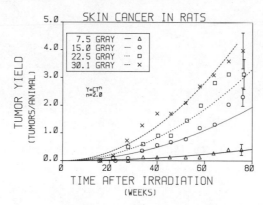

Fig. 1. Examples of temporal tumor onset data
generated in experiments where rat skin
was irradiated with electron radiation
that penetrated about 1.0 mm. The onset
time of each tumor was taken to be the
earliest time of visual detection.
Generally each tumor is examined and
confirmed histologically. Equation 2
(below) was fitted to the data with n = 2
and w = 0.

Analysis of the data alone has so far proved to be inadequate for
specifying the analytic forms of f(D) and g(t). The data are useful for
establishing the generally types of analytic forms, but there is a need for
functions derived from basic biological or statistical considerations. For
compatibility with the multistage theory of carcinogenesis, we have chosen
the following form for g(t) (6, 7):

$$g(t) = c(t-w)^n. \tag{2}$$

This form, sometimes referred to as a Weibull function, has often been used
to fit temporal data, especially data derived from epidemiological studies
of human populations.

While non-integer values of n are conceivable, consistency with the
multistage model model requires the use of integer values. In recent
experiments where the number of animals was greater than 50 there was
upward curvature in the temporal functions indicating an n value greater
than 2. If n is assumed to be 2, then the value of w for a wide range of
data is close to 0 weeks. Thus, we have chosen n to be 2 which gives a w
value of close to 0 weeks.

Examination of the data in Figure 1 indicates that tumors may occur at
any time after irradiation essentially for as long as the animal lives.
Some kind of carcinogenic alteration in the target cells presumably occurs
at the time of or within a few hours after irradiation. If cancer cells
existed at that time, the tumors should be distributed around the median
induction time with the earlier tumors being the more rapidly growing ones,
and the later tumors being the more slowly growing ones. However, tumor
growth rates as a function of the time of detection (generally when the
tumors are about 1 mm in diameter) indicated an equivalent distribution of
growth rates among the late and early tumors (8, 9).

Moreover, the distribution of histological types of tumors was
approximately the same in early and late occurring tumors. These results

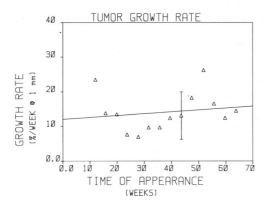

Fig. 2. The means and standard errors of the
growth rates at detection are shown as a
function of detection time measured from
the time of irradiation. Single doses of
electron radiation were applied at 28
days of age. The error bar show is
typical and represents the standard error
of the mean of not less than 10 tumors.

are consistent with the idea that the initial carcinogenic alteration
caused by action of the radiation merely establishes a potential cancer
cell that does not become an actual cancer cell until later. The
conversion of potential cancer cells to actual cancer cells probably
requires more than one step and is related to progression, a process
whereby cells advance in discrete genetic steps to malignancy.

The Dose-Response Function

Perhaps the most widely used analytic form of the dose-response
function, f(D), to describe the biological effect of radiation on cells,
especially cell lethality and chromosomal aberrations, is the so-called,
linear quadratic function derived from the dual action theory (10, 11).
The hypothesis underlying the dual action theory states that the yield of
any biological endpoint requiring two radiation-induced events is
proportional to the square of the radiation dose in a microscopic region of
space that essentially defines the target region with the cell (15). The
form of the expected function is:

$$f(d) = AD + BD^2 \tag{3}$$

Equation 3 is derived from biophysical considerations of the way
radiation dose is distributed statistically in small regions of space or
from various biological hit theories that are predicated on breaks in the
DNA being the primary event in the overall mechanism (15).

In a number of experiments, we have attempted to establish the dose-
response function for radiation carcinogenesis in rat skin.

It is typical of radiation carcinogenesis in several systems that the
dose-response a peak followed by a decline at higher doses. This downturn
of response at higher doses is probably caused by unrepopulated cell
lethality. The downturn is fitted reasonably well by assuming that only
partial repopulation occurs if the lethality is higher than some critical
level. Furthermore, if it is assumed that the alterations relevant to
carcinogenesis are transmitted to daughter cells during repopulative cell

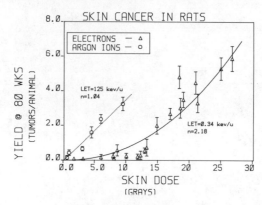

Fig. 3.   Shows the tumor yield as a function of
           surface dose at 80 weeks after
           irradiation for rat skin irradiated at
           28 d of age with monoenergetic electrons
           or argon ions (12, 13, 14, 15). The
           ascending part of the solid curve in
           Figure 4 is equation 3 with A = 0. The
           n values refer to the best fitting power
           function based on a least squares
           calculation. This is perhaps the most
           complete set of data presently available
           on the dose-response function of
           radiation carcinogenesis.

division, then cell lethality should not necessarily reduce the cancer
incidence at doses where complete regeneration has occurred. If
carcinogenically-altered cells participate in the regeneration, there could
be complete compensation for loss of cells at risk.

    Proportionality between the coefficient A and the linear energy
transfer (LET) is one of the more important implications of the linear
quadratic theory. We examined this question by exposing rat skin to an
argon ion beam at the Lawrence Radiation Laboratory Bevalac Accelerator
(16). The LET of this beam is so high (125 kev/µ) that only a few tracks
per nucleus are sufficient to produce several hundred rads of dose. The
results were a striking confirmation of the hypothesis and are also shown
in Figure 3. The dose-response relationship for argon ions is very nearly
linear in the region below about 9 Gy (note: 1 Gy = 100 rads). At higher
doses the skin was unable to compensate for the severe lethality, and the
yield of tumors declined in association with frank ulceration and loss of
tissue. The data from Figure can be used to provide estimates of the
relative biological effectiveness (RBE) for tumor induction as a function
of radiation dose. The results indicate the RBE is about 2.5 at the peak
yield dose and increases as the dose is reduced reaching about 5 at the
lowest dose where data is available (∿100 rads).

Recovery and Repair in Radiation Carcinogenesis of Skin

    Generally mammalian cells are capable of repairing at least part of
the damage caused by the low LET ionizing radiation, and it is important to
establish whether carcinogenic alterations are subject to similar repair
processes. Certainly if multiple events are involved in carcinogenesis, if
one or more events are repaired before subsequent ones occur, the risk of
carcinogenesis may be greatly reduced. Hence, a series of experiments was
designed to attempt to establish experimentally whether proximity of doses

in time was an important factor in radiation carcinogenesis. Such
information would be extremely valuable for extrapolating risks to low
doses and for providing a rational basis for taking dose rate into account
in risk assessment calculations.

An important question for carcinogenesis in general and for radiation
carcinogenesis, in particular, is whether or how the carcinogenic effects
of two or more individual doses add together to produce their overall
effect. The simplest expectation is that multiple doses produce time
functions of tumor yield that are additive in all time increments. That
such a possibility was not the case was found on the basis of results where
two doses of radiation were applied to the rat skin. The timing between
the doses was clearly important and indicated that the tissue was capable
of repairing at least part of the radiation damage relevant to cancer
induction (17). By varying the time between exposures, we estimated that
the repair half-time of the repairing event was about 3 hrs. (18).

A similar degree of repair occurs irrespective of how many individual
doses are given (17). Many individual doses of electrons were given to the
same region of skin. In the first series of experiments a relatively small
numbers of daily fractions (maximum 10) were given. A given dose D was
split into n equal fractions of magnitude D/n. If the time between
fractions is great in comparison to the repair halftime, the expected
yield, Y_n, from n fractions is n times the yield from one fraction Y(D/n),
i.e., Y_n = n x Y(D/n). Since Y_n is a measurable quantity, dividing it by
the fraction number and plotting against the dose per fraction (D/n) gives
Y(D/n) which should show consistency with the results at higher single
doses if the recovery is equally effective irrespective of the number of
fractions.

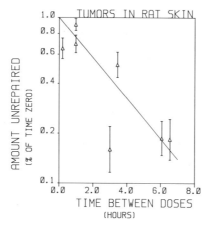

Fig. 4. A plot of the percentage unrepaired (P)
versus time between fractions. P was
determined from the equation: P =
(f(d,0)-f(d,t))/(f(D,0)-f(D,+)), where
f(D,0) is the cancer yield when two equal
doses of magnitude D were given with no
time separating them, f(D,+) is the
response when two exposures were well
separated (greater than 24 hrs.) and
f(D,t) is the tumor response when the two
exposures were separated by time t.

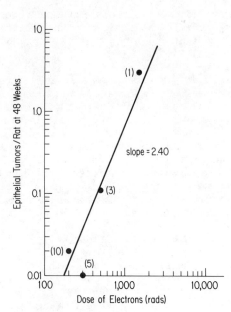

Fig. 5. The tumor yield per fraction at 48 weeks is plotted against the dose of electrons per fraction on a log-log scale. The slope of 2.4 is an estimate of the dose exponent of the second term in equation 3.

In a second series of experiments, the question was addressed whether something fundamentally different happens when the radiation exposures extend to times when the tumors from the early doses are beginning to appear so that cells may be exposed to additional radiation dose as they are progressing to cancer. Radiation doses were given weekly for duration of life.

The increased exponent for the multiple doses is much greater than would be expected if the effects of each individual dose were simply additive in each time increment. Simple additivity an expected exponent of about 3, i.e., 1 or more than about 2, whereas the actual exponent is much greater. For 75 rads per week the exponent was only 2.9, but these data are based on a relatively small number of tumors. Both groups contained about 40 rats so that the 150 rads/week curve is based on about 150 tumors while the 75 rads/week curve is based on less than 12 tumors. In the multistage theory the increased exponent is interpretable either as an increased number of events occurring stochastically in time or as clonal growth of one or more of the intermediate stages.

It is also clear from the data in Figure 6 that split dose repair continued to be operative for at least 52 exposures. In spite of the exponent on the time function being close to 6 for weekly 1.5 Gy doses, the tumor yield was still less than 1.0 tumors/rat at an accumulated dose of 78.0 Gy. A single exposure of 16.0 Gy would produce the same yield (see Figure 2.) which means that about 80% of the carcinogenic effectiveness of the radiation was lost because of repair in the multiple exposures.

The Geometrical Distribution of Dose

A surprising feature of our studies of radiation carcinogenesis in rat skin has been that the yield of tumors is number of cells irradiated (19,

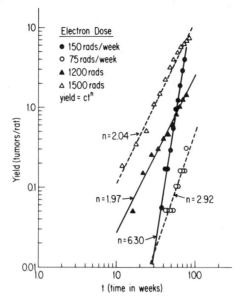

Fig. 6. Tumor yield as a function of time for
doses of 75 and 150 rads per week. Also
included in Figure 8 for comparison are
results for a single dose. The log-log
plot reveals the time exponents to be
about 2 for single doses and more than 6
for the repeated exposures.

20, 21). There are two general explanations of such a finding: (1) either
carcinogenesis does not originate in single cells but rather from clusters
of cells, or (2) the carcinogenic alterations can be repaired or prevented
from being expressed in cells in proximity to unirradiated cells. Since
there is no evidence that carcinogenesis is modifiable by hormones and
other modifiers, the second explanation seems more probable.

To study the effect of geometrical distribution of dose, rat skin was
irradiated with low energy X-rays in either a sieve pattern or in a uniform
patterns. The resulting tumor yields were expressed in units of number of
tumors per unit area of tissue exposed. For the same number of cells
exposed, there was a markedly reduced onset of tumor development when the
radiation was localized in comparison to generalized exposure. Moreover,
when the tissue between the heavily irradiated pores was irradiated with a
low dose, the reduction was eliminated. We interpreted these results to
mean that unirradiated cells near to the irradiated cells were able either
to lower the effective dose possibly by providing diffusible radioprotective compounds or were able to alter the progression of potential
cancer cells. Based on geometrical considerations, the irradiated cells are
protected for a distance of about 0.2 ㎜ from the irradiated region.

Another possibly-related geometrical effect was observed; for a given
surface the yield of tumors declined as the penetration of the radiation
decreased. If the penetration was less than about 180 microns, no tumors
at all were observed (22). If the radiation penetrated deeper than 180
microns, tumors of all histological types, including squamous carcinomas
and adnexal tumors were produced. Overall, the yield of tumors was more
closely related to the dose at about 0.3 mm than to the surface dose.

57

Since the tips of the resting phase hair follicles are located at a depth of about 0.3 mm, the results suggested that the hair follicle may be the target cell population for radiation carcinogenesis in rat skin. A test of this hypothesis by selective irradiation at 0.3 mm with an alpha particle Bragg peak proved to be negative; no additional tumors were induced over the number expected from the Bragg curve plateau region (23). Possibly, the width of the Bragg peak was too narrow to irradiate a sufficient number of cells to produce a detectible yield of tumors, so the question of whether a special target cell population exists at 0.3 mm remains unresolved.

Cell Proliferation and Carcinogenesis

There are several ways that proliferation could play a role in radiation carcinogenesis In addition to the obvious requirement that cancer cells must retain the capacity for cell division, cell division may serve the purpose of converting initial alterations into mutations that can be transmitted to daughter cells (24). Cell division may also promote the progression of potential cancer cells into cancer cells (25). If either of these suggestions is correct, the rate of cell division at the time of and subsequent to irradiation should be an important determinant of the rate of appearance of the cancers.

To test whether the cell proliferation rate affects the tumor yield, rat skin was exposed in the growing phase of the hair cycle when the epithelial cell populations are in a state of rapid proliferation (26). The tumor yield in growing phase skin was only slightly higher than in similarly-exposed resting phase skin in spite of the great differences in the proliferation rates at the time of irradiation. Furthermore, when cell proliferation in the skin was stimulated by plucking the hair repeatedly or by stripping the skin surface with cellophane tape repeatedly, the tumor yield was unaffected. Perhaps not all cells in the hair follicles or the epidermis are at risk for radiation carcinogenesis. If the cells at risk are only a small proportion of the total cells, e.g., the germ cells, proliferation of the entire organ may not reflect proliferation of the relevant subpopulation.

In separate experiments the hair germ cells were stimulated prior to irradiation by plucking hair. Then skin was irradiated at various stages of follicle elongation up to and including the fully mature, hair-producing anagen follicle. The results showed that irradiation of the various stages of follicle elongation had no effect on the skin tumor yield, except that the minimum induction time was reduced slightly in the fully mature anagen phase.

Locating the carcinogenically-sensitive cells in the anagen (growing) phase was attempted by varying the penetration of the radiation (26). The depth found to be most closely correlated with tumor yield was about 0.4 mm; a value not very different from the comparable value found for resting phase skin. In spite of great differences between the depth of anagen (1.0 mm) and telogen resting (0.3 mm) follicles, the location of the sensitive cells did not differ. This can be explained by assuming that the follicular stem cells (the presumptive target cells) remain at about the same level in the skin throughout the entire hair cycle. Such a possibility is plausible because during the transition from the large growing follicle to the smaller resting follicle (a transition known as catagen), the entire follicle below the level of the hair germ cells is resorbed. Presumably cells with carcinogenic alterations existing below the hair germ level in a growing follicle are resorbed before their carcinogenic potential is expressed. Generally the hair growth cycle has a duration of 3 to 4 weeks.

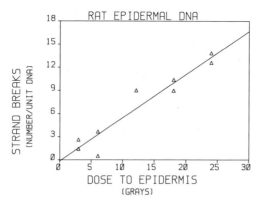

Fig. 7. Single strand breaks in rat epidermis
exposed to single doses of electron
radiation. The straight line is a least
squares fit of the data points.
Measurements were made by means of an
alkaline unwinding procedure.

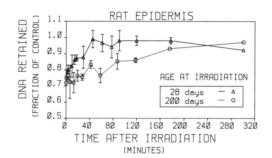

Fig. 8. Repair of single strand breaks in rat
epidermis at 2 ages. Error bars are
standard errors of the mean. The skin
dose was 10 Gray.

DNA Damage and Repair in Relation to Carcinogenesis

There are numerous candidates for the initial lesion in DNA that sets
a cell on the path to cancer. Some of the most frequently cited are DNA
strand breaks, base damage in the form of adducts, base deletion, and DNA-
DNA cross links. Breaks in the deoxyribophosphate strand structure are one
important way that ionizing radiation damages DNA, and we attempted to
determine whether their induction and repair kinetics were correlated with
our knowledge about carcinogenesis in the rat skin (27). If such breaks
occur in only one strand (single-strand breaks), they are readily
repairable, presumably correctly because of the availability of an unbroken
homologous template. However, if breaks occur in both strands (double-
strand breaks), the consequence may be a break in the chromosome which many
not be repairable or may repair in a way that causes chromosomal
rearrangements (28).

Since 2 single strand breaks on opposite strands could produce a
double strand break, it was important to determine whether the kinetics of
single strand break repair correlated with repair of carcinogenically
relevant damage. It was known that mammalian fibroblasts in tissue culture

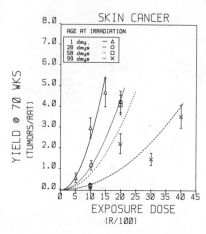

Fig. 9. Cancer yield in rat skin as a function of
x-ray exposure at different ages. Yields
were determined uniformly at 70 weeks
after irradiation. Error bars are
standard deviations estimated from the
total number of tumors.

generally are able to repair radiation-induced single strand breaks with a
halftime of about 20 min. which is much less than the halftime for the
repair of the carcinogenic effect (180 min.). Since the rate of single
strand break repair could differ in vivo, we applied in vitro techniques to
measure the rate of repair of DNA single strand breaks in the rat epidermis
(29). Utilizing alkaline unwinding, we obtained data indicating that
single strand breaks were produced in proportion to dose, and that the
repair halftime was about 21 min. not very different from values found for
a variety of cell lines in vitro. These data are shown in Figures 7 and 8.
The discrepant repair halftimes indicate that single strand breaks are
not consistent with the requirements of an initial lesion in
carcinogenesis.

Age and Radiation Carcinogenesis

In the multistage theory of carcinogenesis, the events necessary to
produce a tumor cell might occur spontaneously which means that they might
accumulate with age. If spontaneously occurring events relevant to
carcinogenesis accumulate with age, one would expect a given dose of
radiation to produce tumors more readily in older animals than in younger
ones. To test this expectation, we exposed rats to single doses of
radiation at various ages. The yield of tumors was determined at identical
times after irradiation (30). The results contradicted the expectation
that spontaneous events accumulate with age. In fact, fewer not more
tumors formed as the rats were irradiated at progressively older ages.
These results are shown in Figure 9.

As a follow up to this observation, the rate of single strand break
repair in the epidermis was measured as a function of age. In parallel
with the reduction in cancer induction, the rate of repair of single strand
breaks also decreased with increasing age. It was noted that other kinds
of repair, namely, wound repair, showed evidence of reduced effectiveness
with increasing age. The relevance of these observations to carcinogenesis
is unknown, but if the carcinogenic repair rate also declines with
increasing age, carcinogenesis may be more closely correlated with repair
potency than with the magnitude of the primary damage.

60

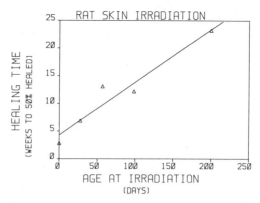

Fig. 10. Healing time of radiation-induced wounds
in rat skin. The skin was exposed to 30
Gray of 0.8 MeV electrons. All wounds
eventually healed, forming contracted
fibrotic scars.

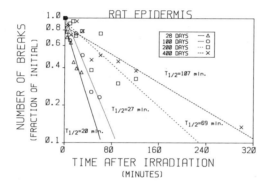

Fig. 11. The repair of radiation-induced single
strand breaks in rat epidermis as a
function of age. Measurements were made
by means of an alkaline unwinding
procedure.

Ultraviolet Carcinogenesis in Combination with Ionizing Radiation

A large part of the skin cancer burden in humans is associated with
exposure to the ultraviolet component of sunlight. However, there is an
indication that humans exposed to both ultraviolet light and ionizing
radiation run a significantly higher risk of developing skin tumors than
individuals exposed to only one of these agents (31, 3). In an attempt to
determine whether rat skin exhibited a similar response synergism, we
exposed rats to single doses of ionizing radiation (electrons) followed by
multiple weekly dose of germicidal (254 nm) or solar spectrum (greater than
290 nm) ultraviolet light (UV). The yield of skin tumors was determined
for at least 18 months after the final radiation dose (32, 33).

As an estimate of dose, we measured pyrimidine dimers in the epidermal
DNA. The pyrimidine dimers were measured by prelabelling the DNA with
[3]HTdR, isolating and digesting the DNA and then separating the bases from
the dimers by paper chromatography. Dimers exhibited a linear dependence
on exposure dose (Figure 12). The UV alone produced a large number of

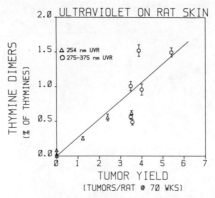

Fig. 12. Thymine dimers in epidermal DNA of rat
skin plotted against he yield of
keratoacanthomas for 2 wavelengths of
ultraviolet radiation. Dimers were
measured by paper chromatography.

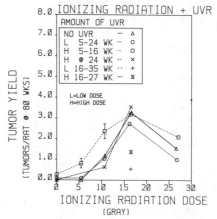

Fig. 13. The yield of malignant tumors in rat
skin exposed to ionizing radiation in
combination with ultraviolet radiation.
Error bars are standard deviations
estimated from the square root of the
total tumor count. The ionizing
radiation was 0.8 MeV electrons. The UV
exposures were given after a single
exposure to ionizing radiation. L = 2 x
10^4 joules/m^2; H = 10 x 10^4 joules/m^2.

benign keratoachanthomas but no malignant tumors. The yield continued to
be proportional to dose.

The data in Figure 13 show the yield of malignant tumors for ionizing
radiation and UV in combination. The addition of UV to the ionizing
radiation yielded more tumors at low doses of ionizing radiation. However,
there were fewer tumors at higher doses of ionizing radiation, where
normally one expects the greatest number of tumors to occur. The reduction
seemed to be a sterilizing effect on the development of small tumors,
because when the UV exposures were stopped, tumors began to appear at about
the same rate as observed earlier in the groups that received ionizing

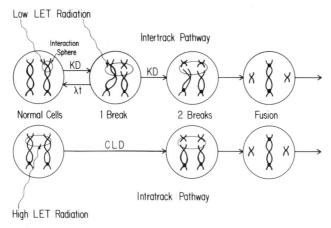

Fig. 14. A model showing how low and high LET radiation might
lead to the same chromosomal lesion by intertrack and
intratrack pathways, respectively. Low LET proceeds in
2 steps with repair, while high LET proceeds in a
single step without repair. The interaction sphere is
the region of the DNA molecule within which radiation
energy must be absorbed to produce a lesion.

radiation without subsequent UV. It was especially interesting that the UV
prevented the onset of all types of tumors including squamous carcinomas
and adnexal (hair follicle) tumors. Since more than 80% of the solar
spectrum UV dose was absorbed in the epidermis, and since virtually none
penetrated to the level of the sebaceous glands, the germ cells receive
little, if any, dose. If the sterilizing effect is a result of direct
action of the UV, one must assume that the presumptive tumor cells were in
or just below the surface epidermis at the time of exposure to the UV.
This result conflicts with the results indicating that critical targets for
radiation oncogenesis can be found about 0.3 mm below the skin surface.

A Model of Radiation Carcinogenesis

One of the major theories concerning the molecular mechanism of
radiation action on living cells is the dual action hypothesis. In this
hypothesis, events or hits resulting in molecular damage are postulated as
the starting point for several measurable endpoints of biological damage.
We have been attempting to explain radiation carcinogenesis data in terms
of a two event or dual action postulate (Figure 14). In this formalism an
interaction is assumed to occur between two primary events somehow forming
an aberrant cell that progresses in a stepwise manner to acquire malignant
properties (34, 35). The interaction is envisioned to proceed quickly when
the events are in close geometrical and temporal proximity. Furthermore,
the events are assumed to be repairable so that an interaction may be
averted if one event is repaired before the second one occurs.
Unfortunately, the identity of the primary event is unknown, although it is
presumably a molecular alteration in a DNA molecule, since the neoplastic
properties must be propagated to daughter cells. As mentioned above, one
plausible candidate is a break in the deoxyribophosphate strand structure
which could be the initial event in a cascade that leads to additional
mutational and karyotypic changes.

Certain conclusions about the nature of the initial events can be derived from information now available. We must assume that the hypothetical events are a direct or indirect result of the molecular absorption events (ionizations) produced by the radiation. This assumption means that the geometrical distribution of the hypothetical lesions in the cells must be directly related to the distribution of the primary ionizations.

Consequently, the distribution of carcinogenic events (hypothetical) is determined by the physical location of the ionizations and the latter can be markedly altered by varying the linear energy transfer (LET) of the radiation. As an ionizing particle, e.g., electron, passes through a cell, it leaves a track of ionizations that are spaced in a manner that depends on the velocity, mass and charge of the particle. The LET is proportional to the number of ionizations per unit length of track. At extremely low LET values, where many individual tracks are necessary to produce a given dose, most ionizations are associated with different particle tracks. For example, high energy electrons produce only about 3 ions in traversing an epidermal nucleus, and as many as 3000 tracks are required to produce a dose of a few hundred rads. As the LET increases the number of tracks necessary to produce a given dose declines proportionally until at very high LET values, e.g., 100 kev/μ or higher, hundreds of rads can be delivered by only one or 2 tracks per nucleus. In the latter circumstance the primary ionizations and any events derived from them follow a geometrical alignment along particle tracks. Consequently, at high LET the chance that members of an interacting pair of events are contained within the same track is quite high. As the LET increases, the chance of events being within an interaction distance of one another increases proportionally, and intratrack interactions are proportional to LET as well as dose. Moreover, since events in a given track are produced essentially simultaneously, intratrack interactions proceed quickly without the possibility of significant repair.

At low LET values, many individual tracks are necessary to produce a given dose, and the two members of any interacting pair of events were likely to be produced by events in different tracks. Since events in different tracks are independent, the probability of two occurring within an interaction distance is the product of the individual occurrence probabilities. Primary events are assumed to be proportional to ionizations (either single ionizations or clusters) and to dose. Hence, the yield of interactions between events in different tracks would be proportional to dose squared. Once two events interact, it is assumed that an irreparable lesion is formed.

Without specifying the nature of the primary events, the above considerations lead to the following dose-response function when the time of exposure is so short that repair during the exposure can be neglected:

$$Y_1(D) = aLD + bD^2 \qquad (4)$$

and to the following function when the dose rate is:

$$Y_2(D) = aLD + (bDr)/c \qquad (5)$$

The similarity of equation 4 with equation 3 derived from the dual action theory is obvious.

Equation 5 is an expression of the expected dose-response function at low dose rates. Equations 4 and 5 mean that the dose-response characteristics of the carcinogenic response to radiation can be specified by 3 constants, a, b, and c. The three parameters are measurable as

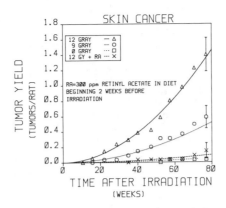

Fig. 15. Skin cancer in rats exposed to single
doses of electron radiation and fed
retigl acetate. The error bars are
standard deviations based on the square
root of the number of tumors.

follows: b in dose-response studies with low LET radiation, a in dose-response studies with high LET radiation and c in fractionation studies with low LET radiation. Such experiments have already been carried out for rat skin and the results are as follows: $a = 2.5 \times 10^{-5}$ tumor μ/rad kev rat, $b = 1.3 \times 10^{-6}$ tumors/rat rad^2 and $C = 0.24$ hr.$^{-1}$. In equation 5, the ratio of aL to b is the dose, D_e, where the linear and dose squared terms make equal contributions to the total response. On the basis of the numerical evaluations above:

$$D_e = (aL)/b = 19L \qquad (6)$$

where L is the LET of the radiation in kev/μ. For argon ions $L = 125$ kev/μ and D_e is 2875 rads, while for electrons $L = 0.34$ kev/μ and D_e is 6 rads.

It is recognized that the approach outlined here is overly simplified in that it neglects a number of potentially important factors, such as, the cytotoxic effect of the radiation and the likelihood that a variety of biological or hormonal factors may modify the expression of neoplastic and potentially neoplastic cells. Certainly cytotoxicity cannot be ignored at doses above the peak yield where further dose increases lead to unregenerated tissue destruction and fewer tumors. Accordingly, the model outlined can only be fitted to data below the peak.

Histology and Growth Characteristics of the Tumors

The skin contains a variety of cell types and the tumors induced by ionizing radiation exhibit a distribution of histological types that reflect the major types of cells found in the skin. For example, the various types of tumors occur with overall relative frequency of occurrence in parentheses as follows: squamous carcinomas (30%), basal cell carcinomas (20%), keratosebaceous tumors (35%), sebaceous tumors (10%), sarcomas (5%). The distribution of tumor types is relatively invariant and does not depend on the type of radiation, the geometrical distribution of the radiation or the temporal pattern of dose application. A slight excess of squamous carcinomas is seen at the doses above the peak yield dose.

Modification of Radiation Carcinogenesis

Retinoids have been found to have considerable antitumor activity against a variety of tumors, including mammary tumors and skin tumors (36). Generally it has been assumed that the retinoids act in the second or promotional phase of tumor development and perhaps even exert their effect on the differentiation in tumor development. Somewhat surprisingly we found that the retinoids act to inhibit mammary tumors when given at about the time of administration of a chemical carcinogen (37). Since the carcinogen employed in these experiments required metabolic activation, the retinoid could have affected that activation. To test for possible inhibition with a direct-acting carcinogen, we gave dietary supplements of retinyl acetate to rats at various times in relation to exposure to carcinogenic doses of ionizing radiation on the skin (37).

The results are shown in Figure 15 which shows the yield of tumors for the non-retinoid exposed animals and for groups exposed to the same radiation dose but also given dietary retinoids at various times as indicated. The group that received the retinoid beginning 2 weeks prior to the radiation exposure and continuing indefinitely thereafter developed only 4 tumors in comparison to 39 tumors in the comparably irradiated controls. Short exposure to the retinoid beginning 2 weeks prior to irradiation and ending 1 week after the irradiation and continuous exposure to the retinoid beginning 1 week after irradiation produced about equal inhibitory effect on the radiation-induced tumors. These results indicate that the development of radiation induced tumors in the skin is subject to the inhibitory action of the retinoids. The degree of inhibition was more marked than has been seen for several indirect acting carcinogens in other tissues (36).

An important question in environmental carcinogenesis is whether and how diverse carcinogens might interact to produce cancer in a given tissue. We examined this question in rats by exposing the skin to single doses of ionizing radiation followed by multiple weekly doses of 7,12 dimethylbenz(a)anthracene (DMBA) (38). DMBA is a polycyclic aromatic hydrocarbon that requires metabolic activation prior to producing its carcinogenic effect. The results are shown in Figure 16. There is a striking difference in the temporal onset patterns. For DMBA the tumor incidence is consistent with a power function with an exponent of about 6, while the same exponent for carrying radiation is much lower, i.e., about 2. This difference is at least partly associated with multiple exposures versus single exposure. Nevertheless, the results are almost exactly additive. The curve showing the tumor yield when the two carcinogens were given to the same animals is almost the exactly the summation of the curves for exposure to only one agent. Certainly prior irradiation with electrons failed to sensitize the skin to exposure to a different carcinogen.

Comparison of Radiation Skin Carcinogenesis in Different Species

The usefulness of experimental animals for estimating hazards and risks for humans is clearly dependent on the validity of the implicit assumption that the mechanisms of action are similar if not identical in different species. At the present time, it is not possible to determine the mechanism of radiation damage in human tissue, but it is possible to draw inferences of similarities between similar species by comparison of dose-response and time-response functions. We have made such a comparison between rats and humans exposed under nearly identical conditions and found a remarkable similarity once the differences of life spans is taken into account (2).

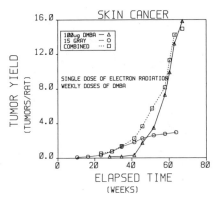

Fig. 16.   Skin cancer rats exposed to ionizing
           radiation (0.8 MeV electrons) followed
           by weekly doses of DMBA in 1.0 ml
           acetone. The combined exposure gave
           almost exactly the same yield as the
           summation of the individual exposures.

On the other hand, a comparison of radiation carcinogenesis in rat and
mouse skin reveals some striking differences which are still unexplained
(39). The tumor yields were compared under conditions of exposure that
were as identical as possible. To compensate for different skin
thicknesses, the penetration of the electron beam was modified in order
that the distribution of dose along the depth of the hair follicles was
proportionally the same in the two species. For the same proportionate
area exposed, the yield of tumors in the rat was about 40 times greater
than that in the mouse.

The great excess of tumors in the rat could be attributed to two
principal factors: (1) the greater size of the rat and (2) the presence of
hair follicle tumors in the rat that were not present in the mouse. By
comparing the results in terms of the tumor yield per unit area, the rat
excess was reduced to about 8 times that of the mouse. While a variety of
epithelial tumors occurred in the rat, squamous carcinoma was the single
predominate tumor in the mouse. Since the latter tumor comprised only
about 30% of the rat tumors, comparison of squamous carcinoma only between
the two species reduced the rat excess to about 2.5.

The rat was more sensitive than the mouse to radiation carcinogenesis,
because it had more cells at risk and because its epithelial cells were at
risk for a variety of additional tumors that were presumably of hair
follicle origin. Neither of these results could have been predicted a
priori and both deserve further study. Such results emphasize the need to
understand mechanisms before making extrapolations between species in
anything other than a qualitative manner.

ACKNOWLEDGEMENT

These studies were partially supported by the following grants:
Department of Energy (COO-3380), National Institute of Environmental Health
Sciences (ES 00260), National Cancer Institute (CA 13343), and American
Cancer Society (00009).

REFERENCES

1. F. C. Bock, Cutaneous carcinogenesis, in: "Advances in Modern Toxicology, Vol. 4," F. N. Marzulli, and H. I. Maibach, eds., John Wiley & Sons, New York (1977), pp. 473-486.

2. R. E. Albert, F. J. Burns, and R. Shore, Comparison of the incidence and time patterns of radiation-induced skin cancer in humans and rats, in: "Late Biological Effects of Ionizing Radiation: Proceeding of a Symposium," Vienna, 13-17 March 1978, Vol. II, International Atomic Energy Agency, Vienna (1978), pp. 499-505.

3. B. Modan, D. Baidatz, and H. Mart, Radiation-induced head and neck tumors, Lancet 1:277-279 (1974).

4. R. E. Albert, W. Newman, and B. Altshuler, The dose-response relationships of beta-ray-induced skin tumors in the rat, Radiat. Res. 15:410-430 (1961).

5. A. Whittemore, and J. Keller, Quantitative theories of carcinogenesis, SIAM Review 20:1-30 (1978).

6. P. Armitage, and R. Doll, The age distribution of cancer and a multistage theory of carcinogenesis, Brit. J. Cancer 8:1-12 (1954).

7. L. Foulds, "Neoplastic Development-2," Academic Press, N.Y. (1975).

8. R. E. Albert, P. Phillips, P. Bennett, F. Burns, and R. Heimbach. The morphology and growth characteristics of radiation-induced epithelial skin tumors in the rat, Cancer Res. 29:658-668 (1969).

9. F. J. Burns, M. Vanderlaan, and R. E. Albert, Growth rate and induction kinetics of radiation-induced rat skin tumors, Radiat. Res. 55:531 (1973).

10. National Academy of Sciences, "The Effects on Populations of Exposure to Low Levels of Ionizing Radiation," Advisory Committee on the Biological Effects of Ionizing Radiation (BEIR), National Research Council, Washington, D.C. (1980).

11. A. Kellerer, and H. A. Rossi, Generalized formulation of dual radiation action, Radiat. Res. 75:471-488 (1978).

12. M. Vanderlaan, F. J. Burns, and R. E. Albert, A model describing the effects of dose and dose rate on tumor induction by radiation in rat skin, in: "Biological and Environmental Effects of Low-level Radiation, Vol. 1," International Atomic Energy Agency, Vienna (1976), pp. 253-263.

13. F. J. Burns, R. E. Albert, and R. Heimbach, The RBE for skin tumors and hair follicle damage in the rat following irradiation with alpha particles and electrons, Radiat. Res. 36:225-241 (1968).

14. R. E. Albert, F. J. Burns, and R. Heimbach, Skin damage and tumor formation from grid and sieve patterns of electron and beta radiation in the rat, Radiat. Res. 30:525-540 (1967).

15. F. J. Burns, R. E. Albert, I. P. Sinclair, and P. Bennett, The effect of fractionation on tumor induction and hair follicle damage in rat skin, Radiat. Res. 53:235-240 (1973).

16. F. J. Burns, and R. E. Albert, Dose-response for rat skin tumors induced by single and split doses of argon ions, in: "Biological and Medical Research with Accelerated Heavy Ions at the Bevalac," University of California (1980).

17. F. J. Burns, R. E. Albert, I. P. Sinclair, and M. Vanderlaan, The effect of a 24-hour fractionation interval on the induction of rat skin tumors by electron radiation, Radiat. Res. 62:478-487 (1975).

18. F. J. Burns, and M. Vanderlaan, Split dose recovery for radiation induced tumors in rat skin, Inter. J. Radiat. Biol. 32:135-144 (1977).

19. R. E. Albert, F. J. Burns, and R. D. Heimbach, Skin damage and tumor formation from grid and sieve patterns of electron and beta radiation in the rat, Radiat. Res. 30:525-540 (1967).

20. R. E. Albert, and F. J. Burns, Tumor and injury responses of rat skin after sieve pattern x-irradiation, Radiat. Res. 67:474-481 (1976).

21. F. J. Burns, R. E. Albert, M. Vanderlaan, and P. Strickland, The dose response curve for tumor induction with single and split doses of 10 Mev protons, Radiat. Res. 62:598-599 (1975).

22. R. E. Albert, F. J. Burns, and R. Heimbach, The effect of penetration depth of electron radiation on skin tumor formation in the rat, Radiat. Res. 30:515-524 (1967).

23. R. Heimbach, F. J. Burns, and R. E. Albert, An evaluation by alpha particle Bragg peak radiation of the critical depth in the rat skin for tumor induction, Radiat. Res. 39:332-344 (1969).

24. M. D. Reuber, Development of preneoplastic and neoplastic lesions of the liver in male rats given 0.025 percent N-2-fluorenyldiacetamide, J. Natl. Cancer Inst. 34:697-723 (1965).

25. F. J. Burns, M. Vanderlaan, and R. E. Albert, Proliferation of early tumor foci in irradiated rat skin, Radiat. Res. 59:18 (1974).

26. F. J. Burns, I. P. Sinclair, R. E. Albert, and M. Vanderlaan, Tumor induction and hair follicle damage for different electron penetrations in rat skin, Radiat. Res. 67:474-481 (1976).

27. M. G. Ormerod, Radiation-induced strand breaks in the DNA of mammalian cells, in: "Biology of Radiation Carcinogenesis," J. M. Yuhas, R. W. Tennant, and J. D. Regan, eds., Raven Press, N.Y. (1976), pp. 67-92.

28. H. P. Leenhouts, and K. H. Chadwick, Radiation-induced DNA double strand breaks and chromosome aberration, Theor. Appl. Genet. 44:167-172 (1974).

29. F. J. Burns, and E. V. Sargent, The induction and repair of DNA breaks in rat epidermis irradiated with electrons, Radiat. Res. 87:137-144 (1981).

30. M. Vanderlaan, P. Strickland, R. E. Albert, and F. J. Burns, Age-dependence of the oncogenicity of ionizing radiation in rat skin, Radiat. Res. 67:629 (1976).

31. R. E. Shore, R. E. Albert, and B. S. Pasternack, Follow-up study of patients treated by X-ray epilation for tinea capitis, Arch. Environ. Health 20:21-28 (1976).

32. P. Strickland, P., "Pyrimidine Dimer Formation in Epidermal DNA and Oncogenesis in Rat Skin Exposed to Ultraviolet Radiation," Ph.D. Thesis, New York University Program in Environmental Health Science (1978).

33. P. Strickland, F. J. Burns, and R. E. Albert, Induction of skin tumors in the rat by single exposure to ultraviolet radiation, Photochem. Photobiol. 30:683-688 (1979).

34. F. J. Burns, and M. Vanderlaan, Split-dose recovery for radiation-induced tumors in rat skin, Int. J. Radiat. Biol. 32:135-144 (1977).

35. F. J. Burns and R. E. Albert, Application of a Linear Quadratic Model with Repair to Rat Skin Carcinogenesis Data, in: "Proceedings of 7th International Congress of Radiation Research," J. J. Broerse, G. W. Barendsen, H. B. Kal, A. J. Van der Kogel, eds., Nijhoff Publishers, (1983), pp. C6-05.

36. R. C. Moon, C. J. Grubbs, and M. B. Sporn, Inhibition of 7,12-dimethylbenz(a)anthracene-induced mammary carcinogenesis by retinyl acetate, Cancer Res. 36:2626-2630 (1976).

37. F. J. Burns, E. V. Sargent, D. McCormick, and R. E. Albert, Retinoid inhibition of radiation-induced rat skin tumors, Proc. Am. Assoc. Cancer Res. 23:89 (1982).

38. F. J. Burns, P. Strickland, and R. E. Albert, The combined carcinogenic action of ionizing radiation and DMBA on rat skin, Radiat. Res. 71:607 (1977).

39. R. E. Albert, F. J. Burns, and P. Bennett, Radiation-induced hair follicle damage and tumor formation in mouse and rat skin, J. Natl. Cancer Inst. 49:1131-1137 (1972).

EXPERIMENTAL RADIATION CARCINOGENESIS*

G. Silini

Secretary, United Nations Scientific Committee on the
Effects of Atomic Radiation (UNSCEAR)
Vienna International Centre
Vienna, Austria

INTRODUCTION

The risk assessment of radiation-induced cancer at the low doses
delivered by environmental and occupational sources would be greatly
facilitated by a more precise knowledge of the shapes of the dose-response
functions. This knowledge is not available at present and is not likely to
be obtained in the near future by direct observations. Two features of the
dose-response relationships are most important for risk evaluation at low
doses: the existence of a dose threshold and the general form of the
curve.

Absence of the threshold is usually assumed if the probability of
tumour induction plotted against dose allows extrapolation to the origin by
eye, or if the calculated regression crosses the abscissa at values which
are not significantly different from zero. Conversely, the presence of a
threshold cannot be excluded when these conditions are not fulfilled.
However, disproving a threshold below the range of direct observation may
be impossible, owing to the statistical fluctuations of the spontaneous
tumur incidence and of the induce response. In practice, therefore,
thresholds are often assumed to be absent, although this condition has
never been proven for any form of radiation-induced malignancy (1) and
should be regarded as a working hypothesis.

In spite of the marked variability between different animal species
and strains, dose-response relationships for various experimental tumours
after single whole-body or localized exposures may be grouped under three
different categories (1):

(a) Tumours showing a progressively higher incidence with
    increasing dose up to a maximum and decline at still higher
    doses (most forms);

(b) Tumours showing a negative correlation between incidence and
    dose (these tumours have normally high spontaneous frequencies);

---

*Opinions expressed in this paper are the author's own and not those of
the UNSCEAR

71

(c) Tumours showing no clear rise of incidence for doses up to
several Gy.

For dose-response relationships of type (a) some regularities have
been pointed out (1) which conform to other radiobiological phenomena
occurring in single cells, such as killing or induction of mutations and
chromosomal aberrations. These are:

(1) RBE values for high-LET radiation relative to x and gamma rays
are higher than 1 and decrease with increasing dose;

(2) For acute doses of high-LET radiation the increase in tumour
incidence is closer to linearity than for low-LET radiation:
this latter usually produces upward concave relationships;

(3) There is little dependence of the tumour yield on dose
fractionation and protraction of high-LET radiation, while for
x and gamma rays the yield usually declines under such
conditions.

Although it is impossible to experimentally reconstruct the form of
the dose-effect relationships at the low doses of practical interest, the
phenomenon of tumour induction shows characteristics which are reminiscent
of other radiation-induced cellular and subcellular effects. It may,
therefore, be asked whether the available evidence for such effects could
throw some light on the nature of the dose-response relationships for
induction of tumours. It is also possible to critically discuss published
models for tumour induction and test their compatibility with available
experimental data. Such exercises could possibly allow generalizations to
be made as to the likely form of the dose-response relationships for some
types of cancer that would minimize the uncertainties of the risk estimates
at the very low dose and dose rates. Although in principle they may be
carried out on both human and animal tumours, in the present paper they
will only be limited to data from animal experiments.

DOSE-RESPONSE RELATIONSHIPS

Radiation-induced cancer is a stochastic phenomenon occurring with a
relatively low probability in a population of irradiated individuals. As
such, it may be analyzed for its dependence on dose and time. The event of
interest may be assumed to occur at the time of diagnosis when tumors are
readily apparent or at the time of death for rapidly lethal tumours. In
experimental work the populations under study usually consist of animals
standardized for species, strain, sex and age, irradiated under controlled
conditions. These animals are followed for a given time or up to natural
death and are appropriately matched with other control non-irradiated
animals treated in exactly the same way. The time of death and ideally
also the cause of death are known for each animal.

Easily diagnosed or rapidly lethal tumours are readily discovered and
for such "manifest" neoplasms mathematical procedures are available to
correct for intercurrent mortality unrelated to tumour incidence. Under
these conditions one speaks of rightly censored data, because for each
individual one either knows the actual time to tumour or assumes that the
hypothetical time to tumour is longer than the time at which the animal
dies or disappears from observation due to other causes. If tumours are
"occult", in the sense that they are incidentally discovered in animals
naturally dying or sacrificed, one speaks of double censored data. In
these cases one knows that the time to tumour is either shorter or longer

than the observed time of death; however, a precise time can never be determined and correcting for competing risks is more complex.

Dose-response curves are functional relationships between an independent and a dependent variable. The independent variable is the specific energy, z, absorbed in the biological structures of interest, commonly expressed as D, the absorbed dose, which is the mean value of z: it should be noted that for the same value of D the values of z can vary greatly, depending on radiation quality. In the present context the following terminology roughly applies:

	Low Dose	Intermediate Dose	High Dose
Low-LET	< 0.2 Gy	0.2 to 2.0 Gy	> 2.0 Gy
High-LET	< 0.05 Gy	0.05 to 0.5 Gy	> 0.5 Gy

For both types of radiation low dose rates are those <0.05 mGy min^{-1}; high dose rates are those >0.05 Gy min^{-1}; intermediate dose rates are those between such limits.

In experimental radiation carcinogenesis the dependent variable, i.e., the response may be variously expressed (1). The simplest and most commonly used responses are the fractions of animals developing tumours (also called the crude tumour incidence) and the mean number of tumours per animal observed after a given dose. At low frequencies the two quantities are equal if tumours occur independently; at high frequencies the two quantities differ. It has been stressed that such ways of expressing the response are unsatisfactory owing to the presence of competing risks and to the different distribution of life times between animals exposed to different doses (2, 3, 4, 5, 6, 7, 8, 9, 10, 11, 12, 13, 14, 15).

Approximate corrections for differences in survival time may be made but results may be misleading when the frequency of tumour appearance varies substantially with post-exposure time. Rigourous corrections for age and intercurrent mortality are possible when the response of the animals is followed throughout life and careful pathology is available at death. The relevant parameter is then the age- or time-dependent rate of tumour appearance (6, 9, 16, 17, 18) or a related cumulative quantity. The basic quantitites in this approach and their risk-corrected estimates for manifest tumours are:

(a)   The tumour rate, as a function of age or time after irradiation. This is the probability at time t of an individual developing a tumour per unit time. Since the actual time of origin of the tumour is unknown, the time when it is first scored is generally used for tumours diagnosed during life time (or the time of death for rapidly lethal tumours). This quantity is obtained by dividing the number of animals developing a tumor, n, by the total number of animals at risk, N, over a given interval of time. For occult tumours observed only incidentally r(t) may not be calculated and the tumour prevalence is used instead.

(b)   The integral tumour rate, R(t). This quantity is less affected by statistical fluctuations and can therefore be calculated more readily. It is defined as the integral of the tumour rate from the time of exposure up to a given time t:

$$R(t) = {}_0\!\int^t r(t)dt$$

This quantity may also be called the mean number of tumours per animal, because it is the expected number of tumours for an animal that is at risk up to time t. The quantity may be corrected for competing risks (19, 20, 9). When multiple non-lethal tumours occur, it is necessary to specify whether the estimate of the integral tumour rate is based on first tumours only or on all observed tumours.

(c)   <u>The acturial incidence or incidence corrected for competing risks, I(t</u>
This is the probability of an animal at risk up to time t to have incurred a tumour. In the absence of competing risks the presence of competing risks may be corrected for in various ways (21). For occult tumours frequently seen in short-lived animals the actuarial incidence (which is then more frequently called <u>prevalence</u>) and the integral tumour rate are more difficult to estimate.

In most experimental studies where tumours are seen in various organs of the same animals, it is usually assumed that such tumours occur independently of each other. It has been shown, however (22), that there may be significant associations between different tumour types, and this possible complication should not be overlooked in the statistical analysis of dose-response relationships.

What has been said so far refers only to acute irradiation. In case of continuous or fractionated long-term exposure additional complexities are introduced. Under such conditions, the dose accrues with time and it may be difficult to separate the two quantities and to identify the relevant value of the cumulated dose. Actually, since induction of a tumour is followed by a period of growth until it becomes observable, the dose received by the target cells during this period is irrelevant to the induction of the tumour. Corrections are, therefore, often applied in order to subtract from the total dose the portion received after the presumed onset of neoplastic growth.

The tumour rate and the integral tumour rate depend on post-irradiation time and on other factors such as age at exposure and absorbed dose. Also, the absorbed dose may change the time dependence of tumour induction in a variety of ways. Temporal relationships, as they reflect in the concept of latency and in risk models, should, therefore, be discussed.

The latent time is the time between irradiation (single acute exposure, in the simplest instance) and manifestation of a tumour. Conceptually, it may be divided into a period of true latency (from initiation to the beginning of growth) and into a further period of growth (until the neoplasm is diagnosed). Latent times are the quantities usually reported in experimental work, since the length of latency may only be inferred by subtracting an estimated period of growth from the sum of the above two periods. There are considerable differences between the mean latent times of various tumours and their distributions. If the follow-up of an experiment is shorter than the minimum latent time, radiation-induced tumors will not be observed. If the distribution of latent times extends significantly beyond the follow-up, the dose-response relationship cannot be based on complete data. In many cases (particularly with continuous long-term irradiation) the distribution of latent times varies with absorbed dose (23, 24): the dose-response relationships derived under these conditions depend critically on the length of the observation period. At low doses, the latent times may exceed the average life span of the animals and practical thresholds may, therefore, result (25, 26, 27, 28). All these factors must by borne in mind in a discussion about the accuracy and reproducibility of dose-response curves: they point to the need to extend the length of follow-up in order that the dose-effect relationships may be assessed with reasonable completeness.

Projection of the incidence or incidence rate beyond the period of follow-up for tumours having long latent times is rarely necessary in experimental work. If necessary, it may be carried out according to two models. The first, called the absolute risk model, assumes that the rates of spontaneous and induced tumours are independent of each other, so that the rate of radiation-induced tumours does not increase in proportion to the age-dependent rate of the spontaneous ones. The second, the relative risk model, assumes that radiation has a multiplicative effect on the spontaneous tumour rate, so that the rate of tumours induced after exposure is a dose-related multiple of the spontaneous rate. Only rarely does the available information allow a decision about which of the two models is closer to reality.

In summary, tumour induction is a stochastic radiation effect that may be analyzed for its dependence on dose and time. The absorbed dose to the relevant tissues is the independent variable in dose-response studies, against which various parameters describing the response may be plotted. These are derived from the observed sequence of tumour appearance and from the number of animals at risk during a given interval. The crude incidence is an unsatisfactory parameter because it neglects differences in life time after exposure and may be affected by intercurrent mortality. Other possible parameters are the tumour rate, $r(t)$, the integral tumour rate, $R(t)$, the actuarial incidence or prevalence $I(t,D)$. Techniques are available for their calculation which are different for manifest or for occult tumours. Knowledge of the latent time is important for the analysis of dose-response curves. When latent times are dose-related, the shape of the relationships depends on observation time: under these conditions practical thresholds may apply at the lowest dose. Projection of the incidence of late-appearing tumours may be carried out according to different action models.

ASSUMPTIONS OF EXISTING MODELS

Owing to insufficent understanding of mechanisms, quantitative predictions about the effect of ionizing radiations (dose, dose rate, quality) may not be derived from basic principles. The formulation of simplified hypotheses under the form of models is the only course of action, because to this end detailed knowledge of mechanisms is not absolutely necessary.

Following the formulation of Berenblum (29), the multistage theory of cancer development has gained wide acceptance (30, 31, 32, 33, 34, 35, 36). Conceptually, it assumes tht cancer starts by initiation of one or a few neighboring cells: direct involvement of DNA has been shown at this level (37, 38, 39), but the actual mechanisms (changes in the DNA base sequence, transposition, deletion, translocation, transfection, activation of oncogenes) remain largely hypothetical (30, 40, 41, 35, 36, 42, 43). Further development of initiated cells into cancerous clones requires probably several stages, which may be promoted, inhibited or reverted by the action of secondary factors: during this long latent period systemic factors (cell division and differentiation, immunological surveillance, hormonal dependence) or exogenous factors may influence the final outcome of the process. Epigenetic factors (dys-differentiation, expression of previously suppressed genes, etc.) may also play some role.

Whatever the nature of initiation, be it somatic mutation induced at the rate of 10^{-5} to 10^{-6} Gy^{-1} of gamma radiation per locus, or any phenomenon similar to cell transformation _in vitro_ occurring at a rate of 10^{-2} to 10^{-4} Gy^{-1} per cell, the yield of malignant tumours per irradiated cell _in vivo_ is probably lower by several orders of magnitude. The theory of sequential development of cancer may explain the discrepancy in the sense that if a sequence of rare events is required to complete the process, the final probability of emergence of a malignant clone would be the product of the probability of each event. Assuming that only the first step (initiation) may be radiation induced, clinical cancer would be expressed at a much lower level of probability. However, the relationship to dose of the final tumour expression would remain similar to that of initiation, as long as the action of the other factors in the sequence would not itself depend on dose, otherwise, the form of the relationship would be distorted.

It is a general weakness of models that they can only describe initiation and cell killing, but not other modifying factors. They are, therefore, mathematical formulations in which mechanisms that cannot at present be described are compounded under the abstraction of symbols and numerical coefficients. The relative importance of these coefficients may be deduced by comparing data with predictions. For descriptive purposes, the following regions of dose may be described in low-LET dose-effect relationships:

(a) 0 - 0.2 Gy. At this level, there are few direct data, but cell killing and damage to tissue functions is considered negligible, so that dose-effect relationships would be close to those predicted by models that do not consider secondary factors.

(b) 0.2 - 2.0 Gy. Tissue damage, cell proliferation and other host factors would not be expected to dominate at this level: therefore, distortions of dose-response relationships would be relative by minor and inconsequential for the purpose of extrapolation.

(c) 2.0 - 10 Gy. Disruption of tissue, immunological and hormonal functions is known to be important and to alter the shape of the relationships in this region of dose. Extrapolation to lower doses must allow for these phenomena.

(d) Above 10 Gy. At this level, severe damage to tissues and organs is the dominating feature: the form of the dose-response could bear no relationship to the initial induction process, and extrapolation to low doses could be meaningless.

A four- to five-fold reduction in the above values might be appropriate for fast neutrons.

The question of whether a malignant clone arises from transformation of a single cell or of several contiguous cells is of critical importance for the formulation of models (44, 45, 46, 32, 47). Chromosomal and biochemical evidence favours at present the uni-cellular hypothesis (48), although most of this evidence is indirect and compatible with the alternative hypothesis that one clone may eventually be selected from among several transformed cells. Conceptually, the initiation of one (as opposed to several) cells should be distinguished from the modifying influence of neighboring cells upon the single transformed one that will eventually start malignant growth. The single- or autonomous-cell hypothesis has been questioned (49, 50, 51) on the basis of experimental data on mammary tumour induction in the rat, but the nature of this system and the arguments themselves of the critique leave some room for doubt. Clearly, such arguments must be resolved by experiments and not by calculations and so far biological evidence against the mono-cellular origin of cancer does not appear to be very solid. The mono-cellular assumption has been incorporated, directly or indirectly, into all models of radiation-induced cancerogenesis. It may be accepted as a working hypothesis, even though other views should not be ignored (52).

The number of cells at risk of transformation in vivo is not known. It is usually argued that in any given tissue the number of cells transformed must be proportional to the number of cells at risk and that this is in turn proportional to the fraction of tissue irradiated. Most models of radiation-induced cancer accept this assumption. From it, one cannot, however, infer that tumour indicence is proportional to the total number of cells in any organ or in the body, because there is no obvious correlation between incidence of tumours and body size in various species. Experiments on the induction of cancer by total and partial irradiation of the mammary tissue in rats (53, 54, 55) and by irradiation of various areas of skin in mice (56, 57, 58) are broadly consistent with the notion that the probability of induction is proportional to the number of irradiated cells at risk, assuming their uniform distribution in the irradiated tissues. However, a study on lung cancer incidence does not fit with this notion (59). It is also argued (26, 27)--and experimental evidence (60, 61) supports this argument--that hot particles are less effective than uniform irradiation for the same total dose to tissues: actually, the high dose delivered to the potentially transformed cells would probably inactivate them, thus resulting in fewer tumours.

To sum up, the pathogenesis of tumours, both spontaneous and radiation-induced, is at present poorly understood. However, carcinogenesis is likely to be a complex multi-stage process between initiation and the final clinical expression. During this long latent time a variety of changes, largely unknown in nature but of very low probability, are thought to take place and numerous endogenous and exogenous factors might accelerate or inhibit the development of potentially cancerous clones. Under such complex circumstances, the use of simplified models may be of help for predictive purposes, even though models cannot at present describe the action of the modifying factors. It may, however, be postulated that at low doses and dose rates the relationship between dose and tumour incidence may reflect that between dose and initial transformation.

Mono-cellular and mono-clonal hypotheses of tumour induction are usually assumed in all models and biological data appear to support in general these notions; however, the mono-cellular origin of cancer should still be treated as a working hypothesis. This hypothesis is critical for model formulation because the alternative one--initiation of interaction between different cells--makes the construction of models difficult or impossible. The number of cells at risk of malignant transformation is assumed, as a rule to be proportional to the fraction of the organ or tissue irradiated. Gross non-uniformity in tissue dose distribution normally results in a lower incidence of tumours than might be expected for the same dose distributed uniformly.

MODELS OF RADIATION-INDUCED CANCER

The bulk of data on the induction of experimental tumours by low-LET radiation is consistent with the generalization that there is a rising incidence at low doses, a peak incidence at some intermediate dose, and a decline at still higher doses. A model of radiation-induced cancer should, therefore, incorporate two opposite trends with dose: an increased induction and then a decline due presumably to killing of potentially transformed cells (62). This may be obtained mathematically by multiplication of an induction function and a cell killing function. The most general formulation of such a model might be as follows:

$$I(D) = (\alpha_1 D + \alpha_2 D^2) \exp - (\beta_1 D + \beta_2 D^2) \qquad (1)$$

where $I(D)$ is some appropriate expression of incidence, α_1 and α_2 are coefficients for a linear and a quadratic term of cancer induction and β_1 and β_2 coefficients for a linear and a quadratic term for cell killing. The term in α_2 will be omitted in a purely linear model, the term in α_1 will be omitted in a purely quadratic one. The exponential term (or parts of it) will be omitted when correction for cell killing is not needed.

The linear model is based on the postulate that each event of energy deposition in a target structure carries some probability of tumour induction. This probability is additive and dose rate or fractionation are not expected to alter the final effect. Since radiation energy is transferred in discrete events, all effects are ultimately linear with dose at low doses when only few cells absorb energy and their number is directly proportional to dose. In spite of the easiness of its formulation, the bulk of information available for low-LET radiation does not conform to this model. Recently, therefore, it has mainly been used for practical purposes, because it is thought to provide an upper boundary of risk for the more likely linear-quadratic model.

For high-LET radiation, the linearity of the initial slope is often distorted by cell killing or saturation phenomena: an exponential killing function may be incorporated to describe this effect. Alternatively, an empirical fit has been used in which the incidence is proportional to the square root of the dose. For systems where bending of the curve is observed, extrapolation to low doses would tend to underestimate the risk; also, dose fractionation and protraction would be expected to enhance tumour induction.

Cell killing or other biophysical phenomena are not the only mechanisms through which linearity of the response could be altered: Mayneord and Clark (26) have discussed the effect of superimposing a log-normal distribution of latent times and an inverse relationship of latency to dose on a purely linear dose relationship. Solution of this model for observation times comparable to human life expectancy results in dose-response functions which are upward concave, sometimes with apparent thresholds.

The linear-quadratic model is based on the observation that for many single-cell systems and many endpoints the form of the dose-response relationship for low-LET radiation is concave upward and the response rises with a power of dose of between 1 and 2. Broadly similar shapes are also observed for systemic effects such as tumour induction. This form of the response is thought to imply the interaction of two elementary types of damage for the occurrence of the final endpoint (63). Repair phenomena and dose-rate effects may be accounted for by the interactions of these sublesions in time and space (64). The same systems, irradiated with high-LET radiation often show linear dose-responses. Under these conditions, the RBE varies frequently as an inverse function of the dose (raised to the power of -0.5).

The most likely target of radiation action appears to be the genome and involvement of DNA in oncogenic transformation has found direct experimental support in cells transformed in vitro by agents that selectively damage DNA (38, 39). The hereditary character of some forms of cancer supports also this contention. It is not surprising, therefore, that models postulating linear-quadratic relationships presuppose a direct action of radiation on DNA or make reference to effects on DNA (chromosome aberrations, mutations) for the derivation of the relevant parameters.

It should be realized, however, that the linear-quadratic model is not a pathogenetic theory; also, the combination of a linear and a quadratic function (perhaps modified further by killing) could fit many data. Thus, on the one hand, a good fit is as such no proof that initiation indeed follows linear-quadratic kinetics and, on the other hand, the great complexity of the basic mechanisms preclude acceptance of the model as a generalized theory of cancer initiation in all tissues and under all circumstances. With these reservations in mind, the model may be applied to study the results of experiments in respect to dose, dose rate, fractionation, protraction and LET.

In order to make use of the model and to test its compatibility with experimental data, there is a need to estimate the values of α_1 and α_2. This may be done by reasonable analogies with other cellular radiobiological effects or by directly deriving the values from empirical studies. The same applies to the cell survival parameters which are known for many lines of cells but may not necessarily apply to specific tumours. Many such exercises have been performed, with different constraints imposed to the fit in order to lower the degrees of freedom involved in deriving so many parameters at the same time (65, 66, 67). The conclusions--for single-dose irradiation and ratios of α_1/α_2 between 0.5 and 2.0 Gy--are that if one totally neglects cell killing one might overestimate the risk by factors of between 2 and 4 in extrapolating down from 2 Gy to 10 mGy. Such differences could not easily be detected in experimental tumour systems.

The quadratic model assumes that for a given endpoint two consecutive primary events are required, or two concurrent events separated in space in such a way that their production by a single track is very unlikely. Proportionality between induction and square of the dose has been noted for a number of experimental tumours (56, 57, 68, 69, 7, 52).

When one fits a quadratic model to experimental data obtained at intermediate or high doses, one finds an effect at low doses which is less than that obtained by linear or linear-quadratic models. For this reason, quadratic relationships have been used (65) to predict the lower boundary of a linear-quadratic dose-response at low doses. Dose-time relationships are difficult to predict for this model and they critically depend on the time function of repair: if repair is very fast dose protraction and fractionation might lead to zero effect.

DOSE-RESPONSE RELATIONSHIPS FOR EXPERIMENTAL TUMOURS

What follows is essentially a selective update of a review published by UNSCEAR in 1977 (1) which contained an examination of many dose-response relationships then available on experimental tumour systems. At that time, the data could not be interpreted by simple mechanisms of action in view of the complex interplay of primary and secondary contributing factors. Observations regarded as a rule low-LET doses in excess of 0.5 Gy and this circumstance prevented an unambiguous definition of the shape of the relationships at low doses. The peculiarities of each system did not allow extensive generalizations, but low-LET radiation delivered at high dose rates seemed more often to produce curvilinear relationships not incompatible with a linear-quadratic model, with one notable exception (9). High-LET radiation, on the other hand, tended to produce more nearly linear relationships. Low dose rate and fractionation tended to decrease the

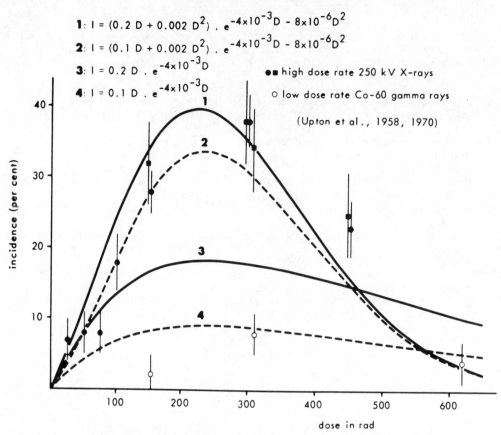

$$1: I = (0.2\ D + 0.002\ D^2) \cdot e^{-4 \times 10^{-3}D - 8 \times 10^{-6}D^2}$$

$$2: I = (0.1\ D + 0.002\ D^2) \cdot e^{-4 \times 10^{-3}D - 8 \times 10^{-6}D^2}$$

$$3: I = 0.2\ D \cdot e^{-4 \times 10^{-3}D}$$

$$4: I = 0.1\ D \cdot e^{-4 \times 10^{-3}D}$$

●■ high dose rate 250 kV X-rays

○ low dose rate Co-60 gamma rays

(Upton et al., 1958, 1970)

Fig. 1. (from ref. 66) Comparison of experimental data on the induction of myeloid leukaemia in RF male mice (data from references 71 and 72) with theoretical models of tumour induction, according to the formulas indicated. Curves 1 and 2 were obtained at high dose rate with 200-300 kV x-rays and cobalt-60 gamma rays, respectively; curves 3 and 4 were obtained with the same radiations but at lower dose rates.

carcinogenic effect of a treatment much more when low-LET radiation was involved (as compared with high-LET); however, changes in the shape itself of the dose-response relationship induced by different regimes of dose administration prevented any precise quantification of such a dose-rate effect. Later (70) the influence of dose distribution in time was examined in 10 different experimental tumour systems: dose-rate effectiveness factors from 1.1 to 6.7 were found, with many of the values actually clustering between 3 and 5.

Myeloid Leukemia

In 1978 Barendsen (66) proposed a linear-quadratic model for tumour induction and derived data for α_1/α_2 and β_1/β_2 from an analysis of data on chromosome aberration induction and reproductive death in mammalian cells. He fitted data by Upton and coworkers (71, 72) on the induction of myeloid leukemia in mice by suitably selected values of such variables and was able to show that the induction of leukemia in vivo by high-dose-rate x- and gamma-radiation could be adequately fitted by this model (Figure 1).

Robinson and Upton (73) reanalysed part of some older data published between 1958 and 1970 on RF mice, correcting for competing risks. About 2000 male mice irradiated with 250-kV X-rays at doses between zero and 4.5 Gy were selected. Early (myeloid leukemia, M, and thymic lymphoma, T) or late (reticulum cell sarcoma, L, or others, R) causes of death were analyzed separately by a non-parametric Kaplan-Meier survival function and its logarithmic transform (the cumulative force of mortality, cum. F. M.). Models were set up for treatment for these two categories, on the assumption of independence between the various causes of death.

For causes M and T, there was a significant decrease of the latent period with dose up to 3 Gy. When the effect of dose on integral tumour rate (which corresponds to the final cum. F.M.) was studied, the form of the relationship for death cause M was peaked with a maximum between 2 and 3 Gy and a further decline up to 4.5 Gy, depending on the age at irradiation of the animals (which was 5-6 weeks for group A and 9-10 weeks for group B). The model used to fit the experimental data was such that the estimate of the final cum. F.M. corresponded to the number of leukemogenic cells per animal. These were assumed to have a linear-quadratic dose dependence for induction and linear-quadratic kinetics for killing. Following Barendsen (66) the authors took an α_1/α_2 ratio of 0.5 Gy and a β_1/β_2 ratio of 3 Gy. The fit of the data actually produced a β_1/β_2 ratio of 2.4, which is in reasonable agreement, considering the assumptions involved. It was concluded that the data were consistent with the postulated linear-quadratic dose-response model.

In a series of papers (68, 52, 74) Mole and collaborators described the induction of acute myeloid leukemia in CBA male mice by x and gamma rays and by fission neutrons. The very low natural incidence of this tumour in control animals and low mortality from competing causes of death give this system some advantage over the one described before (73). Ten single X-ray doses in the range of 0.25-6 Gy were delivered at 0.5 Gy min^{-1}

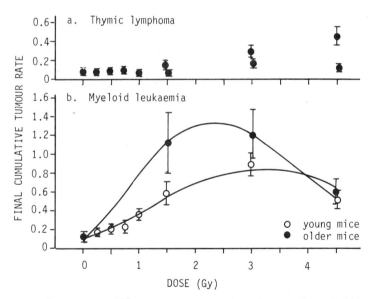

Fig. 2. (from ref. 73) Final cumulative force of mortality ± S.E.)as a function of dose for the induction of (a): thymic lymphoma (cause T) and (b) myeloid leukaemia (cause M) in RF mice. Curve A refers to animals irradiated at 9-10 weeks.

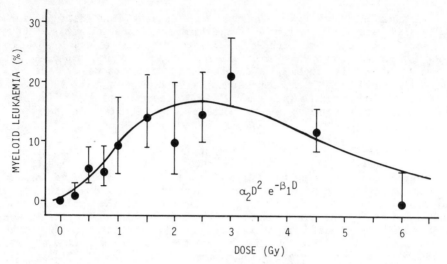

Fig. 3.   (from ref. 74) Percentage incidence of myeloid
          leukaemia ($\pm$ 80% binomial confidence limits) in CBA/H
          male mice exposed to single doses of 250 kVp x rays in
          the range of 0.25 to 6.0 Gy.

and the animals were followed to death. Median survival was similar at all
doses and data were not corrected for intercurrent mortality. There was
essentially no association between latency and dose. The data were fitted
by a four-term polynomial expression similar to (1), as well as by other
simpler models with three or two parameters only. All fits were acceptable
in a statistical sense, but only two of them had all parameters positive
and significantly different from zero. These were I = $\alpha_1 D \exp-(\beta_2 D^2)$ and I
= $\alpha_2 D^2 \exp-(\beta_1 D)$. The former was rejected on the ground that dose-square
cell survival is never found. The observed incidence, on the basis of
various assumptions, could best be fitted by the latter relationship, as
shown in Figure 3. The purely exponential form of the killing function for
hematopoietic cells is not an unreasonable proposition and the value of β_1
derived by Mole is not incompatible with values usually found for such
cells (75). Thus, it has been impossible in this case to estimate
independently and simultaneously four parameters from the data: however,
by assuming a likely exponential shape of the survival function, the
kinetics of initiation for low-LET radiation could be derived and it
appeared to be concave upward with a pronounced dose-square component.

Differences in the induction of myeloid leukemia by treatments with
high (0.25 Gy min^{-1}) or low dose rates gamma rays were studied in this same
system at total doses fo 1.5, 3.0 and 4.5 Gy (76). Protracted exposures
were delivered either as daily fractions (0.25 Gy min^{-1}, 5 days per week
for four weeks) or at constant rates of 0.004-0.11 mGy min^{-1}. The latter
two modes of exposure did not differ in their effectiveness and gave a flat
dose-response at 5-6% incidence. The response observed after protracted
exposure was clearly lower than after acute irradiation by factors of
between 2.2 and 5 at the three total doses mentioned above.

Irradiations with fission neutrons at high dose rate (exposure times
of 2-20 min) were carried out at 7 air-midline kerma values of between 0.02
and 2 Gy (77). The observed incidence of acute myeloid leukemia could be
fitted by an equation of the type I = $\alpha_1 D \exp-(\beta_1 D)$. Neither a purely
linear model without correction for cell killing nor the dose-square model
that fitted the X-ray data could satisfactorily fit the neutron data.

Ullrich and Storer (11) irradiated 10-week-old SPF mice of strain
RFM/Un (both sexes) with gamma rays at 0.45 Gy min^{-1} with doses from 0.1 to
3 Gy. Myeloid leukemia was less frequent in females, where the age-
corrected incidence reached significance over the control level at 1.5 Gy.
Although both a linear and a dose-square model could fit the data
satisfactorily, the dose-square component was not significant and linearity
predominated between zero and 3 Gy. In males, the incidence was
significant over the control level already at 0.5 Gy, and the form of the
relationship was similar to that of females, with a small dose-square term.
The ratio of the linear slopes for the two sexes indicated that males were
more susceptible by about a factor of 5. Lowering the dose rate to 0.083
Gy d^{-1} was very much less effective in the females. After acute and
chronic neutron irradiation, a peak incidence was seen at 0.47 Gy, but this
was not significant over the control value, so that no detailed study of
the dose-response relationship could be made.

Thymic Lymphoma

The studies of Ullrich and Storer (78, 11, 12) in gamma-irradiated
(0.45 Gy min^{-1}) RFM/Un mice were carried out in terms of age-corrected
incidence, standardized to the distribution of ages at death in the
controls. In females (10 weeks old at irradiation) thymic lymphoma was
significantly above the control level of 0.25 Gy or more. No simple model
could describe the response over the entire dose range (0.1 to 3 Gy).
There was a steep rise up to 0.5 Gy, followed by another shallow rise at
higher doses. Over the range of zero to 0.25 Gy a dose-square model fitted
the three experimental points adequately and linearity could be rejected.
From 0.5 to 3 Gy the increase was compatible with linearity. In the males
significance above the control was only obtained at 1 Gy but a linear model
could be fitted up to 3 Gy. Analysis of the shape showed that the linear
component was actually predominating in this sex. Lowering the dose rate
to 0.083 Gy d^{-1} in the females decreased considerably the yield of tumours
and changed the form of the curve from quadratic followed by linear to
linear-quadratic with a negative linear component. Simple linearity could
be rejected. It is quite clear that in the RFM mouse after low-LET
exposure there is no suggestion of the threshold-type response found by
Kaplan and Brown (79) in C57BL mice.

Other data on fast neutron irradiation (0.05 and 0.25 Gy min^{-1} and
0.01 Gy d^{-1}) were reported by the same authors on the same mice (12). In
the range of 0.25-0.5 Gy the RBE with respect to high-dose-rate gamma
irradiation was between 3 and 4 and changed proportionally to the square
root of the dose. For acute neutron treatments the curve was concave
downward, linearity up to about 1 Gy could be rejected and good fit could
be obtained with the square root of the dose. For chronic exposures over
the same range a linear fit described the data adequately and the loss of
efficiency over the acute exposures amounted to about 30%. This finding
is, however, uncertain due to a decrease in susceptibility to lymphoma
induction over a significant portion of life.

Maisin and his group (8) worked on BALB/c mice (male, 12 weeks old)
exposed to single or fractioned (10 equal doses over 9 days) gamma-ray
doses in the range from 0.25 to 6 Gy. A sigmoid-like incidence curve was
found, the incidence rising above control level only at 4 and 6 Gy. Single
doses were more effective at 4 but not at 6 Gy. Neutron irradiation (modal
energy about 23 MeV, doses from 0.02 to 3 Gy) (81) produced an actuarial
incidence of thymic lymphoma which fitted the same type of curve obtained
after gamma irradiation.

Data by Saski and Kasuga (82) on thymic lymphoma induction in neonatal
mice exposed between 200 and 600 R were reported to fit a linear-quadratic

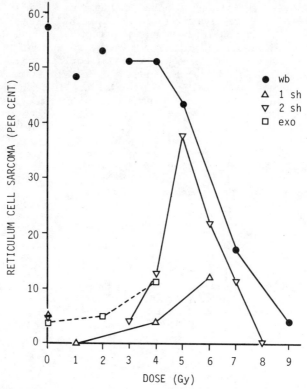

Fig. 4.   (from ref. 84)   Final incidence of "reticulum cell
          sarcoma" as a function of dose under three
          different experimental conditions: (a) whole-body
          irradiation (wb); (b) shielding of one (1 sh) or
          two (2 sh) hind legs; (c) bone marrow
          transplantation in syngeneic chimaeras (exo).

relationship with a negative linear term. Actually, they would probably
fit just as well a threshold-type response such as that of the C57BL (79).

Other Recticular Tumours

     In (C57BL x C3H) hybrid mice irradiated whole-body with 9 Gy of X-rays
and rescued from early death by a homologous bone-marrow graft or by
partial marrow shielding the natural incidence of reticulum cell sarcoma
falls from the spontaneous level of about 50% to a few percent (17, 18).
This effect was attributed to sterilization by the radiation treatment of
the cells giving rise to the tumours. Further studies showed (83) that
irradiation of marrow cells (2 and 4 Gy) prior to their transplantation
into the heavily irradiated hosts provided effective protection against
early death, but resulted in a significantly elevated incidence of
reticulum cell sarcoma at death. When this incidence was expressed per
number of marrow cells injected it was found to be dose-related and to rise
slowly with dose. However, when the data were corrected for an assumed
exponential cell killing, the incidence of tumours rose from 4×10^{-5} to $1 \times$
10^{-4} to 6×10^{-3} per surviving stem cell at zero, 2 and 4 Gy, respectively.
On the assumption that tumours do originate from the injected cells, the
dose-response relationship would be highly curvilinear (concave upwards).

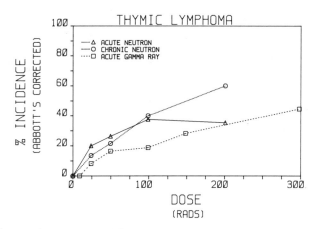

Fig. 5.　(from ref. 12)　Adjusted percentge incidence of
lung adenomas in RFM mice after acute gamma-ray
irradiation (open triangles), acute neutron
irradiation (closed circles) and chronic neutron
irradiation (open circles).

In the same experimental model shielding of marrow in heavily
irradiated mice resulted in its exposure to graded doses of X-rays. In the
shielded animals the incidence of reticular tumours at death increased up
to a maximum at about 6 Gy to the shielded marrow and then declined at
higher doses (84). The final incidence of tumours in the experiments with
exogenous and endogenous marrow is given in Figure 4, showing that in all
instances there is a curvilinear rise with dose.

Ullrich and Storer (78, 11, 12) studied the age-corrected incidence of
reticular tumours in SPF RFM/Un mice irradiated with gamma rays (0.45 Gy
min^{-1} or 0.083 Gy d^{-1}) and in RFM/Un and BALB/c mice irradiated with fast
neutrons (0.05 and 0.25 Gy min^{-1} and 0.01 Gy d^{-1}). All treatments produced
a dose-related decrease of tumours: per unit dose neutrons were more
effective than gamma rays and acute exposure more effective than chronic
ones. The differences between acute and chronic treatments were more
pronounced with gamma than with neutron irradiation. There was an inverse
relationship between the increase of thymic lymphoma and the decrease in
reticulum cell sarcoma, suggestive of some link between the various tumours
of the hematopoietic system, which could itself affect the observed
responses.

Lung Tumours

The induction of lung adenocarcinoma was studied in gamma-irradiated
(0.5 to 2 Gy) SPF BALB/c female mice (10, 11). Both at higher (0.45 Gy
min^{-1}) and at low (0.083 Gy d^{-1}) rates the age corrected incidence could be
fitted by a linear equation whose slope was higher by a factor of 3 at high
dose rates. For neutrons the responses of lung adenomas were peaked at
both high and low dose rate; the different shapes could not be explained by
age-related changes in susceptibility (12) (Figure 5). At high dose rates
the RBE was of the order of 15 to 20. Splitting of the neutron dose into
two fractions separated by 1 or 30 days produced little difference in the
response. On the contrary, splitting of the X-ray doses resulted in
recovery at 1 day only when the total dose was on the dose-square region of
the single-dose response curve. There was no further recovery when the
fractionation interval was increased to 30 days. All these data suggest

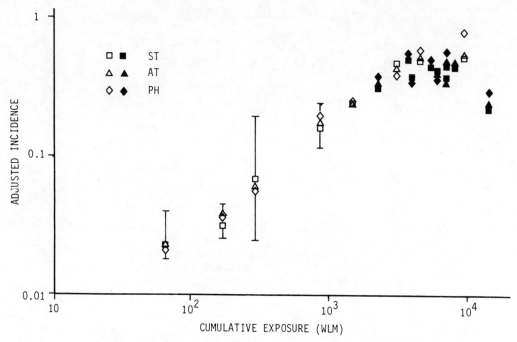

Fig. 6. (from ref. 85) Comparison of the adjusted incidences of malignant lung neoplasms in Sprague-Dawley rats as a function of the inhalation dose of radon-daughters under three models: ST, shifted time model; AT, accelerated time model; PH, proportional hazard model. Open sysmbols refer to low dose rate inhalation (<1600 WLM/month); closed ones to high dose rate inhalation (> 1600 WLM/month).

that the primary mechanisms in the development of lung tumours and in recovery are intracellular in nature (15).

Male Sprague-Dawley rats at 90 days of age were started on a course of exposure to radon in equilibrium with its short-lived daughters. The dose was defined as the product of potential alpha energy concentration and exposure time and expressed in WLM: it varied between zero and 14,000 WLM, in various combinations of exposure levels and times. The prevalence of neoplasms as a function of time was analyzed by non-parametric methods and three models were selected to fit prevalence to dose: a time shift, an accleration and a proportional hazard model: none of these could be discarded on a purely statistical ground. The data in Figure 6 show that the response is linear at first but flattens off at high doses (85). The loss of tumour-free life or "effective period" (1) was studied in these rats as a function of cumulative exposure: also in this case linearity of the response seemed to prevail up to 1000 or 2000 WLM.

Similar methods of analysis were used to study the actuarial incidence of lung carcinoma in Sprague-Dawley rats after whole-body fission neutron irradiation (86). An accelerated-time and a shifted-time model gave similar fits, as shown in Figure 7. The dose-response relationship could be linear up to 0.5 Gy but it appears to flatten at higher doses.

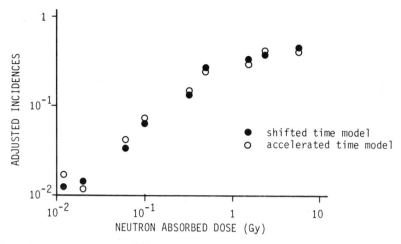

Fig. 7. (from ref. 86) Adjusted incidence of malignant lung
neoplasms in Sprague-Dawley rats as a function of the
fission neutron dose according to a shifted time (ST)
or an accelerated time (AT) model.

Mammary Tumours

Data in the mouse and the rat are available for tumours of the mammary
gland. In the BALB/c mouse the incidence of mammary adenocarcinoma was
studied after exposure to gamma rays (11) and neutrons (13). For gamma
exposure at high (0.40 Gy min^{-1}) or low (0.08 Gy d^{-1}) dose rate, the dose-
incidence relationship could be described as linear, the slope being about
a factor of 2 greater with the high than with the low rate. High (0.05 and
0.25 Gy min^{-1}) and low (0.01 Gy d^{-1}) dose rate neutrons also produced
mammary adenocarcinoma in the same strain, low dose rate being less
effective at low total doses. The changes in susceptibility with age could
not account for the differences. The RBE of neutrons relative to gamma
rays was of the order of 20 or more. The complex shapes of the curves are
shown in Figure 8. In other experiment (87) splitting of fission-neutron
doses of up to 0.5 Gy into two fractions given 1 or 30 days apart had no

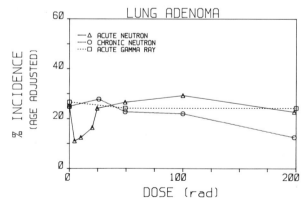

Fig. 8. (from ref. 13) Adjusted percentage incidence
of mammary adenocarcinomas in BALB/c mice as
a function of dose under different conditions
of irradiation as shown.

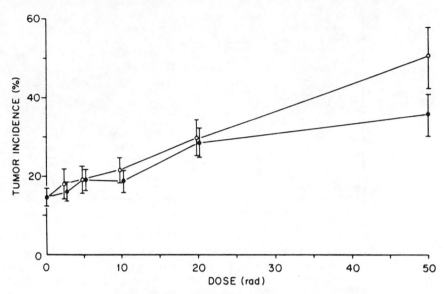

Fig. 9.   (from ref. 87) Incidence of mammary adenocarcinomas in
BALB/c mice as a function of fission neutron dose given as
single exposures and as two equal exposures separated by 24
hours (closed circles) or by 30 days (open circles).

effect on the age-adjusted incidence of mammary adenocarcinoma, as shown in
Figure 9.

Sprague-Dawley female rats were given single 250-kVp X-ray (0.28,
0.56, 0.85 Gy) or 0.43-MeV neutron doses (0.001, 0.004, 0.016, 0.064 Gy) at
two months of age and then followed for the rest of their life for
appearance of mammary adenocarcinoma (AC) or fibroadenoma (FA) (9). In all
irradiated groups the tumour rate increased steeply with time and radiation
acted essentially by shifting forward the spontaneous tumour rate. The
response was expressed for both tumour classes as mortality-corrected
prevalence, I(t), and integral tumour rate, R(t). The FA and total tumour
response was approximately linear with the X-ray dose at all times, while
for neutrons it was concave downward. The AC response was statistically
uncertain but approximately linear. The RBE varied with the square root of
the neutron dose: at the highest doses studied it exceeded a factor of 10
and at the lower end of the scale it approached 100.

In other experiments (88) when females of the same strain were exposed
whole-body to fission neutrons acutely or chronically (doses of 0.02, 0.06
and 0.5 Gy over one month), the prevalence of mammary tumours at 10 months
post-exposure increased relative to single irradiations at all dose levels
tested. Protraction of gamma-ray exposure (150, 300 and 450 R) in a
similar fashion significantly reduced the prevalence seen after
corresponding acute doses. Neutron RBE measured at 20% prevalence was 16
and 68 for acute and chronic irradiation, respectively.

Female animals of another rat strain, the ACI, were also studied for
induction of mammary tumours by X-rays and neutrons (89). They were
irradiated at about three months of age with X-ray doses of 0.37-3.0 Gy or
neutron doses of 0.05-0.36 Gy without any treatment. Other animals
received comparable doses 2 days after implantation of a pellet containing
5 mg of diethylstilbestrol (DES), a hormone which enhances occurrence of
spontaneous and radiation-induced AC in this strain that has a low natural

88

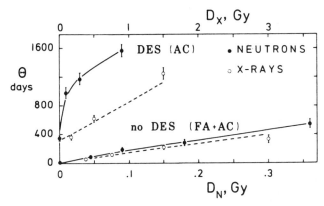

Fig. 10. (from ref. 89) Effect period in days ($\pm$ S.E.) for induction of mammary neoplasms adenocarcinoma (AC) and fibrosarcomas (FA) in ACI rats treated or not with diethylstilbestrol (AES) and irradiated with various doses of x rays (dashed lines) or neutrons (solid lines). Note that the dose scales for the two radiations differ by a factor of 10.

incidence. In the untreated irradiated rats the appearance of tumours was followed to about 750 days post-irradiation. The cumulative rate for all tumor types up to 600 days was a linear function of the X-ray dose. After neutron irradiation the induction of AC was apparently linear but for FA a downward concave shape could not be excluded. For the sum of all tumors over the whole dose range tested the RBE was about 10 in the untreated animals. The DES treatment brought about changes of the neutron dose-response which implied an RBE of about 100 at the low end of the scale, its value changing inversely with the square root of the dose. For both types of radiation and over the whole range of doses tested, the effect period for all tumours in the irradiated animals was a linear function of the dose (Figure 10). Contrary to these effects by DES, irradiation administered during pregnancy, lactation or post-lactation did not result in any change in tumour induction, with respect to the virgin state (90).

Since genetic factors affect the expression of radiation-induced mammary carcinogenesis in the rat (91, 92), it is of interest to compare the response in various strains. Sprague-Dawley, Wag/Rij and BN/BiRIj female rats were used in one such comparison (93, 94) which involved the use of X-rays and monoenergetic neutrons (0.5 and 15 MeV) and single or fractioned doses. Histological examination of the tumours allowed distinction between adenoma and carcinoma. The probability of animals surviving without evidence of tumours was calculated according to a Kaplan-Meir life-table analysis. Weibull functions fitted to the data showed that in Sprague-Dawley and WAG/Rij rats radiation acted essentially by accelerating the appearance of both tumour types. X-ray fractionation (10 fractions of 0.02 Gy given at intervals of 1 month to WAG/Rij animals was marginally less effective than a single dose of 2 Gy. The same could be said of neutron fractionation (10 fractions of 0.025 Gy compared to 1 single dose of 0.25 Gy). For adenomas in the Sprague-Dawley there was no decline of incidence for any of the radiation used up to the highest doses tested (Figure 11). For adenomas in the WAG/Rij the X-ray and neutron curves were linear and concave downward, respectively (Figure 12). For

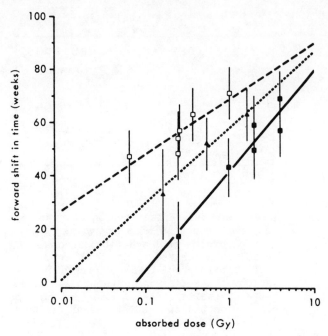

Fig. 11. (from ref. 93) Percentage actuarial incidence (± S.D.)
of benign mammary tumours in Sprague-Dawley rats after
irradiation with x rays (closed squares), 15-MeV
neutrons (closed triangles) or 0.5 MeV neutrons (open
squares). Logarithmic plot.

carcinomas in the same strain the response was practically linear for both
X-rays and neutrons.

Ovarian Tumours

The data of Ullrich et al. (10) on SPF RFM/Un mice showed that acute
whole-body gamma irradiation (0.4 Gy min^{-1}) induced various types of
ovarian tumours and their corrected incidence increased rapidly up to 0.5
Gy. Within this range linear and dose-square non-threshold models could be
rejected. While a linear-quadratic model with a negative linear component
could describe the relationship adequately, a threshold plus dose-square
model (the threshold estimated to be at about 0.12 Gy) proved to fit the
data best up to 0.5 Gy. Lowering the dose rate to 0.08 Gy d^{-1} reduced the
incidence of tumours. An adequate fit was obtained for a threshold-linear
model with a threshold dose of 0.7 Gy. Ovarian tumours in BALB/c mice
showed also a reduction of incidence by a reduced rate of irradiation,
although the data were insufficient for a good description of the curve
(11).

Neutron at low dose rates (12) produced at all doses less tumours than
at high dose rates: this decline could be attributed in part to the
reduction of the rate of exposure and in part to the age-related decrease of
susceptibility. When female BALB/c mice were irradiated whole-body with
fission neutrons either in single or in split exposures (1 or 30 days
intervals) no effect of fractionation could be shown (87).

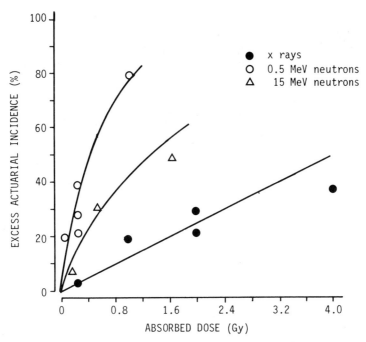

Fig. 12. (from ref. 94) Percentage excess actuarial
incidence (+ S.D.) of fibroadenomas in
WAG/Rij rats after irradiation with x rays
(open circles). Linear plot.

Tumours of the Skin

Highly curvilinear dose-response relationships were reported for the
induction of skin cancer in CBA mice and CD rats by beta particles and
high-energy electrons (56, 57, 95) or by 40-MeV helium ions (95). The
efficiency of cancer production as a function of the depth-dose
distribution and the association of the carcinogenic effect with hair
follicle damage led to the conclusion that skin cancer in the rat
originates from follicle cells. In this species the incidence of tumours
over the ascending part of the curve increased with approximately the
fourth power of the electron dose and the second power of the alpha dose.
The RBE of alpha particles relative to high-energy electrons (at the level
of 1 tumour per animal was about 3 (Figure 13). The response had a peak
incidence at the level of several tens of Gy of sparsely ionizing
radiation.

If, on the basis of the highly curvilinear response, one postulates
the existence of a suboncogenic damage and calculates the time for its
repair (96, 97) one finds a half-time of the order of 4 hours, similar to
that of intracellular sublethal damage. Dose fractionation at 24 hours
with 10-MeV protons also shows (98) that the repair of this damage is
essentially complete by 1 day. In respect to 10 MeV protons, this system
shows a high RBE, which is typical of high-LET radiation, but a high
capacity for recovery, which is characteristics of sparsely-ionizing
radiation.

On the basis of the above results, Vanderlaan et al. (99) proposed a
mathematical model for skin cancer induction by ionizing radiation in the
rat. It envisages the presence of a linear and quadratic component and it
calculates a half-time for the repair of suboncogenic damage of the order

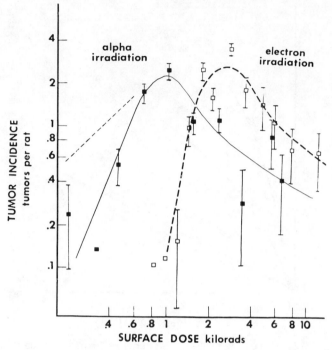

Fig. 13. (from ref. 95) A logarithmic plot of the
number of skin tumours per rat (CD strain) at
76 weeks from irradiation as a function of
alpha and electron surface dose. The dotted
line at the left represents a linear dose-
response relationship.

of 4 hours and a substantial but undetermined dose-rate reduction factor.
Actually, a considerable sparing effect of fractionation for induction of
skin cancer is also confirmed by experiments with 0.8 MeV electrons (100)
showing that 130 Gy in 65 weeks produce the same effect as 15 Gy in a
single exposure.

Hulse et al. (101) studied the induction of dermal and epidermal skin
tumours in CBA/CaH mice after irradiation of large skin areas with beta
particles from ^{204}Tl which do not penetrate the abdominal wall and do not
reach the bone marrow. Surface skin doses ranged from 5.4 to 260 Gy, dose
rate from 2 to 0.017 Gy min^{-1}. Over two-thirds of the tumours were dermal
(fibromas and fibro-sarcomas) and about 60% of all tumors (dermal and
epidermal) were malignant. Most tumours arose within the irradiated area
and only a few at the edge; tumour incidence was expressed per unit area of
skin. Reduction of the dose rate from 1-2 Gy min^{-1} to ten times lower did
not alter the incidence appreciably, but a further drop by a factor of 2
reduced epidermal tumours at all except the highest dose (120 Gy). Dermal
tumours began to increase significantly at about 16 Gy and rose steeply
into a plateau above 60 Gy. Epidermal tumours started at 21 Gy, peaked at
60-120 Gy and fell at still higher doses. The dose-response curves
resembled very much those typical for non-stochastic effects. For
epidermal tumours all non-threshold linear and quadratic models could be
discarded; for dermal tumours all non-threshold and threshold dose-square
models could be discarded. It was suggested (102) that some radioresistant
factor restraining potential tumour cells in the skin was at the origin of
the thresholds and that this factor could be overcome either by high doses
or perhaps also by aging. There were doubts whether the final fall in
tumour yield could at all be related to killing of the potentially

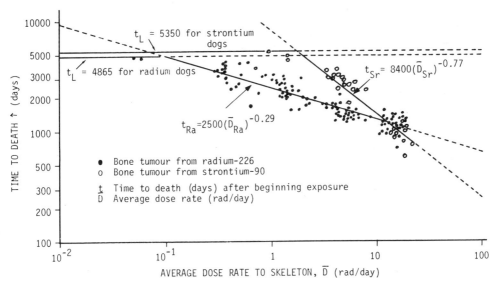

Fig. 14. (from ref. 104) A logarithmic plot of the relationship
between time to death (days) and average skeletal dose rate
(rad/day) for beagle dogs exposed to strontium-90 or to
radium-226. Also shown are the estimated median times to
spontaneous death among the two unexposed control groups.

transformed cells. These data suggest on the whole that extrapolating skin
cancer risk from high doses to low doses would greatly overestimate the
risk in the mouse. Whether such a conclusion might also apply to man
remains, however, an open question.

Bone Tumours

All the data available apply to internal irradiation. The question of
whether there exists a practical threshold for the induction of bone
sarcoma after irradiation by bone-seeking radionuclides was re-addressed
again recently in a study by Raabe et al. (103, 104) who tested the
hypothesis on the basis of data obtained in beagle dogs. Two groups of
animals were given either ^{226}Ra in 8 fortnightly injections of graded
activities at about 1 year of age, to simulate human experience with
radium; or ^{90}Sr by continuous feeding at various rates from midgestation
through 540 days of life, to simulate human contamination from the
environment.

When the survival time of the injected aimals was plotted against the
average dose rate to the skeleton, survival was shown to decline with
increasing dose rats, as in Figure 14. If the relationships fitted hold
down to the lowest dose rates, there must be latency times in the low dose
range far exceeding the normal life span of the animals. If one defines a
practical threshold as the dose rate corresponding to the intersection of
the regression lines minus 3 geometric standard deviations of the control
survival times, this threshold is found to be 0.11 mGy d^{-1} for ^{226}Ra,
amounting to a life-time dose of 0.5 Gy. The corresponding values for ^{90}Sr
may be judged to exceed those for radium by one or two orders of magnitude.
It should, however, be recalled that these are tentative estimates because
many of the animals in the low-dose groups were still alive at the time of
the analysis. There may also be questions concerning the extrapolation of

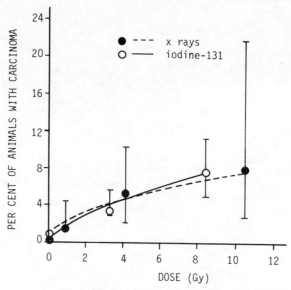

Fig. 15. (from ref. 108) Percentage incidence ($\pm$ 95% C.L.) of thyroid carcinomas in Long-Evans rats as a function of mean thyroid dose from injected iodine-131 and localized x-irradiation.

beagle data to man, in view of inherent differences in the susceptibility to bone sarcoma induction of different species.

Beagle dogs were also studied for induction of osteosarcoma by ^{239}Pu in single injections at 400 and 800 days of age (105). There were 7 injection groups ranging up to 0.11 MBq/kg body weight. The data for incidence rate fitted well a quadratic model and linearity could be rejected if the highest activity level was not included in the calculations on the ground of a possible cell killing effect. The same conclusion was reached when the data were analyzed by a Marshall-Groer model (23). However, here again it should be recalled that the analysis is incomplete and a linear contribution might appear with further follow-up. When the same data were treated by a non parametric proportional hazard relative risk model (106) neither a linear nor a quadratic function could be excluded; however, if the highest injection level was excluded, as in the other analysis (105), the results supported a roughly quadratic rise of the relative risk with injection level.

Liver Tumours

A dose-response relationship between the activity of injected thorotrast and the sum of liver and spleen tumours was obtained in Wistar rats (107). When the raw percentage incidence of all benign and malignant liver neoplasms was plotted against the dose rate a linear dose-response curve was obtained, the intercept of which did not differ significantly from the control incidence.

Liver tumours were also observed in hamster following an administration of ^{239}Pu citrate: the raw cumulative incidence for the few dose points available suggested a rise which was approximately linear up to 2.7 Gy at the time of 50% animal survival. At the highest dose point of 14

94

Gy, the effectiveness of induction per unit dose was appreciably decreased with respect to the next lower point (60).

Tumours of the Thyroid

A study of thyroid tumour induction in female Long-Evans rats after X-ray and ^{131}I irradiation was reported by Lee et al. (108). It aimed at comparing the effectiveness of the two radiation delivered at widely different dose rates (2.8 Gy min^{-1} for X-rays and 1.6 mGy min^{-1}, as a maximum for ^{131}I). Thyroid doses were estimated to be 0.94, 4.1 and 10.6 Gy for X-rays and 0.8, 3.3 and 8.5 Gy for ^{131}I. Tests of the possible role of pituitary irradiation yielded negative results. The incidence of tumours between 6 and 26 months was corrected for the slightly enhanced mortality of the irradiated versus the control animals. Carcinomas were found to increase with a power of dose of less than 1, with no apparent difference in the form of the two relationships nor in the effectiveness of the treatments (Figure 15). This shape of the relationship was attributed to killing of transformed cells. The apparent absence of a dose-rate effect suggested the presence of a strong linear component. Adenomas produced slightly different relationships. These data are apparently at variance with previous ones (reviewed in (109)) suggesting that the effectiveness per unit dose of the X-rays was higher than that of ^{131}I. The discrepancy might be due to the lower doses used in the more recent series (108) which would avoid the occurrence of cell killing or other non-stochastic damage. Although the number of animals used (about 3000) gives this study (108) statistical credibility, it should be emphasized that the data refer only to one sex and one strain.

Tumours of the Pituitary Gland

In female RFM/Un pituitary tumours increased irregularly with dose up to 3 Gy of gamma rays, but up to 2 Gy the age-corrected incidence was not significantly different from control. In male mice the carcinogenic effect was even smaller (10). Lowering the rate (from 0.40 Gy min^{-1} to 0.083 Gy d^{-1}) led to a somewhat less efficient induction (11). Neutrons produced a large number of tumours with a RBE greater than 5; lowering the neutron dose rate (from 0.05 and 0.25 Gy min^{-1} to 0.01 Gy d^{-1}) resulted in less tumours only at doses higher than 0.47 Gy (12).

Tumours of the Harderian Gland

Harderian tumours were induced by gamma rays in male and female REM/Un mice according to a kinetics which was very similar in both sexes. The data on age-adjusted incidence appeared to fit best a linear-quadratic model; only for the females could linearity be excluded (10). Lowering the rate of gamma irradiation reduced substantially the yield and appeared to abolish the dose-square term (11). Harderian gland tumours showed also a marked susceptibility to induction by neutrons: there was an approximately linear increase up to about 0.5 Gy, a plateau at 1 Gy and a decline at 2 Gy. However, no significant effect of the dose rate was observed for neutrons (12).

Combined Tumour Data and Indirect Inferences

Radiation-induced life shortening was reviewed by UNSCEAR in 1982 (91). That analysis concluded that in the low-to-intermediate dose range loss of life was essentially due to tumour induction above the spontaneous level. It does not follow, of course, that the two effects may be directly comparable, because the latency of some tumours varies with dose, dosage, age at exposure, etc.

Life shortening and incidence of various diseases were studied in male BALB/c mice (80) after single exposures of gamma rays, and fractionated exposures split into 10 equal daily fractions. Doses ranged from 0.25 to 6 Gy. Accurate pathology and statistical treatment were reported. Single exposures were generaly more effective than fractionated ones for life shortening. However, over the whole range of doses, leukemias and cancers combined were significantly higher after fractionation. Dose-responses were flat and included a high spontaneous incidence of over 70%. The opposite trend of the two endpoints in respect to fractionation, the high spontaneous cancer incidence and the lack of a clear trend with dose, are all reasons to take these data with some reservations. Whereas the incidence of all carcinomas and sarcomas combined (except lung carcinomas) had a negative trend after single doses of gamma rays, in the same strain of mouse an almost linear increase was reported after single doses of (50)Be neutrons in the range from 0.02 to 3 Gy (81).

Life shortening was also studied in B6CF1 mice following single, fractionated and life-long exposures to gamma rays and fission neutrons (110, 111). Fractionation of a gamma-ray dose over 24 weeks was less effective for survival then the same single dose; the reverse was true of the neutrons. It was argued that neutron fractionation led to an increased incidence of tumours, or to their earlier appearance, or both.

In another experiment life shortening was studied in female BALB/c mice (112) given fission neutrons in single treatments or in split courses at 1 or 30 days. Whole-body doses ranged from 0.02 to 2 Gy. Lifespan was a steep function of dose up to 0.5 Gy following single or fractionated exposures, after which the curve rose to a plateau. Both linear and square-root models fitted the data adequately up to about 0.5 Gy for all modalities of treatment, except the split regime at 30 days where the square-root model could be rejected. In contrast with the data on B6CF1 mice (110, 111), fractionation and protraction of the neutron doses did not enhance life shortening below 0.5 Gy, although it did so at 0.5 and 2 Gy.

CONCLUSIONS

A number of recently published dose-response relationships for a variety of experimental animal tumours have been examined. This data enlarge our knowledge of radiation-induced tumours, particularly at the lower end of the dose scale, down to 150 mGy of gamma rays and to a few tens of mGy of fast neutrons. On the whole, they support the general notion that each tumour model system shows a very specific type of response; however, more precise conclusions about the form of some dose-induction relationships are made possible by the new information.

For sparsely-ionizing radiation most curves appear to be concave upwards and may be fitted by linear-quadratic or quadratic models. In some cases, however, (mammary fibroadenoma in Sprague-Dawley rats, thymic lymphoma in RFM mice, lung adenocarcinoma in BALB/c mice), approximate linearlity could apply. Thymic lymphoma and tumours with a pronounced hormonal dependence (the ovary, for example) show curves with a distinct threshold. This may reflect the role of non-stochastic damage in the development of the tumours, such as the need to inactivate a large proportion of hormonally-active ovarian cells or to inactivate a large number of target cells in the thymus. Also, the induction of skin in the rodent by all types of radiation shows highly curvilinear responses where apparent or real thresholds cannot be excluded.

For neutrons the rising slope of the dose-response relationships is often closer to linearity than for gamma rays. However, in some tumours (lung adenomas in RFM) curvilinearity is suggested, although linearity cannot be excluded. Factors such as dose-related latency might contribute to this curvilinearity. In other cases, neutron-induced tumours rising with a power of dose of less than 1 have been confirmed at low doses. Killing of potentially neoplastic cells may account for this shape of the response.

Dose-rate studies with sparsely-ionizing radiation show almost invariably a decreased tumour incidence with decreasing dose rate. In some instances (lung adenoma in RFM and harderian and pituitary tumours in RFM females) protraction of the dose results in a reduction of the dose-square component in the dose-effect relationship and, therefore, in a more nearly linear response. Dose-rate studies with neutrons show in general less effect on the yield of tumours than would be expected from studies with low-LET radiation at low or intermediate total doses; at high total doses an enhancement of tumour incidence by protraction and fractionation is seen in cases where the response to high dose rates is concave downwards. However, the whole picture is not as simple as cellular data might imply, because at the whole-body level systemic influences may modify the final tumour yield.

Lung carcinoma induced in rats by low-dose-rate radon inhalation or by external neutron irradiation follows a basically linear non-threshold relationship as a function of exposure or dose. High exposure rates to high total exposures to alpha emitting radon daughters are, however, less efficient than low rates. Similarly, the effectiveness of neutrons per unit dose is also decreased at high doses.

Liver tumours produced by internal alpha emitters show a roughly linear rise at low dose rates and a pronounced inverse relationship between latency and dose rate.

Although previous studies of bone sarcoma induction by alpha-emitting bone seekers supported roughly linear relationship between activity and response, recent analyses of more extended data in dogs injected with ^{239}Pu show that such a linear dependence between integral tumour rate and administered activity may be unlikely. The same seems to apply to the relationship between dose rate to cells at risk and tumour rate. Although at present a dose-square component appears to prevail, the appearance of a linear component with more extended follow-up of these experiments cannot, however, be excluded.

The latency of bone sarcoma after incorporation of ^{226}Ra and ^{90}Sr in dogs and mice appears to be inversely related with the average dose rate to the skeleton. This might imply the presence of practical thresholds and under such circumstances linear extrapolation to zero dose of the rate of incidence (and probably also of the life-time incidence) of bone sarcoma would largely overestimate the actual risk.

REFERENCES

1. United Nations, "Sources and Effects of Ionizing Radiation," United Nations Scientific Committee on the Effects of Atomic Radiation 1977 Report to the General Assembly, with Annexes, United Nations Sales Publication No. E.77.IX.I., New York, (1977).

2. M. Faber, Radiation carcinogenesis and the significance of some physical factors, in: "Radiation-Induced Cancer," IAEA, Vienna (1969), pp. 149-159.

3. P. G. Groer, Correction to dose-response curves and competing risks, Proc. Natl. Acad. Sci. USA 76:1524 (1979).

4. P. G. Groer, Dose-response curves and competing risks, Proc. Natl. Acad. Sci. USA 75:4087-4091 (1978).

5. P. G. Groer, Dose-response curves from incomplete data, in: "Late Biological Effects of Ionizing Radiation, Vol. II," IAEA, Vienna (1978), pp. 351-358.

6. D. G. Hoel and H. E. Walburg, Statistical analysis of survival experiments, J. Natl. Cancer Inst. 49:361-372 (1972).

7. R. H. Mole, Pathological findings in mice exposed to fission neutrons in the reactor GLEEP, in: "Biological Effects of Neutron and Proton Irradiations," IAEA, Vienna (1964), pp. 117-128.

8. L. S. Rosenblatt, N. H. Hetherington, M. Goldman, et al., Evaluation of tumour incidence following exposure to internal emitters by application of the logistic dose-response surface, Health Phys. 21:869-875 (1975).

9. C. J. Shellabarger, D. Chmelevsky, and A. M. Keller, Induction of mammary neoplasms in the Sprague-Dawley rat by 430 keV nuetrons and X-rays, J. Natl. Cancer Inst. 64:821-833 (1980).

10. R. L. Ullrich and J. B. Storer, Influence of gamma-ray irradiation on the development of neoplastic disease. II. Solid tumours, Radiat. Res. 80:317-324 (1979).

11. R. L. Ullrich and J. B. Storer, Influence of gamma-ray irradiation on the development of neoplastic disease. III. Dose rate effects, Radiation. Res. 80:325-342 (1979).

12. R. L. Ullrich, M. C. Jernigan, G. E. Cosgrove, et al., The influence of dose and dose-rate on the incidence of neoplastic disease in RFM mice after neutron irradiation, Radiat. Res. 68:115-131 (1976).

13. R. L. Ullrich, M. C. Jernigan, and J. B. Storer, Neutron carcinogenesis. Dose and dose-rate effects in BALB/c mice, Radiat. Res. 72:487-498 (1977).

14. R. L. Ullrich, M. C. Jernigan, and L. M. Adams, Induction of lung tumors in RFM mice after localized exposures to X-rays or neutrons, Radiat. Res. 80:464-473 (1979).

15. R. L. Ullrich, Effects of split doses of X-rays or neutrons on lung tumor formation in RFM mice, Radiat. Res. 83:138-145 (1980).

16. A. M. Kellerer, Radiation carcinogenesis at low doses, in: "Proceedings of the Sixth Symposium on Microdosimetry, Vol. I, Brussels, May 1978," J. Booz and H. G. Ebert, eds., Harwood Academic Publishers Ltd., London (1978), pp. 405-422.

17. V. Covelli, P. Metalli, and B. Bassani, Decreased incidence of reticulum cell sarcoma in whole body irradiated and bone marrow shielded mice, Br. J. Cancer, 31:369-371 (1975).

18. V. Covelli, P. Metalli, G. Briganti, et al., Late somatic effects in syngeneic radiation chimaeras: II. Mortality and rate of specific diseases, Int. J. Radiat. Biol. 26:1-15 (1974).

19. W. Nelson, Theory and applications of hazard plotting for censored failure data, Technometrics 14:945-966 (1972).

20. O. Aalen, Nonparametric inference in connection with multiple decrement models, Scand. J. Stat. 3:15-27 (1976).

21. E. L. Kaplan and P. Meier, Non-parametric estimation from incomplete observations, J. Am. Stat. Assoc. 53:457-481 (1958).

22. J. B. Storer, Associations between tumour types in irradiated BALB/c female mice, Radiat. Res. 92:396-404 (1982).

23. J. M. Marshall and P. G. Groer, A theory of the induction of bone cancer by alpha radiation, Radiat. Res. 71:149-192 (1977).

24. M. P. Finkel, B. O. Biskis, and P. B. Jinkins, Toxicity of radium-226 in mice, in: "Radiation-Induced Cancer," IAEA, Vienna (1969), pp. 369-391.

25. O. G. Raabe, S. A. Book, and N. J. Parks, Bone cancer from radium: canine dose response explains data for mice and humans, Science 208:61-64 (1980).

26. R. V. Mayneord and R. H. Clarke, Carcinogenesis and radiation risk: a biomathematical reconnaissance, Br. J. Radiol. Supplement 12:11-12 (1975).

27. W. V. Mayneord and R. H. Clarke, "Time and Dose in Carcinogenesis," RD/B/N-3940 (1978).

28. W. V. Mayneord, The time factor in carcinogenesis. The 1977 Sievert Lecture, Health Phys. 34:297-309 (1978).

29. I. Berenblum, Theoretical and practical aspects of the two-stage mechanisms of carcinogenesis, in: "Carcinogens: Identification and Mechanisms of Action," A. C. Griffin and C. R. Shaw, eds., Raven Press, New York (1979), pp. 25-36.

30. J. C. Barrett, B. D. Crawford, and P. O. Ts'o, The role of somatic mutation in a multistage model of carcinogens, in: "Mammalian Cell Transformation by Chemical Carcinogens," N. Mishra, et al., eds, Senate Press, New Jersey (1980).

31. J. Cairns, The origin of human cancers, Nature 289:353-357 (1981).

32. E. Farber and R. Cameron, The sequential analysis of cancer development, Adv. Cancer Res. 31:125-226 (1980).

33. R. J. M. Fry, R. D. Ley, D. Grube, et al., Studies on the multistage nature of radiation carcinogenesis, in: "Carcinogenesis, Vol. 7," Hecker et al., eds, Raven Press, New York (1982), pp. 155-165.

34. S. H. Moolgavkar and A. G. Knudson, Mutation and Cancer: A model for human carcinogenesis, J. Natl. Cancer Inst. 66:1037-1052 (1981).

35. H. Rubin, Is somatic mutation the major mechanism of malignant transformation?, J. Natl. Cancer Inst. 64:995-1000 (1980).

36. D. S. Straus, Somatic mutation, cellular differentiation and cancer causation, J. Natl. Cancer Inst. 67:233-241 (1981).

37. P. K. Lemotte, S. J. Adelstein, and J. B. Little, Malignant transformation induced by incorporated radionuclides in BALB/3T3 mouse embryo fibroblasts, Proc. Natl. Acad. Sci. U.S.A. 79:7763-7767 (1982).

38. S. L. Lin, M. Takii, and P. O. P. Ts'o, Somatic mutation and neoplastic transformation induced by (methyl-3H)thymidine, Radiat. Res. 90:142-154 (1982).

39. J. C. Barrett, T. Tsutsui, and P. O. P. Ts'o, Neoplastic transformation induced by a direct perturbation of DNA, Nature 274:229-232 (1978).

40. D. W. van Bekkum and P. Bentvelzen, The concept of gene transfer misrepair mechanism of radiation carcinogenesis may challenge the linear extrapolation model of risk estimation for low radiation doses, Health Phys. 43:231-237 (1982).

41. A. F. Cohen and B. L. Cohen, Tests of the linearity assumption in the dose-effect relationship for radiation-induced cancer, Health Phys. 38:53-69 (1980).

42. L. Siminovitch, On the nature of heritable variation in cultured somatic cells, Cell 7:1-11 (1976).

43. D. G. Scarpelli, Recent developments toward a unifying concept of carcinogenesis, Ann. Clin. Lab. Sci. 13:249-259 (1983).

44. M. N. Gould, Radiation initiation of carcinogenesis in vivo: a rare or common cellular event, in: "Radiation Carcinogenesis, Epidemiology and Biological Implications," J. F. Fraumeni and J. D. Boice, eds., Raven Press, New York (1983).

45. H. Busch, ed., "The Molecular Biology of Cancer," Academic Press, New York (1974).

46. P. J. Fialkow, Clonal origin and stem cell evolution of human tumours, in: "Genetics of Human Cancer," J. J. Mulvihill et al., eds., Raven Press, New York (1977).

47. E. Farber, Chemical carcinogenesis, New Eng. J. Med. 305:1379-1389 (1981).

48. B. Fertil, P. Deschavanne, B. Lachet, et al., Survival curves of neoplastic and non-transformed human cell lines: statistical analysis using different models, in: "Proceedings of the Sixth Symposium on Microdosimetry," J. Booz and H. G. Ebert, eds, Harwood Academic Publishers, London (1978).

49. H. H. Rossi and A. M. Kellerer, Radiation carcinogenesis at low doses, Science 175:200-204 (1972).

50. H. H. Rossi, Biophysical implications of radiation quality, in: "Radiation Research, Biomedical, Chemical and Physical Perspectives," O. Nygaard et al., eds., Academic Press, New York (1975).

51. H. H. Rossi, Interrelation between physical and biological effects of small radiation doses, in: "Biological and Environmental Effects of Low-Level Irradiation," IAEA, Vienna (1976), pp. 245-251.

52. R. H. Mole, Dose-response relationships, in: "Radiation Carcinogenesis: Epidemiology and Biological Implications," J. Fraumeni and J. Boice, eds., Raven Press, New York (1983).

53. C. J. Shellabarger, Modifying factors in rat mammary gland carcinogenesis, in: "Biology of Radiation Carcinogenesis," J. M. Yuhas et al., eds., Raven Press, New York (1976).

54. V. P. Bond, C. J. Shellabarger, E. P. Cronkite, et al., Studies on radiation-induced mammary gland neoplasia in the rat. V. Induction by localized radiation, Radiat. Res. 13:318-328 (1960).

55. C. J. Shellabarger and R. W. Schmidt, Mammary neoplasia in the rat as related to dose of partial-body irradiation, Radiat. Res. 30:497-506 (1967).

56. E. V. Hulse, Incidence and pathogenesis of skin tumours in mice irradiated with single external doses of low energy beta particles, Br. J. Cancer 21:531-547 (1967).

57. E. V. Hulse and R. H. Mole, Skin tumor incidence in CBA mice given fractionated exposure to low-energy beta particles, Br. J. Cancer 23:452-463 (1969).

58. E. V. Hulse, R. H. Mole, and D. G. Papworth, Radiosensitivity of cells from which radiation-induced skin tumours are derived, Int. J. Radiat. Biol. 14:437-444 (1968).

59. J. E. Coggle and D. M. Peel, The relative effects of uniform and non-uniform external radiation on the induction of lung tumours in mice, in: "Late Biological Effects of Ionizing Radiation," IAEA, Vienna (1978), pp. 83-94.

60. A. L. Brooks, S. A. Benjamin, F. F. Hahn, et al., The induction of liver tumours by plutonium-239 oxyde particles in the Chinese hamsters, Radiat. Res. 96:135-161 (1983).

61. C. L. Sanders, G. E. Dagle, W. C. Cannon, et al., Inhalation carcinogenesis of high-fired plutonium-238 oxyde in rats, Radiat. Res. 71:528-546 (1977).

62. L. H. Gray, Cellular radiation biology, in: "Proceedings of the 18th Annual Symposium on Fundamental Cancer Research," Williams and Williams, Baltimore (1965).

63. A. M. Kellerer and H. H. Rossi, The theory of dual radiation action, Curr. Top. Radiat. Res. Quart. 8:85-158 (1972).

64. D. E. Lea, "Action of Radiation on Living Cells," University Press, Cambridge (1962).

65. Committee on the Biological Effects of Ionizing Radiation, "The Effects on Populations of Exposure to Low Levels of Ionizing Radiation," National Academy of Sciences, Washington, D.C. (1980).

66. G. W. Barendsen, Fundamental aspects of cancer induction in relation to the effectiveness of small doses of radiation, in: "Late Biological Effects of Ionizing Radiation," IAEA, Vienna (1978).

67. J. M. Brown, The shape of the dose-response curve for radiation carcinogenesis. Extrapolation to low doses, Radiat. Res. 71:34-50 (1977).

68. I. R. Major and R. H. Mole, Myeloid leukaemia in X-ray irradiated CBA mice, Nature 272:455-456 (1978).

69. R. H. Mole, Bone tumour production in mice by strontium-90: further experimental support for a two-event hypothesis, Br. J. Cancer 17:524-531 (1963).

70. National Council on Radiation Protection and Measurements, "Influence of Dose and Its Distribution in Time on Dose-Effect Relationships for Low-LET Radiations," NCRP Report No. 64 (1980).

71. A. C. Upton, F. F. Wolff, J. Furth, et al., A comparison of the induction of myeloid and lymphoid leukaemias in x-irradiated RF mice, Cancer Res. 18:842-848 (1958).

72. A. C. Upton, M. L. Randolph, and J. W. Conklin, Late effects of fast neutrons and gamma rays in mice as influenced by the dose rate of irradiation: induction of neoplasia, Radiat. Res. 41:467-491 (1970).

73. V. C. Robinson and A. C. Upton, Competing-risk analysis of leukaemia and non-leukaemia mortality in x-irradiated, male RF mice, J. Natl. Cancer Inst. 60:995-1007 (1978).

74. R. H. Mole, D. G. Papworth, and M. J. Corp, The dose-response for X-ray induction of myeloid leukameia in male CBA/H mice, Br. J. Cancer 47:285-291 (1983).

75. J. H. Hendry and B. I. Lord, The analysis of the early and late response to cytotoxic insults in the haemopoietic cell hierarchy, in: Cytotoxic Insult to Tissue," Plotten and Hendry, eds., Churchill and Livingstone, Edinburgh (1984).

76. R. H. Mole and I. R. Major, Myeloid leukaemia frequency after protracted exposure to ionizing radiation: experimental confirmation of the flat dose-response found in ankylosing spondylitis after a single treatment course with X-rays, Leukaemia Res. 7:295-300 (1983).

77. R. H. Mole and J. A. G. Davids, Induction of myeloid leukaemia and other tumours in mice by irradiation with fission neutrons, in: Neutron Carcinogenesis," J. J. Broerse and G. B. Gerber, eds., CEC Report EUR-8084 (1982).

78. R. L. Ullrich and J. B. Storer, Influence of gamma-irradiation on the development of neoplastic disease in mice. I. Reticular tissue tumors, Radiat Res. 80:303-316 (1979).

79. H. S. Kaplan and M. B. Brown, A quantitative dose-response study of lymphoid tumor development in irradiated C57 Black mice, J. Natl. Cancer Inst. 13:185-208 (1952).

80. J. R. Maisin, A. Wambersie, G. B. Gerber, et al., The effects of a fractionated gamma irradiation on life shortening and disease incidence in BALB/c mice, Radiat. Res. 94:359-373 (1983).

81. J. R. Maisin, A. Wambersie, G. B. Gerber, et al., Life shortening and disease incidence in BALB/c mice following a single d(50)Be neutron or gamma exposure, Radiat. Res. 94:374-389 (1983).

82. S. Sasaki and T. Kasuga, Life-shortening and carcinogenesis in mice irradiated neonatally with X-rays, Radiat. Res. 88:313-325 (1981).

83. P. Metalli, G. Silini, V. Covelli, et al., Late somatic effects in syngeneic radiation chimaeras: III. Observations on animals repopulated with irradiated marrow, Int. J. Radiat. Biol. 29:413-432 (1976).

84. P. Metalli, V. Covelli and G. Silini, Dose-incidence relationships of reticulum cell sarcoma in mice. Observations and hypotheses at the cellular level, in: "Late Biological Effects of Ionizing Radiation," IAEA, Vienna (1978).

85. D. Chmelevsky, A. M. Kellerer, J. Lafuma, et al., Maximum likelihood estimation of the prevalence of non-lethal neoplasms, Radiat. Res. 91:589-614 (1982).

86. K. Chmelevsky, A. M. Kellerer, J. Lafuma, et al., Comparison of the induction of pulmonary neoplasms in Sprague-Dawley rats by fission neutron and radon daughters, Radiat. Res. 98:519-535 (1984).

87. R. L. Ullrich, Tumor induction in BALB/c mice after fractionated or protracted exposures to fission spectrum neutrons, Radiat. Res. 97:587-597 (1984).

88. H. H. Vogel, Jr. and H. W. Dickson, Mammary neoplasia following acute and protracted irradiation with fission neutrons and cobalt-60 gamma-rays, (abstract), Radiat. Res. 87:453-454 (1981).

89. C. J. Shellabarger, D. Chmelevsky, A. M. Kellerer, et al., Induction of mammary neoplasms in the ACI rat by 430-keV neutrons, X-rays and diethylstilbestrol, J. Natl. Cancer Inst. 69:1135-1146 (1982).

90. S. Holtzman, J. P. Stone, and C. J. Shellabarger, Radiation-induced mammary carcinogenesis in virgin, pregnant, lactating and postlactating rats, Cancer Res. 42:50-53 (1982).

91. United Nations, "Ionizing Radiation: Sources and Biological
     Effects," United Nations Scientific Committee on the Effects of
     Atomic Radiation 1982 Report to the General Assembly, with
     Annexes, United Nations Sales Publication No. E.82.IX.8, New
     York (1982).

92. H. H. Vogel, Jr. and J. E. Turner, Genetic component in rat
     mammary carcinogenesis, Radiat. Res. 89:264-273 (1982).

93. J. J. Broerse, L. A. Hennen, M. J. van Zwieten, et al., Mammary
     carcinogenesis in different rat strains after single and
     fractionated irradiation, in: "Neutron Carcinogenesis," J. J.
     Broerse and G. B. Gerber, eds., Commission of the European
     Communities Report EUR-8084 (1982).

94. J. J. Broerse, L. A. Hennen, M. J. van Zwieten, et al., Dose-
     effect relations for mammary carcinogenesis in different rat
     strains after irradiation with X-rays and mono-energetic
     neutrons, in: "Biological Effects of Low-Level Radiation,"
     IAEA, Vienna (1984).

95. F. J. Burns, R. E. Albert, and R. D. Heimbach, RBE for skin
     tumours and hair follicle damage in the rat following
     irradiation with alpha particles and electrons, Radiat. Res.
     36:225-241 (1968).

96. F. J. Burns and M. Vanderlaan, Split-dose recovery for radiation-
     induced tumours in rat skin, Int. J. Radiat. Biol. 32:135-144
     (1977).

97. F. J. Burns, R. E. Albert, I. P. Sinclair, et al., The effect of a
     24-hour fractionation interval on the induction of rat skin
     tumours by electron radiation, Radiat. Res. 62:478-487 (1975).

98. F. J. Burns, P. Strickland, M. Vanderlaan, et al., Rat skin tumour
     incidence following single and fractionated exposures to proton
     radiation, Radiat. Res. 74:152-158 (1978).

99. M. Vanderlaan, F. J. Burns, and R. E. Albert, A model describing
     the effects of dose and dose-rate on tumour induction by
     radiation in rat skin, in: "Biological and Environmental
     Effects of Low-Level Radiation, Vol. II," IAEA, Vienna (1976).

100. R. E. Albert, F. J. Burns, and E. V. Sargent, Skin tumorigenesis
     by multiple doses of electron radiation in the rat, (abstract),
     Radiat. Res. 87:453 (1981).

101. E. V. Hulse, S. Y. Lewkowicz, A. L. Batchelor, et al., Incidence
     of radiation induced skin tumours in mice and variations with
     dose rat, Int. J. Radiat. Biol. 44:197-206 (1983).

102. D. G. Papworth and E. V. Hulse, Dose-response models for the
     radiation-induction of skin tumours in mice, Int. J. Radiat.
     Biol. 44:423-431 (1983).

103. O. G. Raabe, N. J. Parks, and S. A. Book, Dose-response
     relationships for bone tumors in beagles exposed to 226-Ra and
     90-Sr, Health Phys. 40:863-880 (1981).

104. O. G. Raabe, S. A. Book, and N. J. Parks, Lifetime bone cancer dose-response relationships in beagles and people from skeletal burdens of 226-Ra and 90-Sr, Health Phys. 44(Suppl. 1):33-48 (1983).

105. A. S. Whittemore and A. McMillan, Osteosarcomas among beagles exposed to Pu-239, Radiat. Res. 90:41-56 (1982).

106. A. V. Peterson, R. L. Prentice, and P. Marek, Relationship between dose of injected 239-Pu and bone sarcoma mortality in young adult beagles, Radiat. Res. 90:77-89 (1982).

107. A. Wesch, G. van Kaick, W. Riedel, et al., Recent results of the German Thorotrast Study. Statistical evaluation of animal experiments with regard to the non-radiation effects in human thorotrastosis, Health Phys. 44(Suppl. 1):317-321 (1983).

108. W. Lee, R. P. Chiacchierini, B. Shleien, et al., Thyroid tumours following iodine-131 or localized x-irradiation to the thyroid and the pituitary glands in rats, Radiat. Res. 92:307-319 (1982).

109. I. Doniach, Effects including carcinogenesis of I-131 and X-rays on the thyroid of experimental animals: a review, Health Phys. 9:1357-1362 (1963).

110. J. F. Thomson, F. S. Williamson, D. Grahn, et al., Life shortening in mice exposed to fission neutrons and gamma rays. I. Single and short-term fractionated exposure, Radiat. Res. 86:559-572 (1981).

111. J. F. Thomson, F. S. Williamson, D. Grahn, et al., Life shortening of mice exposed to fission neutrons and gamma rays. II. Duration-of-life and long-term fractionated exposures. Radiat. Res. 86:573-579 (1981).

112. J. B. Storer and R. L. Ullrich, Life shortening in BALB/c mice following brief, protracted or fractionated exposures to neutrons, Radiat. Res. 96:335-347 (1983).

RADIATION CARCINOGENESIS AND THE HAIR FOLLICLE

I. P. Sinclair
St. Josephs Hospital
Paterson, NJ

F. J. Burns
N.Y.U. Department of Environmental Medicine
New York, NY

INTRODUCTION

Rodent skin has been used extensively as an experimental model for studying radiation carcinogenesis. The advantages of skin for such studies include: radiation beams can be localized in the target tissue without irradiating the whole animal, and tumors can be detected at an early stage of development and followed for long periods of time. The fact that rodent skin has been widely utilzed for testing carcinogenic chemicals permits comparisons of carcinogenesis by radiation and chemicals. The skin of albino rats responds to the carcinogenic action of several known human carcinogens, including, ionizing radiation and ultraviolet light.

RADIATION CARCINOGENESIS - RESTING PHASE SKIN

Experiments were performed to establish dose-response relationships for tumor induction at different penetrations of radiation in resting phase skin (1). The results are shown in Figure 1.

For the deeper penetrations the data are typical for this type of response; initially there is an increase in the number of tumors with dose, followed by a peak and finally a decrease at higher doses. The decrease is associated with the decreased survival of cells from which tumors could arise.

The initial ascending part of the curve can be fitted with a power function with an exponent of 2-3. The data for the lowest penetration show only the initial rise without reaching a peak. Obviously there are substantially different responses at different penetrations when plotted against surface dose. However, the use of surface dose is abritrary, because the location of the sensitive cells is unknown. If the tumor incidence is plotted against dose at other depths, we find a depth (0.27 mm) that reconciles the data into a single curve. To illustrate this the same data are replotted in Figure 2 as a function of the dose at 0.27 mm.

The hair follicle in resting (telogen) stage is about 0.5 mm long and lies at an angle of 30 to 45 degrees to the surface. Thus 0.27 mm is

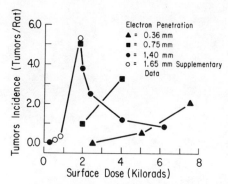

Fig. 1. The yield of tumors per rat as a function
of surface dose for different maximum
penetrations as indicated. The rats
were 28 days of age at the time of
irradiation. The yields are plotted at
80 weeks after irradiation. 1 kilorad
equals 10 Gy.

approximately the depth of the hair germ cells (2). Various energies were
used so that the Bragg peak could be placed at appropriate levels within the
dermis as follows: 0.12, 0.35, and 0.55 mm, corresponding, respectively, to
above, at and below the hair germ cells.

Placing the Bragg peak at a depth which produced maximum dosage to the
hair germ did not elevate the tumor incidence over that which resulted from
the plateau dose. This suggests either that damage to the entire follicle
is a condition for tumor induction or that repair from undamaged parts of
the follicle can reduce tumor formation in the damaged regions.

In these experiments a relationship was established between the number
of atrophic hair follicles produced and the number of tumors (3,4).
Atrophic hair follicles are remnants of hair follicles and are frequently
found in the skin after irradiation. They are seen by examining whole
mounts of the skin epithelium with a dissecting stereo microscope. Whole
mounts are prepared by soaking the skin overnight in 0.25% trypsin. The
dermis is stripped off, and the remaining epidermis and hair follicles are
then stained with hematoxylin and eosin. The results showed a direct
proportionality between the incidence of atrophic follicles and the yield
of tumors. Similar RBE (relative biological effectiveness) values were
observed for tumor and atrophic follicle induction indicating the
proportionality was valid for ionizing radiation with different LET (linear
energy transfer) values.

REPAIR AND MODIFICATION IN RADIATION CARCINOGENESIS

Modifying mechanisms substantially reduce tumor yields for several
types of ionizing radiation, including, protons and electrons in a variety
of grid and sieve patterns. These experiments showed that tumor yields
per unit area were substantially less for localized irradiation than for
larger area irradiations (5,6). The interpretation of the findings was
complicated by a number of effects, such as, electron scatter under the
shields. Nevertheless the experiments established conclusively that tumor
yield depends on the size and shape of the pores and is lowest for the
smallest pore size and greatest pore spacing.

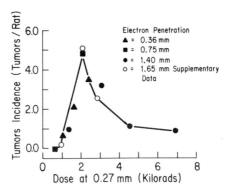

Fig. 2.   Tumor yield in resting phase rat skin as
           a function of dose at 0.27 mm. As in
           Figure 1 the rats were irradiated at 28
           days of age and the tumor yield
           comparisons were made at 80 weeks after
           irradiation. 1 kilorad equals 10 Gy.

        Dose fractionation experiments established the existence of a type of
repair relevant to carcinogenesis (7). One group of animals was given a
dose of radiation which produced a minimal number of tumors, i.e., 7.5 Gy
during the resting phase, and this group together with another unirradiated
group were given graded doses of radiation several weeks later to produce
comparative dose-response curves. The 2 dose-response curves were
displaced horizontally by 6.5 Gy indicating repair of oncogenic damage
equivalent to 5.5 Gy or about 85% of the initial dose. Further studies
established that the repair halftime was about 3 hours (8).

        In summary the effects of irradiation of the resting phase skin
indicate that tumor incidence can be related to the dose delivered to the
base of the follicle and that the minimum dose to the follicle determines
the tumor yield.

        Spared populations, as a partial irradiation of the follicle by sieve
irradiation, can lead to protection against oncogenic effects. Superficial
irradiation yielded essentially no tumors if the penetration was less than
about 200 microns (9).

THE ACUTE HISTOLOGICAL RESPONSE IN GROWING PHASE SKIN

        In the stage of hair growth (anagen stage), the follicle greatly
increases in length and volume as a result of greatly increased mitotic
activity, particularly in the hair germ and matrix regions. In anagen the
follicle extends to a depth of about 1.0 mm below the surface. The energy
of the electrons was varied to provide beams with different penetrations as
shown in Figure 3.

        The deepest penetration delivered a fairly uniform radiation dose to
the entire length of the anagen (growing stage) hair follicle. The dose to
the skin surface was varied from 10 Gy (1000 rads) to about 40 Gy (4000
rads). Several changes in the skin were noted by gross observation
including: suppression of hair growth, loss of hair (epilation) and loss of
the brown scaly material normally present on the skin of male rats. The
skin surface response was evaluated in terms of the amount of desquamation
and ulceration.

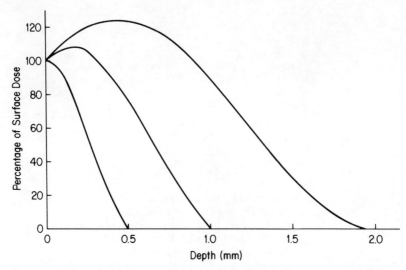

Fig. 3. The depth-dose relationships for the electron beams
utilized in these studies. All measurements were made
with thin-window ionization chambers.

The histological effects were quantified by measuring the relative
size of the various tissue compartments in the skin at various times up to
85 days post-irradiation (10). The compartments were assessed by counting
the number of times a randomly placed spot (intersection of crosshairs in
an eyepiece grid) fell on a given tissue compartment in the microscope
image.

Total DNA measurements were made from biopsy samples taken from
individual rats. The biopsies were performed at 2-day intervals up to 10
days post-irradiation. Loss of total DNA over control levels was equated
to net cell loss, i.e., loss of cells caused by radiation death plus the
cells replaced by repopulation repair. A radioactive label was
incorporated into the DNA by injecting tritiated thymidine after
stimulating hair growth by mechanical depilation. The loss of
radioactivity in the DNA was taken as a measure of cell death irrespective
of repopulation.

At the 2.0 mm penetration the initial rate of loss of radioactivity
was independent of dose. For both 1.0 mm and 2.0 mm penetrations, there
was a reversal after about 8 days, i.e., the amount of radioactivity began
to increase. Histologically the reversal was due to the influx of a large
number of labeled inflammatory cells. The rate of loss of radioactive
label was the same in irradiated and control skin at both penetrations and
all doses. This indicated that the rate of loss of cells was the same as
the normal turnover rate, meaning there was substantial reproductive death.
The decrease in total DNA meant there was little or no repopulation repair
in the first few days post-irradiation.

The histological data on the relative cellularity of the hair follicles is
shown in Figures 4 and 5. The decrease in the number of hits scored in the
controls starting at day 12 reflects the end of the growing phase. The
subsequent increase around day 25 indicates the onset of the next growing
phase. The number of hits in the second growing phase is lower due to the
greater spacing between the follicles in the larger animals. The
significant observation to note in Figure 4 is that there was no
substantial difference between the controls and 20.0 Gy group. For the

110

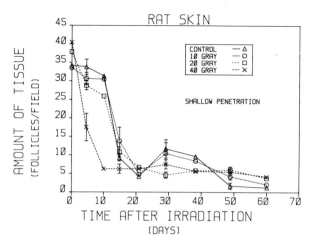

Fig. 4. Relative amount of hair follicle tissue scored as hits per microscope field as explained in the text. Shallow refers to a maximum penetration of 1.0 mm. Rats were irradiated with electrons at 28 days of age.

deep penetration (Figure 5), it should be noted that the initial rates of decrease were the same at all doses; however, the extent of the decline increased with dose until almost complete destruction of the follicle occurred at 40.0 Gy.

The epidermis of the rat consists of a layer of basal cells, a layer of differentiating cells containing granules of kerato-hyaline and an outer, fully-keratinized squamous layer. The effect of the radiation on the epidermis was assessed by measuring its thickness histologically. The essential observation was that the deeper penetration was more effective than the shallower for causing epidermal atrophy by a ratio of 2:1, i.e., 10.0 Gy-2.0 mm was equivalent to 20.0 Gy-1.0 mm, and 20.0 Gy-2.0 mm was equivalent to 40. Gy-1.0 mm.

At 10.0 Gy-2.0 mm there was a transient hyperplasia with a return to normal at 36 days. At 20.0 Gy-2.0 mm there was a complete de-epithelialization at 10 days post-irradiation followed by recovery to an overcompensatory hyperplasia which returned to normal by 86 days post-irradiation.

The sebaceous gland disappeared as a recognizable structure 10 days after irradiation at all doses greater than 10.0 Gy. There was some regeneration, but not all glands regenerated, and those that did were frequently hyperplastic. At 10.0 Gy-1.0 mm there was a decrease in the size of the gland followed by a return to normal. At 10.0 Gy-2.0 mm, there was a more marked decrease in size followed by an overcompensatory hyperplastic regeneration. The effects at 20.0 Gy were accentuated versions of the reactions at 10.0 Gy. In general the more the time of regeneration was delayed the greater the dose and the penetration.

The whole mounts showed that follicle curvival decreased with dose; however, survival was high at 40.0 Gy-1.0 mm which suggests that sparing of the deepest elements of the follicle aids survival of the structure. The number of abnormal follicles peaked between 20.0 and 40.0 Gy at the 1.0 mm

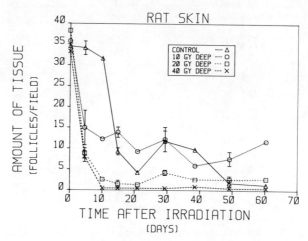

Fig. 5.   Relative amount of hair follicle tissue
scored as hits per microscope field as
explained in the text. Deep refers to a
maximum penetration of 2.0 mm. Rats were
irradiated with electrons at 28 days of age.

penetration and between 10.0 and 20.0 Gy at 2.0 mm penetration. The
decrease at the higher doses was associated with loss of tissue. Earlier
experiments with resting follicles had shown a relationship between
morphological damage (particularly atrophic follicles) and tumor incidence
(3).

CARCINOGENESIS IN THE STAGE OF HAIR GROWTH

Experiments were performed to determine the correlation, if any,
between early histological changes and the subsequent induction of tumors
in rat skin irradiated in the stage of hair growth. The major questions to
be answered were:

1.   What is the sensitivity to tumor induction when the hair follicle
is mitotically active?

2.   Is the tumor yield depth-dependent in the same way as observed in
skin with resting follicles?

In order to correlate tumor incidence with dose at a specific depth
and to ascertain the peak incidence of tumor induction more accurately, rat
skin was irradiated with various doses and penetrations of electron
radiation. The results are shown in Figure 6.

The relationship between tumor incidence and depth was found to match
best at a depth of 0.4 mm (11,12). One can infer that 0.4 mm represents
the location of carcinogenically-sensitive cells. If so, these cells did
not change their location substantially between resting and growing
follicles, even though the growing follicle elongates and extends much
deeper into the dermis than a resting follicle.

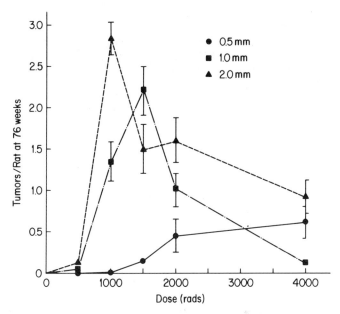

Fig. 6.   Dose-response data for tumor induction in growing phase
rat skin by electron radiation. The maximum
penetration was varied as indicated and the doses refer
to surface doses. the rats were 28 days of age at the
time of irradiation. 1000 rads equals 10 Gy.

    The incidence of skin tumors produced by electron radiation in the
growing phase was compared to the acute histological and gross
morphological changes found in skin. Note in Figure 6 the relatively large
number of tumors produced at 1500 rads-1.0 mm and the small number at 4000
rads-1.0 mm. This is in contrast to what would be expected from the
pattern of acute damage; 1500 rads-1.0 mm had only minimal damage - slight
blanching was the only grossly observable damage. In the histological
study there were only minimal changes, i.e., a slight reduction in the size
of the sebaceous gland followed by a rapid return to normal and no other
significant effects. Whereas 4000 rads-1.0 mm showed severe acute
hypoplasia followed by a relatively persistent epidermal hyperplasia.

    At 1000 rads-1.0 mm, only minimal morphological changes were seen and
yet tumors of all histological types were found. There was, however, a
predominance of the undifferentiated tumors similar to the type commonly
seen in human skin. At 4000 rads-1.0 mm, where there were persistent
hyperplastic sebaceous glands and severe epidermal hyperplasia, there were
no tumors of the keratinizing, kerato-sebaceous or sebaceous type and only
a few undifferentiated tumors.

    At 4000 rads-2.0 mm there was a persistent regenerative hyperplasia,
and yet the incidence of keratinizing tumors was less than at 1000 rads-2.0
mm, where the epidermal hyperplasia was mild and transient. Nor was the
incidence of keratinizing tumors correlated with transient hyperplasia,
since the degree of transient hyperplasia was the same at 2000 rads-1.0 mm
as at 1000 rads-2.0 mm, but the incidence of keratinizing tumors in the
latter group was nearly double the incidence in the former group. On the
basis of these results, no correlation could be established between early
histological changes and tumor incidence.

REFERENCES

1. R. E. Albert, F. J. Burns, and R. D. Heimbach, "The effect of penetration depth on electron radiation onskin tumor formation in the rat," Radiat. Res., 30:515-524 1967.

2. R. D. Heimbach, F. J. Burns, and R. E. Albert, "An evaluation by alpha particle Bragg peak radiation of the critical depth in the rat skin for tumor induction," Radiat. Res. 39:332-344 (1969).

3. R. E. Albert, P. Phillips, P. Bennett, F. Burns, and R. Heimbach, "The morphology and growth characteristics of radiation-induced epithelial skin tumors in the rat," Cancer Res., 29:658-688 (1969)

4. F. J. Burns, R. E. Albert, and R. D. Heimbach, "The RBE for skin tumors and hair follicle damage in the rat following irradiation with alpha particles and electrons," Radiat. Res., 36:225-241 (1968).

5. R. E. Albert, F. J. Burns, and R. D. Heimbach, "Skin damage and tumor formation from grid and sieve patterns of electron and beta radiation in the rat," Radiat. Res, 30:525-540 (1967).

6. R. E. Albert, and F. J. Burns, "Tumor and injury responses of rat skin after seive pattern x-irradiation," Radiat. Res., 67:142-148 (1976).

7. F. J. Burns, R. E., Albert, I. P. Sinclair, and M. Vanderlaan, "The effect of a 24-hour fractionation interval on the induction of rat skin tumors by electron radiation," Radiat. Res., 62:478-487 (1975).

8. F. J. Burns and M. Vanderlaan, "Split dose recovery for radiation induced tumors in rat skin," Intl. J. Radiat. Biol., 32:135-144 (1977).

9. F. J. Burns, R. E. Albert, M. Vanderlaan, and P. Strickland, "The dose-response curve for tumor induction with single and split doses of 10 MeV protrons," Radiat. Res., 62:598 (1975).

10. F. J. Burns and R. E. Albert, "Radiation carcinogenesis in rat skin," In: Radiation Carcinogenesis (eds., A. C. Upton, R. E. Albert, F. J. Burns and R. E. Shore) El sevier, New York, 1986, pp. 199-214.

11. I. P. Sinclair, "The effect of penetration depth on radiation carcinogenesis in growing phase skin." Ph. D. thesis, New York University, 1974.

12. F. J. Burns, I. P. Sinclair, R. E. Albert, and M. Vanderlaan, "Tumor induction and hair follicle damage for different electron penetrations in at skin," Radiat. Res., 67:474-481 (1976).

DOSE-INCIDENCE RELATIONS FOR RADIATION CARCINOGENESIS WITH PARTICULAR

REFERENCE TO THE EFFECTS OF HIGH-LET RADIATION*

A. C. Upton

NYU Institute of Environmental Medicine
550 First Avenue
New York, N.Y. 10016

INTRODUCTION

For many years, radiations of high linear energy transfer (LET) have been known to have a high relative biological effectiveness (RBE) for carcinogenic effects (1), in keeping with their high RBE for most other effects on living organisms (2-7). It has also been known that the RBE of high-LET radiations for carcinogenic effects generally increases with decreasing dose and dose rate (1, 6, 7).

Because the variations in RBE have important implications with respect to fundamental mechanisms of carcinogenesis as well as radiological protection standards, the carcinogenic effects of high-LET radiation have received increasing attention in recent years. Although a comprehensive review of the pertinent literature is beyond the scope of this report, salient observations on dose-effect relationships for radiation carcinogenesis are surveyed in the following.

BIOPHYSICAL AND CELLULAR CONSIDERATIONS

The effects of radiation on cell survival, mutagenesis, and the induction of chromosome aberrations have generally been interpreted in terms of multi-target, multi-hit theories. According to this interpretation, production of such a radiation effect requires either $\underline{n}$ targets within the cell to be hit or a single target to be hit $\underline{m}$ times (2, 8). In the simplest form of the multi-target theory, the relation between the dose (D) and the effect (E) can be described by the expression:

$$E = (1 - \exp -(D/_{Do})^n \qquad (1)$$

---

*Preparation of this report was supported in part by Grant ES 00260 from the National Institute of Environmental Health Sciences, Grant CA 13343 from the National Cancer Institute, and Grant 00009 from the American Cancer Society.

and in the simplest form of the multi-hit theory, it can be described by the expression:

$$E = 1 - \left[1 + \frac{D}{D_o} \frac{1}{2!} \frac{(D)^2}{(D_o)} \cdot \cdot \cdot + \frac{1}{(m-1)!} \frac{(D)^{m-1}}{(D_o)} \right] \exp^{-D/D_o} \quad (2)$$

Both equations can be expanded to give the expression:

$$E = \alpha Dp - \beta Dp^{+1} + \text{higher terms in D}, \quad (3)$$

where p is equal to n or m (9).

The available dose-effect data (e.g., Fig. 1) for low-LET radiation can be described by the expression:

$$E = \alpha_\ell D_\ell + \beta_\ell D_\ell^2 \quad (4)$$

and for high-LET radiation by the expression:

$$E = \alpha_h D_h \quad (5)$$

Hence, the biological effects in question have been postulated to require at least two targets to be hit or two hits to occur in a single target. The two hits are envisaged to occur simultaneously within the track of a single particle in the case of high-LET radiation or in the case of low-LET radiation received at low doses and low dose rates; however, with high doses of low-LET irradiation received at high dose rates, it is envisaged that the two hits may occur within separate particle tracks that traverse a critical volume of the cell in swift succession (represented by the second term in equation 4).

According to the above concepts, and in keeping with the curves in Figure 1, the RBE increases with decreasing dose and dose rate, ultimately

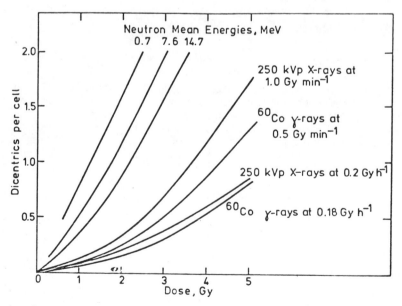

Fig. 1.   Frequency of dicentric chromosome aberrations in human lymphocytes after exposure to high- and low-LET radiations (10).

116

Table 1. Maximum values of the RBE of radiation of different LETs for dicentric aberrations in human lymphocytes.[a]

Radiation	rbe_m
^{60}Co gamma rays	0.4
250 kVp X-rays	1.0
14.7 MeV neutrons	6
7.6 MeV neutrons	10
0.9 MeV neutrons	15
0.7 MeV neutrons	17
Alpha particles < 5 MeV	8
Alpha particles 3-4 MeV	6

[a]From (9), based on data from (10 and 11).

reaching a maximum value that is equivalent to the ratio $\alpha h/\alpha \ell$. Maximum RBE values for radiations of different LETs in the induction of dicentric chromosome aberrations in human lymphocytes have been observed to range from 0.4 with cobalt-60 gamma rays to 17 with 0.7 MeV neutrons (Table 1). For other types of effects, substantially higher maximum values have been reported; e.g., a value of 100 for single locus mutations in plants (5).

To the extent that the cellular mechanisms responsible for radiation carcinogenesis involve mutations or chromosome aberrations, the dose-incidence relationships for radiation-induced cancer should be expected to be comparable to those cited above. Such relationships might be expected to apply, however, only to certain stages of the carcinogenic process and to effects of relatively low doses where they are not confounded by excessive cell and tissue damage. Although the mechanisms of carcinogenesis remain to be determined, it is noteworthy that the dose-incidence data for most radiation-induced neoplasms are in fact consistent with the above relationships.

Overall Relationship between Cancer Incidence and Dose

Induction Period   Cancers induced by radiation are typically preceded by a long induction period, which varies in length with the type of neoplasm in question and age at the time of irradiation. In general, however, the induced cancers tend to occur at the ages when cancers of corresponding types occur in non-irradiated populations. After prenatal irradiation, for example, the increased incidence of leukemia peaks within the first five years of life, in parallel with the incidence of juvenile leukemia in the general population (12, 13). Similarly, the breast cancers induced in women by irradiation during infancy do not appear until more than 30 years later, when the women reach the age at which breast cancers characteristically start to appear in the general population.

The induction period for leukemia is generally shorter than that for other forms of cancer. Most cases of chronic granulocytic leukemia appear within 5-15 years, and few later than 25 years, after irradiation. As a

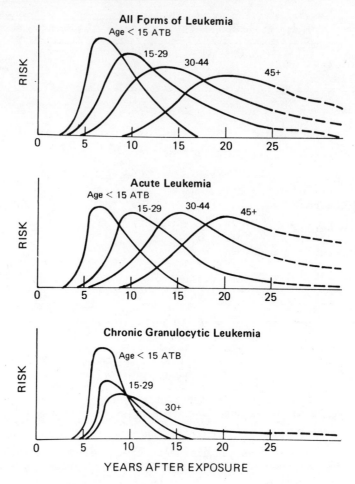

Fig. 2.   Temporal distribution of radiation-induced
           leukemias in a-bomb survivors, in relation to type
           of leukemia and age at the time of irradiation
           (14).

result, the incidence of the radiation-induced cases assumes a wave-like
distribution in time (Figure 2). The patterns for other types of
radiation-induced leukemia, although not identical, are also wave-like
(Figure 2).

     For cancers other than leukemia and osteosarcoma (7), the induction
periods average more than 15-20 years and the cases do not distribute
themselves in wave-like patterns with time after irradiation. It is not
clear whether the annual excess of such cases remains constant after a
certain length of time (i.e., as would be implied by the "absolute risk"
projection model), or whether it continues to increase as a constant
fraction of the underlying baseline incidence (i.e., as would be implied by
the "relative risk" model) (Figure 3). The data evolving from studies of
the atomic bomb survivors (Figure 4) are more compatible with the latter
model than with the former (17, 18), as are the results of experiments in
laboratory animals (Figure 5).

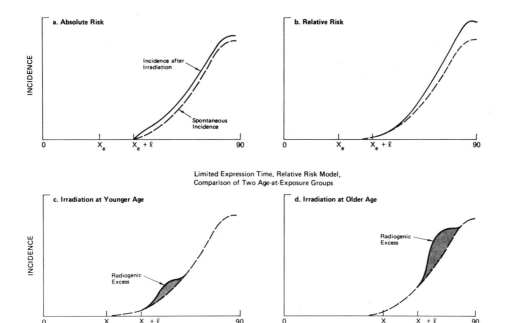

a. Absolute Risk

b. Relative Risk

Limited Expression Time, Relative Risk Model,
Comparison of Two Age-at-Exposure Groups

c. Irradiation at Younger Age

d. Irradiation at Older Age

Fig. 3. Distribution of radiation-induced cancer incidence with time
after irradiation in relation to baseline age-dependent
cancer incidence, as projected for a lifetime by the absolute
risk model (a) or the relative risk model (b); or as
projected for a shorter period by the absolute model (c) or
the relative risk model (d). The symbol x denotes the
minimal latent period. (7).

With chronic irradiation, the median time to tumor appearance, at
least for some forms of cancer, has been shown to vary as a function of the
dose rate according to the Blum-Druckrey model; i.e.,

$$t^n d = C, \qquad (5)$$

where t is the median time to tumor appearance, d is the daily dose of
radiation, and C and n are constants, n being larger than 1 (20).

Dose   Irradiation has been observed to induce many types of neoplasms
in humans and laboratory animals, but all neoplasms are not increased
equally in frequency within a given species or strain (6). Certain
neoplasms are actually decreased in frequency by irradiation (Figure 6).
From the diversity of observed dose-incidence relationships, it is clear
that no one mathematical model for relating incidence to dose is
universally applicable.

For those types of cancer that are known to be induced in humans by
high doses, the dose-incidence relationships at lower doses can be
estimated only by extrapolation. From the existing data, however, it is
not possible to distinguish confidently among alternative extrapolation
models. For this reason, the National Academy of Sciences Advisory
Committee on the Biological Effects of Ionizing Radiation (BEIR Committee)
utilized four different models (Figure 7), to derive a range of risk
estimates, in its latest report (7). The four models all assume a

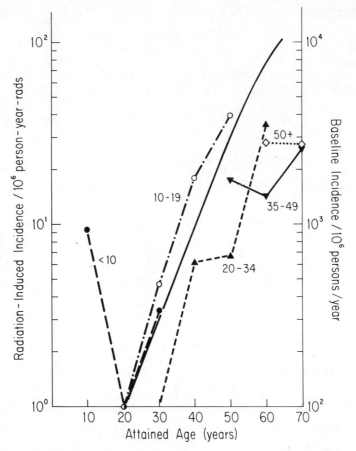

Fig. 4. Incidence of radiation-induced cancer (excluding
leukemia) in relation to attained age in different
birth cohorts of heavily-irradiated Nagasaki a-bomb
survivors, as compared with the baseline incidence in
the general population of Japan. Data for a-bomb
survivors (15) denoted by dashed curves, with age at
time of irradiation of each cohort as indicated. Data
for the general population (16) denoted by the solid
curve (17).

nonthreshold dose-incidence relationship and include: (1) the linear model,
which can be represented by the expression:

$$F(D) = \alpha_0 + \alpha_1 D \qquad\qquad (6)$$

where F(D), the incidence of cancer at dose D, varies as the sum of the
baseline incidence α_0 plus the product of the dose D times a constant risk
coefficient (α_1); (2) the linear-quadratic model, which can be represented
by the expression:

$$F(D) = \alpha_0 + \alpha_1 D + \alpha_2 D \qquad\qquad (7)$$

where F(D), the incidence of cancer at dose D, varies as the sum of the
natural incidence (α_0) plus a linear dose term ($\alpha_1 D$) and a squared dose

120

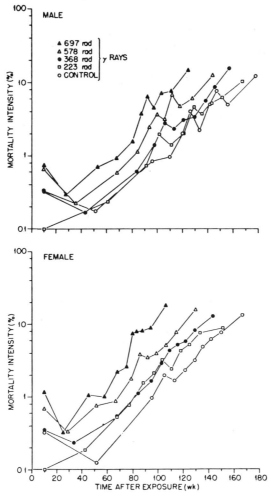

Fig. 5. Death rate in mice, in relation to dose
of whole-body gamma radiation and time
after irradiation (19).

term (α_2D^2); (3) the quadratic risk model, which can be represented by the
expression:

$$F(D) = \alpha_0 + \alpha_2D^2 \qquad (8)$$

where F(D), the excess of cancer at dose D, varies as the sum of the
natural incidence (α_0) plus a squared dose term (α_2D^2); and (4) the linear-
quadratic model in which a negative exponential is included to account for
saturation of the carcinogenic process at high doses, which can be
represented by the expression:

$$F(D) = (\alpha_0 + \alpha_1 + \alpha_2D^2)\exp\,(-\beta_1D-\beta_2D^2), \qquad (9)$$

where the terms are as described above, with the addition of the
coefficients β_1 and β_2.

If the induction of a mutation or chromosome aberration in a single
somatic cell were sufficient to initiate the process of carcinogenesis,

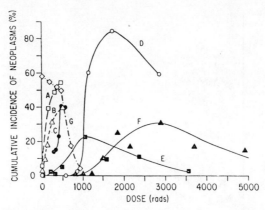

Fig. 6. Dose-incidence curves for different neoplasms in animals
exposed to external radiation: (a) myeloid leukemia in x-
irradiated mice (21); (b) mammary gland tumors at 12 months
in gamma-irradiated rats (22); (c) thymic lymphoma in x-
irradiated mice (23); (d) kidney tumors in x-irradiated rats
(24); (e) skin tumors in alpha-irradiated rats (percentage
incidence X 10 (25); (f) skin tumors in electron-irradiated
rats (percentage incidence X 10) (25); and (g) reticulum cell
sarcoma in x-irradiated mice (26) (from 27).

then the last of the above models would seem more appropriate than the
others on purely radiobiological grounds (7, 28, 29). For leukemia, the
revised data for a-bomb survivors (30) and the data for the mouse (31) are
compatible with this model. For most cancers other than osteosarcoma, the
quadratic model seems incompatible with the data.

For cancer of the female breast, the dose-incidence relationship
appears to be essentially the same in women surviving a-bomb irradiation
(32, 33), women who received radiotherapy to the breast for acute postpartum mastitis (34), women whose breasts were irradiated through repeated
fluoroscopic examinations of the chest in the course of treatment for
pulmonary tuberculosis (35), and luminous dial painters (36). The apparent
constancy of the dose-incidence relationship in the four groups, in spite
of the marked differences in the duration of their exposures, implies that
the linear nonthreshold model is appropriate for carcinogenesis in the
female breast (7, 37, 38).

Evidence favoring a linear nonthreshold model has also been presented
for induction of thyroid cancer by irradiation in infancy (39) and for the
leukemogenic effects of prenatal irradiation (40).

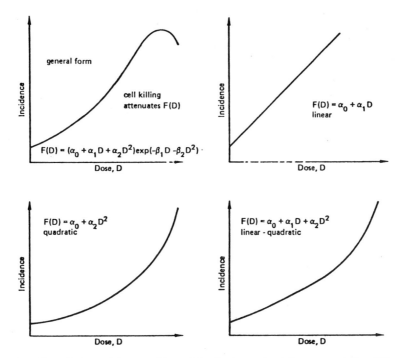

Fig. 7. Alternative mathematical dose-incidence models (7).

Dose Rate   In experimental animals, it has been observed repeatedly that a given dose of x-rays or gamma rays is generally several times less tumorigenic if delivered in many small exposures over a period of days or weeks than if delivered in a single exposure lasting only a few minutes (6, 41).   The effectiveness of high-LET radiation (e.g., neutrons or alpha particles), on the other hand, shows little or no decrease (42), but may increase, with fractionation or protraction of exposure (43), as will be discussed below.

Shortening of the Life Span   In laboratory animals (44) and in a-bomb survivors (45), shortening of the life span from whole-body irradiation is attributable primarily, if not entirely, to increased mortality from neoplasms, at least in the low-to-intermediate dose range (46).   The life-shortening impact of whole-body irradiation thus provides a measure of the carcinogenic effects of radiation on all organs combined.

In mice exposed acutely or chronically to whole-body neutron irradiation, beginning at an early age, the dose-effect relationship is convex upward, the extent of life shortening per unit dose increasing with decreasing dose and dose rate (Figure 8).   This relationship contrasts with the pattern that is typical for gamma-irradiation, in which the extent of life shortening increases linearly with dose in the low-to-intermediate dose range, and the effect per unit dose decreases with decreasing dose rate (Figure 8).   As a result of the differences between the two types of radiation, the RBE of neutrons for life shortening increases with decreasing dose and dose rate (Figure 9) (46).

Leukemia   In mice of the RF (42) and CBA (48) strains, the incidence of myeloid leukemia increases after whole-body neutron-irradiation in the 0.02-2 Gy range.   The dose-incidence curve rises steeply, reaches a maximum at a dose of 1-2 Gy, and is essentially dose rate independent (Figure 10). With x-rays or gamma-rays, on the other hand, the dose-incidence curve

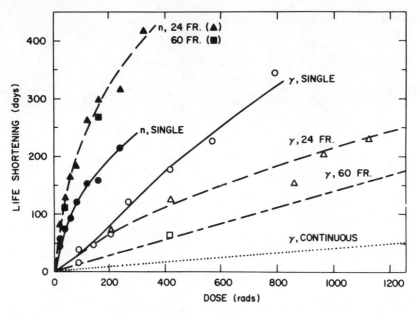

Fig. 8. Shortening of the life span from all causes of death in
         male B6C3F, mice in relation to dose of whole-body
         fission neutron or gamma radiation received in a single
         exposure or in highly fractionated exposure (47).

rises less steeply, reaches a maximum at a higher dose, and decreases
markedly in slope with decreasing dose rate (Figure 10).

The incidence of thymic lymphomas also increases after whole-body
irradiation in mice of the RF strain. With neutron irradiation, the
incidence per unit dose is not reduced by fractionation or protraction of
exposure but may actually be increased, whereas the reverse is generally
true with x- or gamma-irradiation (42).

An increased incidence of leukemia has been observed in persons
injected intravenously with thorotrast (7), but the data do not suffice to
define the relationship between incidence and dose. Although the incidence
of leukemia is also increased in a-bomb survivors, revision of the a-bomb
dosimetry suggests that the neutron component of the dose was not large
enough to have contributed significantly to the leukemogenic effects of a-
bomb irradiation in Hiroshima or Nagasaki (30). Other data on leukemogenesis by high-LET radiation in humans are lacking.

Breast Tumors The rapidity of development and final incidence of
mammary gland tumors in female rats are increased by neutron-irradiation,
to an extent that varies among strains (49, 50). The frequency per unit
dose of benign (Figure 11) and malignant (Figure 12) tumors is higher with
neutrons than with x- or gamma-rays. Furthermore, the tumorigenic
effectiveness of neutrons increases on fractionation or protraction of
exposure, whereas that of gamma rays decreases (Figure 13). The RBE of
neutrons thus increases with decreasing dose and dose rate, exceeding 100
with low-energy neutrons at doses of 0.001-0.05 Gy in rats of some strains
(52, 53). The tumorigenic effectiveness of neutrons and x-rays in some
strains of rats is enhanced to varying degrees by hormonal stimulation,
depending on the conditions of dosage (49).

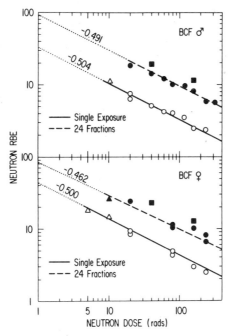

Fig. 9. Relationship between neutron RBE and
neutron dose in male (upper panel and
female (lower panel) B6CF$_1$ mice for
single and fractionated exposures. Open
symbols, single exposures; closed
symbols, 24 weekly fractions. Also
shown (squares) are the points for 60
weekly fractions of neutron radiation,
with similarly fractionated γ exposures
as the standard (47).

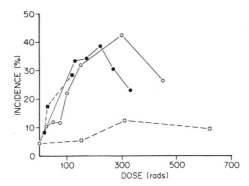

Fig. 10. Incidence of myeloid leukemia in male
mice, in relation to dose and dose rate
of whole body neutron, x- , gamma-
radiation. o single exposure (7-8 x
10^{-2} Gy min^{-1}); □ daily exposures (1-4 x
10^{-6} Gy min^{-1}). Open symbols denote
results with x-rays and gamma rays;
shaded symbols denote results with
neutrons (42).

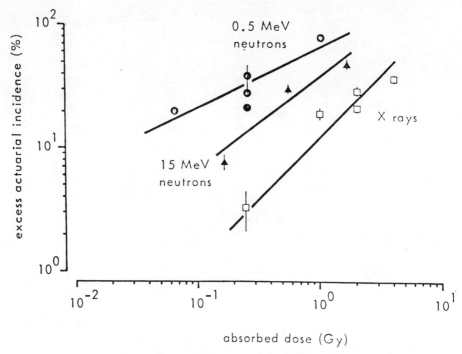

Fig. 11. Actuarial incidence of benign mammary tumours in WAG/Rij
rats after irradiation with x-rays (□), 15 MeV neutrons
(▲), and 0.5 MeV neutrons (●) (50).

Lung Tumors   The incidence of adenocarcinomas of the lung in BALB/c
female mice increases steeply with whole-body fission neutron irradiation,
reaching a maximum and bending over between 0.5 Gy and 2.0 Gy (Figure 14).
The corresponding dose-incidence curve for gamma-irradiation is less steep
and does not bend over until higher doses are reached (Figure 14).   On
fractionation of neutron irradiation, the dose-incidence curve remains
essentially unchanged in the dose region below 0.2 Gy and shows less, if
any, bending over between 0.5 Gy and 2.0 Gy.   On fractionation of gamma-
irradiation, by contrast, the incidence per unit dose is decreased at doses
of 0.5-2.0 Gy (54).

    Inhaled alpha-emitters also increase the incidence of lung cancer in
rats and mice, the dose-incidence curve being convex upward and relatively
dose rate independent (6, 55).   With inhaled beta-emitters, by contrast,
the dose-incidence curve is concave upward and decreases in slope with
decreasing dose rate (6, 55).   In underground hard-rock miners, the
incidence of lung cancer increases with the dose to the respiratory tract
from inhaled alpha emitters.   The dose-incidence curve in miners is convex
upward and steeper than that observed in a-bomb survivors or other
populations exposed to low-LET radiation (7), the difference between the
curves implies an RBE of alpha radiation in the range of 8-15 (7).

    Bone Tumors   In rats, mice, dogs, and humans, the incidence of
osteosarcomas increases with the dose to endosteal cells from locally
deposited alpha-emitters (6, 7).   The dose-incidence curve is characteristically linear in the low-to-intermediate dose range (56) and steeper
than the curve for low-LET radiation, which is characteristically concave
upward in the same range (e.g., Figure 15).   From the ratio of slopes in
the low-to-intermediate dose range, the RBE of alpha radiations has been

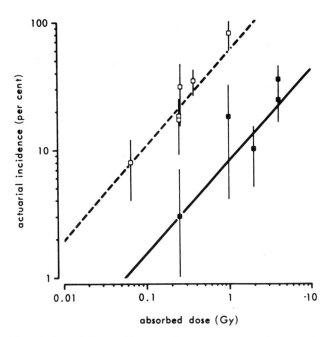

Fig. 12. Actuarial incidence of mammary carcinomas in
WAG/Rij rats after irradiation with x-rays (□) and
0.5 MeV neutrons (●) (50).

estimated to approximate 20 (7). Fractionation of the dose increases the
tumorigenicity of radium-224 alpha irradiation in humans (58).

The dose-incidence curve for irradiation by internally deposited
radium-226 is more complex, conforming to a multistage multihit model in
which there are two initiating steps and one promoting step (59).

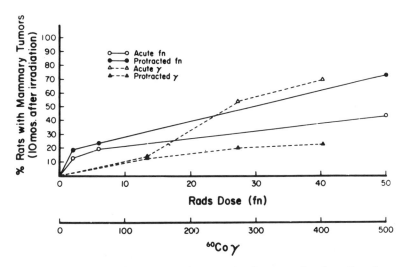

Fig. 13. Incidence of mammary tumors in Sprague Dawley female
rats 10 months after acute or protracted exposures to
fission neutrons (2,6 and 50 rad) or Cobalt-60 gamma-
rays (150, 300 and 450 R). Dose of Cobalt-60 gamma
rays on horizontal scale is 10x fission neutron dose (51).

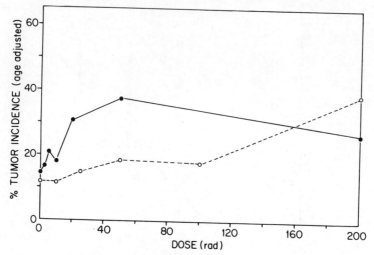

Fig. 14. Incidence of adenocarcinoma of the lung in
BALB/c female mice in relation to dose of
whole-body fission neutron (●) or gamma (o)
radiation received in a single brief exposure
(54).

Other Neoplasms

Dose-incidence data with high-LET radiation are available for a
variety of other neoplasms (6, 60). In general, the data are consistent
with the relationships cited above, which are illustrated schematically in
Figure 16. For certain neoplasms, however, (e.g., ovarian tumors in the
mouse), different patterns are observed, implying differences in the
relevant mechanisms of tumorigenesis (61). In this connection, it is
noteworthy that the induction of ovarian tumors in the mouse is attributed
to sterilization of the ovaries (6), and that RBE of neutrons for the
killing of mouse oocytes is low, implicating cytocidal effects on the
plasma membrane of these cells (63).

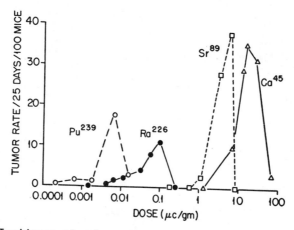

Fig. 15. Incidence of osteosarcoma in mice in relation to dose of
radionuclide injected (57).

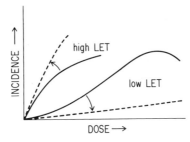

Fig. 16. Schematic dose-response curves for
incidence of tumors in relation to dose
and dose rate of high-LET and low-LET
radiation. (Solid line) High dose
rate; (broken line) low dose rate.

Factors Affecting Susceptibility to Radiation Carcinogenesis

Genetic Background   Although susceptibility to radiation carcinogenesis is shared by all species of mammals studied to date, susceptibility
to the induction of any particular neoplasm varies widely among different
species and strains (6). A striking example is the unusually high sensitivity of the ovary to tumor induction in the mouse. For example, a dose
of 100 rads suffices to induce ovarian tumors in nearly half of the females
in mice of susceptible strains (6, 63) while such tumors are rarely induced
in animals of other species.

In human beings, inherited differences in susceptibility are exemplified in the dramatically increased sensitivity of individuals with retinoblastoma, nevoid basal cell carcinoma syndrome, or certain other hereditary
diseases (64). It is possible that susceptibility may be increased to a
lesser degree in heterozygous carriers of these traits and in heterozygous
carriers of genes for DNA repair defects (65, 66).

The carcinogenic effects of radiation on human populations in
different parts of the world, compared on the basis of the numbers of cases
per 10^6 person years at risk per unit dose, imply that susceptibility
differs little among races or ethnic groups (7). This is not necessarily
true, however, if the different populations are compared on the basis of
relative risks (7).

Differences Among Organs, Tissues, and Cells   Within a given
individual, susceptibility to the carcinogenic effects of radiation varies
markedly among different organs, tissues, and cells. In contrast to
chemical carcinogenesis, where such differences may result from
pharmacokinetic variables, differences in the radiation dose to target
cells and molecules cannot explain the observed variations. Possible
explanations meriting further study include differences in the numbers of
stem cells at risk in different tissues, differences in cell turnover
rates, and differences in repair and renewal capabilities. Whatever the
explanation may be, susceptibility bears no constant relationship to the
baseline incidence of cancer in different organs (Table 2).

Within a given tissue or organ, moreover, not all types of cancer are
induced with equal frequency. For example, the incidence of chronic
lymphocytic leukemia, in contrast to all other types of leukemia, is not
detectably increased by irradiation in any population studied to date (6,
7). Similarly, the thyroid cancers induced by irradiation consist predominantly of well differentiated papillary and follicular adenocarcinomas,
with few tumors of anaplastic types (6, 7).

Table 2. Variation Among Different Human Tissues in Sensitivity to Radiation Carcinogenesis[a]

Site or Type of Cancer	Spontaneous Incidence[b] (per 10^6 yr) male	female	Estimated Radiation Induced Incidence (Excess Cases per 10^6 per yr per rem)
Breast (female)	---	900	
Lung, bronchus	690	230	
Colon	310	340	(> 1)
Stomach	120	70	
Leukemia	80[c]	60[c]	
Thyroid gland	20	60	
Urinary tract	310	130	
Pancreas	105	90	
Lymphoma, multiple myeloma	170	150	
Liver, biliary tract	50	50	
Brain, central nervous system	60	40	(0.1 - 1)
Esophagus	50	20	
Pharynx	15	5	
Salivary glands	10	10	
Skin	>1000	<1000	
Uterus and cervix	---	440	
Ovary	---	140	
Parathyroid gland	<5	<5	
Bone	10	5	(0.01 - 0.1)
Cranial sinuses	<5	<5	
Larynx	80	15	
Mesothelium	<5	<5	
Connective tissue, including heart	35	15	uncertain
Testis	35	---	
Prostate	560	---	
Other	120	120	

[a] From 6, 7, 17
[b] Values represent rounded averages for all ages and races
[c] Excluding lymphatic leukemia

Sex   The susceptibility of endocrine glands and their target organs to radiation carcinogenesis differs between males and females, in keeping with differences in the corresponding baseline tumor rates. Experimental data imply that the differences are attributable primarily to the promoting effects of hormones (67), although unexplained sex differences also exist in the susceptibility of nonendocrine organs to carcinogenesis (6, 7).

Age at Exposure   Susceptibility to the carcinogenic effects of radiation varies markedly with age at the time of irradiation, depending on the neoplasm in question (6, 7). In humans, the relative risk of leukemia is increased more markedly by irradiation before birth than by irradiation later in life (6, 7). The types of leukemia that are induced, however, are also age-dependent; those induced by prenatal irradiation are predominantly acute agranulocytic and stem cell leukemias, whereas those induced by exposure later in life include comparable numbers of acute and chronic granulocytic leukemias (6, 7). With increasing age at irradiation during adult life, the relative risk of all types of leukemia combined remains essentially constant, while the absolute risk increases with age at irradiation (7) (Figure 17).

For cancer of the female breast, susceptibility is higher during adolescence and early adult life than at later ages (7). It is also noteworthy that women irradiated during infancy do not develop radiation-induced breast tumors until they reach the fourth decade, with the result that the susceptibility of this age group has been underestimated heretofore (67, 68). The data imply that carcinogenesis in the breast is initiated by irradiation but that completion of the process depends on promoting effects associated with age-related hormonal stimulation.

SUMMARY

Ionizing radiation is carcinogenic for many, if not most, tissues; however, its carcinogenicity varies, depending on the tissue exposed, conditions of exposure, genetic background, sex, and age of the exposed individual, and other factors. The neoplasms induced by radiation also vary in their types and in their times of onset, depending on the age and sex of the exposed individual. The dose-incidence curve with high-LET radiation characteristically rises more steeply in the low-to-intermediate dose range than the curve with low-LET radiation. The curve with high-LET radiation is also characteristically linear or convex upward in this dose range, whereas the curve with low-LET radiation in the same dose range is characteristically concave upward. With fractionation or protraction of irradiation, the curve with high-LET radiation characteristically remains unchanged or increases in slope, whereas the curve with low-LET radiation characteristically decreases in slope. As a result of these relationships, the RBE of high-LET radiation for carcinogenic effects characteristically increases with decreasing dose and dose rate.

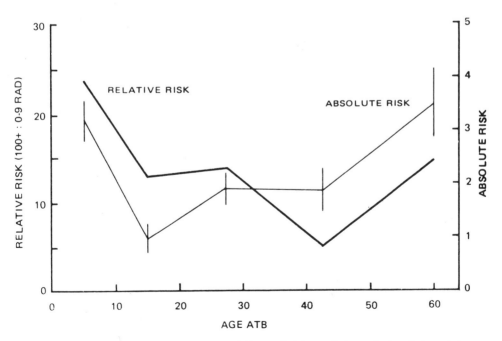

Fig. 17. Estimates of age-specific relative risk and absolute risk (excess deaths per million person-year-rad, with 90% confidence intervals) of leukemia in heavily irradiated a-bomb survivors (45).

ACKNOWLEDGEMENT

The author is grateful to Ms. Kammy Lou Griffin and Ms. Lynda Witte for assistance in the preparation of the manuscript.

REFERENCES

1. International Commission on Radiological Protection, International Commission on Radiological Units, Report of the Committee on RBE, Health Physics 9:357-386 (1963).

2. D. E. Lea, "Actions of Radiation on Living Cells," The MacMillan Co., New York (1947).

3. T. C. Evans, The influence of quantity and quality of radiation on the biologic effect, in: "Symposium on Radiobiology," J. J. Nickson, ed., John Wiley & Sons, Inc., New York (1952), pp. 393-413.

4. R. E. Zirkle, The radiobiological importance of linear energy transfer, in: "Radiation Biology," A. Hollaender, ed., McGraw-Hill, New York (1954), pp. 315-350.

5. International Commission on Radiological Protection, "The RBE of High-LET Radiation with Respect to Mutagenesis," ICRP Publication 18, Pergamon Press, Oxford, England (1972).

6. United Nations Scientific Committee on the Effects of Atomic Radiation, "Sources and Effects of Ionizing Radiation," Publication E.77.IX.1, United Nations, New York (1977).

7. National Academy of Sciences, Advisory Committee on the Biological Effects of Ionizing Radiation, "The Effects on Populations of Exposure to Low Levels of Ionizing Radiation," National Academy Press, Washington, D.C. (1980).

8. A. M. Kellerer and H. H. Rossi, The theory of dual radiation action, Curr. Top. Radiat. Res. Quarterly 8:85-158 (1972).

9. J. A. Dennis, Neutron carcinogenesis and radiological protections: a historical perspective, in: "Neutron Carcinogenesis," J. J. Broerse and G. B. Gerber, ed., Commission of European Communities, Luxembourg (1982), pp. 3-30.

10. D. C. Lloyd and R. J. Purrott, Chromosome aberration analysis in radiological protection dosimetry, Radiat. Protect. Dosimetry 1:19-28 (1981).

11. A. A. Edwards and Lloyd, D. C., Private communication (1984).

12. B. MacMahon, Prenatal X-ray exposure and childhood cancer, J. Natl. Cancer Inst. 28:1178-1191 (1962).

13. R. R. Monson and B. MacMahon, Prenatal X-ray exposure and cancer in children, in: "Radiation Carcinogenesis: Epidemiology and Biological Significance," J. D. Boice, Jr. and J. F. Fraumeni, Jr., Raven Press, New York (1984), pp. 97-105.

14. M. Ichimaru and T. Ishimaru, A review of thirty years study of Hiroshima and Nagasaki atomic bomb survivors. II. Biological effects. D. leukemia and related disorders, J. Radiat. Res. 16(Suppl.):89-96 (1975).

15. T. Wakabayashi, H. Kato, T. Ideda, and W. J. Schull. Studies of the mortality of a-bomb survivors. Report 7. Part III. Incidence of cancer in 1959-1978, based on the tumor registry, Nagasaki, Radiat. Res. 93:112-146 (1983).

16. J. Waterhouse, C. Muir, P. Correa and J. Powell, eds., "Cancer Incidence in Five Continents," Vol. III, IARC Publications No. 15, IARC, Lyon, France (1976).

17. A. C. Upton, The biological basis for assessing carcinogenic risks of low-level radiation, in: "The Role of Chemicals and Radiation in the Etiology of Cancer," E. Huberman, ed., Raven Press, New York, in press.

18. G. W. Beebe, A methodologic assessment of radiation epidemiology studies, Health Physics 46:745-762 (1984).

19. A. C. Upton, A. W. Kimball, J. Furth, K. W. Christenberry, and W. H. Benedict, Some delayed effects of atom-bomb radiation in mice, Cancer Res. 20(No. 8, Part 2):1-62 (1960).

20. R. E. Albert and B. Altshuler, Consideration relating to the formulation of limits for unavoidable population exposures to environmental carcinogens, in: "Radionuclide Carcinogenesis," C. L. Sanders, R. H. Busch, J. E. Ballou and D. D. Mahlum, eds., AEC Symposium Series, CONF-720505, NTIS, Springfield, VA (1973), pp. 233-253.

21. A. C. Upton, F. F. Wolff, J. Furth, and A. W. Kimball, A comparison of the induction of myeloid and lymphoid leukemias in x-radiation RF mice, Cancer Res. 18:842-848 (1958).

22. C. J. Shellabarger, V. P. Bond, E. P. Cronkite, and G. E. Aponte, Relationship of dose of total-body ^{60}Co radiation to incidence of mammary neoplasia in female rats, in: "Radiation-Induced Cancer," IAEA, Vienna (1969), pp. 161-172.

23. H. S. Kaplan and M. B. Brown, A quantitative dose response study of lymphoid tumor development in irradiated C57 Black mice, J. Natl. Cancer Inst. 13:185-208 (1952).

24. P. Maldague, Comparative study of experimentally induced cancer of the kidney in mice and rats with X-rays, in: Radiation Induced Cancer," IAEA, Vienna (1969), pp. 439-458.

25. F. Burns, R. E. Albert, and R. D. Heimbach, RBE for skin tumors and hair follicle damage in the rat following irradiation with alpha particles and electrons, Radiat. Res. 36:225-241 (1968).

26. P. Metalli, V. Covelli, M. DiPaola and G. Silini, Dose-incidence data for mouse reticulum cell sarcoma, Radit. Res. 59:21 (1974).

27. A. C. Upton, Biological aspects of radiation carcinogenesis, in: "Radiation Carcinogenesis, Epidemiology and Biological Significance," J. D. Boice, Jr. and J. F. Fraumeni, Jr., Raven Press, New York, (1984), pp. 9-19.

28. J. M. Brown, The shape of the dose-response curve for radiation carcinogenesis. Extrapolation to low doses, Radiat. Res. 71:34-50 (1977).

29. A. C. Upton, Radiobiological effects at low doses. Implications for radiological protection, Radiat. Res. 71:51-74 (1977).

30. T. Straume and R. L. Dobson, Implications of new Hiroshima and Nagaski dose estimates for cancer risks and RBE, Health Physics 41:666-671 (1981).

31. G. W. Barendsen, Fundamental aspects of cancer induction in relation to the effectiveness of small doses of radiation in: "Late Biological Effects of Ionizing Radiation," IAEA, Vienna (1981), pp. 263-275.

32. C. E. Land, J. D. Boice, Jr., R. E. Shore, J. E. Norman, and M. Tokunaga. Breast cancer risk from low-dose exposure to ionizing radiation: Results of parallel analysis of three exposed populations of women, J. Natl. Cancer Inst. 65:353-376 (1980).

33. C. E. Land and D. H. McGregor, Breast cancer incidence among atomic bomb survivors: implications for radiobiologic risk at low doses, J. Natl. Cancer Inst. 62:17-21 (1979).

34. R. E. Shore, L. Hemplemann, E. Kowaluk, P. Mansur, B. Pasternack, R. Albert, and G. Haughie, Breast neoplasms in women treated with X-rays for acute postpartum mastitis, J. Natl. Cancer Inst. 59:813-822 (1977).

35. J. D. Boice, Jr., M. Rosenstein, and E. D. Trout, Estimation of breast doses and breast cancer risk associated with repeated chest examinations of women with tuberculosis, Radiat. Res. 73:373-390 (1978).

36. K. F. Baverstock, D. Papworth, and J. Venmaro, Risks of radiation at low doses, Lancet 1:430-433 (1981).

37. J. D. Boice, Jr., C. E. Land, R. E. Shore, J. E. Norman, and M. Tokunaga, Risk of breast cancer following low-dose exposure, Radiology 131:589-597 (1979).

38. C. Land, Estimating cancer risk for low-doses of ionizing radiation, Science 209:1197-1210 (1980).

39. R. E. Shore, E. D. Woodward, and L. H. Hemplemann, Radiation-induced thyroid cancer, in: "Radiation Carcinogenesis: Epidemiology and Biological Significance," J. D. Boice, Jr. and J. F. Fraumeni, Jr., eds., Raven Press, New York (1984), pp. 131-138.

40. H. B. Newcombe and J. F. McGregor, Childhood cancer following obstetric radiography, Lancet 2:1151-1152 (1971).

41. National Council on Radiation Protection and Measurements, "Influence of Dose and Its Distribution in Time on Dose-Response Relationships for Low-LET Radiation," NCRP Report No. 64, Washington, D.C. (1980).

42. A. C. Upton, M. L. Randolph, and J. W. Conklin, Late effects of fast neutrons and gamma-rays in mice as influenced by the dose rate of irradiation: induction of neoplasia, Radiat. Res. 41:467-491 (1970).

43. J. R. Thomson, F. S. Williamson, D. Graham, and J. E. Ainsworth. Life shortening in mice exposed to fission neutrons and γ rays. I. Single and short-term fractionated exposures, Radiat. Res. 86:573-579 (1981).

44. Walburg, H. E., Radiation-induced life-shortening and premature aging, Adv. Radiat. Biol. 7:145-179 (1975).

45. G. W. Beebe, H. Kato, and C. E. Land, Studies of the mortality of a-bomb survivors. VI. Mortality and radiation dose, 1950-1974, Radiat. Res. 75:138-201 (1978).

46. United Nations Scientific Committee on the Effects of Atomic Radiation (UNSCEAR), "Ionizing Radiation: Sources and Biological Effects," Report to the General Assembly, with Annexes, United Nations, New York (1982).

47. J. F. Thomson, L. S. Lombard, D. Grahn, F. S. Williamson, and T. F. Fritz, RBE of fission neutrons for life shortening and tumorigenesis, in: "Neutron Carcinogenesis," J. J. Broerse and G. B. Gerber, eds., Commission of the European Communities, Luxembourg (1982), pp. 75-94.

48. R. H. Mole and J. A. G. Davids, Induction of myeloid leukaemia and other tumours in mice by irradiation with fission neutrons, in: "Neutron Carcinogenesis," J. J. Broerse and G. B. Gerber, eds, Commission of the European Communities, Luxembourg (1982), pp. 31-42.

49. C. J. Shellabarger, J. P. Stone, and S. Holtzman, Mammary carcinogenesis in rats: basic facts and recent results in Brookhaven, in: "Neutron Carcinogenesis," J. J. Broerse and G. B. Gerber, eds., Commission of the European Communities, Luxembourg (1982), pp. 99-116.

50. J. J. Broerse, L. A. Hennen, M. J. van Zwieten, and C. F. Hollander, Dose-effect relations for mammary carcinogenesis in different rat strains after irradiation with X rays and monoenergetic neutrons, in: "Proceedings of a Symposium on Biological Effects of Low-Level Irradiation, IAEA, Vienna (1983), pp. 507-519.

51. H. H. Vogel and H. W. Dickson, Mammary neoplasia in Sprague Dawley rats following acute and protracted irradiation, in: Neutron Carcinogenesis," J. J. Broerse and G. B. Gerber, eds., Commission of the European Communities, Luxembourg (1982), pp. 135-154.

52. C. J. Shellabarger, R. D. Brown, A. R. Rae, J. P. Shanley, V. P. Bond, A. M. Kellerer, H. H. Rossi, L. J. Goodman, and R. E. Mills, Rat mammary carcinogenesis following neutron or x-radiation, in: "Proceedings of a Symposium on Biological Effects of Neutron Irradiation," IAEA, Vienna (1974), pp. 391-401.

53. H. H. Vogel, High LET irradiation of Sprague-Dawley female rats and mammary neoplasm induction, in: Proceedings of a Symposium on Late Biological Effects of Ionizing Radiation, Vol. II," IAEA, Vienna (1978), pp. 147-164.

54. R. L. Ullrich, Lung tumor induction in mice: neutron RBE at low doses, in: "Neutron Carcinogenesis," J. J. Broerse and G. B. Gerber, eds., Commission of the European Communities, Luxembourg (1982), pp. 43-56.

55. W. J. Bair, B. B. Boecker, H. Cottier, P. E. Morrow, J. C. Nenot, J. F. Park, J. M. Thomas, and R. G. Thomas, "Annals of the ICRP: Biological Effects of Inhaled Radionuclides," Pergamon Press, Oxford, England (1980).

56. C. W. Mays, Discussion of plutonium toxicity, in: "National Energy Issues, How Do We Decide? Plutonium as a Test Case. A Sympoisum of the American Academy of Arts and Sciences," R. G. Sachs, ed., Ballinger Publishing Company, Cambridge, MA (1980), pp. 127-141.

57. M. P. Finkel, Relative biological effectiveness of internal emitters, Radiology 67:665-672 (1956).

58. H. Spiess and C. W. Mays, Protraction effects on bone sarcoma induction of ^{224}Ra in children and adults, in: "Radionuclide Carcinogenesis," C. L. Sanders, R. H. Busch, J. E. Ballou, and D. D. Mahlum, eds., AEC Symposium Series, CONF-720505, NTIS, Springfield, VA (1973), pp. 437-450.

59. J. M. Marshall and P. G. Groer. A theory of the induction of bone cancer by alpha radiation, Radiat. Res. 71:149-192 (1977).

60. R. J. M. Fry, P. Powers-Risius, E. L. Alpen, E. J. Ainsworth, and R. L. Ullrich, High-LET radiation carcinogenesis, Adv. Space Res. 3:241-248 (1983).

61. R. L. Ullrich, Tumor induction in BALB/c mice after fractionated or protracted exposures to fission-spectrum neutrons, Radiat. Res. 97:587-597 (1984).

62. T. Straume and R. L. Dobson, Neutron RBE for mouse oocyte killing, Radiat. Res. 94:644-645 (1983).

63. A. C. Upton, The dose-response relation in radiation induced cancer, Cancer Res. 21:717-729 (1961).

64. L. C. Strong, Theories of pathogenesis: mutation and cancer, in: "Genetics of Human Cancer," J. J. Mulvihill, R. W. Miller, and J. F. Fraumeni, Jr., Raven Press, New York (1977), pp. 404-414.

65. A. G. Knudson, Genetics and cancer, in: "Cancer: Achievements, Challenges, and Prospects for the 1980's," J. H. Burchenal and H. F. Oettgen, eds., Grune & Stratton, New York (1981), pp. 381-396.

66. M. C. Paterson, Environmental carcinogenesis and imperfect repair of damaged DNA in Homo sapiens: causal relation revealed by rare disorders, in: "Carcinogenesis: Initiation and Mechanisms of Action," A. C. Griffin and C. R. Shaw, eds., Raven Press, New York (1978), pp. 251-276.

67. N. G. Hildreth, R. Shore, and L. Hempelmann, Risk of breast cancer among women receiving radiation treatment in infancy for thymic enlargement, Lancet 1:273 (1983).

68. M. Tokunaga, C. E. Land, T. Yamamoto, M. Asano, S. Tokuoka, H. Ezaki, I. Nishimori, and T. Fujikura, Breast cancer among atomic bomb survivors, in: "Radiation Carcinogenesis: Epidemiology and Biological Significance," J. D. Boice, Jr. and J. F. Fraumeni, Jr., eds., Raven Press, New York (1984), pp. 45-56.

ASSESSMENT OF THE LUNG CANCER RISK FROM RADIATION EXPOSURES DUE TO

AIRTIGHTENING OF DWELLINGS FOR ENERGY CONSERVATION

Werner Burkart

Health Physics Division, Abt. 81
Eidgenoessisches Institut fuer Reaktorforschung
CH-5303 Wuerenlingen, Switzerland

ABSTRACT

In parts of the Swiss Alps, the high radium content of crystalline
rock and soil may produce considerable indoor levels of radon in dwellings
with low air infiltration. Radon measurements in conventional single
family homes in such an area during the winter of 82/83 showed an
arithmetic mean average radon concentration in living quarters and cellars
of 307 Bq/m3 (8.3 pCi/l) and 1410 Bq/m3 (38.1 pCi/l), respectively.
Assuming an increase in the radon concentration of 80% due to air
tightening measures as inferred from a matched pair analysis of Swiss
dwellings, weatherstripping may produce an average increase in the radon
level in the living quarters of 245 Bq/m3 (6.6 pCi/l). Doses to the lung
over a lifetime in such buildings approach or even exceed the doses
encountered by some miner populations with clearly increased lung cancer
risk.

An estimate based on UNSCEAR 82 conversion factors yields an additional
exposure of 0.014 mSv (1.37 mrem) per kWh saved. This value converts to a
risk factor which is several orders of magnitude higher than those from
large scale energy production systems.

INTRODUCTION

Not only activities involved in the production and use of energy but
also modifications in the construction of dwellings implemented to reduce
energy consumption may pose substantial long term hazards to the general
public (1, 2). Airtightening tends to increase indoor pollutants present
in the indoor environment whereas foam insulation contributes a new
toxicant, i.e. formaldehyde. Similar to the risk per unit energy
delivered from an energy producing technology, the risk to human health per
unit energy saved can be estimated (3). In this paper, we try to estimate
the additional exposure of humans to the ionizing radiation from radon and
its short-lived progeny in the indoor air of energy efficient dwellings,
i.e., homes showing lower than average air exchange rates. Contrary to
former purely theoretical consideration (3), these assumptions are based
both on radon measurements in geological regions with high terrestrial

139

radiation and on differences in the indoor radon levels between new or retrofitted dwellings as compared to matched conventional controls (4). The second point is especially important since simultaneous measurements of radon concentration and air exchange rate in dwelling showed that the radon source strength, i.e., infiltration of gas from the soil, may vary in unpredictable ways with the level of airtightness of the home.

As is the case for most indoor pollutants, risk factors for lung cancer induction from radon exposure have to rely mostly on occupational exposures. However, the dose commitment over the human life span from radon and its progeny in the indoor air in high background areas approaches or even exceeds the values of miner populations showing significant increases in the incidence of malignant lung diseases. Although confounding factors like poor control of smoking habits and additional chemical toxicants in mine air do not permit a direct comparison of environmental and occupational exposure risks, both the quality of the radiation involved, i.e., alpha, and the results from occupational epidemiology (5) point to a linear dose effect relationship. Recently, direct epidemiological studies on populations breathing high indoor levels of radon suggest an increase in the lung cancer incidence with elevated environmental radon concentration in Maine and Sweden (6, 7). However, the methodology employed (geographical study) in the former and the small number of lung cancer cases in the latter do not yet allow to establish risk factors from environmental exposure to radon and its decay products.

MATERIALS AND METHODS

Measurements of radon with passive track etch dosimeters type Karlsruhe was described elsewhere (4). The system used cannot detect contributions from radon-220 (thoron). In most cases, three detectors per dwelling were used: one in the cellar (source strength), living room (generally on the ground floor) and a bedroom (mostly on the first floor). Measuring periods varied from 2 to 6 months but fell always into the heating period, i.e., time of lowest air exchange rates.

RESULTS

Indoor Radon Concentrations in the Crystalline Alps

The dwellings were situated in the South-Eastern parts of Switzerland where crystalline basement rock with relatively high uranium and thorium content reaches the surface. The high altitude of the valley floor (St. Moritz 1825 m above sea level) results in a cold climate with 4500 heating grade days (integration of temperature difference inside/outside over heating period) and average July temperature of only 11°C. Historically, trade and now tourism provide the economic basis for tens of thousands of permanent inhabitants at this altitude in Switzerland.

Figure 1 shows the radon concentrations (cellar, ground floor an first floor) in 32 single family homes in this area on a log/probability graph. As expected from the many parameters influencing radon source strength and emanation, the values fit a lognormal distribution fairly well. The geometric mean radon concentration for the living quarters, i.e., living room and bedroom amounts to 255 Bq/m3 (6.9 pCi/ℓ) and 176 Bq/m3 (4.8 pCi/ℓ), respectively. Table 1 shows the numerical values of concentrations and annual effective dose equivalents for the means as well as for the upper 10 and 1 percentiles. The dose commitments are calculated using UNSCEAR 82 conversion factors and a radon daughter equilibrium factor of 0.5 (8).

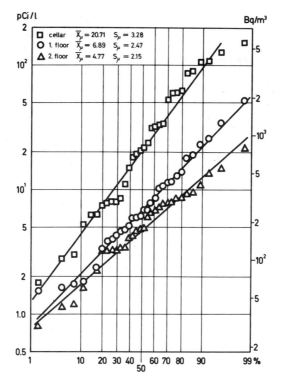

Fig. 1. Distribution of the time averaged indoor radon
concentrations during the winter of 1982/83 in a
sample of 32 single family houses situated in
three alpine valleys of Southeastern Switzerland.

Table 1. Mean values, upper 10 and 1 percentiles for indoor
radon concentrations and resulting annual
effective dose equivalents for a sample of 32
dwellings in the Southeastern Alps of Switzerland
(80% occupancy assumed)

	geometric mean	upper 10 percentile	up. 1 percentile
RADON CONCENTRATIONS in Bq/m3 (pCi/l)			
cellar	766 (20.7)	3'561 (96.2)	12'410 (335.4)
ground floor	255 (6.9)	826 (22.3)	2'091 (56.5)
first floor	176 (4.8)	468 (12.7)	1'030 (27.8)
ANNUAL DOSE IN mSv (mrem)			
living room (a)	7.5 (751)	24.3 (2'433)	61.6 (6'160)
bedroom (b)	5.2 (520)	13.8 (1'379)	30.3 (3'033)
(a + b)/2	6.4 (636)	19.1 (1'906)	46.0 (4'598)

141

The arithmetic mean and its standard deviation, which has to be used to assess the total dose from radon and its progeny to a population amounts to a value of 307 $\pm$ 43 Bq/m3 (8.3 pCi/ℓ) for the living quarters (living room and bedroom weighted each 50%).

An Estimate of Risk from Additional Exposure Due to Airtightening

The most cost-effective measure to achieve energy savings at unchanged temperature settings is to decrease the rate of air exchange. In stone and brick dwellings, this can be achieved by means of weatherstripping and caulking to close airways along windows, doors and blinds. Air exchange rates in occupied buildings are difficult to assess due to their dependence on a multitude of climatic and behavioral parameters. However, central heating and steep increases in the oil price led generally to a strong reduction of air exchange rates over the last decades (7). Since it can be assumed that the indoor radon concentration at an unchanged source term is inversely proportional to the air exchange rate, this energy conservation effort increases the risk from radon and its daughters considerably if the infiltration of the radon gas into the living area is not affected by the retrofitting. The calculation of the additional exposures due to an increase in radon levels resulting from airtightening is depicted in Table 2 for the alpine sample described before. Since exposures and risk should be related to the benefits, the result is compared with the amount of energy saved.

To assess the lung cancer risk from exposure to environmental levels of radon, several assumptions have to be made. Recently, international bodies such as OECD/NEA (10) and UNSCEAR (8) have given reference values for indoor breathing rate radon daughter equilibirium value, time spent indoors, etc. Here, the UNSCEAR 82 conversion factor from radon indoor concentration to annual effective dose equivalent of 29.5 μ Sv/a per Bq/m3 (109 mrem/a per pCi/ℓ) is used. In our calculation, it is inferred that exposure to radon leads to an elevated risk for 20 years (expression period) after a latent period. Using a linear dose-effect relation and a lung cancer risk factor derived from uranium miners of 2.4×10^{-5}/mSv or 6.5×10^{-6}/WLM-a (Figure 2; for a more detailed treatise, see 9, 10), the average exposure in dwellings from the study sample yields a risk of about 3.3×10^{-7} lung cancers per kWh saved due to airtightening. This value is several orders of magnitudes higher than the risk factors per kWh produced in power plants using coal, oil or uranium (3). For the upper 1 percentile, the risk per kWh saved amounts to 1.7×10^{-6} Figure 2 shows how the risk factors used compares to the lung cancer incidences from a multitude of miner populations exposed to a wide range of lung doses.

DISCUSSION

In areas with high radon emanation into buildings, elevated radon concentrations due to the lowering of air exchange rates may lead to annual effective dose equivalents in the range of the limits for occupational exposure or even surpass them. The concomitant risk for lung cancer from a lifetime exposure is estimated for the energy efficient home in Table 2 as follows: a fifty year exposure at 16 mSv/a with a lung cancer risk factor of 2.4×10^{-5} per mSv (total risk over 20 year expression period) yields a 2% chance of dying from lung cancer in a high risk area. This value approaches the risk from heavy smoking. It is often assumed that linear extrapolation to the doses involved may overestimate the effects. In the case of radon and its daughters, however, the high linear energy transfer of the alpha radiation involved and the amount of radiation delivered to the critical tissue, which cannot be considered low at environmental exposure levels, speak against beneficial threshold effects. In some

Table 2. Parameters assumed for the calculation of radon
exposure due to energy conservation by
airtightening (mSv per kWh saved)

Four person-family with 100 m2 of fully heated
living quarters leading to 260 m3 indoor air
volume or 65 m3/person; 4'500 degree-heating days;
225 day heating period/a

	conventional house	airtight house
air exchange rate (h-1)	0.5	0.278
reduced by a factor of	1.8 (4)	
radon indoor concentration Bq/m3(pCi/1)	307 (8.3)	552 (14.9)
radon daughter equilibrium factor	0.5	
time spent indoors	80 %	
effective dose equivalent mSv/a*	9.05	16.29
ADDITIONAL EXPOSURE mSv/a (mrem/a)	7.24 (724)	(1)
air to be warmed up (in 1000 m3/heating period-person)	175.5	97.5
energy needed (in kWh) **	1'181	656
ENERGY SAVED/PERSON-a kWh	525	(2)
EXPOSURE PER kWh SAVED mSv (mrem) (1)/(2)	0.014 (1.38)	

* UNSCEAR82 (8)   ** specific heat of air: 1.005 kJ/kg-°C
density of air: 1.205 kg/m3

dwellings built on ground with elevated radium levels, the lifetime
exposure is in the same range as for some groups of uranium miners having
well-documented risks for lung neoplasms (11).

In addition to radon, other indoor pollutants such as formaldehyde,
cigarette smoke, humidity or allergens may reach critical levels in
buildings with low air exchange rates. The lack of human epidemiological
data prevents the quantification of the long term risks involved. Contrary
to the radon case, however, the indoor concentration levels as compared to
occupational environments are generally low and adjustments to reduce the
source strength are feasible. Therefore, radon has to be considered the
critical indoor toxicant in many cases (13).

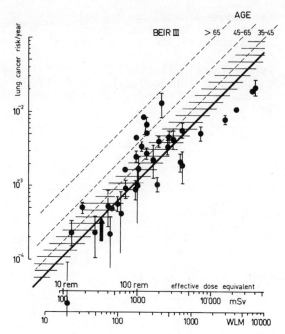

Fig. 2. Risk factors for radon induced lung cancer: each
point denotes a population of miners from the
U.S., Canada, Sweden, United Kingdom or
Czechoslovakia (5)

——————— BEIR I   (1972) 6.5 x 10^{-6}/WLM-a (as used in this
paper)
— — — — BEIR III   (1980) age dependent, up to 50 x 10^{-6}/WLM-a
≡≡≡≡≡   ICRP 32   (1982) 5 - 15 x 10-6/WLM-a (30 year expression
period assumed) (12)
Dose received over 30 years in an indoor environment with
a Rn level of 370 Bq/m3 (10 pCi/1) (based on USCEAR 82
assumptions for breathing rate, lung deposition pattern,
time spent indoors, equilibrium factor)

REFERENCES

1. R. Evans, J. H. Harley, W. Jacobi, A. S. McLean, W. A. Mills, and
C. G. Stewart, Estimate of risk from environmental exposure to
radon-222 and its decay products, Nature 290:98-100 (1981).

2. W. Burkart, Assessment of radiation dose and effects from radon and
its progeny in energy-efficient homes, Nuclear Techn. 60:114-123
(1983).

3. W. Burkart, and S. Chakraborty, Energy conservation: increased
health impact despite source reduction?, in: Comparisons of
Risks Resulting from Major Human Activities, Avignon: SFRP
(1982), pp. 541-548.

4. W. Burkart, C. Wernli, and H. H. Brunner, Matched pair analysis of
the influence of weatherstripping on radon concentration Swiss
dwellings, Rad. Prot. Dos. 7:299-302 (1984).

5. A. F. Cohen, and B. L. Cohen, Tests of the linearity assumption in the dose-effect relationship for radiation induced cancer, Health Phys. 38:53-65 (1980).

6. C. T. Hess, C. W. Weiffenbach, and S. A. Norton, Environmental radon and cancer correlation in Maine, Health Phys. 45:339-348 (1983).

7. O. Axelson, Lung cancer and radon in dwellings, Lancet 2(8253):995-996 (1981).

8. UNSCEAR 82, "Ionizing Radiation: Sources and Biological Effects," Report of the UN Scientific Committee on the Effects of Atomic Radiation, New York (1982).

9. BEIR III-Report, "The Effects on Populations of Exposure to Low Levels of Ionizing Radiation," NRC, Washington (1980), pp. 372-397.

10. OECD/NEA "Dosimetry Aspects of Exposure to Radon and Thoron Daughter Products," NEA Experts Report, Paris (1983).

11. E. Stranden, Radon in dwellings and lung cancer: a discussion, Health Phys. 38:301-306 (1980).

12. ICRP Publication 32, "Limits for Inhalation of Radon Daughters by Workers," Pergamon Press, Oxford (1981).

13. H. Inhaber, Comparative risk of indoor air quality, in: "Indoor Air, Vol. 1, Recent Advances in the Health Sciences and Technology," B. Berglund, T. Lindvall, and J. Sundell, eds., Liber Tryck AB, Stockholm (1984).

CARCINOGENIC EFFECTS OF INHALED RADIONUCLIDES

R. O. McClellan, B. B. Boecker, F. F. Hahn,
B. A. Muggenburg and R. G. Cuddihy

Lovelace Inhalation Toxicology Research Institute
P.O. Box 5890
Albuquerque, NM 87185

ABSTRACT

During the last two decades, a series of studies have been conducted at this Institute to examine the carcinogenic effects of inhaled radionuclides. A number of studies have been conducted with Beagle dogs exposed briefly to aerosols of β-emitters (^{90}Y, ^{91}Y, ^{144}CE and ^{90}Sr) and α-emitters (^{238}Pu and ^{239}Pu) in particles having different in vivo solubilities. The exposure conditions have been varied to produce initial lung burdens ranging downward from those producing acute lethality to levels equivalent to maximum permissible lung burdens for man. Dependent upon the particle size, chemical element and solubility of the particles, the inhalation intakes have resulted in varying degrees of protracted radiation exposure of nasal cavity, lung, lung-associated lymph nodes, liver and skeleton. The animals have been observed for their life span and dose-related increases in cancer have been observed in the most heavily irradiated sites. Although some of the studies are still in progress, sufficient data is at hand to provide cancer risk estimators for a number of radiation exposure scenarios. Some exposed animals are still surviving and may provide material for studies that will aid in providing bridges between observations in molecular and cellular systems, whole animals and people.

INTRODUCTION

Cancer is the main long-term biological effect resulting from exposure to ionizing radiation. These exposures to radiation can result from natural or man-made sources that are either external to the body or deposited within the body. Internally-deposited radionuclides raise a number of questions relating to their dosimetry in different organs and the influence of various physicochemical and biological factors on the resulting dose-response relationships.

Protection of people from workplace and environmental radiation exposures requires adequate knowledge about dose-response relationships and all of the factors that can modify them. The first source of such information is from exposed human populations. Fortunately, there have only been a few groups of people exposed to sufficiently high levels of internally-deposited radionuclides to provide even rudimentary dose-response data. Therefore, for many exposure situations, our knowledge of expected dose-response relationships in people must be derived primarily from life-span studies in laboratory animals. Data from these studies complement and extend the sparse human data currently available. This makes it possible to predict dose-response relationships for many internal exposures such as inhaled fission products or plutonium dioxide for which no current human data exist.

Table 1 summarizes the lifetime risk of cancer in people from various external sources or internally-deposited radionuclides based on currently available data from exposed human populations. The six underlined values represent exposure situations for which human data are not available and, thus, risk estimators must be developed by extrapolation from non-human data. Each risk estimator is expressed as the number of cancers per 10^6 rad of absorbed α or β radiation in the specified organ. Expression of the risk in this manner assumes that a linear dose-response relationship holds over the entire region of interest.

LOVELACE STUDIES

At this Institute, a number of life-span studies are being conducted with Beagle dogs exposed by inhalation to radionuclides (1). One of the important products of such studies is a clear identification of the various organs at risk. As can be seen from Table 2, in vivo solubility plays a key role in determining the relative degree of risk incurred by different body organs from inhaled radionuclides. Relatively soluble fission products irradiate not only the lung, but also the liver, skeleton and nasal cavity. Conversely, radionuclides inhaled in a relatively insoluble form have a prolonged retention in the lung and associated lymph nodes and result primarily in damage to these tissues.

For $^{239}PuO_2$, which is quite insoluble in body fluids, the main organs at risk for long-term effects are also the lung and lung-associated lymph nodes. However, a substantially different mixture of organs at risk has been observed in animals that inhaled aerosols of $^{238}Pu_2$. Apparently, the higher specific activity of the ^{238}Pu compared to the ^{239}Pu produces fragmentation of the deposited particles. This, in turn, leads to substantially enhanced absorption and translocation to other organs, particularly the liver and skeleton.

Each of the studies shown in Table 2 has involved young adult (12 to 14 months old) Beagle dogs who received one brief nose-only inhalation exposure to the specified radionuclide and form. After exposure, periodic whole-body counts and collections of urine and feces were made to determine the patterns of deposition and retention. Parallel serial sacrifice studies were used to measure the changes in tissue distribution as a function of time after exposure. All exposed dogs received frequent clinical observations during their life span and a complete necropsy and histopathological examination at death.

Risk to Lung

Four beta emitters of varying physical half-life, ^{90}Y, ^{90}Sr, ^{91}Y or ^{144}Ce, were incorporated in the same matrix, fused aluminosilicate

Table 1. Cancer risk estimators based on current data from
human populations and laboratory animals (Lifetime
Cancer Cases per 10^6 rads)

Tissue or Organ	Type of Irradiation	Risk Estimator
Tracneobronchial region	Chronic α	1200
Lung	Acute γ and neutron	70
	Acute X ray	120
	Chronic β	<u>50</u>
	Chronic α	<u>1500</u>
Bone	Chronic α, volume seeker	27
	Chronic α, surface seeker	200
		<u>1200</u>
	Chronic β, volume seeker	<u>2-20</u>
Liver	Chronic α	300
	Chronic β	<u>30</u>
Nasal Cavity	Chronic β	<u>10-120</u>

Underlined values are extrapolated from dog data.

Table 2. Studies in dogs exposed by inhalation to beta-
emitting radionuclides

Radionuclide and Form	Nasal Cavity	Lung	TBLN	Liver	Skeleton
I. Soluble β-emitters					
^{137}CsCl	++	++	++	++	++
^{91}YCl$_3$	++	++		++	++
^{144}CeCl$_3$	++	++		+++	++
^{90}SrCl$_2$	++				+++
II. Insoluble β-emitters					
^{90}Y FAP*	+	++	+	+	+
^{91}Y FAP	+	+++	++	+	+
^{144}Ce FAP	+	+++	+++	+	+
^{90}Sr FAP	+	+++	+++	+	+
III. Insoluble α emitters					
^{239}PuO$_2$	+	+++	+++	+	+
^{238}PuO$_2$	+	++	++	+++	+++

*Fused aluminosilicate particles

particles resulting in β-irradiation of the lung that decreased with
effective half-times from a few days to hundreds of days (2). Thus, the
total period over which the lung was irradiated ranged from about two weeks
to around five years.

Two isotopes of plutonium, ^{238}PuO$_2$ and ^{239}PuO$_2$, with different
specific activities were studied (3). During the first ~100 days after
inhalation exposure, similar pulmonary retention occurred for both
isotopes. Beyond this time, the ^{238}Pu left the lung much more rapidly than
did the ^{239}Pu. This resulted in a lung burden of ^{238}Pu that was between

$$\begin{array}{ll} \text{ANNUAL RISK} \\ \text{FACTOR} \\ \text{(RF annual)} \end{array} = \frac{\text{NUMBER OF LUNG TUMORS OBSERVED IN DOGS DYING DURING THE YEAR}}{\begin{array}{l}\text{TOTAL RADIATION DOSES TO THE} \\ \text{LUNG OF ALL DOGS ALIVE} \\ \text{IN THE EXPOSURE GROUP AT} \\ \text{START OF THE YEAR}\end{array}}$$

$$\begin{array}{l} \text{CUMULATIVE} \\ \text{RISK} \\ \text{FACTOR} \end{array} = \sum \left(\text{RF annual} \times \frac{\begin{array}{l}\text{NUMBER OF DOGS SURVIVING} \\ \text{TO START OF YEAR}\end{array}}{\begin{array}{l}\text{TOTAL NUMBER OF} \\ \text{DOGS IN GROUP}\end{array}} \right)$$

Fig. 1.   Computational process for determining annual and cumulative risks of lung cancer in dogs that inhaled beta- or alpha-emitting radionuclides.

one and two orders of magnitude lower than the corresponding lung burden of ^{239}Pu by 1000 days after the inhalation exposure.

Hahn et al. (4) and Cuddihy (5) developed risk factors for lung cancer using data from these studies as illustrated in Figure 1. First, the annual tumor risk factor was calculated by dividing the number of lung tumors observed in all exposed dogs dying in a given year minus the number expected in unexposed dogs by the total absorbed alpha or beta dose to lung for all dogs alive at the start of that year. The cumulative risk factor was then obtained by summing the individual risk factors and adjusting this sum by the fractional survival at the beginning of the year.

All primary lung tumors in dogs dying within a given year were counted regardless of cause of death. Tumors were classified into two general categories, carcinoma and sarcoma. Tumors of different tissue types were counted even though they were found in the same dog, they probably arise independently. Thus, the risk calculated is for a tumor occurring, not the risk of a cancer death. Multiple tumors of the same tissue type in one dog were counted as one tumor.

Cumulative risk factors obtained by this process are shown in Figure 2. Since dogs are still alive in all of these studies, the final cumulative risk factors will change somewhat from those shown. These results illustrate a difference in risk for different insoluble beta emitters depending on the pattern of dose prolongation. The shorter total periods of irradiation produced by ^{90}Y or ^{91}Y seem to be more effective in lung cancer production than the more prolonged irradiation periods from ^{90}Sr or ^{144}Ce. The difference in relative biological effectiveness of alpha emitters versus beta emitters is also evident in Figure 2.

Liver Risk

A similar computational approach was made to determine the risk of liver cancer from internally-deposited beta emitters (6). To date, two of the studies with relatively soluble forms of fission products, ^{144}CeCl$_3$ and ^{137}CsCl, have yielded hepatic tumors that can be used for this purpose. In the study involving inhaled ^{144}CeCl$_3$, 10 hepatic cancers were seen in 41 exposed dogs. The calculated cumulative risk of liver cancer was 84 cancer per 10^6 rad. In the study using intravenously injected ^{137}CsCl, 4 liver

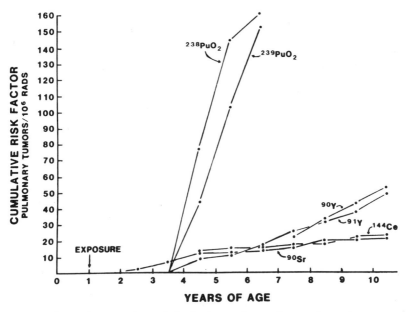

Fig. 2.   Cumulative risk factors for primary lung tumor
           groups of dogs exposed by inhalation to aerosols
           of alpha- or beta-emitting radionuclides.

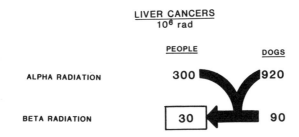

Fig. 3.   Relationship of risk estimates used to estimate
           the risk of liver cancer in people from inhaled
           beta emitters.

cancers were seen in 38 exposed dogs. The resulting cumulative risk of
liver cancer was 99 cancers per 10^6 rads.

    How can one extrapolate these data to possible human exposures? The
strategy we have used is illustrated in Figure 3. The desired unknown
value is the risk of liver cancer from alpha emitters as derived from the
data for people injected with Thorotrast is 300 cancers per 10^6 rad. The
risk of liver cancer from alpha emitters in dogs was estimated from
preliminary data on liver cancers from injected alpha emitters in Beagles
at the University of Utah's Radiobiology Laboratory (8). With our
computational approach, the Utah data yielded a risk of liver cancer in the
dog of 920 cancers per 10^6 rad of absorbed beta dose.

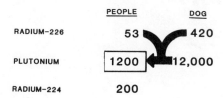

BONE CANCERS
10^6 rad

Fig. 4.   Relationship of risk factors used to estimated the
risk of bone cancer in people from inhaled
plutonium.

The average value for the two studies with beta emitters in dogs was 90
cancers per 10^6 rad. In Figure 3, it can be seen that all of these data
together give a preliminary indication that the dog is ~ 3 times more
radiosensitive in regard to liver cancer than people and that alpha
emitters are about 10 times more effective per rad in producing liver
cancer than are beta emitters. Combining all these factors yields an
estimated risk of liver cancer in people of 30 cancers per 10^6 rad of
absorbed beta dose.

Bone Dose

A similar approach was used to calculate the risk of bone cancer from
inhaled plutonium (3). The flow diagram for this computation is shown in
Figure 4. In this case, the data for internally-deposited ^{226}Ra in people
and Beagles were used as the key link between dog exposures and human
exposures. The human data for ^{226}Ra are derived from the radium dial
painters and chemists while the dog data come from studies at the
University of Utah. The data for bone cancers from plutonium in the dog
come from both studies of injected ^{239}Pu citrate at the University of Utah
and inhaled ^{238}PuO$_2$ at the Lovelace Inhalation Toxicology Research
Institute.

When the relationships among these factors are considered, the
estimated risk of bone cancer from plutonium in people is 1200 cancers per
10^6 rad. An alternate estimate for plutonium-induced bone cancers can be
made by assuming a direct correspondence to the risk of the surface seeking
alpha emitter ^{224}Ra. In this case, the risk is 200 bone cancers per 10^6
rad absorbed alpha dose.

Nasal Cavity Risk

The studies with relatively soluble forms of beta emitters emphasized
another important region at risk within the respiratory tract, the nasal
cavity as reported by Boecker et al. (8). Sinonasal cancers were observed
in dogs in each of the four studies involving relatively soluble beta
emitters. The calculated cumulative risks ranged from 9 to 120 cancers per
10^6 rad of absorbed beta dose. It is of interest that the highest risk
occurred for intravenously injected ^{137}Cs, a radionuclide rather uniformly
distributed throughout the body.

SUMMARY

Table 1 presents our best current estimates of cancer risk estimators for different types of irradiation and organs at risk using both human and laboratory animal data. The key role that life-span studies in laboratory animals play in broadening our knowledge of these dose-response relationships is emphasized by the values underlined. These values, all derived from studies in the dog, fill in important gaps for which no human data are available.

In addition to providing the data necessary for appropriate radiation protection particles and evaluation of existing exposure cases, studies in larger-sized animals like the dog provide the opportunity to follow clinical progression of the induced disease. Also, these animals can provide abundant material for the subsequent study of isolated cells and macromolecules that may be of use in elucidating mechanisms of the carcinogenic process.

ACKNOWLEDGEMENTS

The authors gratefully acknowledge the participation of a large number of ITRI scientific and technical staff in the conduct and analysis of these studies. True teamwork of this kind is a key ingredient in studies of this magnitude and direction. Research performed under U. S. Department of Energy Contract No. DE-AC04-76EV01013. Research conducted in facilities fully accredited by the American Association for the Accreditation of Laboratory Animal Care.

REFERENCES

1. R. O. McClellan, B. B. Boecker, F. H. Hahn, and B. A. Muggenburg, "Lovelace ITRI studies on the toxicity of inhaled radionuclides in Beagle dogs," in "Life-span Radiation Effects Studies in Animals: What Can They Tell Us?", (R. C. Thompson and J. A. Mahaffey, eds.), CONF830951, pp. 7496, 1986.

2. F. F. Hahn, B. B. Boecker, R. G. Cuddihy, C. H. Hobbs, R. O. McClellan, and M. B. Snipes, Influence of radiation dose patterns on lung tumor incidence in dogs that inhaled beta emitters: a preliminary report, Radiat. Res. 96:505-517 (1983).

3. B. A. Muggenburg, J. A. Mewhinney, W. C. Griffith, F. F. Hahn, R. O. McClellan, B. B. Boecker, and B. R. Scott, Dose-response relationships for bone cancers from plutonium in dogs and people, Health Phys. 44:529-536 (1983).

4. F. F. Hahn, B. A. Muggenburg, B. B. Boecker, R. G. Cuddihy, W. C. Griffith, R. A. Guilmette, R. O. McClellan, and J. A. Mewhinney, "Insights into radionuclide-induced lung cancer in people from life span studies in Beagle dogs,"in: "Life-Span Radiation Effects Studies in Animals: What Can They Tell Us?", (R. C. Thompson and J. A. Mahaffey, eds.), CONF830951, pp. 521534, 1986

5. R. G. Cuddihy, Risks of radiation-induced lung cancer, in: "Critical Issues in Setting Radiation Dose Limits," NCRP Proceedings No. 3 (1983), pp. 133-152.

6. B. A. Muggenburg, B. B. Boecker, F. F. Hahn, and R. O. McClellan, "The risk of liver tumors in dogs and man from radioactive aerosols," in: "Life-Span Radiation Effects Studies in Animals: What Can They Tell Us?", (R. C. Thompson and J. A. Mahaffey, eds.), CONF830951, pp. 556563, 1986.

7. BEIR, "The Effects on Populations of Exposure to Low Levels of Ionizing Radiations," National Academy Press, Washington, DC (1980), pp. 372-384.

8. M. E. Wrenn, Research in Radiobiology, in: "Annual Report of Work in Progress in the Internal Irradiation Program," University of Utah, U.S. Department of Energy Report, COO-119-256 (1981).

9. B. B. Boecker, F. F. Hahn, R. G. Cuddihy, M. B. Snipes, and R. O. McClellan, "Is the Human Nasal Cavity at Risk from Inhaled Radionuclides?", in: "Life-Span Radiation Effects Studies in Animals: What Can They Tell Us?", (R. C. Thompson and J. A. Mahaffey, eds.), CONF83091, pp. 564577, 1986.

MECHANISMS OF RADIATION TRANSFORMATION

J. B. Little

Laboratory of Radiobiology
Harvard University School of Public Health
665 Huntington Avenue
Boston, MA 02115

The carcinogenic properties of ionizing radiation were evident within a few years of the discovery of X-rays by Roentgen, when skin cancer began developing in radiation ulcers amongst a number of early radiation workers. This phenomenon has since been confirmed in a number of cellular and animal models, in which it has been shown that radiation will induce cancer in most tissues of most mammalian species. Despite these observations, however, the molecular mechanisms for this effect remain obscure. In order to better elucidate the molecular and cellular events associated with the conversion of a normal cell to a malignant one, recent attention has focused on the induction of malignant transformation of mammalian cells in vitro (1, 2). Such studies have shown that the induction of transformation in vitro is a complex, multi-stage process (1, 3). They have also allowed the correlation of transformation with the induction and repair of specific molecular DNA damage (4), as well as with other cellular effects such as cytogenetic changes (4, 5), and single gene mutations (6, 7). In particular, they have facilitated the design of experiments to test the somatic mutation theory of carcinogenesis; that is, the hypothesis that the initial radiation induced lesion which initiates the process of carcinogenesis is a mutation in a structural gene. It should be remembered, however, that the conversion of a normal cell to one with malignant potential represents but a very early stage in the overall process of the induction of an invasive metastatic tumor in vivo.

Most studies of radiation transformation have been carried out either with primary Syrian hamster embryo cells, or with established lines of mouse embryo fibroblasts. The experiments described in this paper involve the latter system. Such established lines have the advantages of being initially derived from a single cell, of being relatively stable in culture and of possessing a highly density-inhibited, non-transformed phenotype. By the usual experimental protocol, the cells are seeded at low density and treated with the carcinogen. They are subsequently allowed to proliferate for 1-2 weeks until they reach confluence (density-inhibition of growth) and then allowed another 4 weeks in confluence for expression of the transformed foci. These foci of transformed cells are easily recognized and scored overlying the confluent monolayer of normal cells. As a transformation system, these cell lines have the disadvantage of being aneuploid and probably eternal, thus apparently representing cells that have already attained some of the phenotypic characteristics associated with transformation.

Such mouse cell lines may be transformed in a dose dependent manner by X-rays and ultraviolet light; cells isolated from transformed colonies will form tumors in syngeneic animals with high frequency (80-90%) (1). The frequency of transformation following low doses of radiation can be markedly enhanced by post-irradiation incubation of the cells with phorbol ester tumor promoters (8). Likewise, it may be suppressed by incubation with agents such as certain protease inhibitors (9) or retinoic acid derivatives (10) which have also been associated with the suppression of carcinogenesis in experimental animals. Thus, malignant transformation in vitro may be modulated by a number of factors known to influence the induction of cancer in vivo.

In earlier experiments (11), we examined the influence of initial cell density (number of cells at risk) on the yield of transformed foci. These experiments led to the rather unexpected observation that the ultimate yield of transformed foci was largely independent of the number of cells initially at risk over the range of approximately 1 to 300 viable cells. These data are shown as the X symbols in Figure 1. In these experiments, cells were seeded in sufficient numbers such that 1 to approximately 300 viable cells resulted in irradiated cultures allowing for the cloning efficiency of the cells and toxicity of the radiation exposure. Under certain circumstances, transformed foci occurred in a high percentage of cultures derived from a single viable irradiated cell (12); a similar result has been shown for exposure to methylcholanthrene (13, 14). This finding implies that the initial radiation induced event must be a high frequency one, occurring in a large proportion of irradiated cells. It should be noted that following irradiation the single viable cell

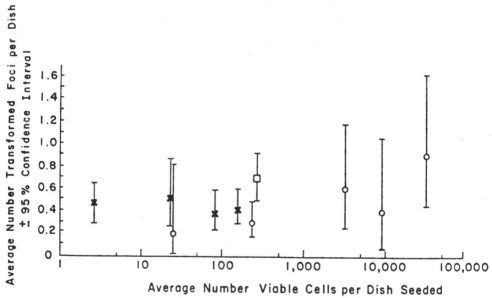

Fig. 1. Independence of yield of transformation in mouse C3H10T1/2 cells on the initial number of cells at risk. (X) - cells seeded at various densities, irradiated with 600 rads, and returned to incubator for 6 weeks to score development of transformed foci; (O) - cells seeded at 300 viable cells per dish, irradiated, allowed to proliferate to confluence, reseeded in new dishes at various dilutions, and returned to incubator for an additional 6 weeks; (□) - undisturbed cultures in dilution experiment. Reproduced from Kennedy et al. (11).

multiplies until a normal appearing confluent monolayer of cells results; transformed foci develop overlying this normal monolayer. Thus, this high frequency event appears to lead to a second low frequency event; that is, the transformation of one or more of the progeny of the irradiated cell. As there are approximately 2×10^6 cells in a culture at confluence, this second event occurs with the frequency of 10^{-6} or less.

This interpretation of the results was confirmed in a second type of experiment (11, 12). In these experiments, cells seeded at low density were irradiated, allowed to proliferate until confluent, and then resuspended and successively subcultured at dilutions of 1:10 to 1:10,000. The diluted cultures were allowed again to reach confluence, and then held for 4 weeks for the development of transformed foci. As is shown in Figure 1 (open circles), the number of transformed foci which developed per dish remained constant despite reseeded cell numbers varying over 4 order of magnitude and were similar to those observed in undisturbed plates. These results suggest that the second event occurred after or soon before confluence was initially reached.

A recent set of experiments was designed to determine more specifically when the proposed second event occurs (15). In these experiments, cells seeded at low density were irradiated and allowed to reach confluence. At this time they were suspended and reseeded in their entirety into one or two dishes. These dishes were returned to the incubator for 4 weeks, and the distribution of transformed foci within a large number of such dishes was determined. The results of a typical experiment are shown in Table 1. The distribution of foci amongst dishes in this experiment is consistent with random occurrence of the second transforming event during the growth of the irradiated cells to confluence. If this is the case, the distribution of foci should follow that calculated for the distribution of mutants under similar conditions by Lea and Coulson (16). As can be seen in Table 2, the experimental data conform very closely to the prediction. This was true of five separate large scale experiments of this type (15). As 75% of the total number of mitoses occurs during the two rounds of cell division prior to reaching confluence, most transforming events would take place just prior to confluence. However, occasional progeny may transform much earlier.

Table 1. Distribution of transformed clone sizes in mouse 10T1/2 cells 8 and 15 days after irradiation

Treatment Group	Number of Transformed Foci in Each Dish	Fraction of Dishes Containing Transformed Foci	Amoung Dishes Containing Foci Average Number of Foci per Dish ± S.E.	
1. 200 rads not reseeded	0,0,0,0,0,0,0,0,0,0,1,1,2	3/13=0.23	1.3	0.33
2. 200 rads reseeded at day 8	0,0,0,0,0,0,0,0,0,0,0,0,0,0, 0,0,0,0,0,0,0,0,0,0,0,1,1,2, 2,2,3,5,7,7,12,15,22	12/37=0.32	6.6	2.7
3. 200 rads reseeded at day 15	0,0,0,0,0,0,0,0,0,0,0,0,0,0,0, 0,0,0,0,0,0,0,0,0,1,1,1,1,1,1,1, 2,2,2,3,4,9,11,12,15,30,35	17/40=0.42	7.7	3.1

Table 2. Comparison of expected and observed distributions of clone sizes for the data presented in Table 2 (pooled results)[1]

	Numbers of Transformed Colonies in Reseeded Groups (r)[2]								
	0	1	2	3–4	5–8	9–16	17–32	33–64	64
Probability that a culture has r transformants (mutants) when the average number (m) of mutants (mutations) per culture is 0.5 (P(0)=0.62) (Lea and Coulson (16), Table 2)	.6065	.1516	.0695	.0648	.0475	.0288	.0155	.0079	.0079
In 77 Dishes Observed	48	8	6	3	3	6	2	1	0
			9				12		
			10.4				8.3		
Expected	46.7	11.7	5.4	5.0	3.7	2.2	1.2	.61	.61

[1] Data from Kennedy and Little (15).

[2] For the chi-square analysis, the categories were grouped as indicated such that no expected or observed numbers were less than 5; with 2 degrees of freedom, $\chi^2=3.3$, $p > 0.10$.

Several other types of experiments have also been performed in order to further study this phenomenon (15). In one series, 350–475 total viable cells were initially seeded representing an approximately 1:2 mixture of irradiated and non-irradiated cells. The resultant yield of transformants was directly proportional to the number of irradiated cells present in the mixture rather than to the total number of cells seeded. This result suggests that transformation occurs only amongst the progeny of irradiated cells, and speaks against the hypothesis that radiation may have activated a virus which spreads throughout the culture when the cells become confluent leading to a constant yield of transformants.

In other experiments, a constant number of irradiated cells were seeded into dishes of varying sizes ranging from 8 to 144 cm^2 in surface area. The yield of transformants was directly proportional to the surface area of the dish and therefore the number of progeny cells present at confluence, rather than to the initial number of irradiated cells. This further confirms the two event hypothesis. Finally, cells from mass cultures were removed at various times during a classical transformation experiment and examined for their ability to grow in soft agar under anchorage independent conditions. No soft agar colonies were observed during the first five days after irradiation, but the ability to produce such colonies occurred as the culture became confluent, and reached a maximum few days later. These results are consistent with a transformational event occurring near confluence as hypothesized above, at which time the ability to grow under anchorage independent conditions appears.

The observation that the initial event in malignant transformation in vitro appears to be a common one involving a large fraction of cells speaks against this event representing a mutation in a specific structural gene or group of genes. Experiments were therefore designed to yield information as to whether DNA damage was specifically involved in the initiation of transformation in vitro. To examination this question, transformation was studied in cells allowed to incorporate Iodine-125 in the form of the DNA precursor [125]IdUrd (17). Iodine-125 decays by electron capture with the release of a shower of very low energy Auger electrons. It has been estimated that approximately 100 electrons volts are deposited with a 10 Å sphere around the site of each disintegration, and that much of the energy deposited in DNA from incorporated [125]IdUrd occurs within a few base pairs of this site (18).   Thus, the radiation exposure from [125]IdUrd incorporated into DNA is not only restricted to the DNA itself but probably to very small regions of the DNA surrounding the site of the decays.

[125]IdUrd was found to be extremely efficient in inducing malignant transformation in vitro (17).   This result is shown graphically in Figure 2 in which the results are shown in comparison with those for [3H]-thymidine. The transformation frequency was enhanced 3-4 fold by doses of ^{125}I which yielded only approximately 20 total disintegrations within the entire genome of each cell. Such doses produced little or no measurable cytotoxicity. A similar frequency of transformation was produced by approximately 400 rads of X-rays; this dose killed approximately 70% of the cells. In separate studies (19), we found that each Iodine-125 disintegration in cellular DNA under frozen conditions led to approximately one DNA double strand break. We have also shown in other experiments (20) that Iodine-125 incorporated into DNA as [125]IdUrd is very efficient in inducing mutations to thioguanine resistance. On the basis of reasonable estimates of the size of the HPRT gene, we calculated that a single Iodine-125 disintegration anywhere within the gene will lead to a mutation (20).

When one considers a rare event such as the occurrence of a HPRT mutation in a population of cells, it is reasonable to expect that, amongst a population in which on the average only 20 DNA lesions are produced in each cell, one of these lesions will occasionally involve this specific gene and thus occasional mutants will arise. In the case of transformation, however, where the initial event appears to occur in a large fraction of the cell, the DNA target would have to be very large. Thus, the iodine-125 results suggest that while DNA damage is indeed involved in the initiation of transformation in vitro, this initial event is unlikely to represent a mutation in a specific structural gene or group of structural genes.

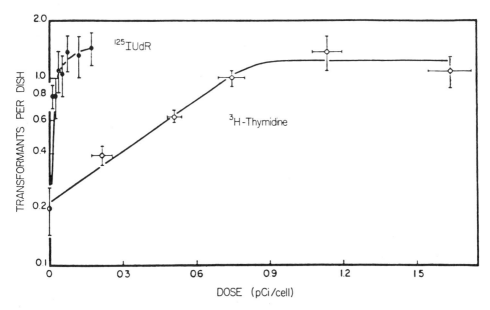

Fig. 2.   Oncogenic transformation induced in mouse BALB/3T3 cells by radionuclides incorporated into cellular DNA during a single S phase of synchronous growth (●) - [125]IdUrd; (○) - [3H]-Thymidine,   Reproduced from LeMotte et al. (17).

The results would suggest, rather, that the cells respond to non-specific DNA damage by the induction of a process which enhances the spontaneous transformation frequency. This second event acts like a mutational one in that it occurs with very low frequency and at random during the growth of the cells. It differs from the usual SOS process in that it cannot be driven by mutagen exposure; that is, exposure to known mutagens during the growth of irradiated cells to confluence does not enhance the frequency of transformation (A. R. Kennedy, unpublished observations). Modifiers of transformation such as tumor promoters or protease inhibitors appear to influence the probability of occurrence of this second event.

These observations and the hypotheses proposed to explain them are certainly unusual in terms of the classical view of mechanisms of transformation. The question arises as to whether they are peculiar to this particular cell system, or whether they might have more general application to radiation carcinogenesis. None of our current knowledge is inconsistent with such a mechanism. To the contrary, there is at least one piece of experimental evidence in vivo which supports such an interpretation. Terzaghi and Nettesheim (21) have shown that chemical carcinogen exposure of rat tracheal epithelium will lead to a low but measurable incidence of tracheal carcinoma. When the treated tracheas are excised, however, and epithelial cells from exposed regions are grown and passaged in culture, it can be shown that a large fraction of such cells are apparently initiated in that they can give rise to transformed progeny. This result suggests that, though only an occasional tumor may arise in a large population of carcinogen exposed cells in vivo, a large fraction of such cells may have carcinogenic potential if allowed to grow under the appropriate conditions. This potential is expressed in terms of the actual transformation of one of their progeny. The unusual characteristics associated with the transformation of mouse embryo fibroblast derived cell lines suggest that the process of radiation transformation is not easily amenable to simple mechanistic models.

REFERENCES

1. J. B. Little, Radiation carcinogenesis in vitro: implications for mechanisms, in: "Origins of Human Cancer, Vol. 4, Book A," H. H. Hiatt, J. D. Watson and J. A. Winston, eds., Cold Spring Harbor Lab., Cold Spring Harbor, New York (1977), pp. 923-939.

2. T. C. H. Yang and C. A. Tobias, Radiation and cell transformation in vitro, Adv. Biol. Med. Phys. 17:417-461 (1980).

3. J. C. Barrett and P. O. P. Ts'o, Evidence for the progressive nature of neoplastic transformation in vitro, Proc. Natl. Acad. Sci. USA 75:3761-3765 (1978).

4. H. Nagasawa, A. J. Fornace, Jr., M. A. Ritter, and J. B. Little, Relationship of enhanced survival during confluent holding recovery in ultraviolet-irradiated human and mouse cells to chromosome aberrations, sister chromatid exchanges, and DNA repair, Radiat. Res. 92:483-496 (1982).

5. A. J. Fornace, Jr., H. Nagasawa, and J. B. Little, Relationship of DNA repair to chromosome aberrations, sister chromatid exchanges and survival during liquid holding recovery in X-irradiated mammalian cells, Mutation Res. 70:323-336 (1980).

6. J. C. Barrett and P. O. P. Ts'o, Relationship between somatic mutation and neoplastic transformation, Proc. Natl. Acad. Sci. USA 75:3297-3301 (1978).

7. G. L. Chan and J. B. Little, Induction of ouabain resistant mutations in C3H 10T1/2 cells by ultraviolet light, Proc. Natl. Acad. Sci. USA 75:3363-3366 (1978).

8. A. R. Kennedy, S. Modal, C. Heidelberger, and J. B. Little, Enhancement of X-ray transformation by 12-0-tetradecanoyl-phorbol-13-acetate in a cloned line of C3H mouse embryo cells, Cancer Res. 38:439-443 (1978).

9. A. R. Kennedy and J. B. Little, Protease inhibitors suppress radiation induced malignant transformation in vitro, Nature 276:825-826 (1978).

10. L. Harisiadis, R. C. Miller, E. J. Hall, and C. Borek, A vitamin A analogue inhibits radiation-induced oncogenic transformation, Nature 274:486-487 (1978).

11. A. R. Kennedy, M. Fox, G. Murphy, and J. B. Little, Relationship between X-ray exposure and malignant transformation in C3H 10T1/2 cells, Proc. Natl. Acad. Sci. USA 77:7262-7266 (1980).

12. A. R. Kennedy and J. B. Little, Investigation of the mechanisms for enhancement of radiation transformation in vitro by 12-0-tetradecanoylphorbol-13-acetate, Carcinogenesis 1:1039-1047 (1980).

13. S. Modal and C. Heidelberger, In vitro malignant transformation by methylcholanthrene of the progeny of single cells derived from C3H mouse prostate, Proc. Natl. Acad. Sci. USA 65:219-255 (1970).

14. A. Fernandez, S. Mondal, and C. Heidelberger, Probabilistic view of the transformation of cultured C3H/10T1/2 mouse embryo fibroblasts by 3-methylcholanthrene, Proc. Natl. Acad. Sci. USA 77:7272-7276 (1980).

15. A. R. Kennedy and J. B. Little, Evidence indicating that the second step in X-ray induced transformation in vitro occurs during cellular proliferation, Radiat. Res. 99:228-248 (1984).

16. D. E. Lea and C. A. Coulson, The distribution of the numbers of mutants in bacterial populations, J. Genet. 49:264-285 (1949).

17. P. K. LeMotte, S. J. Adelstein, and J. B. Little, Malignant transformation induced by incorporation radionuclides in BALB/3T3 mouse embryo fibroblasts, Proc. Natl. Acad. Sci. USA 79:7763-7767 (1982).

18. R. F. Martin and W. A. Hazeltine, Range of radiochemical damage to DNA with decay of Iodine-125, <u>Science</u> 213:896-898 (1981).

19. P. K. LeMotte and J. B. Little, DNA damage induced in human diploid cells by decay of incorporated radionuclides, <u>Cancer</u> <u>Res</u>. 44:1337-1342 (1984).

20. H. L. Liber, P. K. LeMotte, and J. B. Little, Toxicity and mutagenicity of X-rays, [125]IdUrd or ^{3}H-TdR incorporated in the DNA of human lymphoblast cells, <u>Mutation</u> <u>Res</u>. 111:387-404 (1983).

21. M. Terzaghi and P. Nettesheim, Dynamics of neoplastic development in carcinogen exposed tracheal mucosa, <u>Cancer</u> <u>Res</u>. 39:4003-4010 (1979).

THE RADIOBIOLOGY OF <u>IN VITRO</u> NEOPLASTIC TRANSFORMATION

J. B. Little

Laboratory of Radiobiology
Department of Cancer Biology
Harvard School, Public Health
Boston, MA

INTRODUCTION

The carcinogenic properties of ionizing radiation became evident within a few years of the discovery of X-rays by Roentgen, when the development of cancer in radiation ulcerations of the skin was observed in a number of early radiation workers. This phenomenon has since been confirmed in many cellular and animal models, in which it has been shown that radiation will induce cancer in most tissues of most mammalian species. Despite these observations, however, the molecular mechanisms for this effect remain obscure.

There are four general characteristics which appear to be common to the process of radiation carcinogenesis. First, carcinogenesis requires time. The latent period from radiation exposure to the appearance of a recognizable tumor is variable but may take as long as 30 to 40 years in human beings. Some animal studies indicate that the duration of the latent period is related to radiation dose, but in all cases an absolute minimum latent period appears to exist. Second, the effect appears to be heritable; that is, the initial cellular changes that trigger carcinogenesis are transmitted to daughter cells. Indeed, many cell divisions may elapse between exposure to radiation and the development of recognizable malignant changes. Third, carcinogenesis requires a cell proliferation. In some cases, agents or treatments that stimulate cell proliferation appear to enhance the process. Fourth, carcinogenesis can be influenced by non-carcinogenic secondary factors. This phenomenon has been shown classically in two-stage carcinogenesis experiments in mouse skin. In this system, the incidence of skin papillomas produced by a small dose of a primary carcinogen can be greatly enhanced by subsequent repeated applications of croton oil. The phorbol esters, which are the active agents in croton oil, are not carcinogenic by themselves but have the ability to "promote" carcinogenesis induced by an "initiating" agent such as radiation or chemical carcinogens.

These observations led many years ago to the formulation of the somatic mutation theory for carcinogenesis; that is, a somatic mutation in a structural gene represents the initial heritable change in neoplastic cells. By its nature, this would be a rare event occurring in only occasional cells within a given tissue. This phenomenon thus appeared

163

consistent with the observations that cancer is a rare event in terms of the large number of cells present in any given tissue. This theory is given further support by two other observations. First, cytogenetic studies have provided evidence that many tumors appear to be descended from a single cell; that is, cancer represents the growth of a single family of abnormal cells. Second, DNA is clearly the critical cellular target in carcinogenesis. Radiation and most chemical carcinogens are mutagens which produce DNA damage and induce enzymatic DNA repair processes.

On the other hand, it must always be kept in mind that the process of carcinogenesis in vivo is a complex, multi-stage one. The long time period between exposure to the carcinogen and the appearance of a clinically recognizable cancer is associated with the step-wise evolution of cytologic and pathologic changes by which cells become progressively more anaplastic. Such changes are characteristic of neoplastic development and progression. Furthermore, the initial changes which accompany the conversion of a normal cell to a malignant cell are also complex.

It is largely within the past decade that suitable cell systems have been developed which allow the study of the conversion of normal mammalian cells in vitro to those which possess the characteristic phenotype of cancer cells. This process has been termed malignant or neoplastic transformation. During this process, potentially transformed cells undergo a constellation of morphologic and physiologic changes which differentiate them from normal cells. Transformed cells show prominent changes as regards the control of growth in vitro. These include the loss of density-dependent "contact" inhibition of growth, and the development of the ability to grow in suspension. The latter phenomenon is sometimes termed the loss of anchorage dependence. The cells also undergo morphologic changes in terms of their growth pattern and cytologic features. Whereas normal cells have a limited proliferative lifespan in vitro before the cells cease dividing and die, transformed cells are immortal. Finally, transformed cells will form malignant tumors upon reinjection into syngeneic animals. This latter characteristic is generally considered as the ultimate criterium for the complete transformation of a cell.

Transformed cells also show other prominent characteristics such as changes in surface charge, the appearance of surface antigens, increased proteolytic enzyme activity, and various membrane changes. Indeed, the variety of the changes associated with the process of transformation indicate the complexity of the neoplastic process. These observations lead to the natural question as to which of these changes are essential to the process of carcinogenesis in vivo.

Studies with cultivated cells in vitro have shown that the induction of neoplastic transformation is a complex, multi-stage process (1, 2). They have also allowed the correlation of transformation with the induction and repair of specific molecular DNA damage, as well as with other cellular effects such as cytogenetic changes and single gene mutations. In particular, they have facilitated the design of experiments to test the somatic mutation theory of carcinogenesis; that is, the hypothesis that the initial radiation-induced lesion which initiates the process of carcinogenesis is a mutation in a structural gene.

Transformation System

Most quantitative studies of radiation transformation have been carried out with rodent cell systems; in particular, primary Syrian hamster embryo cells (3) or established lines of mouse embryo fibroblasts (4, 5). The hamster embryo system has the advantage of employing stable diploid cells with a low frequency of spontaneous transformation. However, transformation is scored by a colony assay; that is, carcinogen treated cells are seeded at low density and the individual colonies which grow up are observed under the microscope to determine the fraction of these which show phenotypic evidence of transformation. Such a system has the disadvantages of observer bias as well as the logistics of individually scoring many colonies to determine a rare event.

The mouse embryo fibroblast derived cell lines commonly in use include the BALB/3T3 and C3H/10T1/2 systems. Such established cell lines have the advantages of being initially derived from a single cell, of being relatively stable in culture, and of possessing a highly density-inhibited, non-transformed phenotype. They are, however, aneuploid and immortal, and have thus already acquired certain characteristics of transformation. Transformation is usually scored by a focus assay. By the usual experimental protocol, the cells are seeded at low density and treated with the carcinogen. They are subsequently allowed to proliferate for 1-2 weeks until the cells reach confluence (density-inhibition of growth), and then allowed another 4 weeks in confluence for expression of the transformed foci. These foci of transformed cells are easily recognized as dense, piled-up colonies of cells overlying the normal confluent monolayer. The appearance of such a focus is shown in Figure 1. Cells isolated from such foci form malignant tumors (fibrosarcomas) with high frequency upon reinjection into syngeneic mice.

Radiation Transformation in vitro: Total Dose, Dose-rate and LET

The radiation dose response relationship for the induction of neoplastic transformation shows two important characteristics. At low

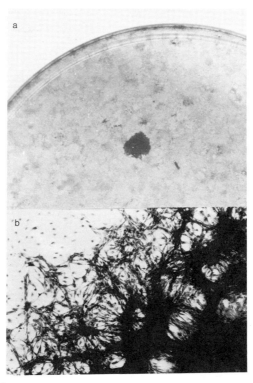

Fig. 1.   (A) Section of Petri dish with transformed focus of mouse C3H 10T1/2 cells. (B) High power view of edge of focus. Note normal monolayer on upper left.

doses, the yield of transformants increases with dose reaching a maximum at approximately 400-600 rads. At higher radiation doses, the yield of transformants reaches a plateau; that is, the frequency of transformation shows no further increase with increasing radiation dose. These characteristics are shown in Figure 2, in which dose response curves for the induction of transformation by X-rays and neutrons are compared with those for ultraviolet light and the chemical carcinogen dimethyl-benzanthracene (DMBA) (6). As can be seen in Figure 2, the biphasic nature of the dose response curve is common to both physical and chemical carcinogens. This latter observation may at least partially explain why high radiation doses in some in vivo studies have not proven to be as carcinogenic as might be predicted based on lower dose exposures.

Two physical parameters have received considerable attention in studies of radiation transformation. These are the effect of radiation quality or linear energy transfer (LET), and of dose rate. The effects of 430 kV neutrons were initially studied in SHE cells (7) and fission spectrum neutrons in mouse 10T1/2 cells (8). In both cases, the resultant dose response curves were compared with those for transformation induced by X-rays. The results of these two studies were similar; there was a rapid increase in transformation induced by neutron irradiation occurring at significantly lower doses than was observed for X-rays. This effect can be seen in the fission neutron dose response curve shown in Figure 2. The

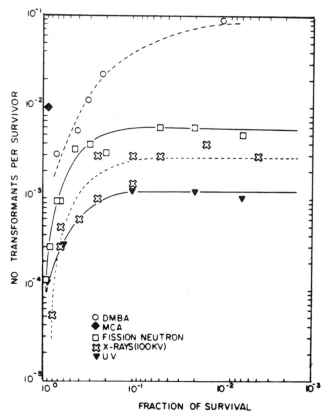

Fig. 2. Dose-response curves for neoplastic transformation of mouse 10T1/2 cells by various physical and chemical carcinogens. Reproduced from Yang et al. (6) where sources of original data can be found.

plateau on the dose response curve was reached at about 200 rads rather than approximately 600 rads. The transformation frequency on the plateau, however, was only slightly elevated as compared with that observed for X-rays. A generally similar results has been observed for high LET alpha radiation (9), and for accelerated particles (6). One of the most striking findings, however, has been the observation that exposure to fission-spectrum neutrons at low dose-rates apparently leads to a marked enhancement in malignant transformation, particularly in the dose range below 100 rads, as compared with single high dose-rate neutron exposure (10). This observation could have considerable significant in terms of the evaluation of risks to the human population of fission-spectrum neutrons, and possibly of other high LET radiations.

Most of these studies of the effects of high LET radiation have been carried out with exponentially growing cells. An interesting result has emerged from one study in which cells were irradiated with alpha particles from a plutonium-238 source while in the density inhibited, stationary phase of growth (9). Following x-irradiation of stationary cultures of the mouse 3T3 cells used in these experiments, cell survival was significantly enhanced and transformation markedly reduced when the cells were held in stationary growth for periods up to 9 days after irradiation. This phenomenon presumable results from recovery or repair processes which are active in non-proliferating cells. Following alpha radiation, however, prolonged holding in the stationary phase had no influence on the ultimate survival or yield of transformation in these cultures. Thus, when transformation was compared in non-proliferating cells irradiated with either X-rays or alpha particles and held in stationary growth for long periods of time, the transformation frequency was 50 to 100-fold higher in the alpha irradiated cultures. Thus, the relative biological effectiveness (RBE) for transformation by alpha particles which appeared to be only 2-3 in exponentially growing cells was 20-40 in cells irradiated and held in stationary growth. This observation could have significant implications in terms of the RBE of alpha particles in critical cell populations in vivo.

Borek and Hall (11) first reported that irradiation of Syrian hamster embryo cells irradiated with a total dose of either 50 or 75 rads split into two equal fractions with 5 hours between them yielded a transformation frequency about 2-fold higher than when the same total dose was given as a single fraction. Shortly thereafter, Terzaghi and Little (12) reported that the transformation frequency was significantly reduced when total doses of 300 or 800 rads were split into two equal fractions in mouse 10T1/2 cells. These authors found no difference when cells were exposed to 150 rads either in a split dose or single dose protocol. These apparently conflicting results were resolved by Miller and Hall (13) who studied the phenomenon in mouse 10T1/2 cells over the entire dose range from 30 to 800 rads total dose. They observed a biphasic response. With total doses below about 150 rads, transformation was enhanced by a factor of about 2 when the dose was split into two equal fractions separated by 5 hours. With doses above 200 rads, on the other hand, the transformation frequency was suppressed when the dose was split. Almost identical results were subsequently obtained by Little (14) with mouse BALB/3T3 cells.

As these results suggested that transformation produced by low doses of ionizing radiation might be enhanced following low dose-rate exposure, experiments were designed specifically to measure the effect of dose-rate on transformation. Hall and Miller (15), in keeping with their expectations based on the split dose results, observed an enhancement in transformation following exposure to continuous low dose-rate irradiation as compared with the same total dose given as an acute exposure. On the other hand, Han and coworkers (16) observed that a reduction of the dose-rate resulted in a marked reduction in transformation frequency. Although

167

these findings remain in apparent conflict, it should be noted that the irradiation conditions including the proliferative status of the cells differed considerably between the two experiments.

Modulation of Radiation-Induced Transformation

There is a significant body of evidence which suggests that the initiation of transformation involves DNA damage, and is modulated by molecular DNA repair processes (1). These include the observations that transformation may be induced by a direct perturbation of DNA either by a combination of 5-bromodeoxyuridine plus X-rays or near UV light exposure, or from radioactivity incorporated into cellular DNA. There have also been a number of correlative type experiments in which the production and removal of specific DNA adducts is associated with changes in the frequency of transformation, as well as liquid holding experiments in which the kinetics of cellular and cytogenetic changes have been compared with molecular repair processes following X-ray or ultraviolet light irradiation. However, this initial DNA damage must eventually be expressed in terms of the oncogenic transformation of the cell or one of its progeny. This expression period includes the time period between exposure to the carcinogen and the development of fully transformed, tumorigenic cells.

There is accumulating evidence that the expression of oncogenic transformation can be markedly modulated by noncarcinogenic secondary factors including environmental conditions and exposure to specific chemical agents (17). Cell proliferation is one of these factors. Sufficient capacity for cell division amongst target cell populations, as well as appropriate stimuli to proliferation, appear to be necessary for the phenotypic expression of transformation. These in vitro observations are consistent with the long understood importance of cell proliferation in both clinical and experimental cancer. For example, wounding increases the frequency of carcinogen-induced skin cancer, and partial hepatectomy can markedly increase the frequency of liver cancer induced by certain chemical agents. One of the particularly interesting findings to emerge from recent studies of radiation transformation is that the frequency of trans-formations, particularly that induced by low doses of radiation, can be markedly enhanced by post-irradiation incubation with the phorbol ester tumor promoting agents. The question had been raised heretofore whether the effect of these promoting agents might be restricted to the mouse skin.

The effect of post-irradiation treatment with a phorbol ester tumor promoter is shown in Figure 3. As can be seen, its greatest relative enhancing effect on transformation occurred following the lower doses of X-rays. The primary effect of phorbol ester tumor promoters on X-ray transformation in vitro occurs during the proliferative phase of expression (18). Previously, it was a commonly held opinion that tumor promoters enhanced carcinogenesis primarily by stimulating cell proliferation. Although the action of these agents may be associated with the stimulation of cell proliferation, the in vitro studies have shown clearly that this factor by itself is insufficient to explain their promoting effect. Promoting agents are also effective in vitro at long times after exposure of the cells to primary carcinogens, as is the case in vivo. Incubation with tumor promoters beginning after 10-15 rounds of cell division post-irradiation is still effective in enhancing transformation in vitro (18).

Since the initial observation that X-ray induced malignant transformation could be considerably enhanced by post-irradiation incubation with phorbol ester tumor promoters (18), there has been considerable interest in the modification of transformation by various other non-carcinogenic agents. Kennedy and Little (19) showed that certain inhibitors of proteolytic enzymes markedly suppress X-ray induced

168

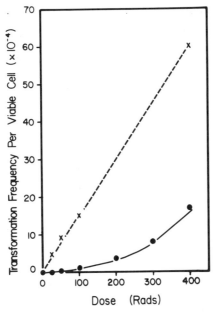

Fig. 3.   Effect of phorbol ester tumor promoter TPA on X-ray induced transformation in mouse 10T1/2 cells. ●——●, X-ray exposure alone. X----X, X-ray exposure followed by incubation with TBA. Reproduced from (17).

transformation _in vitro_ as well as transformation enhanced by the phorbol ester tumor promoters. Harisiades et al. (20) showed that radiation transformation can be suppressed by post-irradiation incubation with certain vitamin A analogues. The effects of such agents may be complex, however, and their mechanisms of action are still not clear. For example, superoxide dismutase or catalase may either enhance or suppress transformation depending upon when the cells are incubated with them. Of particular interest in this respect, is the emerging evidence that tumor promoters may act at the cell surface through a free radical mediated mechanism (21, 22).

Mechanisms of Radiation Transformation

The classical view of the initiation of transformation, embodied in the somatic mutation theory, is that radiation induces a mutation in a specific structural gene or group of genes in an occasional cell in the population. This cell proliferates to form a microcolony of potentially transformed cells at confluence; this microcolony eventually develops into a recognizable transformed focus. It thus appeared appropriate to express the yield of transformants in terms of a transformation frequency per viable irradiated cell, similarly to the way the frequency of mutations is commonly expressed. This phenomenon would presume that the ultimate yield of transformed foci per dish for a given treatment would be directly related to the initial cell density or number of viable cells present in the dish at the beginning of the experiment; the frequency of transformation per viable cell would therefore be independent of the initial cell density. However, this has not proven to be the case. When the influence of initial cell density on the yield of transformed foci was studied in mouse 10T1/2 cells, the rather unexpected observation emerged that the ultimate yield of transformed foci was largely independent of the number of cells initially at risk over the range of approximately 1 to 300 viable cells (23).

In these experiments, cells were seeded in sufficient numbers such that one to 300 viable cells resulted in irradiated cultures allowing for the cloning efficiency of the cells and the toxicity of the radiation exposure. The results of experiments in which the cells were irradiated with 400 rads are shown in Figure 4. The X symbols represent the data for various initial cell densities. As can seen, approximately 0.4 transformed foci developed per dish despite approximately two orders of magnitude difference in the initial cell density. This phenomenon implies that the use of the frequency of transformation per initial viable cell as a means of quantifying transformation is a meaningless parameter. As the yield of transformants per dish induced by a given radiation exposure remained approximately constant despite two or more orders of magnitude variation in the initial number of viable cells, marked differences in the apparent "transformation frequency" could be obtained simply by varying the initial number of cells at risk.

Under some circumstances, transformed foci have developed in a high percentage of cultures derived from a single viable irradiated cell (24). This finding implies that the initial radiation induced event must be a high frequency one which occurs in a large proportion of the irradiated cells. It should be noted that following irradiation the single viable cell multiplies until a normal appearing confluent monolayer of cells results; transformed foci develop everlying this normal monolayer. Thus, this high frequency event appears to lead to a second low frequency event, that is, the transformation of one or more of the progeny of the irradiated cell. As there are approximately 2×10^{-6} cells in a culture at confluence, this second event occurs with the frequency of 10^{-6} or less.

This interpretation of the results was confirmed in a second type of experiment (23, 24). In these experiments, cells seeded at low density

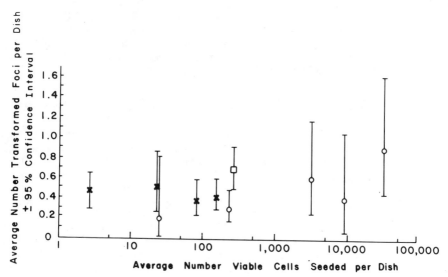

Fig. 4. Effect of initial cell density on ultimate yield of transformed foci in mouse 10T1/2 cells irriadiated with 400 rads. (X) various initial seeding densities. (O) Cell densities in reseeded cultures. (□) undisturbed dishes in reseeding experiments. Reproduced from (23).

were irradiated, allowed to proliferate until confluent, and then resuspended and successively subcultured at dilutions of 1:10 to 1:10,000. The diluted cultures were allowed again to reach confluence, and then held for 4 weeks for the development of transformed foci. As is shown in Figure 4 (open circles), the number of transformed foci which developed per dish remained constant despite reseeded cell numbers varying over 4 orders of magnitude, and were similar to those observed in undisturbed plates. These results suggest that the second event occurred after or soon before confluence was initially reached.

In these initial studies (23), it was assumed that the second step occurred after the cultures had become confluent, because only then did its consequences become detectable. However, it was subsequently shown that transformed cells can arise soon after initiation (25), and some clones of transformed cells may already be present by the time initiated cultures become confluent (26). Thus, studies were carried out to determine specifically the timing of the proposed second event by measuring the distribution of transformed clone sizes present after the multiplication of cultures initiated by x-irradiation (27, 28). In these experiments, cells seeded at low density were irradiated and allowed to reach confluence. At this time they were suspended and reseeded in their entirety into one or two dishes. These dishes were returned to the incubator for 4 weeks; the number of transformed foci which developed should reflect the number of potentially transformed cells in the dish upon reseeding. By this method, the distribution of transformed clone sizes within a large number of initial dishes was determined.

The results of a typical experiment are shown in Table 1. The distribution of foci amongst dishes in this experiment appears consistent with the random occurrence of the second transforming event during the growth of the irradiated cells to confluence. If this is so, the distribution of foci among the reseeded dishes should follow that calculated for the distribution of mutants under similar conditions by Lea and Coulson (29). As can be seen in Table 2, the experimental data conform very closely to the prediction. This was true of five separate large scale experiments of this type (28). As 75% of the total number of mitoses occurs during the two rounds of cell division prior to reaching confluence, most transforming events would take place just prior to confluence. However, occasional progeny may transform much earlier.

Table 1. Distribution of transformed clone sizes in mouse 10T1/2 cells 8 and 15 days after irradiation[1].

Treatment Group	Number of Transformed Foci in Each Dish	Fraction of Dishes Containing Transformed Foci	Among Dishes Containing Foci Average Number of Foci per Dish S.E.
1. 200 rads not reseeded	0,0,0,0,0,0,0,0,0,0,1,1,2	3/13 = 0.23	1.3 ± 0.33
2. 200 rads reseeded at day 8	0,0,0,0,0,0,0,0,0,0,0,0,0,0, 0,0,0,0,0,0,0,0,0,0,0,1,1,2, 2,2,3,5,7,7,12,15,22	12/37 = 0.32	6.6 ± 2.7
3. 200 rads reseeded at day 15	0,0,0,0,0,0,0,0,0,0,0,0,0,0, 0,0,0,0,0,0,0,0,1,1,1,1,1,1, 2,2,2,3,4,9,11,12,15,30,35	17/40 = 0.42	7.7 ± 3.1

[1]Data from Kennedy and Little (28).

Table 2. Comparison of expected and observed distributions of clone sizes for the data presented in Table 1 (pooled results)[1].

Numbers of Transformed Colonies in Reseeded Groups (r)[2]

	0	1	2	3-4	5-8	9-16	17-32	33-64	64
Probability that a culture has r transformants (mutants) when the average number (m) of mutants (mutations) per culture is 0.5 (P(0) = 0.62) (Lea and Coulson (29), Table 2)	.6065	.1516	.0695	.0648	.0475	.0288	.0155	.0079	.0079
In 77 Dishes Observed	48	8	6 ⎱ 9	3	3 ⎱ 12	6	2	1	0
Expected	46.7	11.7	5.4 ⎱ 10.4	5.0	3.7 ⎱ 8.3	2.2	1.2	.61	.61

[1]Data from Kennedy and Little (28).

[2]For the chi-square analysis, the categories were grouped as indicated such that no expected or observed numbers were less than 5; with 2 degrees of freedom, $\chi^2 = 3.3$, $p > 0.10$.

Several other types of experiments were also performed in order to further study this phenomenon (28). In one series, 350–475 total viable cells were initially seeded representing an approximately 1:2 mixture of irradiated and non-irradiated cells. The resultant yield of transformants was directly proportional to the number of irradiated cells present in the mixture rather than to the total number of cells seeded. This result suggests that transformation occurs only amongst the progeny of irradiated cells, and speaks against the hypothesis that radiation may have activated a virus which spreads throughout the culture when the cells become confluent leading to a constant yield of transformants.

In other experiments, a constant number of irradiated cells were seeded into dishes of varying sizes ranging from 8 to 144 cm^2 in surface area. The yield of transformants was directly proportional to the surface area of the dish, and therefore the number of progeny cells present at confluence, rather than to the initial number of irradiated cells. This further confirms the two event hypothesis. Finally, cells from mass cultures were removed at various times during a classical transformation experiment and examined for their ability to grow in soft agar under anchorage independent conditions. No soft agar colonies were observed during the first five days after irradiation, but the ability to produce such colonies occurred as the cultures became confluent, and reached a maximum a few days later. These results are consistent with a transformation event occurring near confluence as hypothesized above, at which time the ability of the cells to grow under anchorage independent conditions appears.

The observation that the initial event in malignant transformation in vitro appears to be a common one involving a large fraction of cells speaks against this event representing a mutation in a specific structural gene or group of genes. Experiments were therefore designed to yield information as to whether DNA damage was specifically involved in the initiation of transformation _in vitro_. To examine this question, transformation was studied in cells allowed to incorporate Iodine-125 in the form of the DNA precursor [125]IdUrd (30). Iodine-125 decays by electron capture with the release of a shower of very low energy Auger electrons. It has been estimated that approximately 350 electrons volts are deposited within a 10 Å sphere around the site of each disintegration, and that much of the energy deposited in DNA from incorporated [125]IdUrd occurs within a few base pairs of this site. Thus, the radiation exposure from [125]IdUrd incorporated into DNA is not only restricted to the DNA itself, but most likely to very small regions of the DNA surrounding the site of decay.

[125]IdUrd was found to be extremely efficient in inducing malignant transformation _in vitro_ (30). This result is shown graphically in Figure 5 in which the results are shown in comparison with those for ^{3}H-thymidine. The transformation frequency was enhanced 3-4 fold by doses of ^{125}I which yielded only approximately 20 total disintegrations within the entire genome of each cell. Such doses produced little or no measurable cytotoxicity. A similar frequency of transformation was produced by 400 rads of X-rays; this dose killed about 70% of the cells. In separate studies (31), each Iodine-125 disintegration in cellular DNA under frozen conditions led to approximately one DNA double strand break. It was also shown in other experiments (32) that Iodine-125 incorporated into DNA as [125]IdUrd is very efficient in inducing mutations to thioguanine resistance. On the basis of reasonable estimates of the size of the HPRT gene, it was calculated that a single Iodine-125 disintegration anywhere within the gene will lead to a mutation (32).

When one considers a rare event such as the occurrence of a HPRT mutation in a population of cells, it is reasonable to expect that, amongst a population in which on the average only 20 DNA lesions are produced in each cell, one of these lesions will occasionally involve this specific gene and thus occasional mutants will arise. In the case of transformation, however, where the initial event appears to occur in a large fraction of the cells, the DNA target would have to be very large. Thus, the iodine-125 results suggest that while DNA damage is indeed

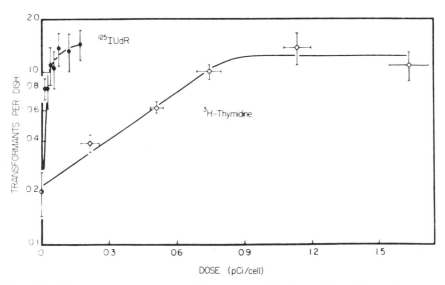

Fig. 5. Dose-response curves for neoplastic transformation of mouse BALB/3T3 cells by [125]Iododeoxyuridine (●) and ^{3}H-thymidine (○).

involved in the initiation of transformation in vitro, this initial event is unlikely to represent a structural gene mutation.

The second step in transformation behaves like a mutational event in that it takes place at random during the growth of the cells, and occurs at a frequency of approximately 10^{-6} or less in the progeny of irradiated cells. The nature of the first event remains obscure. Because it occurs in such a high proportion of irradiated cells, it is unlikely to be the result of a mutation in a specific structural gene or group of genes. The results would suggest, rather, that the cells respond to non-specific DNA damage by the induction of a process which enhances the spontaneous transformation frequency amongst their progeny. This process differs from the usual SOS process in that it cannot be driven by mutagen exposure; that is, exposure to known mutagens during the growth of irradiated cells to confluence does not enhance the frequency of transformation (A. R. Kennedy, personal communication). The involvement of chromosomal rearrangements or gene amplification in this process remain to be determined. A schematic representation of the events in transformation is shown in Figure 6. As is indicated, modifying factors such as tumor promoters or protease inhibitors appear to influence the probability of occurrence of this second event.

These observations and the hypotheses proposed to explain them are certainly unusual in terms of the classical view of mechanisms of transformation. The question arises as to whether they are peculiar to this particular cell system, or whether they might have more general application to radiation carcinogenesis. None of our current knowledge is inconsistent with such a mechanism. To the contrary, there are now several studies in animals which support such an interpretation (33). These involve studies of the malignant potential of carcinogen treated rat tracheal epithelial cells (34), mouse mammary cells (35, 36) and thyroid cells (37). Each of these studies indicate that a large proportion of the population of carcinogen treated cells (of the order of 5-10%) possesses malignant potential in terms of their ability to give rise to either transformed progeny in vitro or malignant tumors in vivo. In other words, though only an occasional tumor may arise in a large population of carcinogen exposed cells if they are left in situ, a large fraction of such cells may have carcinogenic potential if allowed to grow under the appropriate conditions. This potential is expressed in terms of the actual transformation of one or more of their progeny. Thus, the unusual characteristics associated with the transformation of mouse embryo

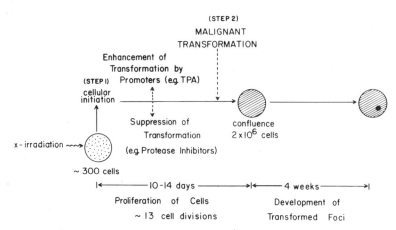

Fig. 6.   Schematic representation of events in transformation of mouse 10T1/2 cells by radiation.

fibroblast derived cell lines do not appear to be an isolated phenomenon. Rather, these findings suggest that the process of radiation transformation is not easily amenable to simple mechanistic models.

Human Diploid Cell Transformation

As has been described above, rodent cells are readily transformed by radiation in a dose dependent manner. Transformation can be easily scored by either a colony morphology or focus assay; the cells isolated from such foci will form progressively growing malignant tumors upon reinjection into syngeneic hosts. It has become clear during the past decade, however, that the complete transformation of human diploid fibroblasts is very difficult to induce in vitro. This appears to be because the process of immortalization is an extremely rare event in human cells. Immortality is, however, one of the prime characteristics which differentiates tumor cells from normal diploid cells which have a limited proliferative capacity in vitro. The process of immortalization appears to be an early and frequent event in many rodent cells, occurring either spontaneously or as the result of carcinogen treatment. Established mouse embryo cell lines such as BALB/3T3 and C3H/10T1/2 are already immortal and aneuploid, this process having occurred spontaneously when the cells lines were established in culture.

This investigation reported in this section was undertaken to gain further information concerning the mechanisms for the transformation of human diploid fibroblasts by radiation, in particular those factors which might be related to the process of immortalization. This section is drawn from a more detailed review to be published elsewhere (38).

Chromosomal rearrangements are associated with most human and rodent tumors. The low efficiency of complete transformation of cultured human cells has been ascribed to the stability of human chromosomes. We have therefore focused on chromosomal aberrations and rearrangements induced by X-irradiation. The experimental approach has been to irradiate cultures at early passage, and to follow them throughout their normal lifespan by subculturing them regularly at 1:4 dilutions. Chromosome rearrangements were studied by obtaining G-banded karyotypes at regular intervals. Evidence was sought for: (1) the induction and persistence of chromosomal rearrangements in X-irradiated cells; (2) the emergence of abnormal clones of cells during proliferation; and (3) changes in the lifespan of irradiated cultures. Our eventual goal was to relate specific chromosomal rearrangements to characteristics of transformation, in particular immortalization.

Whereas the complete transformation of human diploid fibroblasts occurs rarely and has proven very difficult to induce in vitro (39), several investigators have shown that certain characteristics of transformation may be more readily induced in human fibroblasts (40-43). These include the ability to grow under anchorage independent conditions, which is occasionally associated with the appearance of changes in growth pattern and morphology resembling focus formation. Cells isolated from anchorage independent colonies may form small tumor nodules when injected into nude mice, though these nodules rarely grow to more than 1 cm in diameter and usually regress (41, 44). Moreover, the environmental conditions in which the cells are grown and assayed must be very carefully controlled to maintain a low frequency of spontaneous anchorage independent growth, as well as a measurable induced frequency. These findings suggest that the induction of anchorage independent growth may be an early carcinogen-induced change in normal human fibroblasts that might result from a mutation controlling certain membrane functions or perhaps a change in gene expression.

Although the induction of gross chromosomal aberrations in mammalian cells by ionizing radiation has been widely studied, surprisingly little information is available concerning the frequency of non-lethal chromosomal rearrangements in X-irradiated human diploid cells. We, therefore, examined the change in the frequencies of X-ray induced chromosomal rearrangements in human diploid fibroblasts as a function of subculture time (45). The cells were regularly subcultivated at a 1:4 dilution and followed throughout their lifespan in vitro; metaphase spreads and G-banded karyotypes were examined at regular intervals. Evidence was sought not only for the induction of chromosome rearrangements but also for their stability in cultures allowed to proliferate for long periods after irradiation.

The frequency of gross chromosomal aberrations was examined in metaphase spreads in cells irradiated with 400 rads of X-rays while in the confluent, density-inhibited phase of growth. A series of dishes was regularly subcultured at a 1:4 dilution, while others were maintained in confluence without subculturing for up to 43 days. Chromosome-type aberrations including dicentrics, rings and fragments were measured at various times after irradiation. As can be seen in Figure 7, the frequency of gross chromosomal aberrations declined rapidly in cells allowed to proliferate after radiation exposure. Few aberrations were observed at the second subculture, and none were present at subculture 5. This rapid decline in chromosomal aberrations with subcultivation suggests that the presence of such aberrations at mitosis is lethal to the cells; the cells containing aberrations are thus lost from the population.

The frequency of aberrations in first division metaphases declined rapidly with holding periods of 4-24 hrs in cells not subcultured after irradiation but maintained under density inhibited conditions (no proliferation). Thereafter, however, the aberration frequency remained stable at a level of 30-40% of the initial frequency up to 43 days after

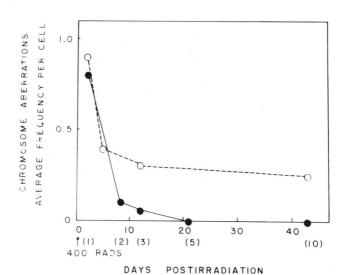

Fig. 7. Change in frequency of gross chromosomal aberrations with time in human diploid fibroblasts irradiated with 400 rads. ●————●, cells subcultured regularly; post-irradiation subculture number show in parenthesis. ○----○, cells maintained in density-inhibition of growth (no proliferation) until indicated time.

176

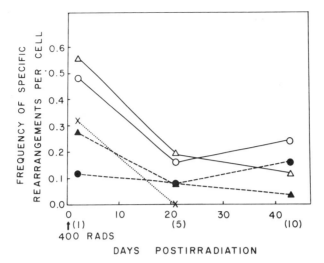

Fig. 8. Changes in frequency of various chromosomal rearrangements
with time in human diploid fibroblasts irradiated with 400
rads and subcultured regularly (subculture number in
parenthesis). △———△ , all deletions or fragments.
▲- - -▲ , cells with deletions or fragments only.
all translocations. ○———○ , cells ●- - -● with
translocations only. ✕- - -✕ , all chromosomal
aberrations.

irradiation. The kinetics of this decline in chromosomal aberrations with
short confluent holding periods corresponds exactly to those previously
described for the repair of potentially lethal damage in X-irradiated cells
(46). These results suggest that a certain amount of the damage which
results in chromosomal aberrations at the first mitosis is rapidly repaired
following radiation exposure. However, a significant fraction of this
damage persists for long periods of time in nonproliferating cells. When
the cells are allowed to proliferate, the presence of the aberrations which
occur at mitosis are lethal to the cells, and these cells are lost from the
population.

The changes in the frequency of various chromosomal rearrangements
during the growth of irradiated cells examined on G-banded karyotypes are
shown in Figure 8. Data are presented for translocations, dicentrics and
rings, fragments or deletions, and inversions in cells irradiated with 400
rads and examined at the first, fifth and tenth subcultivation after
irradiation. As was seen in Figure 7, the frequency of gross chromosomal
aberrations (dicentrics and rings) declined to 0 after the first
subcultivation. The frequency of translocations (open circles) remained at
about 50% of the initial value at subcultures 5 and 10. However, a certain
number of the cells which contained translocations will also contain
chromosomal aberrations which are lethal to the cells such as dicentrics,
inversions and deletions. Data on the persistence of translocations in
cells which contained no other visible chromosomal damage are also shown in
Figure 8 (closed circles). As can be seen, the frequency of such cells did
not change significantly from the first through the tenth subcultivation.
Similar results were seen in cells initially irradiated with 600 rads.
These results suggest that in cells containing X-ray induced translocations
alone, these translocations persist over many cell generations. Such
chromosomal rearrangements thus appear to be very stable. The apparent
decline in the overall frequency of translocations with subculture observed

in Figure 8 reflects the death of cells which also contained deletions and dicentrics.

Nonrandom chromosomal changes, particularly translocations, have been recognized in cells from a number of human cancers. Cells with specific chromosomal rearrangements form abnormal clones, and it has been suggested that the formation of such clones may be an important factor in the development of cancer. The finding that stable translocations are induced by radiation in cultured human diploid fibroblasts, and that these translocations persist over many generations of replication, led us to examine whether certain of these cells might gain a selective growth advantage such that clonal populations of cells containing specific marker chromosomes emerged as apparently occurs in human tumors (47).

In order to examine this question, cultured human diploid fibroblasts were exposed to single or multiple radiation exposures, subcultivated thereafter at regular intervals at a 1:4 dilution, and followed throughout their lifespan. G-banded metaphase preparations were examined microscopically at each subcultivation for the presence of marker chromosomes suggesting the presence of abnormal clones. Such clones contained stable chromosomal rearrangements including translocations, deletions or inversions. The term "clone" was used only when the following conditions were satisfied: (1) at least three metaphases containing identical structural chromosomal rearrangements were found; and (2) one cell type was observed in at least two different passages.

No abnormal clones were observed in four nonirradiated control cultures, whereas clones did emerge in two out of eight cultures exposed to single doses of 400 or 600 rads of X-rays. Because the initial frequency of chromosomal rearrangements is highly dependent upon radiation dose, several cultures were exposed to several doses of radiation at successive subcultivations. Multiple abnormal clones developed in five out of six cultures exposed to sequential radiation doses. Typically, these clones appeared between the 30th and 50th mean population doubling (MPD). Earlier appearing clones disappeared from the population at later times, as the clonal cells apparently became senescent. Some later appearing clones persisted in the mass population until complete senescence. At certain times during its lifespan, 80% of more of the cells in the entire population might belong to a single abnormal clone. In two cases, the terminal cell population consisted entirely of a single clone of cells.

Evidence of clonal succession, that is the appearance and disappearance of successive clones of cells over the lifespan of the culture, was observed in several of these cultures. Such clonal succession probably represents the sequential emergence and attenuation of clones which initially attain a selective growth advantage and then undergo early senescence. An example of clonal succession in such a culture is shown in Table 3. Three different clones possessing unique chromosomal rearrangements were first observed at subculture 6 after irradiation. One of these (clone C) a bearing several translocations became predominant in the culture between subcultures 11-16, comprising over 50% of the population at subculture 15. This clone disappeared from the population after subculture 16. Three other clones also emerged during these later times. One of these (clone F) bearing a chromosome 1:18 translocation became predominant from subculture 17 until the culture senesced. By this time, the population consisted primarily of cells derived from this single clone.

These results indicate that certain cells bearing stable chromosome rearrangements may gain a selective growth advantage, permitting clonal expansion to the point where single clones of cells bearing specific

178

Table 3. Emergence and attenuation of cytogenetically distinct abnormal clones in X-irradiated human diploid fibroblasts followed throughout their lifespan *in vitro*[1]

Post-Irradiation Sub culture no.	no. of Metaphases examined	Abnormal Clones[2]					
		A	B	C	D	E	F
6	20	1(5)	1(5)	1(5)	0	0	0
8	29	4(14)	2(7)	2(7)	0	0	0
11	22	0	3(14)	4(18)	2(9)	0	0
13	35	0	0	5(14)	8(23)	7(20)	3(9)
15	29	0	0	15(52)	0	0	4(14)
16	18	0	0	4(22)	1(5)	1(5)	4(22)
17	40	0	0	3(6)	0	0	30(60)
19	9	0	0	0	0	0	7(78)

[1] Data from Y. Kano and J.B. Little (Submitted)

[2] Number (percentage) of cells in each clone.

rearrangements can be recognized as comprising a significant fraction of the mass population. It is not known whether an increased probability of clonal expansion is related to certain specific rearrangements which confer a selective growth advantage to the cells, or whether clonal expansion is a random phenomenon independent of the rearrangements present. No specific pattern of rearrangements has thus far evolved amongst the various abnormal clones we have observed in different cultures. Should the emergence of abnormal clones with specific chromosomal rearrangements be a necessary step in the development of the transformed phenotype, the results described above indicate that radiation exposure can facilitate the development and expansion of such clones.

These observations on the emergence of abnormal clones in irradiated cultures led us to examine whether such cells might show any changes in lifespan *in vitro* (48). In these experiments, cultures were exposed to single or multiple doses of radiation and followed throughout their lifespan with regular subcultivation. The lifespan (mean population doublings) of 46 irradiated cultures were compared with those of 9 nonirradiated control cultures. The results are shown in Table 4. The mean lifespan of 44 of the irradiated cultures was slightly significantly prolonged as compared with 9 control cultures (58.4 vs. 53.0 MPD, $p < 0.05$). As the cytotoxic effect of radiation was not included in the calculation of MPD, the actual lifespan of surviving irradiated cells was significantly greater than 58.3.

In the two remaining irradiated cultures, cell strains emerged with a considerably prolonged lifespan (Table 4). In one of these, several abnormal clones emerged at earlier passages and eventually disappeared, but the clone which appeared at MPD 44 expanded to include the entire population by MPD 57. Subsequent to MPD 57 this culture has consisted entirely of monoclonal cells; the mass culture senesced at MPD 47. This culture is currently surviving at MPD 84. However, this clone of cells must have undergone another 20 MPD during clonal expansion from a single cell to include the entire population (2×10^6 cells/dish), as well as at least 10 additional MPD during the repopulation of cultures following

179

Table 4. Lifespan of control and irradiated human diploid
fibroblasts[1]

| | No. of Cultures | Lifespan (MPD)[2] | |
		Mean	Range
Controls	9	53.0	48-57
Irradiated Single doses	26	57.3	51-66
Irradiated, Multiple doses	18	59.7	51-67
Irradiated, Prolonged lifespan	2	76[3] 82[3]	- -

[1]Data from Kano and Little (submitted). Strain AG1522 used in all experiments.
[2]The increased number of population doublings surviving cells must undergo in irradiated cultures to repopulate the dish not included in calculations of lifespan. Thus, the actual lifespan measured in terms of MPD of surviving irradiated cells will be greater than the figure shown.
[3]Abnormal clones. Actual MPD thus greater by about 20 (see text).

irradiation (each dose of 600 rads kills more than 95% of the cells). Thus, the cells in this clone have undergone at least 114 MPD, more than twice the mean lifespan of control cells or of the other cells in the mass culture.

The karyotype of these monoclonal cells was highly abnormal showing a variety of stable chromosomal rearrangements, including a deletion in the short arm of chromosome 1 (p22, p32), and a translocation between chromosome 11:12. The human N-ras and B-lym oncogenes have been mapped to the short arm of chromosome 1 in the vicinity of the breakpoints of the deletion. The karyotype of the other clone of cells with a prolonged lifespan (Table 4, 76 MPD) showed two translocations involving chromosome 22 (1;22 and 6;22). The sis oncogene has been mapped to chromosome 22 (22q12-q13), the region of the breakpoint in the chromosome 6;22 translocation. These observations have led us to hypothesize that the prolonged lifespan of this clone of cells might be related to oncogene activation. Interestingly, the morphology of the cells in both of these cultures was normal, and they did not grow in soft agar. Thus, the prolonged lifespan was not associated with the acquisition of characteristics of morphologic transformation.

The low frequency of immortalization of human fibroblasts by radiation as compared with rodent cells has been ascribed to the chromosomal stability of human cells. The results described above indicate that irradiation of normal human diploid cells in vitro induces stable chromosomal rearrangements including deletions and translocations which are passed on to their progeny and persist throughout their lifespan. Occasionally, cells containing specific rearrangements may gain a selective growth advantage and be recognized within the population as an abnormal clone. Such clones may expand to include the majority of the population, although they usually senesce and disappear. The life history of heavily irradiated cultures of human diploid fibroblasts therefore appears to be characterized by clonal succession; that is, the successive emergence and disappearance of several abnormal clones of cells. Occasionally, such cells have a significantly prolonged in vitro lifespan. Under these conditions, the clone expands until it includes 100% of the population. Whether this increased lifespan is related to the specific chromosomal rearrangements characteristic of the clone, or whether it is related to some other factor independent of these rearrangements, is not at present evident.

Amongst nearly 100 human diploid fibroblast cultures followed throughout their post-irradiation lifespan in vitro, including those in Table 4, none have given rise to truly immortal cells. On the other hand, morphologic transformation including changes in growth pattern, focus formation and a high frequency of anchorage independent growth has occurred in several cases.

On the basis of these findings, we hypothesize that morphologic transformation and immortalization are separate and distinct steps in the process of transformation of human cells. Immortalization is a very rare event which is induced at extremely low frequencies in human diploid fibroblasts, whereas characteristics of morphologic transformation may be induced quite easily. This is in contradistinction to the process in rodent cells, in which immortalization is an early and frequent occurrence.

REFERENCES

1. J. B. Little, Radiation transformation in vitro: implications for mechanisms of carcinogenesis, in: "Advances in Modern Environmental Toxicology, Vol. 1," N. Mishra, V. Dnukel, and M. Mehlman, eds., Senate Press, Inc., New Jersey (1981), pp. 383-426.

2. J. C. Barrett and P. O. P. Ts'o, Evidence for the progressive nature of neoplastic transformation in vitro, Proc. Natl. Acad. Sci. USA, 75:3761-3765 (1978).

3. Y. Berwold and L. Sachs, In vitro transformations of normal cells to tumor cells by carcinogenic hydrocarbons, J. Nat. Cancer Inst. 35:641-661 (1965).

4. C. A. Reznikoff, J. S. Bertram, D. W. Brankow, and C. Heidelberger, Quantitative and qualitative studies of chemical transformation of cloned C3H mouse embryo cells sensitive to post-confluence inhibition of cell division, Cancer Res. 33:3239-3249 (1973).

5. T. Kakunaga, A quantitative system for assay of malignant transformation by chemical carcinogens using a clone derived from BALB/3T3, Int. J. Cancer 12:463-473 (1973).

6. T. C. H. Yang and C. A. Tobias, Radiation and cell transformation in vitro, Adv. Biol. Med. Phys. 17:417-461 (1980).

7. C. Borek, in: "Particle Radiation Therapy," V. P. Smith, ed., Am. Coll. Radiology, Philadelphia, PA (1975), pp. 284-301.

8. A. Han and M. M. Elkind, Transformation of mouse C3H 10T1/2 cells by single and fractionated doses of X-rays and fission-spectrum neutrons, Cancer Res. 39:123-130 (1979).

9. J. B. Robertson, A. Koehler, J. George, and J. B. Little, Oncogenic transformation of mouse BALB/3T3 cells by plutonium-238 alpha particles, Radiat. Res. 96:261-274 (1983).

10. C. K. Hill, F. M. Buonaguro, C. P. Myers, A. Han, and M. M. Elkind, Fission-spectrum neutrons at reduced dose rates enhance neoplastic transformation, Nature 298:67-69 (1982).

11. C. Borek and E. J. Hall, Effect of split doses of X-rays on neoplastic transformation of single cells, _Nature_ 252:499-501 (1976).

12. M. Terzaghi, and J. B. Little, Oncogenic transformation _in vitro_ after split dose X-irradiation, _Int. J. Radiat. Biol._ 29:583-587 (1976).

13. R. Miller and E. J. Hall, X-ray dose fractionation and oncogenic transformation in cultured mouse embryo cells, _Nature_, 272:58-60 (1978).

14. J. B. Little, Quantitative studies of radiation transformation with the A31-11 mouse BALB/3T3 cell line, _Cancer Res._ 39:1478-1484 (1979).

15. E. J. Hall and R. C. Miller, The how and the why of _in vitro_ oncogenic transformation, _Radiat. Res._ 87:208-223 (1981).

16. A. Han, C. K. Hill, and M. M. Elkind, Repair of cell killing and neoplastic transformation at reduced dose rates of ^{60}Co gamma-rays, _Cancer Res._ 40:3328-3332 (1980).

17. J. B. Little, Influence of noncarcinogenic secondary factors on radiation carcinogenesis, _Radiat. Res._ 87:240-250 (1981).

18. A. R. Kennedy, G. Murphy, and J. B. Little, The effect of time and duration of exposure to 12-0-tetradecanoyl-phorbol-13-acetate (TPA) on X-ray transformation of C3H 10T1/2 cells, _Cancer Res._ 40:1915-1920 (1980).

19. A. R. Kennedy and J. B. Little, Protease inhibitors suppress radiation induced malignant transformation _in vitro_, _Nature_ 276:825-826 (1978).

20. L. Harisiadis, R. C. Miller, E. J. Hall, and C. A. Borek. A vitamin A analogue inhibits radiation-induced oncogenic transformation, _Nature_ 274:486-487 (1978).

21. H. Nagasawa and J. B. Little, Factors influencing the induction of sister chromatid exchanges in mammalian cells by 12-0-tetradecanoyl-phorbol-13-acetate, _Carcinogenesis_ 2:601-607 (1981).

22. I. Emerit and P. A. Cerutti, Tumor promoter phorbol 12-myristate-13-acetate induces a clastogenic factor in human lymphocytes, _Proc. Natl. Acad. Sci. USA_ 79:7509-7513 (1982).

23. A. R. Kennedy, M. Fox, G. Murphy, and J. B. Little, Relationship between X-ray exposure and malignant transformation in C3H 10T1/2 cells, _Proc. Natl. Acad. Sci. USA_ 77:7262-7266 (1980).

24. A. R. Kennedy and J. B. Little, Investigation of the mechanisms for enhancement of radiation transformation _in vitro_ by 12-0-tetradecanoyl-phorbol-13-acetate, _Carcinogenesis_ 1:1039-1047 (1980).

25. J. M. Backer, M. Boerzig, and I. B. Weinstein, When do carcinogen-treated 10T1/2 cells acquire the commitment to form transformed foci?, _Nature_ 299:458-460 (1982).

26. E. J. Hall, H. H. Rossi, M. Zaider, R. C. Miller, and C. Borek, The role of neutrons in cell transformation research: II, experimental, in: "Neutron Carcinogenesis," J. J. Broerse and G. B. Gerber, eds., Commission of the European Communities, Luxembourg (1982), pp. 371-395.

27. A. R. Kennedy, J. Cairns, and J. B. Little, Timing of the steps in transformation of C3H 10T1/2 cells by X-irradiation, Nature 307:85-86 (1984).

28. A. R. Kennedy and J. B. Little, Evidence that a second event in X-ray induced oncogenic transformation in vitro occurs during cellular proliferation, Radiat. Res. 99:228-248 (1984).

29. D. E. Lea and C. A. Coulson, The distribution of the numbers of mutants in bacterial populations, J. Genet. 49:264-285 (1949).

30. P. K. LeMotte, S. J. Adelstein, and J. B. Little, Malignant transformation induced by incorporated radionuclides in BALB/3T3 mouse embryo fibroblasts, Proc. Natl. Acad. Sci. USA 79:7763-7767 (1982).

31. P. K. LeMotte and J. B. Little, DNA damage induced in human diploid cells by decay of incorporated radionuclides, Cancer Res. 44:1337-1342 (1984).

32. H. L. Liber, P. K. LeMotte, and J. B. Little, Toxicity and mutagenicity of X-rays, (^{125})dUrd or (^{3}H)TdR incorporated in the DNA of human lymphoblast cells, Mutation Res. 111:387-404 (1983).

33. A. R. Kennedy, Evidence that the first step leading to carcinogen-induced malignant transformation is a high frequency common event, in: "Cell Transformation Assays: Application to Studies of Mechanisms of Carcinogenesis and to Carcinogen Testing," J. C. Barrett, ed., Raven Press, New York, in press.

34. M. Terzaghi and P. Nettesheim, Dynamics of neoplastic development in carcinogen-exposed tracheal mucosa, Cancer Res. 39:4003-4010 (1979).

35. S. P. Ethier and R. L. Ullrich, Detection of ductal dysplasia in mammary outgrowths derived from carcinogen-treated virgin female BALB/c mice, Cancer Res. 42:1753-1760.

36. K. H. Clifton, K. Kamiya, R. T. Mulcahy, and M. N. Gould, Radiogenic neoplasia in the thyroid and mammary clonogens: progress, problems and possibilities, in: "Symposium Proceedings, Estimation of Risk from Low Doses of Radiation and Chemicals: A Critical Overview," Brookhaven National Laboratory (May 20-23, 1984).

37. R. T. Mulcahy, M. N. Gould, and K. H. Clifton. Radiogenic initiation of thyroid cancer: a common cellular event, Int. J. Radiat. Biol. 45:419-426 (1984).

38. J. B. Little, Mechanisms of malignant transformation of human diploid cells, in: "Carcinogenesis: A Comprehensive Survey, Vol 10; The Role of Chemicals and Radiation in the Etiology of Cancer," E. Huberman, ed., Raven Press, New York (1985), pp. 337-353.

39. T. Kakunaga, Neoplastic transformation of human diploid fibroblast cells by chemical carcinogens, Proc. National Acad. Sci. USA 75:1334-1338 (1978).

40. G. Milo and J. A. DiPaolo, Neoplastic transformation of human diploid cells in vitro after chemical carcinogen treatment, Nature (Lond.) 275:130-132 (1978).

41. K. C. Silinskas, S. A. Kateley, J. E. Tower, V. M. Maher, and J. J. McCormick, Induction of anchorage-independent growth in human fibroblasts by propane sultone Cancer Res. 41:1620-1627 (1981).

42. C. Borek, X-ray-induced in vitro neoplastic transformation of human diploid cells, Nature(Lond.) 283:776-778 (1980).

43. R. J. Zimmerman and J. B. Little, Characterization of a quantitative assay for the in vitro transformation of normal human diploid fibroblasts to anchorage independence by chemical carcinogens, Cancer Res. 43:2176-2182 (1983).

44. R. J. Zimmerman and J. B. Little, Characteristics of human diploid fibroblasts transformed in vitro by chemical carcinogens, Cancer Res. 43:2183-2189 (1983).

45. Y. Kano and J. B. Little, Persistence of X-ray-induced chromosomal rearrangements in long-term cultures of human diploid fibroblasts, Cancer Res. 44:3706-3711 (1984).

46. A. J. Fornace, Jr., H. Nagasawa, and J. B. Little, Relationship of DNA repair to chromosome aberrations, sister chromatid exchanges and survival during liquid holding recovery in X-irradiated mammalian cells, Mutation Res. 70:323-336 (1980).

47. Y. Kano and J. B. Little. Mechanisms of human cell neoplastic transformation: X-ray-induced abnormal clone formation in long-term cultures of human diploid fibroblasts. Cancer Res. 45:2550-2555 (1985).

48. Y. Kano and J. B. Little. Mechanisms of human cell neoplastic transformations: relationship of specific abnormal clone formation to prolonged lifespan in X-irradiated human diploid fibroblasts. Int. J. Cancer. 36:407-413 (1985).

INDUCTION OF CHROMOSOME ABERRATIONS AND MALIGNANT TRANSFORMATION
IN DIFFERENT CELL LINES BY
PHOTONS AND MONOENERGETIC NEUTRONS

J. Zoetelief, J.J. Broerse and G.W. Barendsen

Radiobiological Institute TNO
Rijswijk, The Netherlands

ABSTRACT

The relations among different types of cellular effects, i.e. cell reproductive death, chromosome aberrations and malignant transformation caused by ionizing radiation of different quality are essential in studies of mechanisms in radiobiology.

The induction of cell reproductive death and of chromosome aberrations (primarily dicentrics and centric rings) were studied in three lines of mammalian cells (R-1,M; RUC-2 and V-79). Cell survival curves and dose-effect relations for transformation were investigated in C3H/10T1/2 cells. In addition, some information is provided on the use of induction of chromosome aberrations in (human) peripheral lymphocytes as a biological dosimetry system in case of total body irradiation.

For studies on chromosome aberrations, irradiations of plateau phase cultures containing 70 to 80 percent of cells in the G_0 or prolonged G_1 phase were carried out with ^{137}Cs γ rays, 300 kV X-rays and 0.5, 4.2, and 15 MeV neutrons. The data on cell transformation were obtained for the same neutron energies and 300 kV X-rays and the results pertain to standardized value of 10^3 clonogenic cells per culture flask of 25 cm^2 area.

The dose-response relationships were analyzed for neutrons in terms of a linear dose coefficient only, while the results for photons required analysis in terms of linear and quadratic coefficients. The effectiveness per unit of dose for cell inactivation is greater than that for the induction of dicentrics and centric rings by factors of about 5 to 9. These factors are relatively constant within one cell line. Correction for cells in other phases than G_0, G_1, and including acentric fragments in the scoring of chromosome aberrations, results in ratios for induction of cell reproductive death to induction of gross chromosome aberrations of 1.2 to 1.6. Cell transformation is induced much less frequently than cell reproductive death. The ratios of corresponding linear dose coefficients are in the order of 10^{-3}.

The largest relative biological effectiveness (RBE) values are found for 0.5 MeV neutrons, which range at low doses from 8 to 13 for all types of effect investigated. For 4.2 and 15 MeV neutrons the low dose RBE values are about 4 to 9 and 3 to 6, respectively. The RBE values for the R-1,M cells are lower than for the relatively resistant V-79 and RUC-2 cells.

INTRODUCTION

In many models and hypotheses that have been developed for the interpretation of dose-effect relationships, it is assumed that the relative biological effectiveness (RBE) for different biological endpoints depends in a similar way on radiation quality. For instance, in the theory of dual radiation action (1), it is assumed that the production of two sublesions within a site with a diameter of about 1 μm is the fundamental cause of a wide range of cellular effects. Other investigators (2) have stressed that in addition to the energy deposition patterns, the precise chemical nature of primary biomolecular changes has to be considered. This latter point of view is supported by radiobiological studies involving different cell types (3) where differences were found in intrinsic radiosensitivities as well as in RBE values of neutrons. Therefore, the determination of accurate dose-response relationships under standardized experimental conditions for the induction of various cellular effects by ionizing radiation and their dependence on radiation quality (e.g. characterized by the linear energy transfer (LET) or average lineal energy ($\bar{y}$)), is considered essential in studies of mechanisms in radiobiology. Analysis of such data can provide insight into basic biophysical processes involved in the induction of various biological effects such as cell reproductive death, chromosome aberrations, mutations and malignant transformation. These insights are required as bases for risk estimates to be applied for radiation protection purposes.

Interest in studies on chromosome aberrations and cell reproductive death as biological endpoints is based in part on the suggestion that chromosomal aberrations are the major cause of cell reproductive death. However, no general agreement exists on the type of chromosome damage involved in cell inactivation. In studies with X-rays, some investigators (7, 8), observed a strong correlation between loss of chromosome fragments and loss of reproductive capacity, whereas the formation of anaphase bridges was found not to be an important cause of cell inactivation. Experiments of other investigators (5, 9) led to the conclusion that gross chromosome aberrations (di- and polycentrics, centric rings and acentric fragments) are likely to cause cell inactivation. In the latter studies (9), the formation of anaphase bridges was found to be an important cause of cell reproductive death. More recently, it was suggested (10) that in addition to gross chromosome aberrations other types of damage must play an important role in cell reproductive death. It is evidently of interest to obtain information on both types of damage in the same types of cells irradiated under the same conditions and for different qualities of radiation.

The induction of chromosome aberrations in cells can be used as a biological dosimetry system for ionizing radiation (4, 5). The majority of investigators (4, 5), employ human peripheral blood lymphocytes. This system seems especially useful for dose estimates in case of accidental whole body irradiation. For partial body irradiation, a system based on the induction of chromosome aberrations in human skin fibroblasts seems advantageous.

The development of cancer after irradiation is the result of a complex sequence of events initiated by energy deposition from ionizing radiation and influenced by many physical, chemical, and biological factors. Chromosome aberrations might play an important role in carcinogenesis. In

the sequence of events involved in carcinogenesis, malignant transformation
of cells is a very important step for the initiation of unrestrained
growth. Information on transformation of cells in culture is relevant to
carcinogenesis since it has been shown that clones with altered
morphological characteristics can develop into tumours after inoculation in
syngeneic hosts. Results from studies on in vitro transformation can
therefore provide a basis for the interpretation of data on carcinogenesis in
vivo.

In this contribution, results are presented on induction of cell
reproductive death and of chromosome aberrations in three cell lines after
irradiation with ^{137}Cs γ rays, 300 kV X-rays and 0.5, 4.2, and 15 MeV
neutrons. The use of induction of chromosome aberrations in cells as a
biological dosimetry system is briefly summarized. Information on cell
transformation in C3H/10T1/2 cells for several neutron energies is given in
relation to induction of cell reproductive death.

SOME EXPERIMENTAL ASPECTS OF SCORING OF CHROMOSOME ABERRATIONS, CELL REPRODUCTIVE DEATH AND MALIGNANT TRANSFORMATION

As stated before, it is of importance to study cellular effects in
several types of cells, because of reported differences in radiosensitivity
between different cell lines. When the results of different cellular
effects are to be compared, however, this should be done only for the same
cell line irradiated under similar experimental conditions including type of
radiation, dose rate, fractionation, oxygenation, temperature and
distribution of cells in the cell cycle.

With tissue culture techniques, it is possible to take pieces from
normal tissues or from a tumour, cut these specimens into small pieces,
separate out the individual cells and prepare a suspension of single cells.
Most of these cells will grow in vitro for only a few weeks, but some may
continue to grow for many years. Examples of lines of these latter cells,
the so-called established cell lines, are e.g., rat rhabdomyosarcoma cells
(R-1,M), rat ureter carcinoma cells (RUC-2) and Chinese hamster cells
(V-79) (11).

When cultured cells are exposed to ionizing radiation, three types of
chromosomal aberrations can occur depending on their cell cycle stage at
the time of irradiation, namely, chromosome, chromatid and subchromatid
aberrations (Figure 1). Most studies are restricted to chromosome type
aberrations, as these are the most easily scored. This effect is also a
very important endpoint, since the cell population at risk in humans is
generally not rapidly proliferating, i.e., most cells will be in the G_0 or
prolonged G_1 phase of the cell cycle where the majority of chromosomal
aberrations induced will be of the chromosome type. To arrive at a
population of cultured cells having a large number of cells in G_1, plateau
phase cultures are commonly used. In Figure 2, the culture characteristics
are shown for three cell lines. Given are the growth curves as a function
of time after plating together with the fractions of cells in the $G_{0,1}$
phase of the cell cycle versus time after plating. The fractions of cells
in G_0 or G_1 determined by measurements of the DNA content distributions of
the cells using a flow cytofluorometer were 0.75, 0.7, and 0.8 for R-1,M;
V-79 and RUC-2 cells, respectively, after 6 days of culture in falcon
flasks (25 cm^2 growth area).

With in vitro techniques, the fraction of cells which retain the
capacity for unlimited proliferation is determined by the number of
colonies formed (13). The clonogenic capacity of irradiated cells is
generally assayed by counting the number of clones of more than 30 cells

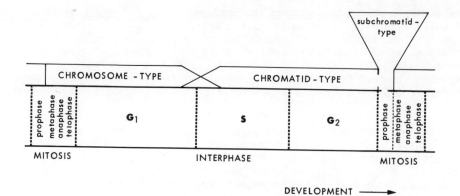

Fig. 1. Relation between type of chromosomal aberration induced by radiation and stage in the cell replication cycle at the time of irradiation (UNSCEAR, 1969 (12)).

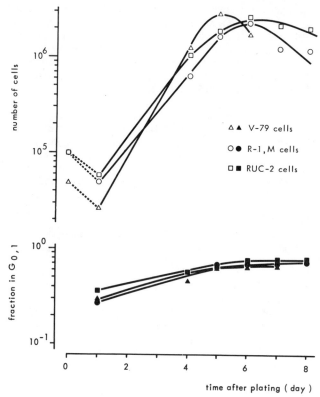

Fig. 2. Culture characteristics of three cell lines. Upper part of the figure: growth curves as a function of time after plating. Lower part: fraction of cells in the $G_{0,1}$ phase of the cell cycle versus time after plating.

which develop from single cells plated in culture flasks. The clones are commonly scored after culturing in a medium at 37°C for a period of about 12 days following irradiation. Control plating efficiencies have to be

determined. These were about 70, 60 and 70 per cent for R-1,M; RUC-2 and
V-79 cells taken from the plateau phase cultures, respectively.

For studies on induction of chromosome aberrations it is essential to
collect cells in the first mitosis postirradiation. Investigations on T-1
cells of human origin showed relative numbers of aberrations of 1.0, 0.5,
and 0.26 for first, second and third mitosis postirradiation, which is in
qualitative agreement with the observation of Carrano (9). Following
irradiation in $G_{0,1}$ phase of the cell cycle, cells should be stimulated to
induce progression through the cell cycle. Cells can be halted in mitosis
by e.g., colcemid (a spindle poison) and can be obtained by shaking them
off from the culture flasks. It is essential that the total population of
irradiated cells is accumulated in mitosis. Radiation induced mitotic
delay influences the time required by cells to reach the first mitosis, but
is, for X-rays, less for G_1 cells than for cells in other phases (14).
Collected mitotic cells are swollen by adding a hypotonic solution for
several minutes at 37°C and then fixed. Metaphase spreads are prepared by
dropping the fixed cells onto microscope slides which are stained.

The induction of chromosome aberrations in cells can be used as a
biological dosimetry system for ionizing radiation. Most investigators
employ (human) peripheral blood lymphocytes (4, 5). The technique of
lymphocyte cytogenetic dosimetry requires small samples of heparinized
blood, from which lymphocytes are separated and stimulated to enter the
mitotic cycle. After culturing for, e.g., 48 hours the cells are fixed,
dispensed onto microscope slides and stained. The culturing techniques
employed for (human) lymphocytes irradiated in vivo as well as the
sampling times are of considerable importance (15, 16). The dose estimate
for in vivo conditions is made on the basis of the observed yield of
chromosome aberrations produced in vitro.

A schematic diagram showing the different types of chromosome
aberrations which can be observed in metaphase is given in Figure 3. The
chromosome as seen in the metaphase of cell division consists of two
parallel threads; those composing one chromosome are termed sister

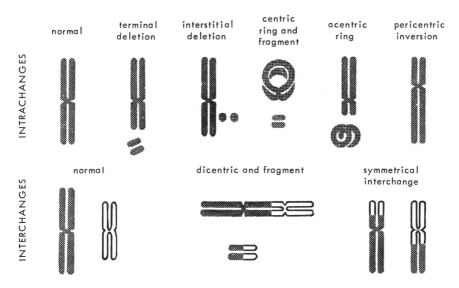

Fig. 3. Chromosome-type aberrations that can be distinguished
          cytologically at the metaphase of the cell replication cycles
          (12).

chromatids. In each chromosome, the sister chromatids are held together at a specific point, the centromere. In studies of chromosome-type aberrations, a distinction is made between intrachanges which are produced within single chromosomes and interchanges which involve an exchange of parts between different chromosomes. In scoring chromosome aberrations, terminal deletions, interstitial deletions and centric rings (Figure 3) are generally referred to as acentric fragments, although the mechanisms of production are different.

Dicentrics and centric rings are the easiest recognizable aberrations and can be scored unambiguously (Figure 4). Acentric fragments cannot be scored unambiguously because of their variable size. With the commonly employed homogeneous staining techniques (Figure 4), pericentric inversions and reciprocal translocations are not detectable, since, apart from the chromosome threads, only the centromeres and gaps are visible. Fortunately though, the frequencies of induction of pericentric inversions and reciprocal translocations could be expected to be the same as those for centric rings and dicentrics, respectively. This expectation of equal frequencies is based on the assumption that symmetrical aberrations have probabilities of occurrence equal to their asymmetrical counterparts (17).

For normal cells, cultured in vitro, growth ceases, e.g., by contact inhibition when a monolayer of cells completely fills the culture flask or dish. Cell cultures derived from tumours show usually a less restricted irregular pattern of growth; the cells tend to pile up. The visible patterns of cell growth give the first indication for cell transformation. The development of malignant tumours upon inoculation of transformed cells in syngeneic hosts provides the ultimate confirmation that transformation is malignant. The cell lines most often used for in vitro transformation studies are short-term cultures of Syrian hamster embryo cells (18) and the C3H10T1/2 (clone 8) mouse cell line developed by Reznikoff et al. (19).

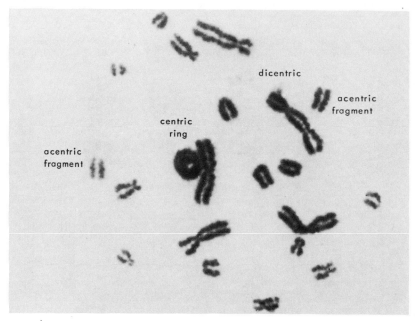

Fig. 4.   Different types of chromosome aberrations as observed in a metaphase spread of V-79 cells.

The Syrian hamster cell system has an advantage, a relatively high sensitivity for transformation enabling effects of very low doses of radiation to be studied. However, the cells are usually developed from fresh embryos for each experiment and comprise a mixture of all the body tissue cells. The cells do not adapt completely to in vitro conditions and usually survive only for about 30 generations. Transformations are scored typically 8 to 14 days after irradiation by microscopic examination of individual colonies of cells. Depending on the visible growth patter, each colony is scored as either normal or transformed. Transformed colonies are characterized by piling up of cells with criss-crossing at their edges. The transformation frequency is taken as the ratio of the number of transformed clones to the total number of clones.

The C3H10T1/2 cell system (19) has a very regular growth pattern which provides a suitable background against which abnormal growth patterns can be recognized. Transformation is characterized in this system by piled up 'foci' which can be distinguished when the cells have grown to cover the entire flask, i.e., typically 5 to 6 weeks after irradiation. The transformation frequency is taken as the number of foci relative to the number of surviving (i.e., colony forming) cells. It is essential that the transformation frequencies pertain to a standardized number of clonogenic cells per culture flask of specified area (e.g, 10^3 viable cells on a flask of 25 cm^2 area, since the transformation per surviving cell increases by a factor of about 20 when the number of viable cells per cm^2 decreases from about 25 to about 3 (20).

DOSE-EFFECT RELATIONS FOR CELL INACTIVATION AND CHROMOSOME ABERRATIONS IN THREE CULTURED CELL LINES FOR IRRADIATION WITH PHOTONS AND MONOENERGETIC NEUTRONS

When a cell retains and expresses its capacity for unlimited proliferation in tissue culture, it is scored as a surviving cell. Cell survival curves for a specific type of radiation represent the relationship between the fraction of surviving cells (S) and the absorbed dose of

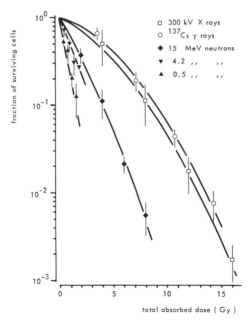

Fig. 5. Survival curves for V-79 cells subjected to various types of radiation.

radiation (D). The survival curves for V-79 cells are given in Figure 5, for irradiation with ^{137}Cs γ rays, 300 kV X-rays and 0.5, 4.2, and 15 MeV neutrons. The results for neutrons are presented as a function of total absorbed dose. The error bars in the figure refer to the standard deviations from at least 4 independent experiments. It is concluded from Figure 5 that 0.5 MeV neutrons are most effective, 4.2 and 15 MeV neutrons are intermediate and photons have the lowest effectiveness. No significant differences in effectiveness between the two types of photon radiation are observed. The dependence on radiation quality for R-1,M and RUC-2 cells is qualitatively similar to that of V-79 cells (21). However, the three cell lines show appreciable differences in sensitivity to ionizing radiation. For all types of radiation, R-1,M cells show the highest sensitivity, V-79 cells are intermediate, and RUC-2 cells show the lowest sensitivity (21). This indicates the importance of the investigation of cellular effects for different cell lines.

The fractions of dicentrics and centric rings per cell versus total absorbed dose are plotted in Figure 6 for V-79 cells, for the five types of radiation employed. The uncertainties indicated in the figures refer to the standard deviations assuming a Poisson distribution of dicentrics and centric rings between cells. Similar to the situation for impairment of clonogenic capacity, the effectiveness for induction of dicentrics and centric rings is greatest for 0.5 MeV neutrons, intermediate for 4.2 and 15 MeV neutrons and least for photons. Important differences are observed between the sensitivities of the three cell lines with respect to the induction of dicentrics and centric rings (21).

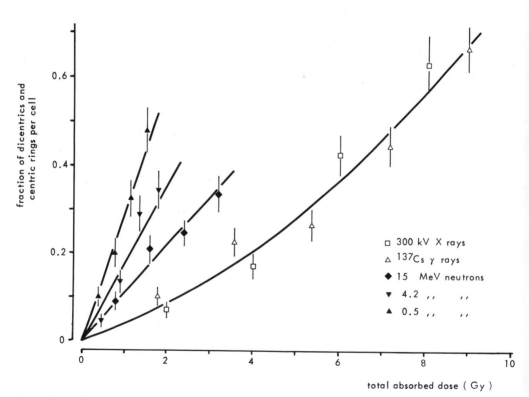

Fig. 6. Induction of dicentrics and centric rings per cell in V-79 cells by various types of radiation as a function of total absorbed dose.

192

A number of models has been developed for the interpretation of cell survival curves (22). The simplest survival curve is represented by the equation:

$$S(D) = e^{-k_d D} \tag{1}$$

where the subscript d refers to cell reproductive death, $S(D)$ is the surviving fraction after a single absorbed dose D, and k_d is the inactivation constant. As a model for inactivation, the inactivation constant k_d represents the net sensitivity of each cell and may be associated with a net target volume. Another shape of survival curves shows an increase of effect per unit dose throughout the range of observation (22). In practice, these curves are approximated by:

$$S(D) = e^{-(\alpha_d D + \alpha_d D^2)} \tag{2}$$

The linear and quadratic dose terms can be interpreted by assuming that primary biomolecular lesions can be induced by either energy deposition from a single ionizing particle or by that deposited by two particles crossing one or more critical sites or structures in the cell that are involved in cell inactivation.

The frequency of induction of chromosome aberrations $Y(D)$ is commonly fitted by a polynomial:

$$Y(D) = \alpha_a D + \beta_a D^2 + \gamma_a D^3 + \dots . \tag{3}$$

where the subscript "a" refers to chromosome aberrations.

For induction of chromosome aberrations by high LET radiation, $Y(D)$ increases linearly with the dose:

$$Y(D) = k_a D \tag{4}$$

For X and gamma rays g$Y(D)$ increases more rapidly than proportionally with the dose. In practice, most data on chromosome aberrations can be adequately analyzed by taking into account only linear and quadratic dose terms (5):

$$Y(D) = \alpha_a D + \beta_a D^2 \tag{5}$$

The linear and quadratic dose terms can be interpreted similarly as those in equation 2 for cell survival, being related to energy depositions from one ionizing particle and to those from two particles.

The dose-effect relationships for impairment of clonogenic capacity and for induction of dicentrics and centric rings were analyzed according to models with linear and quadratic dose terms. For the various relations the coefficients were obtained from least-squares fits to the experimental data using a computer code (23). To obtain the uncertainties in the coefficients, a series of fits was made to each set of experimental data according to a specially developed computer program (Hennen, personal communication); the principle used is that the amount of biological effect at each dose is specified by a mean value and its standard deviation (as indicated in Figures 5 and 6 by points and error bars, respectively). Furthermore, it is assumed that the possible variation in the amount of biological effect at each dose is governed by the Poisson distribution. For each set of experimental data, point values for the amount of biological effect at each dose were selected according to the Poisson distribution and these point values were used to obtain the parameter

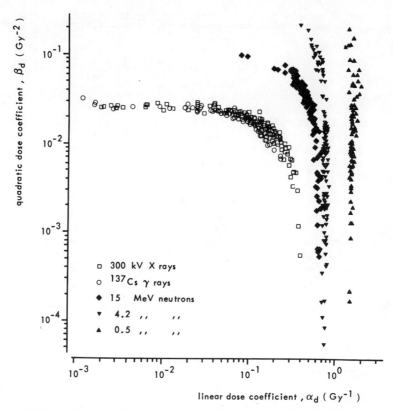

Fig. 7. Mutual dependence of variations in the linear and quadratic
dose coefficients of α_d and β_d for analysis of survival curves
for V-79 cells exposed to various types of radiation.

values by a least-squares fit. The quoted uncertainties refer to the
standard deviations in the dose coefficients from 126 fits to each
experimental dose-effect relation. For interpretation of the uncertainties
in the coefficients derived with the two parameter model, it has to be
realized that the uncertainties are not independent. An example of the
relation between the linear and quadratic dose coefficients as analyzed
with the computer fitting procedure is given in Figure 7 for induction of
cell reproductive death in V-79 cells by the different types of radiation
employed. The density of the points in this figure provides information
about errors. It can be concluded from Figure 7 that the neutron survival
curves can adequately be described by a linear dose term only, whereas for
photons, an appreciable contribution from the quadratic dose coefficient is
observed. Furthermore, the figure shows that, e.g., a relative low α_d is
correlated with a relatively high β_d value.

The results of the computations of parameters for the different cell
lines and various types of radiation are given in Table 1 for induction of
cell inactivation and in Table 2 for induction of dicentrics and centric
rings. For photons, the analysis of the data is given in terms of a linear
and a quadratic dose term for both cell inactivation and chromosome
aberrations. For all experiments with 4.2 and 0.5 MeV neutrons, the

Table 1. Analysis of reproductive death induced in three cell lines by various types of radiation

Function:	$S=\exp(-k_d D)$	$S=\exp\{-(\alpha_d D+\beta_d D^2)\}$		
Parameter:	$k_d(\mathrm{Gy}^{-1})$	$\alpha_d(\mathrm{Gy}^{-1})$	$\beta_d(\mathrm{Gy}^{-2})$	$\alpha_d\beta_d^{-1}(\mathrm{Gy})$
Type of radiation				
V-79 cells				
300 kV X-rays	—	0.15 ± 0.09	0.016 ± 0.007	9^{+17}_{-6}
^{137}Cs gamma rays	—	0.07 ± 0.05	0.020 ± 0.005	4^{+4}_{-3}
15 MeV neutrons	0.63 ± 0.03	0.5 ± 0.1	0.03 ± 0.02	17^{+43}_{-9}
4.2 MeV neutrons	0.74 ± 0.03	—	—	—
0.5 MeV neutrons	1.4 ± 0.1	—	—	—
RUC-2 cells				
300 kV X-rays	—	0.08 ± 0.07	0.016 ± 0.007	$5^{+12}_{-4.5}$
^{137}Cs gamma rays	—	0.09 ± 0.07	0.014 ± 0.007	6^{+17}_{-5}
15 MeV neutrons	0.43 ± 0.04	0.3 ± 0.1	0.022 ± 0.021	15^{+39}_{-10}
4.2 MeV neutrons	0.4 ± 0.1	—	—	—
0.5 MeV neutrons	1.05 ± 0.06	—	—	—
R-1,M cells				
300 kV X-rays	—	0.28 ± 0.09	0.04 ± 0.02	7^{+12}_{-4}
^{137}Cs gamma rays	—	0.27 ± 0.09	0.04 ± 0.01	7^{+5}_{-3}
15 MeV neutrons	0.87 ± 0.03	0.80 ± 0.06	0.027 ± 0.022	30^{+142}_{-15}
4.2 MeV neutrons	1.09 ± 0.07	—	—	—
0.5 MeV neutrons	2.42 ± 0.06	—	—	—

Table 2. Analysis of induction of dicentrics and centric rings in three cell lines by various types of radiation

Function:	$Y=k_a D$	$Y=\alpha_a D+\beta_a D^2$		
Parameter:	$k_a(\mathrm{Gy}^{-1})$	$\alpha_a(\mathrm{Gy}^{-1})$	$\beta_a(\mathrm{Gy}^{-2})$	$\alpha_a\beta_a^{-1}(\mathrm{Gy})$
Type of radiation				
V-79 cells				
300 kV X-rays	—	0.02 ± 0.01	0.008 ± 0.002	3^{+2}_{-2}
^{137}Cs gamma rays	—	0.04 ± 0.01	0.003 ± 0.001	13^{+12}_{-5}
15 MeV neutrons	0.11 ± 0.01	0.10 ± 0.01	0.002 ± 0.004	$50^{+\infty}_{-35}$
4.2 MeV neutrons	0.17 ± 0.04	—	—	—
0.5 MeV neutrons	0.29 ± 0.03	—	—	—
RUC-2 cells				
300 kV X-rays	—	0.016 ± 0.009	0.005 ± 0.002	3^{+5}_{-2}
^{137}Cs gamma rays	—	0.013 ± 0.007	0.003 ± 0.001	4^{+6}_{-2}
15 MeV neutrons	0.12 ± 0.01	0.08 ± 0.02	0.014 ± 0.009	6^{+14}_{-4}
4.2 MeV neutrons	0.11 ± 0.01	—	—	—
0.5 MeV neutrons	0.19 ± 0.02	—	—	—
R-1,M cells				
300 kV X-rays	—	0.053 ± 0.008	0.003 ± 0.004	$18^{+\infty}_{-12}$
^{137}Cs gamma rays	—	0.056 ± 0.009	0.003 ± 0.005	$19^{+\infty}_{-13}$
15 MeV neutrons	0.10 ± 0.01	0.098 ± 0.007	0.002 ± 0.004	$49^{+\infty}_{-34}$
4.2 MeV neutrons	0.10 ± 0.01	—	—	—
0.5 MeV neutrons	0.37 ± 0.04	—	—	—

analysis was made by using a linear dose term only. The analysis of the results for 15 MeV neutrons is presented both by using a linear and a quadratic dose term and by assuming a linear dose term only. From Table 1, it can be concluded that the coefficients of the quadratic dose terms for irradiation with photons are not significantly different for the three cell lines, although the values for R-1,M cells tend to be the highest. For 15 MeV neutrons at doses below 5 Gy, the contribution from the quadratic dose term might be neglected. For induction of dicentrics and centric rings by photons (Table 2), it can be concluded that, for RUC-2 and V-79 cells, a quadratic dose term is present, while for R-1,M cells in the investigated dose range, this contribution is not significantly different from zero. Since the number of doses is limited to four or five, the results will be discussed by assuming for all experiments with photons a linear and a quadratic dose coefficient and taking for neutrons a linear dose term only.

COMPARISON OF DOSE-EFFECT RELATIONS FOR INDUCTION OF CELL REPRODUCTIVE DEATH WITH THOSE FOR INDUCTION OF CHROMOSOME ABERRATIONS IN THREE CELL LINES

The underlying assumption for a comparison of the two types of cellular effects under the same irradiation conditions is that a given dose of radiation produces a number of lesions distributed at random over a population of cells. Cells without a lethal lesion are survivors and this fraction depends on the Poisson distribution. It has been suggests (5) that there is a direct correlation between cell survival and gross chromosome aberrations according to the following equation:

$$S(D) = e^{-Y(D)} \qquad (6)$$

Consequently, the parameters derived from survival curves and from dose-effect relations for induction of chromosome aberrations pertaining to the yield of lethal lesions and the yield of aberration can be directly compared.

To obtain insight into the relation between induction of cell reproductive death and the induction of chromosome aberrations for the three cell lines and for various types of radiation, the ratios of the dose coefficients for these two endpoints are given in Table 3. For photons, the relative effectiveness for induction of the two endpoints is determined by $\alpha_d \cdot \alpha_a^{-1}$ (at low doses) and $\beta_d \cdot \beta_a^{-1}$ (at high doses). For neutrons, the values of $k_d \cdot k_a^{-1}$ indicate the relative effectiveness for induction of cell reproductive death as compared with that for chromosome aberrations. Within the individual cell lines, the values for $k_d \cdot k_a^{-1}$ show relatively small variations, whereas the $\alpha_d \cdot \alpha_a^{-1}$ and $\beta_d \cdot \beta_a^{-1}$ values show larger differences. For irradiations with photons, the $\alpha_d \cdot \beta_d^{-1}$ values for induction of cell reproductive death in the different cell lines (Table 1) are not significantly different; a mean value of about 6 Gy can be taken as a common ratio. For induction of chromosome aberrations by photons, a ratio of 6 Gy between linear and quadratic dose coefficients is also within the uncertainty limits (Table 2), but the uncertainties are so large that further conclusions are not considered justifiable. Therefore in Table 3, the average of $\alpha_d \cdot \alpha_a^{-1}$ and $\beta_d \cdot \beta_a^{-1}$ is given as a measure for the ratio of induction of cell reproductive death to induction of chromosome aberrations for irradiations with photons. It can be concluded from Table 3 that values for the average of $\alpha_d \cdot \alpha_a^{-1}$ and $\beta_d \cdot \beta_a$ for each cell line show relatively small differences from the means of $k_d \cdot k_a^{-1}$. This suggests within one cell line a constant ratio between induction of cell reproductive death and induction of chromosome aberrations, independent of the type of radiation. However, the mean $k_d \cdot k_a^{-1}$ value for R-1,M cells (about 9) is larger than those for V-79 and RUC-2 cells (about 5). The $k_d \cdot k_a^{-1}$ values are larger than 1; this indicates that dicentrics and centric rings cannot be the only cause for cell reproductive death.

If the assumptions of Carrano (9) and Lloyd et al (5) are accepted, then acentric fragments should also be taken into account in the

196

Table 3. Ratio of dose coefficients for induction of reproductive
death to that for induction of dicentrics and centric rings

Cell line	V-79 cells		RUC-2 cells		R-1,M cells	
	$\alpha_d\alpha_a^{-1}$	$\beta_d\beta_a^{-1}$	$\alpha_d\alpha_a^{-1}$	$\beta_d\beta_a^{-1}$	$\alpha_d\alpha_a^{-1}$	$\beta_d\beta_a^{-1}$
300 kV X-rays	$7.5^{+7.5}_{-5.5}$	2^{+2}_{-1}	$5.0^{+12.4}_{-4.6}$	$3.3^{+4.5}_{-1.9}$	$5.3^{+2.6}_{-2.5}$	$13^{+\infty}_{-12}$
^{137}Cs gamma rays	$2^{+2}_{-1.7}$	7^{+5}_{-3}	$6.9^{+20}_{-5.9}$	$6.7^{+5.8}_{-2.9}$	$4.8^{+2.5}_{-2.0}$	$13^{+\infty}_{-9}$

	V-79	RUC-2	R-1,M
Average of $\alpha_d\alpha_a^{-1}$ and $\beta_d\beta_a^{-1}$	4·6	5·5	9·0
	$k_dk_a^{-1}$	$k_dk_a^{-1}$	$k_dk_a^{-1}$
15 MeV neutrons	$5.7^{+0.9}_{-0.7}$	$3.6^{+0.7}_{-0.6}$	$8.7^{+1.3}_{-1.0}$
4·2 MeV neutrons	$4.3^{+1.6}_{-0.9}$	$3.6^{+1.4}_{-1.1}$	$10.9^{+2.0}_{-1.6}$
0·5 MeV neutrons	$4.8^{+1.0}_{-0.7}$	$5.5^{+1.0}_{-0.8}$	$6.5^{+1.0}_{-0.7}$
Mean $k_dk_a^{-1}$	4·9	4·2	8·7

Table 4. Ratio of dose coefficients for induction of cell reproductive
death to that for induction of chromosome aberrations

	Cell line		
	R-1,M	V-79	RUC-2
average of $\alpha_d \cdot \alpha_a^{-1}$, $\beta_d \cdot \beta_a^{-1}$ and $k_d \cdot k_a^{-1}$	9	5	5
fraction of cells in $G_{0,1}$	0.75	0.7	0.8
$\dfrac{\text{acentric fragments}}{\text{dicentrics + centric rings}}$	4	1.8	1.4
$\dfrac{\text{cell inact.}}{\text{gross chrom. aber.}}$	1.3	1.2	1.6

interpretation of cell survival studies. Therefore, the scoring of
dicentrics and centric rings has been extended in a number of experiments
by scoring acentric fragments. The ratios of acentric fragments to
dicentrics and centric rings found in these additional studies are given in
Table 4. In addition, it must be borne in mind that dicentrics and centric
rings can be induced only in cells irradiated in the $G_0 + G_1$ phases of
the cell cycle. The fractions of cells in the $G_0 + G_1$ phases of the cell
cycle are also given in Table 4. The resulting ratios for induction of
cell inactivation to induction of gross chromosome aberrations (dicentrics,
centric rings and acentric fragments) are close to one (Table 4). This
indicates that induction of gross chromosome aberrations might explain an
appreciable part of induction of cell reproductive death. In addition, it
must be recognized that scoring of acentric fragments is not unambiguous
because of their variable size. It can, however, not be excluded that in
addition to gross chromosome aberrations other types of damage play a
significant role as concluded by Tremp (10).

RBE-LET RELATIONS FOR INDUCTION OF CELL INACTIVATION AND CHROMOSOME
ABERRATIONS FOR SMALL RADIATION DOSES

The RBE values for neutrons obtained for both biological endpoints are
presented in Table 5 for the different cell lines employed. The results

for levels of effect corresponding to different doses of 300 kV X-rays are given. Corrections for the contributions of the photon components of the neutron beams are not included in this table. It can be seen from the table that the RBE values decrease with increasing dose of X-rays. Significant differences are not observed between the RBE values for the different biological endpoints. The largest RBE values (average for cell death and chromosome aberrations) are found for 0.5 MeV neutrons, which show values of about 8, 12, and 12 at low dose levels for R-1,M; RUC-2, and V-79 cells, respectively.

For 4.2 MeV neutrons, the mean RBE values at low dose levels are about 3, 6, and 7 for R-1,M; RUC-2, and V-79 cells, respectively. However, for the experiments with neutrons of this energy, the relative photon contribution to the total dose was rather high (26%). Correction for the photon contribution will increase the RBE values to about 4, 8, and 9 for 4.2 MeV neutrons alone. The mean RBE values at low doses for 15 MeV

Table 5. RBE of neutrons as a function of dose of 300 kV X-rays for induction of cell inactivation and chromosome damage

Dose of X-rays (Gy)	15 MeV neutrons		4·2 MeV neutrons		0·5 MeV neutrons	
	cell death	chrom. aberr.	cell death	chrom. aberr.	cell death	chrom. aberr.
R-1,M cells						
0·001	3·1 {4·7 / 2·3}	1·9 {2·5 / 1·2}	3·9 {6·1 / 2·8}	1·9 {2·5 / 1·2}	8·6 {13 / 6·4}	7·0 {9·2 / 4·4}
1	2·7 {4·3 / 2·0}	1·8 {2·4 / 1·2}	3·4 {5·5 / 2·5}	1·8 {2·4 / 1·2}	7·6 {12 / 5·8}	6·6 {9·1 / 4·4}
2	2·4 {3·9 / 1·9}	1·7 {2·4 / 1·2}	3·0 {5·0 / 2·3}	1·7 {2·4 / 1·2}	6·7 {11 / 5·2}	6·3 {9·0 / 4·4}
5	1·8 {3·1 / 1·5}	1·5 {2·4 / 1·2}	2·3 {4·0 / 1·8}	1·5 {2·4 / 1·2}	5·0 {8·6 / 4·1}	5·4 {8·8 / 4·4}
RUC-2 cells						
0·001	5·4 {47 / 3·1}	7·5 {16 / 4·6}	5·0 {50 / 2·7}	6·9 {15 / 4·2}	13·0 {110 / 4·4}	11·0 {36 / 7·1}
1	4·5 {13 / 3·7}	5·7 {11 / 3·8}	4·2 {10 / 4·0}	5·2 {9·7 / 3·4}	11·0 {32 / 8·8}	9·0 {17 / 5·8}
2	3·8 {8·3 / 3·1}	4·6 {7·7 / 3·2}	3·6 {6·4 / 3·4}	4·2 {7·1 / 2·9}	9·4 {21 / 7·5}	7·3 {13 / 4·9}
5	2·7 {4·1 / 2·2}	2·9 {4·3 / 2·2}	2·5 {3·1 / 2·3}	2·7 {4·0 / 2·0}	6·5 {10 / 5·1}	4·6 {7·0 / 3·4}
V-79 cells						
0·001	4·2 {11 / 2·5}	5·5 {14 / 3·7}	4·9 {13 / 3·2}	8·5 {25 / 4·8}	9·3 {25 / 6·3}	15·0 {38 / 9·6}
1	3·8 {8·6 / 2·1}	3·9 {8·3 / 2·9}	4·5 {10 / 2·5}	6·1 {15 / 3·7}	8·4 {20 / 4·6}	10·0 {23 / 7·5}
2	3·5 {6·8 / 2·1}	3·1 {5·9 / 2·3}	4·1 {8·0 / 2·4}	4·7 {10 / 3·0}	7·7 {16 / 4·5}	8·1 {16 / 6·1}
5	2·7 {4·2 / 1·9}	1·8 {3·1 / 1·5}	3·2 {4·9 / 2·2}	2·8 {5·5 / 2·0}	6·1 {9·5 / 4·0}	4·8 {8·3 / 3·9}

† The results presented are the means with maximum and minimum values corresponding to the standard deviations.

neutrons are about 2.5, 6, and 5 for R-1,M; RUC-2 and V-79 cells, respectively. It can be concluded that the mean RBE values for R-1,M cells are lower than those for the relatively resistant RUC-2 and V79 cells, which are similar. The RBE values for these latter cells lines extrapolated to levels corresponding to low doses of X-rays are in good agreement with relevant Q values (25).

Recently, Roberts and Holt (24) reported an RBE value for the induction of chromosome aberration in V-79/4(AHI) cells of 6.4 for 2.1 MeV neutrons at low dose levels. This value is somewhat but not significantly smaller than our RBE value of 4.2 MeV neutrons for V-79 cells. Our RBE values at low doses are considerably smaller than those found for human lymphocytes (5) irradiated with neutrons of different energies. However, the RBE values found in our studies at levels of effect corresponding to 2 Gy of reference radiation are in good agreement with those of Lloyd et al. (5). This observation which was also made by Roberts and Holt (24) requires further investigation.

For risk analysis, use is generally made of the expression (26):

$$E = \alpha D + \beta D^2 \tag{7}$$

where E denotes the biological effect and D the absorbed dose. For radiation protection purposes at low doses (up to about 50 mGy for photons) and low dose rates (up to about 50 mGy a^{-1} for photons), the linear dose term is predominant. Therefore, the linear dose coefficients for induction of cell inactivation and chromosome aberrations are presented as a function of radiation quality in Figures 8 and 9, respectively. As measure for the radiation quality, the frequency averaged lineal energies, $\overline{y_F}$, are used. The choice of $\overline{y_F}$ is arbitrary, since the appropriateness of the different parameters for the specification of radiation quality has not yet been established. The values for $\overline{y_F}$ are taken from a review of microdosimetric parameters (27). The linear dose terms for neutrons are corrected for the relative photon contributions to the total absorbed dose.

It can be concluded from Figures 8 and 9 that the uncertainties in the estimation of the RBE values for neutrons are mainly due to the uncertainties in the results obtained for photons. For investigation of cell reproductive death, information is also available for exponentially growing cell cultures (Figure 8). No significant differences in the results for the different modes of cell culture were observed, but for the experiments with exponentially growing cells, smaller uncertainties in the fitting parameters were found. Between the two types of photon radiation, large variations in the linear dose components can occur within the experimental uncertainties. Therefore, it is not possible to draw a conclusion on the dependence of the linear dose coefficient on $\overline{y_F}$ in this region. Experiments with fractionated or protracted irradiation will allow a more accurate assessment of the linear dose term for photons, as indicated in Table 6. For neutrons an increase in the linear dose coefficients is observed with increasing $\overline{y_F}$, for both types of effect, although the dependence for induction of cell inactivation seems somewhat different from that for induction of chromosome aberrations. In the investigated $\overline{y_F}$ region, an increasing linear dose term with increasing $\overline{y_F}$ is generally observed.

For induction of chromosome aberrations in single dose experiments, maximum RBE values for neutrons at a 67% confidence level are about 15, 20, 40 for 15, 4.2, and 0.5 MeV neutrons, respectively. When the uncertainties for X-rays for the exponentially growing cultures are used, similar maxima are observed for induction of cell inactivation. For a more accurate

Table 6.   Analysis of induction of dicentrics and centric rings in V-79 cells

$$Y = \alpha_a D + \beta_a D^2$$

Type of radiaton	$\alpha_a (Gy^{-1})$	$\beta_a (Gy^{-2})$	
300 kV X rays	0.02 ± 0.01	0.008	single dose
^{137}Cs γ rays	0.04 ± 0.01	0.003	
300 kV X rays	0.021 ± 0.005	0.0007	split dose
^{137}Cs γ rays	0.023 ± 0.005	0.0008	

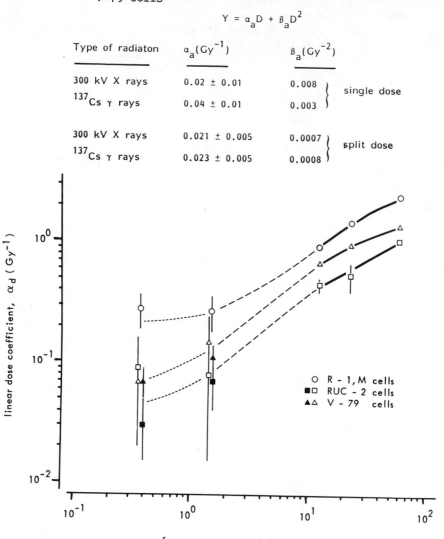

O R - 1, M cells
■□ RUC - 2 cells
▲△ V - 79 cells

Fig. 8. Effectiveness per unit of dose at small doses for induction of cell inactivation in different cell lines as a function of the mean values of the frequency distributions of the lineal energy, $\bar{y}_F$. Only the linear dose coefficients, α_d, are taken into account in the presentation of the results. Open symbols, plateau phase cells; closed symbols, exponentially growing cells. The site diameter for the $\bar{y}_F$ values is 1 μm in unit density tissue.

assessment of RBE values at low doses, modern flow cytometry techniques allowing large numbers of cells to be scored should be used in the future.

DOSIMETRY BASED ON INDUCTION OF CHROMOSOME ABERRATIONS

The induction of chromosome aberrations in cells can be used as a biological dosimetry system. Most investigators (4, 5) employ human

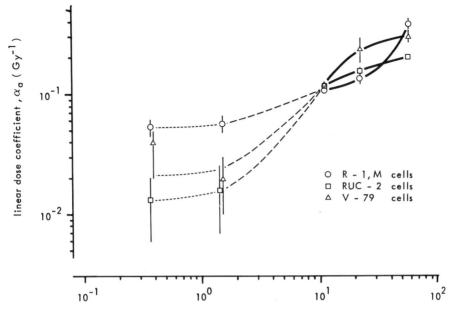

Fig. 9. Effectiveness per unit of dose at small doses for induction of
dicentrics and centric rings in different cell lines as a
function of the mean values of the frequency distributions of
the lineal energy, $\overline{y_F}$. Only the linear dose coefficients, α_a,
are taken into account in the presentation of the results.
The site diameter for the $\overline{y_F}$ values is 1 μm in unit density
tissue.

peripheral blood lymphocytes. The system seems particularly useful for
estimating doses received by people in accidental whole body irradiation.
The detection limits for this application correspond to about 0.05 Gy of X-
rays, 0.1 Gy of gamma rays, and 0.01 Gy of fission neutrons (16). The
technique is summarized in Section 2. The dose estimate for in vivo
conditions is made on the basis of the observed yield of chromosome
aberrations produced in vitro. In general, metaphases are analyzed for
gross chromosome aberrations. In Table 7 a summary of the yield of
dicentrics per cell for different types of radiation is given. It can be
concluded from the table that the yield of dicentrics shows a considerable
variation with the quality of the radiation employed.

In many situations of exposure to ionizing radiation, the dose
distribution over the body will be highly inhomogeneous (especially in
radiotherapy) and lymphocytes from unirradiated and irradiated regions are
mixed, thus giving rise to an underestimation of the absorbed dose (34).
To overcome this problem, a method of estimating the irradiated blood
volume was suggested (35) by testing whether the dicentric distribution in
the cells deviates from a Poisson distribution which could be expected
after homogeneous irradiation. This method seems applicable for photons
(36) but not for example, for neutron irradiation, since even for uniform
irradiation the dicentrics are overdispersed (30). A study of chromosome
damage in patients after therapy with d+T neutrons (34) shows that the
aberration yield in lymphocytes has a significant correlation with the
therapeutic dose. Cytogenetic dosimetry is in principle feasible when
correction factors for specific partial body irradiations are determined.

Table 7. Values of coefficients α_a and β_a for induction of dicentrics in human lymphocytes by different types of radiation *

Type of radiation	dose rate (Gy.min^{-1})	$\alpha \times 10^2$ ($\pm$ st.dev.) (Gy^{-1})	$\beta \times 10^2$ ($\pm$ st.dev.) (Gy^{-2})	reference
^{60}Co γ rays	0.003	1.8 $\pm$ 0.8	2.9 $\pm$ 0.5	28
^{60}Co γ rays	0.5	1.6 $\pm$ 0.3	5.0 $\pm$ 0.2	28
15 MeV electrons	1	0.6 $\pm$ 1.1	5.7 $\pm$ 0.6	29
fission neutrons ($\bar{E}$ = 0.4 MeV)	0.002-0.07	90 $\pm$ 7	-	5
fission neutrons ($\bar{E}$ = 0.7 MeV)	0.5	83 $\pm$ 1	-	5
^{252}Cf neutrons ($\bar{E}$ = 2.13 MeV)	$\sim$ 0.0025	60 $\pm$ 2	-	5
d(16.7)+Be ($\bar{E}$ = 7.6 MeV)	0.3	48 $\pm$ 3	6 $\pm$ 2	5
d + T ($\bar{E}$ = 14.7 MeV)	0.3	26 $\pm$ 4	9 $\pm$ 3	5
d + T ($\bar{E}$ = 15 MeV)	0.12	14.1 $\pm$ 0.7	3.8 $\pm$ 0.1	30
650 MeV neutrons ($\bar{E}$ = 250 MeV) "build-up"	0.003	15 $\pm$ 3	25 $\pm$ 7	31
650 MeV neutrons ($\bar{E}$ = 250 MeV) "build-up"	0.1	7 $\pm$ 4	57 $\pm$ 9	31
650 MeV α rays (peak)	-	14.1**	2.25**	32
Π^- (peak)	$\sim$ 0.02	23 $\pm$ 2	4.8 $\pm$ 0.9	33
Π^- (plateau)	$\sim$ 0.0125	13 $\pm$ 2	2.8 $\pm$ 1.1	33

*doses range generally from about a few tenth of a Gy upto a few Gy

**for 95 percent confidence zones, see reference

A formalism for calculation of the dose to lymphocytes in external beam therapy is available (37).

For partial body irradiations, chromosome aberrations in skin fibroblasts might be used for dose assessments (38). These cells exist for long time periods in the skin and can be stimulated to divide in culture. Chromosomal aberrations have been detected from skin biopsies after therapeutic irradiation (39). The main disadvantages of this technique are the time required for in vitro cell growth between biopsy and cytological examination and the requirement for chromosome banding techniques, since the surviving aberrations are principally symmetrical chromosomal types (38).

CELL TRANSFORMATION IN VITRO BY X-RAYS AND FAST NEUTRONS IN COMPARISON WITH INDUCTION OF CELL INACTIVATION

The available dose-effect relations for the induction of cell reproductive death, chromosome aberrations, morphological transformation and specific mutations in mammalian cells after exposure to radiation of different linear energy transfer (LET) have been reviewed by Barendsen (40). The quantitative evaluation of differences in dose-effect relations for the above mentioned cellular responses is hampered by the fact that the amounts of effects observed can be influenced considerably by various experimental factors including types of cells, cell density, distribution of cells in the cell replication cycle, time interval between irradiation and determination of biological response and criteria employed for the assessment of the biological effect. It could be concluded, however, that cell transformation is much less frequently induced than chromosome aberrations and cell reproductive death by factors ranging from 50 to 100, while mutations are less frequently induced than transformation by factors ranging from 30 to 100.

Cell survival curves and dose-effect curves for transformation have been obtained for C3H10T1/2 cells irradiated with fast neutrons with energies of 0.5 MeV, 4.2 MeV, and 15 MeV and with 300 kV X-rays. The dose-effect relations have been analyzed in terms of values α_t, β_t, α_d and β_d in the equations:

$$F(D) = \alpha_t D + \beta_t D^2 \quad \text{(transformation)} \tag{8}$$

and

$$S(D)/S(0) = \exp-(\alpha_d D + \beta_d D^2) \quad \text{(survival)} \tag{9}$$

The values of the four parameters are presented in Table 8. The estimated accuracy of the RBE values ranges from 10 to 30 percent, mainly due to the uncertainties in estimates of α_d and α_t for X-rays. The values of the parameters were derived as averages from at least three separate experiments. The results obtained from neutrons can be analyzed adequately in terms of linear dose coefficients α_d and α_t only, whereas for photons also the use of quadratic coefficients is required.

The results show that RBE values of neutrons of various energies obtained as ratios of α_d values or α_t values for neutrons relative to those for X-rays are similar for the induction of reproductive death and transformation. Although RBE values for induction of cell transformation and induction of cell reproductive death are similar, in general, a factor of 1000 between frequency of induction of the two types of effect is found.

The results of 0.5 MeV neutrons obtained for C3H10T1/2 cells are less than a factor 2 different from comparable data on fission neutrons published by others (41). This agreement might be fortuitously, considering the differences in exposure conditions.

Table 8. Analysis of induction of cell inactivation and of transformation *in vitro* in C3H/10T1/2 cells by various types of radiation

survival

Type of radiation	α_d (Gy^{-1})	β_d (Gy^{-2})	RBE for α_d
300 kV X rays	0.25	0.036	1
15 MeV neutrons	0.82	0	3
4 MeV neutrons	1.55	0	6
0.5 MeV neutrons	3.26	0	13

transformation

Type of radiation	α_t (Gy^{-1})	β_t (Gy^{-2})	RBE for α_t
300 kV X rays	2×10^{-4}	0.5×10^{-4}	1
15 MeV neutrons	9×10^{-4}	0	5
4 MeV neutrons	13×10^{-4}	0	7
0.5 MeV neutrons	24×10^{-4}	0	12

CONCLUSIONS

o It is essential to study cellular effects of ionizing radiation in different cell lines because of differences in intrinsic radiosensitivity.

o Standardized experimental conditions are required to allow a quantitative intercomparison of frequencies of induction of different types of biological effects.

o The dose-effect relationships for neutrons can, in general, be described adequately by a linear dose term only, whereas for photons, an appreciable contribution from the quadratic dose coefficient is observed.

o Induction of gross chromosome aberrations can explain an appreciable part of induction of cell reproductive death. Particularly when it is taken into account that acentric fragments cannot be scored unambiguously because of their variable size.

o The use of induction of chromosome aberrations in human peripheral blood lymphocytes as a biological dosimetry system in case of total body irradiation requires standardized experimental conditions with regard to cell culturing and growth stimulation. For partial body exposures (human) skin fibroblast systems seem advantageous.

o RBE values of neutrons of specified energy for the various cellular endpoints seem quite similar although variation among different cell lines are considerable. The largest RBE values are observed for 0.5 MeV neutrons, showing a value, at low doses, of about 13.

o Risk estimates, related to effects at small doses of ionizing radiation, should be made on the basis of linear dose terms obtained from dose-effect relations employing modern flow cytometry techniques allowing the scoring of large numbers of cells.

ACKNOWLEDGEMENTS

The experimental studies at TNO have been supported by the Commission of the European Communities under Contract Number BIO-A-300-81-NL. Figures 5, 6, and 7 have been reproduced from the Int. J. Radiat. Biol. with permission from Taylor and Francis publishers. The efficient assistance of Messrs. A. C. Engels, C. J. Bouts and N. J. P. de Wit in the neutron and photon irradiations and of Messrs. W. C. Kuypers and J. F. Gaiser in the biological experiments, of Mrs. J. Smit in the typing of the manuscript and of Mr. J.Ph. de Kler in the preparation of the figures is gratefully acknowledged.

REFERENCES

1. A. M. Kellerer and H. H. Rossi, RBE and the primary radiation action, Radiat. Res. 47:15-34 (1971).

2. G. W. Barendsen, C. J. Koot, G. R. van Kersen, D. K. Bewley, S. B. Field, and C. J. Parnell, The effect of oxygen on impairment of the proliferative capacity of human cells in culture by ionizing radiations of different LET, Int. J. Radiat. Biol. 10:317-327 (1966).

3. J. J. Broerse, G. W. Barendsen, J. F. Gaiser, and J. Zoetelief, The importance of differences in intrinsic cellular radiosensitivity for the effectiveness of neutron radiotherapy treatments, in: "Radiobiological Research and Radiotherapy, Vol. 2," IAEA, Vienna, (1977), pp. 19-29.

4. N. Vulpis, L. Tognacci, and G. Scarpa, Chromosome aberrations as a dosimetric technique for fission neutrons over the dose range 0.2-50 rad, Int. J. Radiat. Biol. 33:301-306 (1978).

5. D. C. Lloyd, R. J. Purrott, G. W. Dolphin, and A. A. Edwards, Chromosome aberrations induced in human lymphocytes by neutron irradiation, Int. J. Radiat. Biol. 29:169-182 (1976).

6. R. Sager, Transposable elements and chromosomal rearrangements in cancer - a possible link, Nature 282:447-448 (1979).

7. S. J. Grote, Radiation-induced lethality and genetic damage in mammalian cells, Thesis, University of London (1971).

8. S. J. Grote, G. P. Joshi, S. H. Revell, and C. A. Shaw, Observations of radiation-induced chromosome fragment loss in live mammalian cells in culture, and its effect on colony-forming ability, Int. J. Radiat. Biol. 39:395-408 (1981).

9. A. V. Carrano, Chromosome aberrations and radiation-induced cell death, Mutat. Res. 17:341-366 (1973).

10. J. Tremp, Chromosome aberrations and cell survival in irradiated mammalian cells, Radiat. Res. 85:554-566 (1981).

11. G. W. Barendsen, H. C. Janse, B. F. Deys, and C. F. Hollander, Comparison of growth characteristics of experimental tumours and derived cell cultures, Cell Tissue Kinet. 10:469-475 (1977).

12. United Nations Scientific Committee on the Effects of Atomic Radiation, in: "Radiation-induced Chromosome Aberrations in Human Cells," General Assembly 24th Session, No. 13, (A/7613), Annex C, United Nations, New York (1969).

13. T. T. Puck, P. J. Marcus, and S. J. Cieciura, Clonal growth of mammalian cells in vitro, J. Exp. Med. 103:273-283 (1956).

14. M. W. Kooi, J. Stap, and G. W. Barendsen, Proliferation kinetics of cultured cells after irradiation with X-rays and 14 MeV neutrons studied by time-lapse photography, Int. J. Radiat. Biol. 45:583-592 (1984).

15. P. P. W. van Buul and A. T. Natarajan, Chromosomal radiosensitivity of human leucocytes in relation to sampling time, Mutat. Res. 70:61-69 (1980).

16. R. J. Purrott, N. Vulpis, and D. C. Lloyd, Chromosome dosimetry: The influence of culture media on the proliferation of irradiated and unirradiated human lymphocytes, Radiat. Prot. Dos. 1:203-208 (1981).

17. P. P. W van Buul, R. Ricordy, F. Spirito, and A. D. Tates, The symmetry of radiation-induced chromatid exchanges in Chinese hamster cells in vivo and in vitro, Mutat. Res. 50:377-382 (1978).

18. C. Borek, E. J. Hall, and H. H. Rossi, Malignant transformation in cultured hamster embryo cells produced by X-rays, 430 keV monoenergetic neutrons and heavy ions, Cancer Res. 38:2997-3005 (1978).

19. A. C. Reznikoff, J. S. Bertram, D. W. Brankow, and C. Heidelberger, Qualitative and quantitative studies of chemical transformation of cloned C3H mouse embryo cells sensitive to postconfluence inhibition of cell division, Cancer Res. 33:3239-3249 (1973).

20. M. Terzaghi and J. B. Little, X-radiation-induced transformation in a C3H mouse embryo-derived cell line, Cancer Res. 36:1367-1374 (1976).

21. J. Zoetelief and G. W. Barendsen, Dose-effect relationships for induction of cell inactivation and asymmetrical chromosome exchanges in three cell lines by photons and neutrons of different energy, Int. J. Radiat. Biol. 43:349-362 (1983).

22. ICRU, Report 30, "Quantitative Concepts and Dosimetry in Radiobiology," ICRU, Washington (1979).

23. P. R. Bevington, "Data Reduction and Error Analysis for the Physical Sciences," McGraw-Hill, New York (1969).

24. C. J. Roberts and P. D. Holt, The production of chromosome aberrations in Chinese hamster fibroblasts by gamma and neutron radiation, Int. J. Radiat. Biol. 41:645-656 (1982).

25. J. Zoetelief, B. Hogeweg, and J. J. Broerse, Radiation quality and absorbed dose at different positions in the primary beam and around the shielding of a neutron generator, in: "Proc. 6th Symposium on Microdosimetry, EUR 6064," J. Booz and H. G. Ebert, eds., Commission of the European Communities (1978), pp. 615-627.

26. ICRP Publication 26, "Annals of the ICRP," Pergamon Press, Oxford (1977).

27. J. Booz, Mapping of fast neutron radiation quality, in: "Proc. 3rd Symposium on Neutron Dosimetry in Biology and Medicine, EUR 5848," G. Burger and H. G. Ebert, eds., Commission of the European Communities (1978), pp. 499-514.

28. D. C. Lloyd, R. J. Purrott, G. W. dolphin, D. Bolton, A. A. Edwards, and M. J. Corp, The relationship between chromosome aberrations and low LET radiation dose to human lymphocytes, Int. J. Radiat. Biol. 28:75-90 (1975).

29. R. J. Purrott, E. J. Reeder, and S. Lovell, Chromosome aberration yield in human lymphocytes by 15 MeV electrons given at a conventional dose rate and in microsecond pulses, Int. J. Radiat. Biol. 31:251-256. (1977).

30. E. Schmid and M. Bauchinger, Chromosome aberrations in human lymphocytes after irradiation with 15.0 MeV neutrons in vitro II: Analysis of the number of absorption events and the interaction distance in the formation of dicentric chromosomes, Mutat. Res. 27:111-117 (1975).

31. N. Vulpis and M. Bianchi, Chromosome aberrations induced in human lymphocytes by 600 MeV neutrons, Radiat. Prot. Dos. 3:103-106 (1982).

32. N. Parmentier, M. Guichard, M. T. Deloy, and J. Brenot, Modele biophysique applique a la survie des cellules tumorales et a la formation d'abberations chromosomiques dans les lymphocytes humains, in: Proc. 5th Symposium on Microdosimetry, EUR 5452," J. Booz and H. G. Ebert, eds. Commission of the European Communities, Luxembourg (1975), pp. 719-740.

33. R. J. Purrott, Chromosome aberrations yields in human lymphocytes exposed to fractionated doses of negative pi mesons, Int. J. Radiat. Biol. 28:599-602 (1975).

34. E. Schmid, J. Dresp, M. Bauchinger, H. D. Franke, G. Langendorff, and A. Hess, Radiation induced chromosome damage after tumour therapy with 14 MeV, DT neutrons, Int. J. Radiat. Biol. 38:691-695 (1980).

35. G. W. Dolphin, D. C. Lloyd, and R. J. Purrott, Chromosome aberration analysis as a dosimetric technique in radiological protection, Health Phys. 25:7-15 (1973).

36. S. Kuttner-May and H. Traut, Strahlentherapeutisch induzierte chromosomenaberrationen: Untersuchungen zur 'Biologischen Dosimetrie', Strahlentherapie 157:607-612 (1981).

37. K. E. Ekstrand, R. L. Dixon, S. Plunkett, and M. Raben, The calculation of dose to human lymphocytes in external beam radiation therapy, Radiat. Res. 85:399-407 (1981).

38. D. Couzin, Frequency changes with time in vivo of radiation-induced chromosomal aberrations in skin fibroblasts, Mutat. Res. 60:367-380 (1979).

39. J. K. R. Savage and T. R. L. Bigger, Aberration distribution and chromosomally marked clones in X-irradiated skin, in: "Mutagen-induced Chromosome Damage in Man," H. J. Evans and D. C. Lloyd (Edinburgh University Press, Edinburgh (1978), pp. 155-159.

40. G. W. Barendsen, Dose-effect relationships for various responses of mammalian cells to radiation of different linear energy transfer, J. Soc. Radiol. Prot. 4:143-152 (1984).

41. H. M. Elkind, A. Han, and C. K. Hill, Error-free and error-prone repair in radiation-induced neoplastic cell transformation, in: "Radiation Carcinogenesis: Epidemiology and Biological Significance," J. D. Boice and J. F. Fraumeni, Raven Press, New York (1984), pp. 303-318.

RADIATION INDUCED TRANSFORMATION IN PRIMARY DIFFERENTIATED THYROID CULTURES

C. B. Seymour and C. Mothersill

Saint Luke's Hospital
Rathgar, Dublin 6, Ireland

ABSTRACT

A technique has been developed where long-term differentiated cell cultures can be established from human and animal (sheep) thyroid glands. The cultures retain morphological and functional characteristics of _in vivo_ thyroid tissue. These include iodide trapping, T_4 production and PAS positive follicle development. The cultures have been irradiated and subcultured to provide data on survival following exposure to various doses of ^{125}Iodide or ^{60}Cobalt. More recently, a technique has been developed which allows the development of several endpoints of _in vitro_ transformation to be monitored in the irradiated cultures.

The system provides one of the first opportunities to study radiation transformation in primary differentiated cultures of epithelial origin.

INTRODUCTION

One of the major problems limiting research into the mechanisms of radiation transformation is the lack of suitable models for study. Most available cellular transformation systems use rodents cell lines which are undifferentiated and of fibroblast origin. While quantitative data can undoubtedly be obtained using these systems, they are obviously not ideal for the study of human cancer induction by radiation. An essential requirement for this would appear to be an epithelial cell system since the great majority of human cancers are of epithelial origin. Other advantageous properties would be differentiated characteristics, lack of spontaneous transformation and a susceptibility for the intact organ to develop cancer following irradiation.

A system which fulfills most of these requirements was developed in our laboratory some years ago (O'Connor et al. 1980; Mothersill et al. 1981, 1984 a,b; Murphy et al. 1983). Using sheep or human thyroid glands, cultures can be established which retain a large number of characteristics of the _in vivo_ gland.

The thyroid is an organ of particular interest in the study of radiation effects on tissue for several reasons, e.g., the well documented association between childhood irradiation and increased incidence of thyroid tumours (Duffy & Fitzgerald, 1955; Simpson & Hempelmann, 1957; Rooney & Powell, 1959), the increased incidence of thyroid cancer among A-bomb survivors from Hiroshima and Nagasaki (Parker et al. 1973; Ezaki et al. 1983) and the occurrence of significant levels of airborne [125]Iodine in accidental emissions from nuclear power plants. These factors and the availability of a good basic culture system led us to try to develop a technique for the study of radiation transformation in thyroid cultures.

METHODS

Primary Culture of Thyroid Glands

The method used for the primary culture of sheep and human thyroid cells has been described in detail previously (O'Connor et al. 1980; Mothersill et al. 1984).

The growth medium normally used is Basal Medium (Eagle's (BME) with added insulin, hydrocortisone and TSH (40 mIU/ml). Other basic media successfully used include the following: Dulbecco's Modified Medium, Nutrient Mixture F-12 (Ham's), Modified Essential Medium (Eagle's), McCoy's Medium and Leibowitz Medium. These were all found to give cultures similar to those obtained with BME, provided the additives remained constant (Murphy et al. 1983.)

Iodide Trapping and T_4 Production

Iodide trapping and T_4 production were measured as described previously (Mothersill & Seymour 1984). Results were corrected for passive diffusion of iodine using the non thyroid established CHO-KI line.

Radiation Survival Curves and Transformation Assay

Survival of irradiated thyroid cells was determined using the clonogenic technique of Puck & Marcus (1956). Monolayer cultures were irradiated after 10-15 days. Cells were removed from the dishes immediately using trypsin (0.25%) and versene (1 mM 1:1 V/V). The resulting cell suspension was counted using a Coulter counter and an appropriate number of cells was added to fresh medium such that the expected number of survivors was 50-100 cells. The cells were allowed to plate and grow to form macroscopic colonies which were counted after 10 days and used to calculate the surviving fraction.

The transformation assay is performed on the same or similar cultures used for radiation survival experiments but new flasks were seeded with 0.5 x 1.0 x 10^6 cells. These were repeatedly allowed to grow to confluence and then subcultured using the same procedure.

The development of transformed characteristics was monitored during the repeated subculturings of the irradiated cell population. After 3-4 subcultures the control cells senesced. The irradiated cells continued to grow and were monitored for reduced serum dependence (ability to grow in medium containing 1% serum) and ability to grow in soft agar at the third and subsequent passages. The technique used for determination of growth in soft agar was that described by Kruse and Patterson (1973).

Tests performed to ensure that the cells were epithelial are described in Mothersill & Seymour (1984).

RESULTS

Survival Studies

The effect of increasing doses of Cobalt γ-rays on the survival of differentiated human and sheep thyroid cells is shown in Figure 1. Human thyroid cells are in general more sensitive than sheep but both have Do values in the usual range for mammalian cells, i.e., 1.0 - 1.6 Gy for human and ∿2.0 Gy for sheep.

When a single dose of radiation is split, the results for sheep (Figure 2) indicate that a recovery factor of approximately 5 is obtained. This is unexpectedly high in view of the extrapolation number of approximately 2 obtained for the single dose survival curve.

An important source of radiation damage to the thyroid is radioactive iodine. In experiments using long-term exposure to ^{125}I as a radiation source in this culture system a characteristic β particle survival curve with no shoulder was produced (Figure 3). Using a standard form of dose

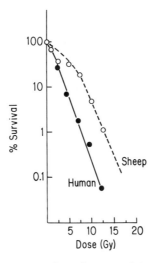

Fig. 1. Survival curves for sheep and human thyroid cells irradiated as a 10 day old monolayer.

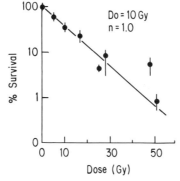

Fig. 2. Recovery curve for sheep thyroid cells irradiated as a 10 day old monolayer.

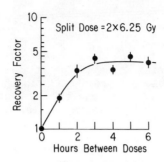

Fig. 3. Survival curve for sheep thyroid cells irradiated
over 7 days with ^{125}I

calculation the Do was calculated to be 10 Gy, representing a reduced RBE
(by a factor of 5). However, the iodine was left on the cultures for seven
days, in order to better simulate the in vivo situation, and this probably
makes it difficult to reconcile the γ and ^{125}I doses for this particular
culture system. These results represent the first attempts in vitro to
produce a survival curve using radioactive iodine.

TRANSFORMATION STUDIES

Development of Transformed Characteristics by Irradiated Cells

Application of the transformation technique to differentiated cultures
of sheep thyroid cells irradiated to 10 Gy with gamma rays 10 days after
plating resulted in the development of three of the four transformation
endpoints within four subcultures. The first indication of transformation
is non-senescence or 'immortalization'. Unirradiated controls senesced
after 3-4 subcultures.

The frequency of 'immortalization' as an event in irradiated cultures
was examined by plating cells (10,000-50,000) at each passage and counting
the number which gave rise to clones. The results (Table 1) indicate that
the control unirradiated cells show a decline in cloning efficiency at
passage 3 and have senesced by passage 4. Irradiated cells maintain a
cloning efficiency of ∿1% from passage 1 through passage 4.

Irradiated flasks containing the non-senescent cells were divided into
two groups. Half were maintained as confluent monolayers in an air

Table 1. Cloning efficiency for thyroid cells at each passages from 1-
4 after irradiation as primary differetiated cultures.
Results expressed as mean ± S.E. (n = 3)

Radiation Dose (Gy)	Cloning efficiency % (Passage Nos. 1-4)			
	1	2	3	4
0	1.57±0.3	1.75±0.35	0.43±0.06	0
2.5	1.45±0.2	1.9 ±0.2	1.5 ±0.2	1.2 ±0.15
5.0	0.77±0.1	0.96±0.15	1.0 ±0.15	0.68±0.08
7.5	0.23±0.03	0.73±0.1	0.65±0.06	1.14±0.2

incubator at passage 4 or 5 with twice weekly medium changes. These developed loss of contact inhibition, shown by characteristic piled up foci after 2-3 weeks. The foci develop on an epithelial like monolayer and have edges corresponding to the epithelial foci described by Klein (1976). The average number of foci detected per flask (n = 100) in a typical experiment was 8 with a range over the hundred flasks of 1-13. After counting the foci the cells were trypsinized, shaken vigorously and filtered through fine mesh to ensure a single cell suspension. They were then plated on soft agar at a density of 1 x 10^4. Plates were maintained in a CO_2 incubator and supplementary growth medium (1.5 ml) was added on day 7. After about 12 days soft agar colonies $\sim$0.5 mm diameter could be seen. The average transformation frequency determined over four separate experiments by expressing the number of colonies as a per cent of the initial cell number plated is 0.0035. This should be taken as an upper limit, as irradiated but non-transformed cells will probably have senesced before soft agar growth is apparent in the transformed population. The growth rate of the transformed cell population could also be expected to exceed the growth of non-transformed cells.

To check for serum dependence the remaining half of the cultures were subcultured regularly into medium containing 1% serum. Low serum tolerance developed after loss of contact inhibition and anchorage dependence at passage 7-8.

Development of Transformation Markers in the Irradiated Population

Irradiated and control cells were screened at each passage for the development of an oncogene product (P53) and for shifts in the LD isozyme pattern, characteristics which are often associated with malignant cells.

Primary results (Table 2) indicate that the LD pattern does shift towards the more anaerobic profile following a high radiation dose. No effect of irradiation on P53 production was noted.

DISCUSSION

One of the major advantages of this system is that it allows both radiation survival and transformation to be monitored on the same cell population. Using the technique it can be shown that the survival of both sheep and human thyroid cells exposed to ionizing radiation lies within the range obtained for other mammalian systems. The few human samples examined show a very high sensitivity to radiation with Do's in the range 1-1.6 Gy with very little evidence of a shoulder on the survival curve.

The technique described here allows four characteristics of transformed cells to be detected in thyroid cultures and should prove useful in the study of transformation in primary epithelial cell lines and primary differentiated cultures. The first indication of transformation is non-senescence or 'immortalization'. This is described by Newbold et al. (1982) as a rare but early event in Syrian hamster embryo fibroblast transformation and has been shown to be an essential prerequisite for transformation with certain ras oncogenes (Land et al. 1983; Newbold & Overell 1983). Our system would appear to show that immortalization is a very frequent event among the clonogenic subpopulation of differentiated thyroid cell cultures since the cloning efficiency of irradiated cells at passage 4 is close to that of controls prior to senescence. This would support other work using radiation as a carcinogen. It has been shown using both the C3H 10T1/2 transformation system (Hall et al. 1982; Kennedy & Little 1984) and the in vivo rat thyroid system (Mulcahy et al. 1984) that the first step in the process leading to transformation is a very

Table 2. Relative amounts of isoenzymes of lactate dehydrogenase (LD) detected in irradiated and control
thyroid cells at passages 1-3

Passage	Dose	LD1	LD2	LD3	LD4	LD5
1	0	0.8	13.6	47.0	37.0	–
	10 Gy	–	13.1	56.9	30.0	–
2	0	–	14.0	47.3	38.7	–
	10 Gy	1.71	28.8	28.2	15.5	10.5
3	0	3.4	15.8	60.8	20.0	–
	10 Gy	1.3	8.6	31.9	35.4	22.8

common event following irradiation. Senescence occurs early in control thyroid cultures, confirming results published by Dumont et al. (1980) showing that thyroid cells in the animal or human normally undergo only about 15 divisions. The occurrence of senescence at an early stage makes the assay useful where quantitative correlation is desired between the carcinogenic stimulus and the transformation endpoint. The development of several piled up foci occurs at the first passage after senescence of the controls. The foci are similar to the characteristic epithelial foci described by Klein (1976) and unlike the fibroblast foci do not show criss-crossing at the edges. Anchorage independence shown by soft agar growth occurs at the passage where focus formation occurs but it is interesting that the reduced serum dependence does not occur for several passages after that. This finding is in contrast to that of Newbold (personal communication, 1983), who found reduced serum dependence to be an early indication of transformation in hamster dermis cultures.

Since there is considerable evidence that transformation is a multi-stage process (Albert & Burns 1977), the technique should prove useful as it allows the factors controlling several transformation endpoints to be independently studied. This is in contrast to many other transformation assays (Martin & Anderson 1976; Reznikoff et al. 1973). These assays use mainly rodent fibroblast cells which spontaneously transform eventually (Paul 1975) and generally only demonstrate one transformation endpoint which can be easily monitored under experimental conditions (Klein 1976). This leads to the possibility that peculiarities of the system are involved in addition to basic transformation mechanisms.

Further development of the technique will include attempts to produce tumours in nude mice by inoculation of potentially transformed thyroid cells and the study of tumour marker production as the transformation process develops.

REFERENCES

1. R. E. Albert, F. J. Burns, Carcinogenic atmospheric pollutants and the nature of low level risk, in: "Origins of Human Cancer, Vol. 4, Book A," H. H. Hiatt, J. D. Watson, and J. A. Winsten, eds., Cold Spring Harbor Lab., Cold Spring Harbor, New York (1977), pp. 289-292.

2. B. J. Duffy, Jr. and P. J. Fitzgerald, Cancer of the thyroid in children, a report of 28 cases. *Journal of Clinical Endocrinology* 10: 1296 (1955).

3. J. E. Dumont, J. F. Malone, and A. J. Van Herle, "Irradiation and Thyroid Disease: Dosimetric, Clinical and Carcinogenic Aspects," Commission of the European Communities Publication No. Eur 6713 en. (1980).

4. T. Ezaki, K. Yaguwa, Y. Hayashi, T. Nishida and T. Ishmaru, *J. Jap. Pract. Surg. Soc.* 144(9): 1127 (1983).

5. E. J. Hall, H. H. Rossi, M. Zaider, R. C. Miller, and C. Borek, *in*: "Neutron Carcinogenesis," J. J. Broerse and G. B. Gerber, eds., Commission of the European Communities, Luxemburg (1982), pg. 381-405.

6. A. R. Kennedy, J. Cairns, and J. B. Little, Timing of the steps in transformation of C3H 10T1/2 cells by X-irradiation, *Nature* 307:85-86 (1984).

7. J. C. Klein, The use of *in vitro* methods for the study of X-ray induced transformation, *in*: "Biology of Radiation Carcinogenesis," J. M. Yuhas, R. W. Tennant, and J. D. Regan, eds., Raven Press, New York (1976), p. 301.

8. P. F. Kruse and M. K. Patterson, "Tissue Culture: Methods and Applications," Academic Press, New York (1973).

9. R. Land, L. F. Parada, and R. A. Weinberg, Tumorigenic conversion of primary embryo fibroblasts requires at least two cooperating oncogenes, *Nature* 304:597-602.

10. R. G. Martin and J. L. Anderson, Death and transformation, *in*: "Biology of Radiation Carcinogenesis," J. M. Yuhas, R. W. Tennant, and J. D. Regan, eds, Raven Press, New York (1976), p. 287

11. C. Mothersill, A. Murphy, M. K. O'Connor, C. B. Seymour, and J. F. Malone, A role for lactate in the differentiation of cultured sheep thyroid cells, *Cell Biol. Int. Reports* 5(9):877-886 (1981).

12. C. Mothersill, C. B. Seymour, and J. F. Malone, Maintenance of differentiated sheep thyroid cells in culture for 3 months, *Acta Endocrinologica* 107:54-59 (1984).

13. C. Mothersill, C. B. Seymour, M.J. Moriarty and M.J. Cullen, Longterm culture of human differentiated thyroid cells, *Acta Endocrinologica*, 108:192199 (1985).

14. C. Mothersill and C. Seymour, Development of transformed characteristics by sheep thyroid cells irradiated as differentiated primary cultures, *Cell Biol. Int. Reports*, 8(10):887896 (1984).

15. R. T. Mulcahy, M. N. Gould, and K. H. Clifton, Radiogenic initiation of thyroid cancer: a common cellular event, *Int. J. Radiat. Biol.* 45(5):419-426 (1984).

16. A. Murphy, C. Mothersill, M. K. O'Connor, J. F. Malone, M. J. Cullen, and J. K. Taaffe, An investigation of the optimum culture conditions for a differentiated culture of sheep thyroid cells, Acta Endocrinoligica 104:431-436 (1983).

17. R. F. Newbold and R. W. Overell, Fibroblast immortality is a prerequisite for transformation by EJ c-Ha-ras oncogenes, Nature 304:648-651 (1983).

18. R. F. Newbold, R. W. Overell, and J. F. Connell, Induction of immortality is an early event in malignant transformation of mammalian cells by carcinogens, Nature 229:633-635 (1982).

19. M. K. O'Connor, M. J. Cullen, and J. F. Malone, Long-term culture of sheep thyroid cells, Acta Endocrinol. 93, Suppl. 231 (1980).

20. L. N. Parker, J. L. Belsky, T. Mandai, W. Blot and R. Kawate, Serum thyrotropin level and goitre in relation to childhood exposure to atomic radiation. J. Clin. Endocrinol. & Metab. 37: 797 (1973).

21. J. Paul, "Cell and Tissue Culture, 5 Edition," Churchill Livingstone, Edinburgh, New York and London (1965).

22. T. T. Puck and P. I. Marcus, Action of X-rays on mammalian cells, J. Exp. Med. 103:653-666 (1956).

23. C. A. Reznikoff, J. S. Bertram, D. W. Brankow, and C. Heidelberger, Quantitative and qualitative studies of chemical transformation of cloned C3H mouse embryo cells sensitive to post-confluence inhibition of division, Cancer Res. 33:3239 (1973).

23. E. R. Rooney and R. W. Powell, Carcinoma of the thyroid in children after Xray therapy in early childhood. J. Am. Med. Assoc. 169: 1 (1959).

24. C. L. Simpson and L. H. Hemplemann, The association of tumours and Roentgen ray treatment of the thorax in infancy. Cancer 10: 42 (1957).

THE INDUCTION AND REPAIR OF ULTRAVIOLET LIGHT DAMAGE IN MAMMALIAN CELLS

A. M. Rauth

Physics Division
Ontario Cancer Institute
Department of Medical Biophysics
University of Toronto
500 Sherbourne Street
Toronto, Ontario M4X 1K9
Canada

INTRODUCTION

Ultraviolet light (UV) has been extensively used as a damage inducing agent in mammalian cells in in vitro cell cultures. The wavelengths studied have been primarily in the range of 200-300 nm where deoxyribonucleic acid (DNA) absorbs most strongly. In the present article a review will be made of the major effects of UV in this wavelength range on such in vitro systems in terms of: (1) damage production; (2) cell survival and mutation; (3) the role of various repair processes in modifying the induced damage; and, finally, (4) the carcinogenic process. An attempt will be made to indicate to some degree where these effects of UV differ from those of ionizing radiation and to point out some unique features of mammalian cells compared to bacterial systems where the models for understanding UV effects have originated. Due to the breadth of the material covered, extensive reference has been made to review articles which summarize the original work. The references cited are in no way complete and only represent an introduction to the original literature. In particular, extensive use of the following reviews has been made (1-11).

Basic Energy Absorption Processes - Ionizing Radiation Compared to UV Radiation

When a monoenergetic beam of electrons passes through a thin plastic film, approximating biological material, it loses energy. If the film is thin enough (10 nm) and the beam energetic enough (20 Kev), the electrons, on the average, undergo only a single energy loss event with the electrons in the film. The most probable energy loss event is around 20 ev; few energy losses occur below 5 ev and there is a finite but diminishing probability of higher energy losses (12) (Figure 1). Thus, the initial energy loss events are large relative to the energy of chemical bonds, proportional to the electron density of the specimen and random throughout the sample. In the case of DNA in an aqueous solution, primary energy loss events can occur directly in the DNA or in the water surrounding the DNA. The energy losses in the water can produce reactive water radicals ($OH^{\cdot}$, e_{aq}^{-}

217

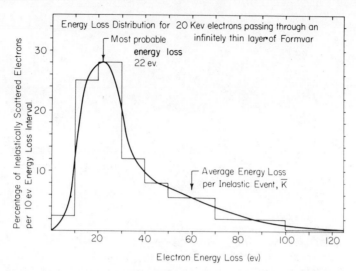

Fig. 1. The "first-collision" energy loss distribution of
electrons passing through a "biologically equivalent"
solid, redrawn from reference 12.

and H·) which can diffuse and react with DNA. As a result of these
processes, strand breaks and base damage occur (13).

In contrast, UV in the range 200-300 nm, far UV, or 300-400 nm, near
UV, deposits energy in absorbing chromophores in the range of 6-3 ev. In
the case of DNA in aqueous solution, absorption of photons in the range of
200-300 nm results in the excitation of pyrimidine bases to a singlet state
which can react directly with water to form pyrimidine hydrates or the
excited singlets can undergo intrasystem crossing to a longer lived triplet
state. Reactions from the triplet state with neighbouring pyrimidines can
give rise to pyrimidine dimers of the cyclobutane dimer type (thymine-
thymine, cytosine-thymine, or cytosine-cytosine) (Figure 2) as well as
other dimer linkages (14). Because of their chemical stability, these
dimers remain in the DNA and can be directly measured. The hydrates are
much more unstable and can dehydrate, resulting in the return to the
original pyrimidine or in the case of cytosine a deaminated derivative
(14). The reaction of excited pyrimidines with other molecules such as
amino acids can occur in model systems and evidence for DNA-protein
crosslinks in cells has been obtained (15, 16). Nevertheless, the initial
lesion that has been most extensively monitored in biological systems is
the cyclobutane pyrimidine dimer. Thus, the initial lesions formed in
biological material by ionizing radiation and UV radiation are quite
different in both their type and distribution throughout the cell. This
difference is reflected in differences in the cellular and molecular
behavior of cells exposed to these radiations.

Exposing Cells to Ultraviolet Light Radiation

Ultraviolet light is strongly absorbed by most glass and plastics, and
in the growth medium used for mammalian cells. Thus for cell irradiations
where absolute dosimetry is important, it is necessary to either suspend or
cover cells with aqueous buffer with no absorption in the UV range of
interest or carry out appropriate dosimetry to correct for absorption by
the medium (17, 18). It may also be necessary to consider the absorption
and scattering of UV light by the mammalian cells themselves. A single
cell with a diameter of 10-20 microns, a thousand fold the volume of a
typical bacterium, can have a decrease in UV intensity within it due to

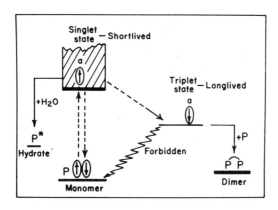

Fig. 2. Schematic diagram of the excitation of pyrimidine
         (P) by UV light to yield dimers and hydrates.

absorption by nucleic acid and protein. This can cause a decrease in dose
through the cell of 20-40% for UV wavelengths of 265 nm (2, 17). This
problem is diminished when cells are irradiated as monolayers and the cell
is flattened out. The UV source used for most irradiation is a low
pressure mercury lamp (germicidal lamp) with over 90% of its output at
253.7 nm in the UV range (18). The most common way of varying dose rate is
to vary the distance of the cells from UV light or the use of neutral
filters.

Survival of Mammalian Cells Exposed to UV Light

     In contrast to bacteria, mammalian cells are slower growing with
typical doubling times of 10-30 hours. Their interphase cell cycle can be
divided into G_1, S, G_2, and M phases on the basis of when DNA is being
synthesized during the cell cycle. For many mammalian cells the DNA
synthetic phase, S, is 6-8 hours long, mitosis, M, 0.5-1.0 hours, G_2, the
post DNA synthetic phase, 2-4 hours long with the balance of the cell cycle
being taken up by the pre-DNA synthetic G_1 phase.

     When asynchronous populations of mammalian cells are exposed to UV
irradiation and the survival of their colony forming ability determined, a
survival curve is obtained with a shoulder and an exponential final slope
when plotted on a log survival versus dose scale. Representative D_0's for
such curves are in the range of 2-6 J/m^2 (17). However, these D_0's are
typically those of the most resistant subpopulations. When survival is
determined for synchronized cell populations, a substantial degree of
variation occurs throughout the cell cycle. For several different cell
lines, this is seen as cells early in S phase being most sensitive to
radiation and cells in late S phase being most resistant and increasing
sensitivity occurring through G_2, M, and G_1 to early S phase (17). The
major delays in cell progression about the cell cycle appear to be in the
passage of damaged cells through S phase (17). In general, this pattern of
sensitivity is not the same as seen for ionizing radiation and there is
little evidence of G_2 delays for UV irradiated cells that are seen for
ionizing radiation (19).

     The production of pyrimidine dimers can be directly measured in
mammalian cells by a variety of techniques (20). Over the dose range used
for most biological studies with mammalian cells, dimers are produced
linearly with dose. At high UV doses, an equilibrium is established
between dimer formation and reversal by UV light. The equilibrium is
wavelength dependent (14). There have been reports of increased production

of dimers in S phase compared to G_1 or G_2 phase (21-23) but this is not always seen (24). In general, the variations in dimer production about the cell cycle do not appear adequate to explain the difference in survival seen (25). It is usually assumed that pyrimidine dimers are produced at random in the DNA of UV irradiated cells but it has been pointed out that the measurements do not distinguish between a true random distribution and local damage in regions that are themselves randomly distributed (1).

The relative effectiveness of different wavelengths of UV light to inactivate the colony forming ability of a variety of rodent and human cells in vitro has been measured by a number of different groups. The work has recently been reviewed and summarized (2). One can express the relative response per photon as a function of the wavelength of the mono-chromatic light used to irradiate the cells. It is concluded that in the wavelength region, 230-302 nm, cell killing for the cell lines studied irradiated either in the growing or quiescent "growth arrested" state can be associated with damage to DNA. In particular, there is a very close correspondence between the action spectra for pyrimidine dimer production and mammalian cell inactivation. It might be noted, however, that, to the degree that the lethal damage produced arises from an initial excitation of pyrimidine bases, the reaction of such excited bases with other cellular components such as proteins might equally well explain the lethal effects of radiation. The action spectra for such other products have not been determined.

Early indirect evidence for the occurrence of repair of UV damage in mouse L cells was obtained by using caffeine, a known inhibitor of bacterial repair processes (7). Ultraviolet light irradiated cells, plated for their colony forming ability in the presence of millimolar amounts of the drug, had a much lower survival than control cells. The major effect of caffeine was to reduce the shoulder of the survival curve. For this cell line, little effect of caffeine was seen on the survival of cells exposed to ionizing radiation (26). By carrying out experiments in which caffeine was added to or withdrawn from irradiated cells at various times after UV irradiation, the conclusion was reached that the time at which caffeine acted was when the UV damaged cell passed through its first S phase after UV irradiation. This implied that an S phase dependent recovery process was sensitive to the presence of caffeine. Some subsequent studies with other mouse cell lines showed similar effects with caffeine. However, the effect of caffeine is far from universal for all cell lines (7). Some Chinese hamster lines and many human cell lines failed to show a potentiation of UV damage at the level of cell survival when post-irradiation incubation was carried out in the presence of caffeine. Thus, in various cell lines there appears to be either a differential sensitivity of an S phase dependent recovery process to caffeine or a differential balance between two or more repair processes, one sensitive and one resistant to caffeine (7).

More recently, it has become apparent that caffeine can also alter the sensitivity of a variety of human and mouse cell lines to ionizing radia-tion but this effect appears to be quite different in its mechanism and cycle specificity than the effect of caffeine on UV irradiated cells (27). It appears that at lower levels of caffeine (1-2 mM) its effect is to inhibit the repair of X-ray induced lesions that are expressed in G_2 phase. This might occur either due to an inhibition of the radiation induced mitotic delay decreasing the time for lesion management or direct inhibi-tion of a repair process (28, 29). Inhibition of this delay by caffeine results in decreased cell survival and an increased production of chromo-some aberrations even after high linear energy transfer radiation (30).

Additional evidence for an S phase specific recovery from UV damage

can be demonstrated in rodent cells by irradiating synchronized populations
of cells at various points in the cell cycle and testing the response of
surviving cells to a second dose of radiation at various times after giving
the first dose. Recovery from damage, as indicated by a return of the
normal shoulder on the cell survival curve, requires the cell to progress
through S phase (31-33).

Overview of Repair Mechanisms

Three major modes of repair of pyrimidine dimers have been looked for
and found to varying degrees in mammalian cells (1, 4, 5). They are
photoreactivation, excision repair and post replication repair. They are
illustrated in Figure 3. Photoreactivation appears absolutely specific for
cyclobutane pyrimidine dimers produced by UV light. The photoreactivation
enzyme binds to dimers and in the presence of visible light monomerizes
them to their original pyrimidine state (34). Placental mammals have low
levels of the enzyme in comparison to more primitive cells. The low levels
of the enzyme and/or inappropriate conditions to demonstrate
photoreactivation activity in many commonly used mammalian cell lines has
limited its usefulness in determining the possible roles of pyrimidine
dimers in causing cell killing and mutation in these cells.

The proposed scheme of excision repair is analogous to that for which
more detailed evidence exists in prokaryotic systems (1, 4, 5). It involves
the removal of the dimer containing section of DNA and then repair
synthesis using the intact DNA strand as template for restoring the gap.
At least four enzyme activities are required: (1) a specific endonuclease
to cut the DNA strand by the dimer; (2) a second nuclease to remove the
damage; (3) a polymerase to synthesize DNA in the gap; and (4) a ligase to
restore the continuity of the DNA strand. If successful, this process
should result in error free repair. These enzymes have not been well
characterized in mammalian cells. In addition, the organization of DNA in
mammalian cells is much more complex than in bacteria. The nucleosome model
of DNA involves DNA-protein interactions not present in bacteria as well as
extensive higher order folding and organization (1). The role that such
tightly bound proteins may play in limiting the accessibility of chromatin
to repair enzymes is a subject of current study (35). In this regard, it
has been noted, at least in one system, that the initial production of
dimers is higher in the nucleosome core than in linker DNA (36).

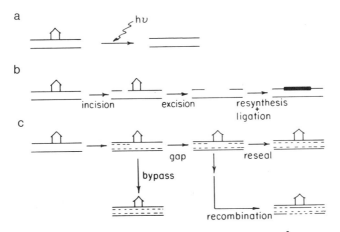

Fig. 3. Models for the repair of pyrimidine dimer (⇧) damage in DNA.

Post replication repair models again stem from concepts derived from bacterial models (4, 5). In some of the cases illustrated, repair may be a misnomer in that damage is not being eliminated but is being bypassed or tolerated. If a dimer is present in the DNA when it is to be replicated during normal DNA synthesis, several things may happen. The new DNA synthesis may stop at the dimer and then start again downstream from the dimer leaving a gap. This gap may be closed by a filling-in of the gap at a later time by new synthesis in a potentially error prone process. The gap may be effectively eliminated by a repair in which recombination occurs with a 50% probability of transferring the dimer to the newly synthesized strand or of it remaining in the parent strand (5). A second general possibility is that when new DNA synthesis reaches a dimer, it slows down but bypasses the dimer in a continuous fashion by either a copy choice mechanism or by direct insertion of bases (4, 5). Both these mechanisms are potentially error prone. Thus, in comparison to the excision repair mechanism, the post replication repair mechanisms are much more subject to errors.

As in excision repair, the complexity of the mammalian cell chromosome adds additional degrees of complexity to designing and interpreting experiments to study post replication repair based on these models. The above models have their origin primarily in work with bacteria such as E. coli. The E. coli chromosome has one unique origin of replication and replicates its 4×10^6 base-pair circular chromosome bidirectionally (4). In contrast, a mammalian cell chromosome has many origins of replication separated by 50-200,000 base-pairs. Synthesis occurs bidirectionally from these replication origins to termination sites or until replication forks meet each other (4, 37). These units of replication are called replicons. Thus, mammalian cell replicons are much smaller than the single replicon of bacteria, and at biological doses of UV, only a few dimers per replicon would be produced (4). In mammalian cells these replicons only initiate once during cell duplication and they initiate at specific times during S phase. In addition, in asynchronous populations of mammalian cells, approximately one-half the cells will be in S phase at any one time.

Excision Repair

Comparisons of the rate and extent of removal of pyrimidine dimers from different types of established cell lines as well as primary explants of mammalian cells have demonstrated a great range. Although initially it was thought that rodent cells were deficient in excision of dimers while human cells were much more proficient, it has become apparent that there can be a wide range within a given species, e.g., hamster or human, such that there can be considerable overlap within the two species (38). Comparisons between established lines of cells suggest that the degree of dimer excision is not always correlated with cell survival, suggesting the presence of alternative repair pathways (17) and/or differences in the cells used such that the same technique is not equally efficient in measuring rate and extent of removal of dimers (39). In this regard, it is also clear that different techniques for measuring dimer removal can give different results for the same cell line in terms of rate and extent of dimer removal (40). Thus, further comparisons of technologies is warranted.

Despite these problems with established cell lines of different species, there have been interesting correlations of extent of dimer excision and species type for primary fibroblasts. It has been demonstrated that there is a direct correlation between maximum life span and extent of excision repair in a number of placental mammals (41, 42). To what degree this is correlated with accumulation of damage in these cells is not yet clear.

One approach to obtaining accurate comparisons of the extent and rate of dimer excision in human cells is to use human diploid fibroblasts which can be maintained in culture in a quiescent non-dividing state for long periods of time (1 year) (43). In these cases, cell identity does not change (no cell growth) and normal DNA replication is minimized. Repair of pyrimidine dimers is observed and appears to be the sum of two first order reactions characterized by a fast (1.7 day^{-1}) and a slow (0.25 day^{-1}) rate constant. One suggestion is that the two components could be related to two fractions of DNA damage, perhaps linker versus core DNA although other possibilities are discussed. That the repair observed is biologically significant is indicated by the elimination of the loss of colony-forming ability and mutagenic effects of UV in such non-dividing cells (44). The initial rates of dimer excision appear identical with those measured in proliferating normal cells in culture (44, 45). This suggests that the rate and extent of repair is independent of the cell cycle or phase of cell growth.

Perhaps the strongest evidence for the role of excision of pyrimidine dimers in mammalian cell survival and mutation comes from the use of repair deficient mutants. A widely used material has been cells from patients with xeroderma pigmentosum (3, 8). This human genetic disease is autosomal recessive. Patients with this disease are sensitive to sunlight and have a high probability of skin cancer. Fibroblasts from these patients have a D_0 for UV sensitivity up to one-tenth that of normal fibroblasts. By somatic cell hybridization techniques at least 8 complementation groups have been identified (8). All groups have the defect that they fail to remove dimers from their DNA at normal rates, i.e., they are defective in the incision step of repair. The most obvious explanation is that these cells are deficient in an active endonuclease activity. However, studies of extracts of xeroderma pigmentosum cells indicate that they incise UV damaged DNA normally but fail to incise UV damage in chromatin (4). This has led to the suggestion that these cells may lack a protein that allows dimer damage to be made accessible to endonuclease action. A third possibility is that these cells are defective in some regulatory step of DNA repair.

When comparisons are made of the UV survival and mutability of normal human fibroblasts and xeroderma pigmentosum strains of complementation group A, it was observed that on an equal dose basis xeroderma pigmentosum cells were hypermutable. However, if the comparisons were made not on an equal dose basis, but on an equal survival level, it was found that the same number of mutants occurred in both normal and xeroderma pigmentosum lines (46). This suggested strongly that the deficiency in excision repair was a deficiency in an error-free process. However, recent experiments of a similar nature with xeroderma pigmentosum cells from complementation group C has indicated that even on an equi-survival basis the repair deficient cells are hypermutable (47). Whether this difference is due to the different cells used or details of the mutation assays is not clear.

The xeroderma pigmentosum mutants are sensitive to a number of chemical agents as well as UV light (10) but have the same sensitivity to ionizing radiation as normal cells under aerobic irradiation conditions. However, under hypoxic irradiation, they show a degree of deficiency in repair compared to normal cells, suggesting some overlap between ionizing radiation damage formed under hypoxic irradiation conditions and UV damage (48).

Besides the incision defective xeroderma pigmentosum strains, there is also the xeroderma pigmentosum variant. It appears to have normal levels of excision repair but is thought to have a deficit in another aspect of repair, post replication repair (4). Interestingly, it is sensitive to caffeine inhibition both in terms of its colony forming ability and in the synthesis of new DNA (4).

Although initially the xeroderma pigmentosum lines were the only widely used and available mammalian cell repair deficient mutants, more recently somatic cell mutants in established mammalian cell lines have been isolated. An example of one group of such mutants is the Chinese hamster cell AA8-4 mutants (49). After selection of a number of mutants on the basis of their sensitivity to UV light, it was found that they were also deficient in their ability to carry out the incision step for UV damage. Hybridization studies have identified at least four complementation groups (50). When survival and mutation studies were carried out on cells from one of the complementation groups, again the repair deficient mutant was hypermutable relative to the wild type parent. However, in contrast to at least some of the xeroderma pigmentosum results, some degree of hypermutability remained even when the comparison was made on an equal cell survival basis (25, 51). This was interpreted to indicate that the defect in repair was not in a completely error-free process, although again details of the mutation assay used might be involved (51). These UV repair deficient cells are also sensitive to a variety of chemical agents and, like xeroderma pigmentosum cells, are normal in their resistance to ionizing radiation delivered under aerobic conditions and slightly sensitive when irradiated under hypoxic irradiation conditions (52), suggesting some anoxic radiation lesions are UV like. Synchronized populations of a related Chinese hamster cell mutant have been exposed to UV at various positions in the cell cycle and have very little variation in response compared to wild type cells (25). Thus, it appears that the cell cycle variations in UV light sensitivity are primarily mediated by differences in the repair of UV damage throughout the cell cycle.

Post Replication Repair

Exposure of mammalian cells to UV light results in an initial increasing inhibition of DNA synthesis over the first thirty minutes to one hour after irradiation and then a gradual recovery of synthetic ability, the rate of which is inversely related to UV dose (1, 4, 5). The interpretation of these results is complicated by the fact that cells are continually moving into and out of the DNA synthetic phase. UV irradiation at the lower doses appears to primarily slow the passage of cells through S phase without strongly altering their rate of movement through other points of the cell cycle. This results in an increase in the fraction of the cells in S phase (4). Even with this increase in cells in S phase, the total rate of DNA synthesis decreases in the culture. Because of the complexities of DNA synthesis in mammalian cells, the relatively small size of the replicons and the many points of initiation of DNA synthesis, the interpretation of this inhibition is not straightforward. Several possibilities exist to explain this inhibition (4): (1) The initiation of new replicons is reduced; (2) the rate of elongation of nascent strands is reduced either due to the presence of pyrimidine dimers which block the synthesis of new DNA or sequestering of polymerases at the damaged site; (3) normal DNA synthesis and repair synthesis are coordinated in such a way that normal synthesis slows down to allow repair to take place; or (4) UV induces new modes of DNA synthesis. Extensive studies have been carried out by a number of workers using a variety of techniques to analyze the nature of the newly synthesized DNA. Although not all in complete agreement, the consensus of opinion that appears to emerge from these studies (4) is as follows. Replicon initiation is not the major factor affecting DNA synthesis at higher UV doses although it may be at low doses (53). The initial reduction of DNA synthesis is due to a temporary blockage of the DNA replication fork at the site of unexcised pyrimidine dimers. At this point, a variety of possibilities can occur but the favoured result is that after some delay DNA synthesis occurs in a continuous fashion by the dimer. The expected result from bacterial studies was that gaps would occur opposite dimers and they would be closed by recombination repair. Some evidence for such a process has recently been obtained in mammalian cells but it seems to involve a small percent of the total dimer sites (54). The mechanisms by which the synthesis of DNA past the dimer might occur, e.g., copy choice and direct insertion of bases have been summarized in detail elsewhere (4). However, because of the complexity of the mammalian cell DNA replication system, definite evidence has been hard to come by. A possible approach to this problem is to use UV irradiated viruses as substrates of known structure to probe the DNA repair mechanisms of infected cells (55). Recent work using DNA replication synchronized SV40 virus infecting monkey kidney cells indicates that both DNA stand exchange and trans-dimer synthesis may be occurring at dimer sites during the viral DNA replication (56). It will be important to see to what degree these viral results reflect what may be going on in host cell DNA.

New Directions for Repair Studies

New and powerful DNA technologies have been applied recently to uncover some of the molecular details of UV light repair and mutagenesis in bacterial systems (57). Using UV irradiated DNA substrates of defined sequence, the action of two UV-specific endonucleases, one purified from the bacterium M. luteus and one encoded by phage T4 have been studied. It appears that both enzymes have two distinct activities, a dimer-specific N-glycosylase activity and a pyrimidinic (AP) endonuclease activity which cleaves a phosphodiester bond 3' to the newly created AP site. Subsequent excision steps might require removal of the terminus, excision of the dimer and resynthesis followed by DNA ligation. In contrast, the excision activity in E. coli encoded by uvrA, uvrB and uvrC genes appears to be quite different (58). Action of this enzyme complex results in incision on both sides of the pyrimidine dimer and the removal of a fragment 12-13 nucleotides long that contains the dimer site. Subsequent action of a polymerase and ligase would repair the incision site. Certain features of repair deficient mutants of mammalian cells suggest that similar molecular processes might take place.

One of the approaches which allowed the detailed enzymology of the uvrA, uvrB and uvrC gene products to be worked out in bacteria was the molecular cloning of the individual repair genes so that gene products could be purified from strains that overproduce the protein (58). It has recently been reported that one can transfect and clone a repair gene from a mammalian cell (59, 60). The success of this technology opens up a whole new area of experimentation using mammalian cell repair systems. The general outline of the experiments for gene transfection is of particular interest as a useful strategy for isolating a repair gene before attempting cloning (59). In the DNA transfection experiments an excision repair deficient mutant of Chinese hamster ovary (CHO) cells was used as a recipient and donor DNA from excision proficient human HeLa cells was isolated. The Chinese hamster cell, as well as being sensitive to UV, was extremely sensitive to mitomycin C. Thus, mitomycin C resistance was even a better selection agent for transformants than UV. The presence of human donor DNA in CHO cells could be detected by the presence of highly repetitive human DNA sequences (Alu sequences). To reduce the chance of selecting a CHO cell DNA repair revertant, a clonal bacterial gene was transfected with the HeLa cell DNA and a coselection was made for both repair proficiency and drug resistance phenotypes. Because of its striking sensitivity to mitomycin C, the CHO mutant repair proficiency was assessed as ability to survive in low concentrations of mitomycin C. After isolation of primary transfectants, DNA was isolated from this cell type to transfer to the CHO mutant to obtain secondary transfectants. The resulting transformant demonstrates a common set of human DNA sequences and resistance to UV and mitomycin C. Approaches similar to this approach, except the drug resistant marker was ligated to the human DNA, have been used by other workers to generate similar secondary transfectants (60). DNA from these secondary transfectants was used to construct a cosmid recombinant library in E. coli. A probe for the drug resistant marker was used to select 7 clones. Although all these cosmids could induce drug resistance, only one transferred resistance to UV and mitomycin C (60). The molecular cloning of this repair gene from HeLa cells should allow studies of its role in repair in comparison with xeroderma pigmentosum cells as well as in more general repair studies.

UV Carcinogenesis

It is apparent from the foregoing that UV irradiation can produce pyrimidine dimers in mammalian cell DNA. It has been noted that the action spectra for mammalian cell transformation measured by neoplastic transformation or anchorage independent cell growth also are similar to the action spectrum for pyrimidine dimer production (2). By photoreactivation or excision repair, such damage can be removed under at least some conditions in error-free fashion. However, if the damage is not removed before DNA replication is attempted, mistakes can be made either by aberrant DNA synthesis trying to bypass the dimer or attempts at error prone forms of repair. Thus, damage that fails to be removed before DNA synthesis may act as a trigger for mutation and perhaps cell death. However, in the complex mammalian cell systems, a mistake in DNA replication need not be expressed immediately. The gene in which it occurs may not be transcribed or only transcribed at a low level. In addition, in the complexity of tissue renewal systems, the cell may be in a "quiescent state", not dividing until a proper stimulus arises. Such models fit the classical mutation-promotion concepts of carcinogenesis (Figure 4) (61).

In this context it is useful to consider that not all cells in human tumours are clonogenic. That is, neoplasms may be regarded as stem cell systems in which a minority of cells may have the proliferation capacity to maintain tumour growth and a majority of cells display varying degrees of differentiation (62). Recent studies of the molecular biology of neoplasia

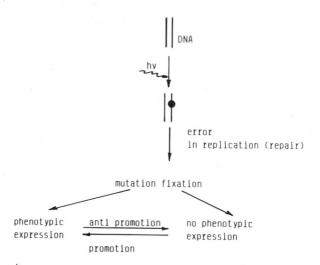

Fig. 4. Possible role of unrepaired UV damage in the carcinogenic process (after Trosko and Chang, 1981).

have indicated that the growth of at least some human tumors is controlled by the expression of oncogenes. In some cases, cellular growth factors normally regulate these oncogenes. The inappropriate or over-expression of these oncogenes can be related to point mutations in these genes or in genes regulating their expression. Thus, the ultimate expression of DNA damage may be in the form of the production of mutations in a minority stem cell population such that they lose their regulatory controls that determine normal self-renewal or cell cycle entry (62).

It is apparent that the understanding of DNA repair processes for UV and other forms of damage is progressing rapidly at the molecular level. The challenge will continue therefore to relate these molecular events to *in vitro* cellular endpoints such as cell survival and mutation. As has been pointed out earlier (5), it will also be important to relate these molecular and cellular events to the *in vivo* situation where aberrations in the control of cell division and differentiation are underlying factors in the carcinogenic process.

ACKNOWLEDGEMENTS

Appreciation is expressed for support from the Ontario Cancer Treatment and Research Foundation, the Medical Research Council of Canada and the National Cancer Institute of Canada.

REFERENCES

1. J. E. Cleaver, DNA repair and its coupling to DNA replication in eukaryotic cells. Biochim. Biophys. Acta 516:489-516 (1978).

2. T. P. Coohill, Action spectra for mammalian cells *in vitro*, in: "Topics in Photomedicine," K. C. Smith, ed., Plenum Press, New York and London (1984), pp. 1-37.

3. C. Friedberg, U. K. Ehmann, and J. I. Williams, Human diseases associated with defective DNA repair, Adv. Radiat. Biol. 8:85-174 (1979).

4. J. D. Hall and D. W. Mount, Mechanisms of DNA replication and mutagenesis in ultraviolet-irradiated bacteria and mammalian cells, Prog. Nucleic Acid Res. 25:53-126 (1981).

5. P. C. Hanawalt, P. K. Cooper, A. K. Ganesan, and C. A. Smith, DNA repair in bacteria and mammalian cells, Ann. Rev. Biochem. 48:783-836 (1979).

6. R. R. Hewitt and R. E. Meyn, Applicability of bacterial models of DNA repair and recovery to UV-irradiated mammalian cells, Adv. Radiat. Biol. 7:153-179 (1978).

7. B. A. Kihlman, "Caffeine and Chromosomes," Elsevier Scientific Publishing Co., Amsterdam, New York, Oxford (1977).

8. M. C. Paterson, N. E. Gentner, M. V. Middlestadt, and M. Weinfeld, Cancer predisposition, carcinogen hypersensitivity, and aberrant DNA metabolism, J. Cell. Physiol. Suppl. 3:45-62 (1984).

9. T. Lindahl, DNA repair enzymes, Ann. Rev. Biochem. 51:61-87 (1982).

10. R. B. Setlow, Repair deficient human disorders and cancer, Nature (London) 271:713-717 (1978).

11. J. J. Roberts, The repair of DNA modified by cytotoxic, mutagenic, and carcinogenic chemicals, Adv. Radiat. Biol. 7:211-436 (1978).

12. A. M. Rauth and J. A. Simpson, The energy loss of electrons in solids. Radiat. Res. 22:643-661 (1964).

13. M. Fielden, Initial chemical lesions, in: "Radiation Carcinogenesis and DNA Alterations," F. J. Burns, A. C. Upton, and G. Silini, eds., Plenum Press, New York (1986). Submitted.

14. S. Y. Wang, "The Photochemistry and Photobiology of Nucleic Acids," Academic Press, New York (1976).

15. A. J. Varghese, Photochemical addition of amino acids and related compounds to nucleic acid constituents, in: "Aging, Carcinogenesis, and Radiation Biology," K. C. Smith, ed., Plenum Publishing Co., New York (1976), pp. 207-223.

16. A. J. Fornace and K. W. Kohn, DNA-protein cross-linking by ultraviolet radiation in normal human and xeroderma pigmentosum fibroblasts, Biochim. Biophys. Acta 435:95-103 (1976).

17. A. M. Rauth, Effects of ultraviolet light on mammalian cells in culture, in: "Current Topics of Radiation Research, 6," M. Ebert and A. Howard, eds., North-Holland Publishing Co., Amsterdam, London (1970), pp. 195-248.

18. J. Jagger, "Introduction to Research in Ultraviolet Photobiology," Prentice-Hall, New Jersey (1967).

19. M. M. Elkind and G. F. Whitmore, "The Radiobiology of Cultured Mammalian Cells," Gordon and Breach, New York (1967).

20. E. C. Friedberg and P. C. Hanawalt, "DNA Repair, A Laboratory Manual of Research Procedures, Volume 1," Marcel Dekker Inc., New York and Basel (1981).

21. D. L. Steward and R. M. Humphrey, Induction of thymine dimers in synchronized populations of Chinese hamster cells, Nature (London) 212:248-300 (1966).

22. J. E. Trosko, M. Kosschau, L. Covington, and E. H. Y. Chu, UV-induction of pyrimidine dimers during different phases of the cell cycle of mammalian cells, Radiat. Res. 27:535 (1966).

23. A. R. S. Collins, C. S. Downes, and R. T. Johnson, Cell-cycle related variations in UV damage and repair capacity in Chinese hamster (CHO-K1) cells, J. Cell. Physiol. 103:179-191 (1980).

24. J. M. Clarkson, The induction of thymine dimers by UV light as a function of cell state, Int. J. Radiat. Biol; 34:583-586 (1978).

25. R. D. Wood and H. J. Burki, Repair capability and the cellular age response for killing and mutation induction after UV, Mutat. Res. 95:505-514 (1982).

26. A. M. Rauth, Evidence for dark-reactivation of ultraviolet damage in mouse L cells, Radiat. Res. 31:121-138 (1967).

27. P. M. Busse, S. K. Base, R. W. Jones, and L. J. Tolmach, The action of caffeine on x-irradiated HeLa cells. II. Synergistic lethality, Radiat. Res., 71:666-677 (1977).

28. S. K. Das, C. C. Lau, and A. B. Pardee, Abolition by cycloheximide of caffeine-enhanced lethality of alkylating agents in hamster cells, Cancer Res. 42:4499-4504 (1982).

29. K. Hanssen, B. A. Kihlman, C. Tanzarella, and F. Palitti, Influence of caffeine and 3-amino-benzamide in G_2 on the frequency of chromosomal aberrations induced by thiotepa, mitomycin C and N-methyl-N-nitro-N'-nitrosoguanidine in human lymphocytes, Mutation Res. 126:251-258 (1984).

30. C. Lücke-Huhle, L. Hieber, and R. D. Wegner, Caffeine-mediated release of alpha-radiation-induced G_2 arrest increases the yield of chromosome aberrations, Int. J. Radiat. Biol. 43:123-132 (1983).

31. R. M. Humphrey, B. A. Sedita, and R. E. Meyn, Recovery of Chinese hamster cells from ultra-violet irradiation damage, Int. J. Radiat. Biol. 18:61-69 (1970).

32. P. Todd, Fractionated ultraviolet light irradiation of cultured Chinese hamster cells, Radiat. Res. 55:93-100 (1973).

33. M. Domon and A. M. Rauth, Cell cycle specific recovery from fractionated exposures of ultraviolet light, Radiat. Res. 55:81-92 (1973).

34. B. M. Sutherland, Photoreactivation in mammalian cells, Int. Rev. Cytol. Suppl. 8:301-334 (1978).

35. P. C. Hanawalt, P. K. Cooper, A. K. Ganesan, R. S. Lloyd, C. A. Smith, and M. E. Zolan, Repair responses to DNA damage: Enzymatic pathways in E. coli and human cells, J. Cell. Biochem. 18:271-283 (1982).

36. R. M. Snapka and S. Linn, Efficiency of formation of pyrimidine dimers in SV40 chromatin in vitro, Biochemistry 20:68-72 (1981).

37. R. Sheinin, J. Humbert, and R. E. Pearlman, Some aspects of eukaryotic DNA replication, Ann. Rev. Biochem. 47:277-316 (1978).

38. A. Collins, C. Jones, and C. Waldren, A survey of DNA repair incision activities after ultraviolet irradiation of a range of human, hamster, and hamster-human cell lines, J. Cell Science 56:423-440 (1982).

39. J. E. Cleaver, Structure of repaired sites in human DNA synthesized in the presence of inhibitors of DNA polymerases alpha and beta in human fibroblasts, Biochim, Biophys. Acta, 739:301-311 (1983).

40. J. M. Clarkson, D. L. Mitchell, and G. M. Adair, The use of an immunological probe to measure the kinetics of DNA repair in normal and UV-sensitive mammalian cell lines, Mutat. Res. 112:287-299 (1983).

41. R. W. Hart and R. B. Setlow, Correlation between deoxyribonucleic acid excision repair and life span in a number of mammalian species, Proc. Natl. Acad. Sci. (USA) 71:2169-2173 (1974).

42. K. Y. Hall, R. W. Hart, A. K. Benirschke, and R. L. Walford, Correlations between ultraviolet-induced DNA repair in primate lymphocytes and fibroblasts and species maximum achievable life span, *Mechanisms of Aging and Development* 24:163-173 (1984).

43. G. J. Kantor and R. B. Setlow, Rate and extent of DNA repair in nondividing human diploid fibroblasts, *Cancer Res.* 41:819-825 (1981).

44. V. M. Maher, D. J. Dorney, A. L. Mendrala, B. Konze-Thomas, and J. J. McCormick, DNA excision-repair processes in human cells can eliminate the cytotoxic and mutagenic consequences of ultraviolet radiation, *Mutat. Res.* 62:311-323 (1979).

45. M. C. Paterson, B. P. Smith, P. H. M. Lohman, A. K. Anderson, and L. Fishman, Defective excision repair of x-ray-damaged DNA in human (ataxia telangiectasia) fibroblasts, *Nature (London)* 260:444-447 (1976).

46. V. M. Maher and J. J. McCormick, Effect of DNA repair on the cytotoxicity and mutagenicity of UV irradiation and of chemical carcinogens in normal and xeroderma pigmentosum cells, *in*: "Biology of Radiation Carcinogenesis," J. M. Yuhas, R. W. Tennant, and J. D. Regan, eds., Raven Press, New York (1976), pp. 129-145.

47. J. G DeLuca, D. A. Kaden, E. A. Komives, and W. G. Thilly, Mutation of xeroderma pigmentosum lymphoblasts by far-ultraviolet light, *Mutat. Res.* 128:47-57 (1984).

48. R. B. Setlow, F. M. Faulcon, and J. A. Regan, Defective repair of gamma-ray-induced DNA damage in xeroderma pigmentosum cells, *Int. J. Radiat. Biol.* 29:125-136 (1976).

49. L. H. Thompson, J. S. Rubin, J. E. Cleaver, G. F. Whitmore, and K. Brookman, A screening method for isolating DNA repair-deficient mutants of CHO cells, *Somat. Cell Genet.* 6:391-405 (1980).

50. L. H. Thompson, D. B. Busch, K. Brookman, C. L. Mooney, and D. A. Glaser, Genetic diversity of UV-sensitive DNA repair mutants of Chinese hamster ovary cells, *Proc. Natl. Acad. Sci. (USA)* 78:3734-3737 (1981).

51. L. H. Thompson, The use of DNA-repair-deficient mutants of Chinese hamster ovary cells in studying mutagenesis mechanisms and for testing for environmental mutagens, *in*: "Induced Mutagenesis, Molecular Mechanisms and their Implications for Environmental Protection," D. W. Lawrence, ed., Plenum Press, New York, London (1981), pp. 217-246.

52. J. S. Rubin and G. F. Whitmore, DNA repair-deficient Chinese hamster ovary cell exhibiting differential sensitivity to rays under aerobic and hypoxic conditions, *Radiat. Res.* 101:528-534 (1985).

53. J. E. Cleaver, W. K. Kaufmann, L. N. Kapp, and S. D. Park, Replicon size and excision repair as factors in the inhibition and recovery of DNA synthesis from ultraviolet damage, *Biochem. Biophys. Acta* 739:207-215 (1983).

54. A. J. Fornace, Recombination of parent and daughter strand DNA after UV-irradiation in mammalian cells, *Nature (London)* 304:552-554 (1983).

55. M. J. Defais, P. C. Hanawalt, and A. P. Sarasin, Viral probes for DNA repair, Adv. Radiat. Biol. 10:1-37 (1983).

56. J. M. Clark and P. C. Hanawalt, Replicative intermediates in UV-irradiated simian virus 40, Mutat. Res. 132:1-14 (1984).

57. W. A. Haseltine, Ultraviolet light repair and mutagenesis revisited, Cell 33:13-17 (1983).

58. A. Sancar and W. D. Rupp, A novel repair enzyme: uvR ABC excision nuclease of E. coli cuts a DNA strand on both sides of the damaged region, Cell 33:249-260 (1983).

59. J. S. Rubin, A. L. Joyner, A. Bernstein, and G. F. Whitmore, Molecular identification of a human DNA repair gene following DNA-mediated gene transfer, Nature (London) 306:206-208 (1983).

60. A. Westerveld, J. H. J. Hoeijmakers, M. van Duin, J. deWit, H. Odijk, A. Pastink, R. D. Wood, and D. Bootsma, Molecular cloning of a human DNA repair gene, Nature (London) 310:425-429 (1984).

61. J. E. Trosko and C.-G Chang, The role of radiation and chemicals in the induction of mutations and epigenetic changes during carcinogenesis, Adv. Radiat. Biol. 9:1-36 (1981).

62. R. N. Buick and M. N. Pollak, Perspectives on clonogenic tumor cells, stem cells and oncogenes, Cancer Res. 44:4909-4918 (1984).

ALTERATIONS IN BENZO(A)PYRENE METABOLISM AND ITS DNA ADDUCT FORMATION IN

SKIN OF MICE CHRONICALLY EXPOSED TO ULTRAVIOLET-B RADIATION

H. Mukhtar, M. Das and D. R. Bickers

Department of Dermatology, University Hospitals of Cleveland
Case Western Reserve University and Veterans Administration
Medical Center
Cleveland, Ohio 44106

ABBREVIATIONS

AHH, aryl hydrocarbon hydroxylase; EH, epoxide hydrolase; ECD, 7-ethoxycoumarin O-deethylase; GST, glutathione S-transferase; BP, benzo(a)pyrene; 3-OH BP, 3-hydroxybenzo(a)pyrene; BP-4,5-oxide, benzo(a)pyrene 4,5-oxide; BPDE-I, $7\beta,8\alpha$-dihydroxy-$9\alpha,10\alpha$-epoxy-7,8,9,10-tetrahydrobenzo(a)pyrene; UVB, ultraviolet B, CDNB, 1-chloro 2,4-dinitrobenzene; NADH nicotinamide adenine dinucleotide reduced; NADPH, nicotinamide adenine dinucleotide phosphate reduced; SCC, squamous cell carcinoma; PAH, polycyclic aromatic hydrocarbon; PBS, phosphate buffered saline; ELISA, enzyme linked immunoabsorbent assay.

ABSTRACT

Cutaneous xenobiotic metabolizing enzymes including aryl hydrocarbon hydroxylase (AHH), 7-ethoxycoumarin O-deethylase (ECD), epoxide hydrolase (EH) and glutathione S-transferase (GST) activities were examined in SKH hairless mice chronically irradiated with UVB to induce squamous cell carcinoma (SCC). Enzyme activities in irradiated tumor-bearing skin were compared to those present in the skin of non-irradiated control animals as well as in unirradiated non-tumor bearing skin sites of the SCC-bearing mice. The inducibility of skin AHH and ECD in each set of animals was assessed following a single topical application of coal tar (1 ml/100 gm). Enzyme-mediated binding of ^{3}H-benzo(a)pyrene (BP) and its metabolite $7\beta,8\alpha$-dihydroxy-$9\alpha,10\alpha$-epoxy-7,8,9,10-tetrahydrobenzo(a)pyrene (BPDE-I) to epidermal DNA was also evaluated. Basal AHH and ECD activities in microsomes for UVB-irradiated SCC-bearing dorsal skin were 4.6 and 4.8-fold lower than those in dorsal skin of non-irradiated control animals. Enzyme activities in non-tumor bearing ventral skin from the UVB-irradiated SCC-bearing mice also were 2.2-2.8-fold lower as compared to activities in the non-irradiated control animals. The reduction in AHH activity paralleled the levels of enzyme-mediated binding of radiolabelled BP metabolites and of BPDE-I to epidermal DNA. GST activity was found to be increased (173% in non-tumor bearing ventral skin of UVB-irradiated mice whereas no difference in activity between SCC-bearing dorsal skin and dorsal skin of

control animals could be detected. EH activity was unchanged in each group
of animals. Treatment with topically applied coal tar resulted in higher
inducibility of AHH and ECD in both SCC-bearing (13-fold) as well as in
non-tumor skin sites (6-fold) of UVB-irradiated mice than in skin of
control animals (3-fold). Coal tar application also increased the covalent
binding of ^{3}H-BP and of the metabolite BPDE-I to skin DNA. This was
greater in SCC-bearing dorsal skin (119-129%) than in non-irradiated skin
of control animals (48-62%). Our studies suggest that the metabolism of BP
by cutaneous cytochrome P-450 dependent monooxygenases is impaired in skin
of mice irradiated chronically with UVB. These studies also illustrate the
complex interrelationship that exist in target tissue simultaneously
exposed to chemical and physical oncogens in the environment.

INTRODUCTION

     Cancer of the skin is by far the most common type of human neoplasm.
Of the approximately 1.25 million new cancers diagnosed annually in the
United States at least 400,000 originate in the skin (1). Epidemiologic
studies have clearly shown that basal cell and squamous cell carcinomas
originate primarily on body surfaces which are directly exposed to the
environment (2, 3). Skin is a major interface between the body and its
environment and is continuously exposed to physical agents such as solar
radiation, which includes the oncogenic mid range ultraviolet between 290-
320 nm, known as the UVB (2). It is apparent from both animal and human
studies that the relationship between UV radiation and skin cancer is not
simplistic; in the majority of experimental systems employed to study
carcinogenesis several etiologic factors appear to be at work both
sequentially and/or simultaneously (2, 3). Thus, it is now known that
tumor formation in the skin occurs as a result of a two-stage process
defined as initiation and promotion (4).

     Some studies on the mechanism of cancer induction have focused
primarily on a search for the detection of differences in biochemical
markers between normal and neoplastic cells or for variations in the
patterns of enzyme activity in the target tissues which might be suitable
markers for neoplastic transformation. One such enzyme system is known as
the microsomal cytochrome P-450 dependent monooxygenase which catalyzes the
metabolism of various drugs, chemical carcinogens and other xenobiotics
(5). Of the cytochrome P-450 dependent monooxygenases, AHH has been among
the most extensively studied marker for neoplastic change (6, 7). For
example, higher inducibility of this enzyme appears to correlate with
enhanced risk of tumor susceptibility of PAHs in several inbred mouse
strains (8). Other studies have shown that cytochrome P-450 dependent
xenobiotic metabolizing enzymes are either lowered or undetectable in most
types of neoplasms (6, 9, 10). For example, Adamson and Fouts (10)
compared the Novikoff hepatoma with hepatoma 5123 (11) for their ability to
metabolize various drugs and concluded that the enzyme activity was not
detectable in either type of hepatoma. Sultatos and Vessell (6) have also
shown that ethylmorphine N-demethylase and aniline hydroxylase activities
are lowered in hepatic and mammary carcinomas. On the other hand, Mason
and Okey have shown that the cytochrome P-450 content is elevated in one
type of mammary carcinoma (7). While it is well known that the skin is
directly exposed to both physical and chemical carcinogens in the
environment virtually nothing is known about the interaction of these
oncogens for skin. In this paper we provide evidences that prolonged
exposure of mouse skin to UVB radiation produces major changes in the basal
levels and in the inducibility of these enzymes.

234

MATERIALS AND METHODS

Chemicals

(3)BP-4,5-oxide (specific activity 289 mCi/mmol) and unlabelled BP-4,5-oxide were provided by the Cancer Research Program of the National Cancer Institute, Division of Cancer Cause and Prevention (Bethesda, MD). (G-^{3}H)-BP (specific activity 25 Ci/mmol) was purchased from Amersham Searle (Chicago, IL). Standard coal tar solution (USP) was used. All other chemicals used were of the highest purity commercially available.

Tumor Protocol

The dorsal skin of groups of randomly selected male SKH-1 hairless mice, obtained from Temple University Health Sciences, The Skin and Cancer Hospital, Philadelphia at 8 weeks of age, were radiated using from a bank of four Westinghouse FS-40-T-12 fluorescent sunlamps. The mice were exposed three times weekly on alternate days for 25 minutes for 22 weeks to UVB (2.0-2.2 x 10^{-4} W/cm^2) at a distance of 9 inches. Control non-irradiated animals were kept in the same room in a separate area protected from the light source. Neoplasms developed only on the dorsal skin beginning after 17-18 weeks of exposure. Gross skin tumors appeared after 20-22 weeks of exposure to UVB light at which time the animals were withdrawn for metabolic studies.

Treatment of Animals

For the studies of basal enzyme activity control (non-irradiated), non-tumor skin sites and SCC-bearing skin of UVB-irradiated mice were evaluated. Enzyme induction was assayed after a single topical application of USP coal tar solution (1 ml/100g) 24 hours before sacrifice. Non-coal tar treated animals received the same volume of acetone. For the determination of the in vivo binding of BP-metabolites to DNA, animals received a single topical application of 1 nmol ^{3}H-BP (in 100 l acetone) 2 hours prior to sacrifice. BPDE-I-DNA adduct formation was assessed using an ELISA assay.

Enzyme Source

The animals were killed by decapitation. Tissues were removed and rinsed thoroughly with ice cold 0.1 M phosphate buffer pH 7.4. All subsequent operations were carried out at 0-4°C. The skin was scraped with a sharp scalpel blade to remove subcutaneous fat and muscle. The tissues were minced with scissors in 0.1 M phosphate buffer pH 7.4 containing 10 mM EDTA. The minced tissue was homogenized with a Polytron Tissue Homogenizer. Microsomes were prepared as described previously (12), suspended in homogenizing media, and were used as the enzyme source for measuring EH and monooxygenase activity. Cytosolic fractions were used as the enzyme source for measuring GST activity.

DNA Extraction and Estimation of Total BP Adducts

The DNA From tissue homogenates was extracted essentially as described earlier (13). The purified DNA was then dissolved in 5.0 ml of 0.1 M sodium chloride pH 7.0 and estimated by measuring its absorption at 260 nm. Aliquots were counted on a Packard TriCarb 460 CD liquid scintillation spectrometer to determine the amount of ^{3}H-BP metabolites bound to tissue DNA.

Enzyme-linked Immunosorbent Assay for PDE-I-DNA Adducts

DNA from the skin was prepared as described above and BPDE-I adducts quantitated by a competitive enzyme-linked immunoassay (14) using a recently developed monoclonal antibody (5D11) which recognizes BPDE-I modified DNA.

Enzyme Assays

AHH and ECD activities were determined as described earlier (12). EH activity in the microsomal fractions was assayed using radiolabelled BP-4,5-oxide as substrate as described previously (12). GST activity in cytosol was assayed by the procedure of Habig et al. (15) using CDNB as a substrate. Protein was determined according to the procedure of Lowry et al. (16).

RESULTS

Cutaneous Xenobiotic Metabolism in UVB-induced SCC-bearing Mouse Skin

In Table 1 a comparison of the basal activities of xenobiotic metabolizing enzymes in SCC-bearing dorsal skin and in non-tumor bearing ventral skin of UVB-irradiated mice and in the skin of non-irradiated control mice is shown. AHH and ECD activities in microsomes prepared from SCC-bearing dorsal skin were 5.6 and 4.8 fold lower than those of the

dorsal skin of non-irradiated control animals. Non-tumor bearing ventral skin of SCC-bearing mice also showed 2.2-2.3 fold lower AHH and ECD enzyme activities as compared to dorsal skin of non-irradiated controls (Table 1). Basal enzyme activity as well as inducibility by topically applied coal tar on cytochrome P-450 dependent monooxygenases did not differ in dorsal and ventral skin of unirradiated mice (data not shown). Microsomal EH activity was similar in each of the group (Table 1). Cytosolic GST activity was found to be elevated (173%) in non-tumor bearing ventral skin of UVB-irradiated SCC-bearing mice as compared to controls but no difference in enzyme activity was observed between SCC-bearing skin of the UVB-irradiated animals and in the non-irradiated controls (Table 1).

Effect of Topical Application of Coal Tar on Xenobiotic Metabolism in UVB-induced SCC-bearing Mouse Skin

Studies of Miyake et al. (17) have shown that cytochrome P-450 monooxygenases in Morris hepatomas are not induced by treatment with conventional inducers of cytochrome P-450. Other studies have indicated that the drug metabolizing enzyme activities of various hepatomas are induced by 3-methylcholanthrene and phenobarbital (9). Our prior studies have shown that a coal tar preparation widely used in dermatologic practice, is a potent inducer of cutaneous and hepatic cytochrome P-450 monooxygenases (18). In the present study we investigated the effect of topical application of coal tar on AHH and ECD activities in skin of control and UVB-irradiated SCC-bearing mice. Data in Table 2 depicts the inducibility of AHH and ECD following topical application of coal tar to the tumor-bearing dorsal skin. Coal tar treatment resulted in a 14-fold induction of AHH and ECD activities in SCC-bearing dorsal skin of UVB-irradiated mice (Table 2). The inducibility of these enzymes by coal tar in non-tumor bearing ventral skin of UVB-irradiated mice and skin of non-irradiated controls was 6 and 3-fold, respectively.

236

Table 1. Skin drug and carcinogen metabolizing enzyme activities in non-irradiated controls and of UVB-irradiated squamous cell carcinoma bearing hairless mice

Enzyme activities[*]	Dorsal skin of non-irradiated controls	Non-tumor bearing ventral skin of UVB-irradiated mice	SCC-bearing dorsal skin of UVB-irradiated mice
AHH	10.56 ± 0.12	4.71 ± 0.09^a	1.89 ± 0.04^b
ECD	12.39 ± 0.10	4.30 ± 0.07^a	2.56 ± 0.04^b
EH	110 ± 10	112 ± 18	90 ± 10
GST	53.83 ± 0.9	93.14 ± 2.13^a	54.84 ± 3.81^c

[*]All enzyme activities are expressed as p mol product/min/mg protein with the exception of GST which is given as nmol/min/mg protein. Data represent mean $\pm$ SEM of four indiviudal values.

a - statistically significant from control skin ($p < 0.05$)

b - statistically significant from control and non-tumor bearing skin of UVB-irradiated mice ($p < 0.05$)

c - statistically significant from non-tumor bearing skin of UVB-irradiated mice ($p < 0.05$)

Covalent Binding of Benzo(a)pyrene Metabolites to DNA in UVB-induced SCC-bearing Mouse Skin

Table 3 depicts the in vivo covalent binding of total BP metabolite and of BPDE-I to skin DNA. First the binding of total BP-metabolites to skin DNA was assessed by measuring the amount of isotopically labelled BP metabolites bound to tissue DNA after topical application of the hydrocarbon. The covalent binding of BP metabolites to skin DNA was 2.2-fold and 1.9-fold lower in SCC-bearing dorsal skin and non-tumor bearing ventral skin of UVB-irradiated mice, respectively when compared to non-irradiated controls (Table 3). Interestingly, the binding of BP metabolites to skin DNA was found to be enhanced following topical application of coal tar to non-irradiated control animals and to SCC-bearing dorsal skin of UVB-irradiated mice (Table 3). The enhancement of binding to BP metabolites to skin DNA evoked by coal tar was higher in SCC-bearing dorsal skin of UVB-irradiated mice (2.3 fold) while that in non-irradiated control animals was enhanced 1.6-fold. However, the capacity of BP metabolites to bind covalently to skin DNA did not increase by coal tar treatment in non-tumor bearing ventral skin of UVB-irradiated mice.

The covalent binding of BPDE-I to skin DNA was then evaluated using monoclonal antibodies directed against BPDE-I modified DNA in an ELISA assay. The covalent binding of BPDE-I to skin DNA was found to be appreciably lower in SCC-bearing dorsal skin of UVB-irradiated mice (35%) and in non-tumor bearing ventral skin of UVB-irradiated mice (40%) as compared to non-irradiated controls (Table 3). The binding of BPDE-I to skin DNA was also found to be induced by topical application of coal tar to control non-irradiated skin (48%) and to SCC-bearing dorsal skin of UVB-irradiated mice (119%). The binding of BPDE-I to skin DNA was unaffected in non-tumor bearing skin of the UVB-irradiated mice.

Table 2. Inducibility of skin drug and carcinogen metabolizing enzyme activities by topically applied coal tar in non-irradiated controls and of UVB-irradiated squamous cell carcinoma bearing hairless mice

Enzyme activities[*]	Dorsal skin of non-irradiated controls	Non-tumor bearing ventral skin of UVB-irradiated mice	SCC-bearing dorsal skin of UVB-irradiated mice
AHH			
Control (acetone)	9.56 ± 0.11	3.53 ± 0.08^a	1.63 ± 0.04^b
Coal tar induced	31.41 ± 0.64	20.28 ± 0.49^a	21.84 ± 0.51
ECD			
Control (acetone)	10.48 ± 0.14	3.80 ± 0.10^a	2.33 ± 0.04^b
Coal tar induced	35.41 ± 0.70	22.06 ± 0.51^a	30.67 ± 0.71^c

[*]Expressed as pmol product/min/mg protein and represent mean $\pm$ SEM of four individual values.

a - statistically significant from control skin ($p < 0.05$)

b - statistically significant from control and non-tumor bearing skin of UVB-irradiated mice ($p < 0.05$)

c - statistically significant from non-tumor bearing skin of UVB-irradiated mice ($p < 0.05$)

DISCUSSION

The effect of chronic UV irradiation on skin enzymes that metabolizes drugs and carcinogens including PAHs was assessed. Prior studies have demonstrated that in several types of malignancies cytochrome P-450 dependent xenobiotic metabolizing enzymes are either lowered or nondetectable (6, 9, 10). Our findings indicate that basal activities of cytochrome P-450 dependent xenobiotic metabolizing enzymes are greatly diminished in the skin of hairless mice chronically irradiated with UVB for the induction of cutaneous SCC. It is of particular interest that the non-tumor bearing ventral skin of the irradiated animals also showed diminished basal AHH and ECD activities with values intermediate between those in non-irradiated controls and those in the SCC-bearing dorsal skin of the same animals. The decrease in cutaneous xenobiotic metabolizing enzymes of SCC-bearing skin might be due to a loss of, or at least a decrease in microsomal enzyme protein which could metabolize xenobiotics such as the PAHs. Since we did not observe any change in liver enzyme activities it is unlikely that any circulating inhibitors or activators stimulated by UVB could account for the differences observed in the skin. Adamson and Fouts (10) have shown that the loss of mixed function oxidase activity in hepatic tumors was due neither to a deficiency of cofactors such as NADPH and glucose-6-phosphate nor to the presence of inhibitors of xenobiotic metabolizing enzymes. LePage and Henderson (19) suggested that the biochemical mechanisms of carcinogenesis might best be explored by means of the "deletion hypothesis". The deletion theory of carcinogenesis suggests a relationship between the development of neoplastic cells and the loss of some enzymes found in normal cells (20). The theory could explain the reduction of xenobiotic metabolizing enzyme activity in SCC-bearing skin as observed in this study.

The inhibition of cutaneous monooxygenases in SCC-bearing skin of UVB-irradiated animals was paralleled by a decrease in observed covalent binding of BP metabolites to DNA. The topical application of coal tar to

Table 3. Effect of coal tar application on cutaneous BP-DNA and BPDE-I-DNA adducts formation in control and UVB-irradiated squamous cell carcinoma bearing hairless mice

DNA-adduct formation	Dorsal skin of non-irradiated controls	Non-tumor bearing ventral skin of UVB-irradiated mice	SCC-bearing dorsal skin of UVB-irradiated mice
BP-adducts[a]			
Control (acetone)	1.74	0.93	0.80
Coal tar induced	2.81	0.95	1.83
BPDE-I adducts[b]			
Control (acetone)	0.40	0.24	0.26
Coal tar induced	0.59	0.20	0.57

Data from a typical experiment repeated thrice with identical results.

a - pmol BP metabolites bound/mg DNA. Estimated by determining the radioactivity bound to DNA

b - pmol BPDE-I bound/mg DNA. Estimated by enzyme linked immunoabsorbent assay as described in 'Materials and Methods'.

non-irradiated control mice and to UVB-irradiated SCC-bearing skin by coal tar was greater than that occurring in non-irradiated control skin which correlated with enzyme activity.

The chronic use of coal tar medications for extended periods of time has been associated with the development of skin cancer in human populations. Hodgson (21) reported that an individual treated twice daily for 7 years with applications of a drug containing large amounts of coal tar developed cutaneous squamous cell carcinoma. Epidemiologic and occupational studies have clearly shown the relationship of chronic skin exposure to coal combustion products to the development of human skin cancer (22). There is evidence to suggest that tumor formation is associated with one or more of the several PAHs present in coal tar (23). The PAHs require metabolic activation by the cytochrome P-450-dependent mixed-function oxidase system commonly known as AHH (5). The precise relationship between AHH activity, inducibility of the enzyme in target tissues, and susceptibility to chemical carcinogenesis by PAH remains controversial (24). It was earlier hypothesized that AHH activity is a major determinant of the carcinogenic risk of PAHs (8). More recently, it has become clear that the binding of bay-region diol-epoxides of PAHs to cellular DNA plays a critical role in tumor induction by PAHs (5). For example, the tumorigenicity of BP appears to involve its metabolism to BPDE-I and the subsequent binding of this metabolite to DNA (5).

Our data indicate that exposure of the skin of SCC-bearing UVB-irradiated mice to coal tar results in greater induction of AHH and higher levels of binding of BP metabolites, especially BPDE-I to DNA. This suggests that chronically UVB-irradiated skin of these animals may be at higher risk for tumor induction by environmental chemicals such as PAHs. This may explain the known tendency of human skin cancers to occur more frequently in individuals with prior skin malignancies (3, 25).

ACKNOWLEDGEMENTS

    Supported in part by NIH Grants CA 38028 and ES-1900 and funds from
the Veterans Administration and Skin Cancer Foundation. Thanks are due to
Ms. Sandra Evans for preparing the manuscript.

REFERENCES

1. D. R. Bickers, in: "Current Concepts in Cutaneous Toxicity," V. A.
    Drill and P. Lazar, eds, Academic Press, New York (1980), pp. 95-
    126.

2. E. A. Emmett, CRC Critical Rev. Toxicol. 2:211-255 (1973).

3. G. M. Findlay, Lancet 24:1070-1073 (1928).

4. R. K. Boutwell, in: "Carcinogenesis, A Comprehensive Survey, Vol. 2,"
    Raven Press, New York (1978), pp. 49-58.

5. A. H. Conney, Cancer Res. 42:4875-4917 (1982).

6. L. G. Sultatos and E. S. Vessell, Proc. Natl. Acad. Sci. USA 77:600-
    603 (1980).

7. M. E. Mason and A. B. Okey, Cancer Res. 41:2778-2782 (1981).

8. D. W. Nebert, F. M. Goujon, and J. E. Gielen, Nature (Lond.) 236:107-
    110 (1972).

9. L. G. Hart, R. H. Adamson, H. P. Morris, and J. R. Fouts, J. Pharmacol.
    Exp. Ther. 149:7-15 (1965).

10. R. H. Adamson and J. R. Fouts, Cancer Res. 21:667-672 (1961).

11. H. P. Morris, H. Sidransky, B. P. Wagner, and H. M. Dyer, Cancer Res.
    20:1252-1254 (1960).

12. H. Mukhtar and D. R. Bickers, Drug Metab. Disp. 9:311-314 (1981).

13. H. Mukhtar, B. J. Del Tito, Jr., M. Das, E. P. Cherniack, E. A.
    Cherniack, and D. R. Bickers, Cancer Res. 44:4233-4240 (1984).

14. R. Santella, C. D. Lin, W. L. Cleveland, and I. B. Weinstein,
    Carcinogenesis 5:373-378 (1984).

15. W. H. Habig, M. J. Pabst, and W. B. Jakoby, J. Biol. Chem. 249:7130-
    7139 (1974).

16. O. H. Lowry, N. J. Rosebrough, A. L. Farr, and R. J. Randall, J.
    Biol. Chem. 193:265-275 (1951).

17. Y. Miyake, J. L. Gaylor, and H. P. Morris, J. Biol. Chem. 249:1980-
    1987 (1974).

18. H. Mukhtar, C. M. Link, E. Cherniack, A. M. Kushner, and D. R. Bickers,
    Toxicol. Appl. Pharmacol. 64:541-549 (1982).

19. G. A. LePage and J. F. Henderson, in: "Progress in Experimental Tumor
    Research, Vol. 1" Kargar, Basel/New York, (1960) pp. 440-476.

20. V. R. Potter, Cancer Res. 21:1331-1333 (1961).

21. G. Hodgson, Brit. J. Dermatol. 60:282-284 (1948).

22. S. A. Henry, Brit. Med. Bull; 4:389-401 (1947).

23. W. E. Poel and A. G. Kammer, J. Natl. Cancer Inst. 18:41-55 (1957).

24. G. Kellerman, G. R. Shaw, and N. Luyten-Kellerman, N. Engl. J. Med. 289:934-937 (1972).

25. J. H. Epstein, F. J. Sullivan, and W. L. Epstein, J. Invest. Dermatol. 36:73-77 (1961).

IMMUNOSUPPRESSION BY ULTRAVIOLET RADIATION; POSSIBLE ROLE OF CIS-UROCANIC ACID, A PRODUCT OF UV IRRADIATION

Frances P. Noonan, Edward C. De Fabo and Harry Morrison

Flinders University of South Australia

Dermatology Department
George Washington University
Washington, D.C.

Department of Chemistry
Purdue University
Indiana

INTRODUCTION

Ultraviolet radiation has a suppressive effect on the immune system in vivo which appears to be a critical step in ultraviolet carcinogenesis, preventing the immunologic rejection of the highly antigenic UV-induced tumours.

We have studied the mechanism by which UV radiation initiates immune suppression; the wavelengths responsible (250-320 nm) do not penetrate beyond the skin, suggesting than an immunosuppressive photoproduct may be formed in the skin after UV radiation. From our studies which established an action spectrum or wavelength dependence for immunosuppression (De Fabo and Noonan, 1983, J. Exp. Med., 157:84-98), we put forward the hypothesis that UV-induced immune suppression is initiated by an interaction between UV radiation and urocanic acid, (deaminated histidine), one of the major UV-absorbing component of the stratum corneum. Urocanic acid undergoes an isomerization of UV irradiation from naturally occurring trans form to the cis form. We have investigated the premise that cis-urocanate interacts with the immune system.

Previous studies had indicated that UV irradiation in vivo depresses antigen presentation. Antigen presentation is a function of specialized cells of the reticuloendothelial system which have the function of processing antigen and presenting it to T lymphocytes thus triggering an immune response. Antigen presenting cells express on their surface a glycoprotein-Ia antigen, recognition of which by the T lymphocyte is essential for successful antigen presentation. Expression of the Ia antigen is labile, and represents an important control point of the immune response.

The epidermis contains antigen-presenting cells called Langerhans cells. We investigated if cis-urocanate alters the immunologic properties of these cells. Epidermal sheets from Balb/c mice were cultured with cis or trans urocanate in cell culture medium. The cultured sheets were then stained with one of four stains, and the number of Langerhans cells counted. A decrease of 25-35% in the number of Langerhans cells was found in epidermal sheets cultured with cis but not with trans urocanate, compared with control cultures, when either a fluorescein linked or a peroxidase linked stain for Ia antigen was used. In parallel cultures the number of Langerhans cells detectable was unchanged by cis urocanate if the sheets were stained for ATPase (detecting a membrane enzyme) or for the - glucuronidase (a cytoplasmic enzyme). It was necessary to culture the epidermal sheets for 3 days to demonstrate this effect, which was shown in two strains of mice bearing different alleles of the Ia antigen - Balb/c mice (Ia^d), and C3H mice (Ia^k). The effect appeared to be energy dependent as it did not occur at 4C, and was not due to interference by cis-urocanate with the binding of anti-Ia antibody to the Ia antigen since addition of cis urocanate to the anti-Ia antibody staining for Ia antigen had no effect.

These findings are consistent with an effect of cis-urocanate on a subset of Ia positive epidermal Langerhans cells, and are thus consistent with the hypothesis for a role of cis urocanate in modulating the immune response.

DNA DAMAGE AND CHROMOSOME ABERRATIONS

K. H. Chadwick and H. P. Leenhouts

National Institute for Public Health and Environmental
Hygiene, Bilthoven
and Association Euratom-ITAL Wageningen
The Netherlands

INTRODUCTION

Recent work in Medical Cytogenetics has demonstrated not only the close association between specific chromosome alterations and specific forms of cancer (81, 22, 34), but has also shown that oncogenes can be found to be involved in these specific chromosome alterations (17, 25, 2, 15). The suspected role of oncogenes in cancer has been strengthened by the very exciting developments in molecular biology which have shown the close homology between some cellular oncogenes and some viral genes and have examined the activity of oncogenes in cell transformation studies (6, 20, 78). There are indications of increased oncogene activity in transformed cells (45, 37), of the presence of mutated oncogenes in transformed cells (49, 47, 65), of the association between the oncogene protein product and platelet derived growth factor (76, 19) and that the loss of controlling genes possibly leads to the increased activity of oncogenes (4, 35) in retinoblastoma and neuroblastoma. These malignancies which occur predominantly in children and are to some extent hereditary, have been used by Knudsen (30) to support his two mutation theory of cancer induction. Other evidence supporting the mutation "theory" comes from the very close association between the mutagenic activity of certain chemical and physical agents and their known carcinogenic activity (38) and from the fact that medical syndromes associated with an increased susceptibility to cancer also are associated with decreased ability to repair DNA damage (63).

There is no doubt that some alteration or alterations to the nuclear DNA can transform a cell from a normal state to a malignant state, but there does not yet appear to be any general explanation which ties together all the different pieces of information in one coherent theory of the origin and cause of malignancy.

DNA damage and chromosome alterations are clearly part of the story and in this presentation we wish to discuss the association between DNA double strand breaks and chromosomal aberrations. We will also show that our assumption that the same radiation induced molecular lesion may lead to different biological end-points implies direct correlations between the end-points and present examples of these correlations.

The Unineme Structure of Chromosomes

It is now generally accepted that the unreplicated chromosome has as its backbone one continuous length of double helix DNA running from one end of the chromosome to the other. This has not always been the case and, although several lines of evidence pointed towards this so-called unineme structure of the chromosome, it was only with the DNA molecular weight determinations of Drosophila chromosomes by Kavenoff and Zimm (1973) that the concept became accepted.

The very long thin thread of DNA seems to be organized into a chromosome structure via the histone "beads" (31). The DNA is wrapped round the outside of the histone "beads" and a few base pairs of DNA form a linkage from one "bead" to another. The beads are then formed into a fibre and the fibre is spiralized to form the chromosome structure which becomes visible in mitotic cells (Figure 1). It now appears that the unspiralized interphase chromosome, invisible in the light microscope, is controlled in the cell nucleus by regular contact points with a cellular matrix structure.

Two well-known theories of chromosomal aberration formation, the Classical theory (59-61, 33) and the Exchange theory (51-54) were both developed prior to the general acceptance of the unineme structure of the chromosome.

The Classical Theory

Sax (59-61) concluded from a study of radiation induced chromosomal aberrations in Tradescantia that the breaks in the chromatid arms of the chromosome arose from a "one-hit type of event" and that the dose response relationship for chromatid breaks was linear. He proposed that sometimes two breaks interacted with each other leading to an exchange of chromosome material. These exchanges were thus expected to be related to the square of the dose, and this was close to what he found for X-rays. With more densely ionizing radiation, however, the exchanges were proportional to dose. Thus, it was concluded that the exchanges could only be formed when

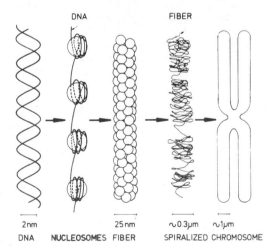

Fig. 1.   A schematic representation of how the very long DNA double helix molecule is organized in the chromosome so that it runs continuously from one end to the other forming the backbone of the chromosome.

the two breaks were close together so that both breaks might sometimes be induced by the same event and these exchanges would be proportional with dose. The more densely ionizing the radiation, the larger the proportion of exchanges induced linearly with dose. Lea and Catcheside (1942) proposed that the yield of exchanges should be described by a linear-quadratic dose relationship

$$Y = aD + bD^2 \qquad\qquad (1)$$

where "a" represents the one-hit component and "b" the two-hit component (Figure 2).

The Classical theory predicts that breaks should be linear with dose and also be plentiful in comparison with exchanges. Although the experimental work of Lea, Catcheside and Thoday (33, 69-70, 11) appeared to support these predictions, later work by Revell (1966) confirmed the results of Sax and suggested much fewer breaks compared with exchanges and a "two-hit component" in the dose relationship for the breaks. The "breaks" measured by Lea, Catcheside and Thoday are now thought to have been achromatic gaps and not true breaks at all.

In terms of the much later developed unineme structure of the chromosome and the double-helix model of DNA (77), the chromatid break can be equated with a DNA double strand break so that the Classical theory would now suggest that a simple break or deletion arose from one DNA double strand break and exchange arose from the interaction of two double strand breaks. Bender, Griggs and Bedford (1974) have more or less proposed that chromosome aberrations from cells irradiated in the G_1, pre-DNA replication, phase arise in this way from DNA double strand breaks induced completely by radiation, however, for aberrations arising in cells irradiated in S or G_2 phase they propose that some unrepaired single strand breaks may be converted to double strand breaks by the action of a single-strand nuclease enzyme.

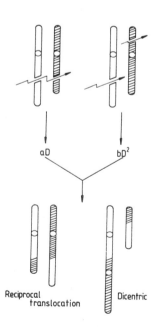

Fig. 2. Classical representation of the formation of chromosomal exchanges from two chromosome breaks and the derivation of the yield-dose equation.

The Exchange Theory

As a consequence of experimental measurements on chromatid aberrations in Vicia faba, Revell suggested an alternative theory of aberration formation in order to explain the low frequency of breaks compared to exchanges and also the non-linear dose relationship of the breaks. Revell suggest (51-54) that all chromatid aberrations, both breaks and exchanges, were formed from an exchange process and he also suggested that chromatid-arm breakage was "probably not the primary form of damage". He invoked a "primary event of damage" in a chromatid arm which could interact with another neighboring primary event to achieve "exchange initiation" which then led to the chromatid exchange. It is interesting to note that he compared the exchange process for aberration formation with meiotic recombination.

Revell's exchange theory is defined only for chromatid aberrations because it was developed as a result of observations of this G_2 type of aberration. There appears to be no reason why the theory should also not be applied to chromosome aberrations. The important differences with the Classical theory are that the Exchange theory predicts that all aberrations including breaks arise from an exchange type of process and should have linear-quadratic dose kinetics and that the exchange process is an active process, initiated by radiation events which lead to the breakage and exchange of chromatid arms.

The question that remains relates to the nature of the "primary event of damage" seen in terms of the unineme structure of the chromosome. Is it a DNA single strand break, a single strand base damage or is it a DNA double strand lesion?

The Molecular Theory of Aberration Formation

The molecular theory has been developed from the following postulates:

1. The dose relationship for the induction of DNA double strand breaks has in general a linear-quadratic form;

2. In the unineme concept of chromosome structure a DNA double strand break is a chromatid-arm break;

3. All chromosomal aberrations, breaks and exchanges found at the first mitosis after irradiation arise from one radiation induced chromatid-arm break and the cells attempt to repair that break;

4. All chromosomal aberrations will, therefore, exhibit a linear-quadratic dose relationship in general.

According to these proposals, some form of incorrect repair of the chromatid-arm break has to be invoked in order to be able to derive all the various aberration configurations which are normally found in irradiated cells.

It will become clear later that the repair process we prefer as an explanation of the formation of aberrations from a single chromatid-arm break, a recombination process, bears a close resemblance to the exchange process proposed by Revell so that the theory we propose can almost be envisaged as a modification and modernization of the exchange theory.

In order to explain the formation of chromosomal aberrations from one chromatid-arm break, we originally proposed that a broken chromatid end could join with a normal telomere (36). At that time, very little was known about the nature of the telomere and all the chromosome aberrations could be readily explained in this way. However, as Savage (1975) has correctly pointed out, the process of telomere-break rejoining can only lead to the formation of chromatid aberrations if some disturbance of the normally close sister chromatid pairing occurs; this is not usual and we agree with Savage that the telomere-break rejoining process is unlikely to be involved in the formation of chromatid aberrations.

When we wrote our book in 1979 (12), we discussed the possibility that the telomere-break rejoining process might be responsible for some chromosome aberrations. At the time, several pieces of information from chromosome banding studies of irradiated cells and in medical cytogenetics seemed to indicate a possible involvement of the chromosome ends in the formation of aberrations. Even the famous Philadelphia chromosome, associated with chronic myeloid leukemia, was thought to be formed by the translocation of a fragment from chromosome 22 to the end of the long arm of chromosome 9 (55-56, 18, 79, 48). Very recently, it has been shown, using molecular biological techniques that a minute piece of DNA from the end of the long-arm of chromosome 9 is reciprocally translocated to chromosome 22 so that this aberration is not formed by telomere-break rejoining (2). This result has made us review our ideas on telomere-break rejoining and conclude that although we do not discount the process completely, we do attach much more importance to the formation of aberrations via the recombination repair process. However, it is perhaps worth mentioning that if all the aberrations which we reviewed previously as evidence for telomere-break rejoining do arise from an exchange process, it would appear that the telomeres are rather active in this type of exchange.

Recombinational Repair of DNA Double Strand Breaks

The repair of DNA double strand breaks after radiation has been adequately demonstrated in recent years. Resnick (1976) proposed a model to explain how the radiation induced DNA double strand breaks could be repaired. Although Resnick's model was not originally developed to explain the formation of chromosomal aberrations, it was immediately clear to us that it provided a potential explanation for the formation of all the normal aberration configurations (13).

The essence of the Resnick model is that the repair of a DNA double strand break can be achieved by making use of a homologous undamaged DNA helix and the process of recombination. Sometimes the repair is not perfect and leads to an exchange of DNA pieces.

The model is summarized in Figure 3 and runs as follows:

a. and b. radiation induces a DNA double strand break;

c. enzyme activity causes partial degradation of one of the two strands at each of the two ends to leave single stranded "tails";

d. the single stranded "tails" are recombinogenic with an undamaged homologous DNA helix;

e. an endonuclease nick in one strand of the undamaged DNA helix permits the strand to pair by matching complementary bases with one of the single stranded regions at the break, forming a heteroduplex;

f. further unwinding of the undamaged helix permits a second heteroduplex to be formed between the second single strand "tail" and the other strand of the undamaged DNA helix;

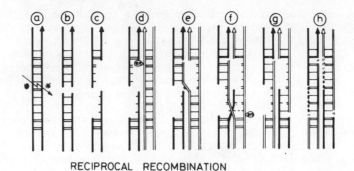

RECIPROCAL RECOMBINATION

Fig. 3.   Schematic representation at the DNA level of reciprocal
            recombination proposed by Resnick (1976) as one
            consequence of the repair of a DNA double strand break.

g. an endonuclease nick in this strand of the originally undamaged
    homologous DNA helix permits a reciprocal recombinational exchange of
    the DNA double helices;

h. DNA synthesis, polymerase and ligase, seal the small single strand gaps
    which remain.

    The reciprocal recombinational repair of one DNA double strand break
leads to an exchange of double helices and this can be envisaged as an
exchange of chromatid-arms.   The process of Figure 3 is re-drawn in terms
of the chromosomes in Figure 4 which shows how the process results in
areciprocal translocation.   We have thus two DNA double strand breaks or
chromatid-arm breaks involved in the exchange but only one is caused by
radiation.   The second arises enzymatically as a result of a repair
process.   All chromosomal aberration configurations apparently arising from
two chromatid-arm breaks can be explained quite rationally by this process.

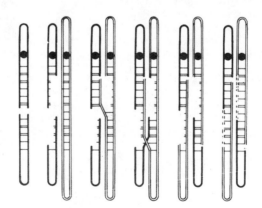

RECIPROCAL TRANSLOCATION

Fig. 4.   The translation of the molecular process of
            Resnick to the situation at the chromosomal level
            using the unineme concept of chromosome structure.
            This figure shows that at this level reciprocal
            recombination can lead to the formation of a
            reciprocal translocation.   Other configura- tions
            can easily be derived from the same process.

However, the process depends completely on the close association between the DNA double helix carrying the radiation induced DNA double strand break and a homologous undamaged DNA helix. At first sight it would appear that this repair would only be possible between sister chromatids or homologous chromosomes. Fortunately, the repair process proposed by Resnick only requires homology between the two DNA double helices in the region around the double strand break and this short range homology can, in principle, be provided by any other chromosome. A large proportion of the eukaryotic chromosomal DNA is made up of highly repetitive and closely homologous DNA sequences (7, 16, 71) distributed throughout the genome. This repetitive DNA means that the recombinational repair of a DNA double strand break can occur quite readily between non-homologous chromosomes and provides us with a general model to describe chromosomal aberration configurations as a logical consequence of the cell's attempt to repair one DNA double strand break. A detailed drawing of how the different configurations are formed as a consequence of this repair process has been provided previously and readers are referred to our book (pages 68-69) (12).

A good comparison can now be made between our proposals and the Exchange theory of Revell. Both theories invoke an exchange or recombination type of process between two chromatid-arms, the only real difference being that Revell proposed a "primary event of damage" in each chromatid-arm giving "exchange initiation", whereas we propose one radiation induced lesion--a double strand break--in one chromatid-arm with homologous association with an undamaged second chromatid to give "exchange initiation". With the recent developments in molecular biology, we are able to identify our radiation induced lesion and define via Resnick's model the molecular processes involved in the exchange process.

One consequence of our model is that the repetitive DNA sequences should be preferentially involved in chromosomal aberration formation in the region of the break-points and, although the repetitive DNA is distributed throughout the genome, it does appear to be concentrated in certain regions such as centromeres, telomeres, and heterochromatin. This would mean that, although the initiating double strand breaks might be randomly distributed over the genome, those occurring in regions of repetitive DNA would be more likely to be found involved in aberration formation and thus the "break-points" determined in radiation cytology may be expected to be non-randomly distributed in the genome. There is experimental evidence that this does happen and non-random distributions of "break-points" have been reported with over-representation in centromeric, telomeric, and hetero-chromatin (9-10, 26, 32, 62, 73, 1, 8, 14, 21, 43-44, 57, 24, 80).

A Model for Meiotic Recombination

As a consequence of a review of the extensive genetic analysis of meiotic recombination and a study of yeast transformation using E. coli plasmids with part of a yeast chromosome carrying a double stranded gap, Szostak et al. (1983) have proposed a new model to explain meiotic recombination which is based on the repair of a DNA double strand break. The double strand break is considered to be the initiation site for recombination which can lead to either gene conversion or crossing over (Figure 5). As can be seen, the model bears a very strong resemblance to that of Resnick and contains the same basic features. In a later paper, Sugawara and Szostak (1983) consider the possibilities of recombination occurring between repetitive DNA in non-homologous chromosomes. They find some restriction in this type of recombination possibly by an aspect of higher order chromosome structure, although this restriction appeared to be less severe when the recombining plasmid contained a centromere. It was

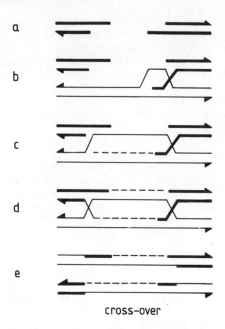

a

b

c

d

e

cross-over

Fig. 5.   The double strand break repair model of
Szostak et al. (1983) mainly developed to
explain meiotic recombination but showing a
lot of similarity to the model of Resnick.

also found that this recombination in yeast depended on the RAD 52 gene
which is associated with the repair of DNA double strand breaks and lack of
which renders yeast very sensitive to ionizing radiation.

These recent results and the consequent model of Szostak et al.
suggest that the repair of a DNA double strand break can lead to the
exchange of chromatid-arms and thus the formation of chromosome
aberrations. In our opinion, there is now considerable experimental
evidence both in E. coli and yeast, to support our proposal that one
chromatid-arm break can, by way of a recombinational repair process, lead
to chromosomal aberrations in eukaryotic cells.

Experimental Evidence on the Role of DNA Double Strand Breaks in the
Formation of Chromosomal Aberrations

Probably the most direct evidence for the crucial role of DNA double
strand breaks in the formation of chromosomal aberrations is to be found in
the series of publications by Natarajan and Obe (41-44). These
publications describe a set of elegant experiments in which Neurospora
endonuclease (NE) was introduced into Chinese Hamster Ovary cells after
irradiation. Neurospora endonuclease is known to be specific for single
stranded DNA and converts a single strand break into a double strand break.
Natarajan and Obe determined the numbers of chromatid aberrations in G_2
cells with and without the endonuclease treatment after X-ray and UV
exposure (1978). They demonstrated a substantial increase (more than
factor 2) in both the number of chromatid breaks and exchanges after X-
rays. The endonuclease did not affect the UV induced aberrations.

They later showed a similar effect after X-ray treatment of G_1 cells,
although these results were somewhat confused by the appearance of
chromatid-type of aberrations in the G_1 irradiated cells as a result of the

endonuclease treatment (42). They also investigated the repair time of the single strand breaks in G_2 cells by delaying the endonuclease treatment and showed that after 30 minutes the endonuclease only increased the number of breaks and not of exchanges. This was interpreted to indicate that, although the single strand breaks remained open, under the experimental conditions used, and could be converted to breaks, the time for the breaks to be converted to exchanges was too short prior to the mitosis. This paper also presents direct evidence that the endonuclease does convert single strand breaks to double strand breaks by reporting measurements of DNA molecular weight distributions after X-rays with and without the endonuclease treatment. The last paper in this series reports on the endonuclease induced increase in aberrations after X-ray and neutron irradiation and shows the the enzyme has less effect on the neutron induced aberrations than on those from X-rays. This is also logically explained by the relative number of single strand breaks and double strand breaks, as neutrons, because of their more densely ionizing tracks, are expected to produce relatively more double strand breaks than X-rays.

All these experiments are interpreted by the authors to demonstrate that "(a) the basic structure involved in chromosome aberrations is DNA; (b) double strand breaks lead to chromosome aberrations".

In addition, we note that in all the data reported by Natarajan et al. on the effect of Neurospora endonuclease the relative increase in the number of breaks is very closely similar to the relative increase in the number of exchanges. In terms of the Classical hypothesis this is not what would be expected as the breaks are proposed to be straight-forward breaks and the exchanges should arise from the interaction between two breaks. Thus, all things being equal, according to the Classical hypothesis, the relative increase in the number of exchanges should be the square of the relative increase in breaks; this is obviously not the case.

Although the relative increase in the number of double strand breaks caused by the endonuclease treatment is also reported to be around 2 (42) close to the value for breaks and exchanges, we do not think that this can be taken as serious evidence in favour of our proposal that one DNA double strand break gives a chromosomal exchange as the X-ray doses and the experimental conditions used for the DNA measurements were quite different from those used for the chromosomal studies.

Nevertheless, these results provide compelling evidence in favour of a direct association between DNA double strand breaks and chromosomal aberrations.

Another set of experiments which provide direct evidence that the target for the induction of chromosomal aberrations must be very small indeed are those which have studied the formation of chromosomal aberrations after irradiation with very soft X-rays (74-75, 67-68, 23). These experiments used carbon X-rays (0.28 keV) which produce electron tracks depositing all their energy in less than 7 nm, to produce exchange aberrations (dicentries, centre rings) in lymphoxytes, V 79 Chinese hamster cells and human fibroblasts. In all cases, the C X-rays were very efficient in producing these aberrations at low radiation doses where the " " term dominated the dose effect relationship and where the aberrations must have arisen from single tracks (Figure 6). The results lead the authors to conclude: "if DNA is assumed to be the target molecule (dimension 2 nm) ... either that only one DNA helix needs to be damaged by the radiation for an exchange to occur between it and an undamaged helix where they are virtually in contact" (Goodhead et al., 1980). The results of Natarajan, et al., clearly indicate that this DNA damage must be a DNA double strand break.

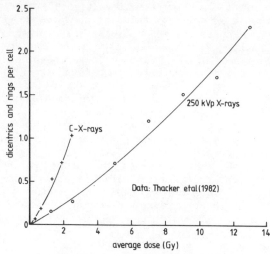

Fig. 6. A comparison of the dose-effect relationships for the induction of dicentrics and rings in plateau-phase V 79 Chinese hamster cells for 0.28 keV carbon X-rays and 250 kVp X-rays showing the high efficiency of the soft C X-rays at low doses (redrawn from Thacker et al., 1982).

The BUdR Experiment

In a series of ingenious experiments Kihlman and Natarajan have tried to investigate the formation of chromosomal aberrations by using the 5-bromodeoxyuridine labelling method (BUdR) (28-29, 42). By allowing cells to replicate for one or two rounds in BUdR, the chromatids in the cells were not only made more sensitive to X-rays but also could be differentiated from each other at the scoring because of the different staining properties of the labelled and unlabelled chromatids. The most important experiments concerned the use of Vicia faba root cells in the G_2 phase (28-29) as they led to the interpretation that two lesions on separate chromatid arms were necessary to produce a chromatid exchange, a conclusion in direct contradiction with our hypothesis. In the following, we discuss the results of these experiments and offer our alternative interpretation.

The protocol of the experiments is shown in Figure 7. After one round of DNA synthesis in BUdR the two chromatids each have one strand of the DNA normally loaded with thymidine (T) and the other strand partially loaded with BUdR (B); a second round of DNA synthesis in BUdR leads to one chromatid with both strands loaded with BUdR (BB) one chromatid of TB constitution. Alternatively, a second round in normal medium leads to one chromatid with both strands unloaded (TT) and the other of TB constitution. After the two rounds of synthesis the cells were exposed either to long UV light (320-380 nm) or to X-rays and were gathered at mitosis for scoring. The differential staining permitted an investigation of whether exchanges occurred predominately between the more sensitive chromatids (e.g., TB constitution) or between TB and TT chromatids.

The long UV experiment was done because exposure of TT type chromatids does not cause any aberrations, whereas exposure of TB chromatids causes aberrations which are very similar to those normally induced by X-rays.

254

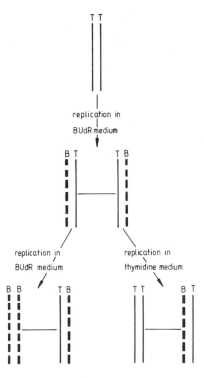

Fig. 7. A schematic representation of the
protocol of BUdR loading of chromosomes
and the constitution of the chromatids
for the comparative treatments used by
Kihlman et al. (1978).

This experiment offered the possibility of investigating, in cells of TT/TB
constitution, whether exchanges occurred between the damaged TB chromatids
and the undamaged TT chromatids.

What Kihlman et al. (1978) found is shown in Table 1. In addition,
Kihlman et al. claim only to find 4 TT-TB exchanges out of a possible 71
per 100 cells and they conclude that although the 4 TT-TB exchanges do show
that the Resnick repair process might be possible, it is only a rare event.
However, in making up the numbers Kihlman et al. exclude completely the 12
isochromatid breaks, which would also indicate interaction between TT and
TB chromatids and they ignore the small excess of SCE, i.e., 0.6/cell,

Table 1. Total aberrations and SCE's found by Kihlman et al. (1978)
after exposure of TT-TB chromosomes of Vicia faba to long UV
light

Treatment	Aberrations per 100 cells				SCE per cell
	Chromatid breaks	Isochromatid breaks	Sub-chromatid exchanges	Chromatid exchanges	
BUdR + UV	14	12	43	28	22.9
BUdR − no UV	0	0	0	0	22.3

found in the light experiment. The isochromatid breaks are excluded because they are supposed to be associated with an SCE, although only 2 of them could definitely be associated with an SCE.

An estimate of the probability for this association for the Classical or Exchange two-lesion model of isochromatid break can be made as follows.

Vicia faba has 12 chromosomes and at 23 SCE per cell as found by Kihlman et al. (1978) we have 2 SCE per chromosome.

Assume 10% of a chromatid is involved in an SCE (we feel this is overestimated) then the probability that the first lesion for the isochromatid break falls by the SCE is 2 x 1/10. The probability that the second lesion falls at the same place on the other chromatid is the probability that it falls on the same chromosome (1/12) multiplied by the probability it occurs by the SCE (1/10) = 1/120.

Total probability for the isochromatid break at exactly the same place as the SCE is 2/10 x 1/120 = 1/600. With an expectancy of 1:600, the exclusion of 12 TT-TB exchanges in a total of 83 exchanges per 100 cells is not justified mathematically.

According to our one lesion model, the chance that the lesion coincided with an SCE would be 2/10, which is comparable with the 2 out of 12 reported.

The 0.6 SCE/cell excess in the light experiment is ignored by Kihlman et al. as an average of 22.9 is not considered significantly different from 22.3 without light. However, in each case of four experiments the light exposure induced more SCE's. We think these SCE's are induced by the light in an exchange process as shown in Figure 8. If this is the case, we would have to add a further 60 TT-TB exchanges per 100 cells to the numbers quoted by Kihlman et al.

We now conclude that what Kihlman et al. really found were 71 - 4 = 67 TB-TB exchanges and 4 + 12 + 60 = 76 TT-TB exchanges and that the TB-TT exchange, between a damaged and undamaged chromatid is far from rare and occurs to about the same extent as TB-TB exchanges.

In the X-ray experiment Kihlman et al. (1978) irradiated G_2 cells of Vicia faba having TT-TT, TT-TB, TB-TB, and TB-BB constitution with 40 R and measured the frequency and types of chromosomal aberrations induced (Table 2). They showed an increasing sensitivity with increased chromosomal loading with BUdR. They then used the collection times of the cells with TT-TB constitution and analyzed whether breakage or exchange occurred in TT or TB chromatids (Table 3). They then concluded that, as there were $\sim$3 times more breaks in TB than in TT chromatids (27:10) according to the two lesion model for exchanges there should be $(3)^2$ = 9 times as many exchanges between TB-TB chromatids as between TT-TT chromatids with 6 times as many exchanges between TT-TB chromatids. They compared their expected values 1:6:9 with the experimental values 1:9.4:9.6 and concluded that two lesions must be involved in an exchange, though they found an overrepresentation of TT-TB exchanges. Two things are extremely important here, the first is that Kihlman et al. (1978) in making this comparison used $\sim$100 exchanges but chose to ignore completely over 50 isochromatid breaks, presumably TT-TB exchanges, on the grounds that they must be associated with SCE's, though no evidence for this was presented. The second important point is that, by deriving the increased sensitivity value of $\sim$3 from the breaks and calculating the value of 9 for exchanges, Kihlman et al. (1978) automatically, though possibly not consciously, adopted the Classical theory of aberration formation. The Exchange theory predicts all breaks are a result of exchange, thus the sensitivity increase for the breaks

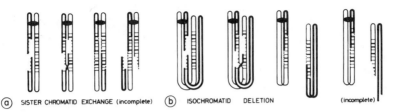

Fig. 8.   Schematic representation to show how the Resnick model
          for repair of a DNA double strand break can lead to the
          formation of sister chromatid exchanges without the
          necessity of the DNA synthesis phase.

Table 2.   Types and frequencies of aberrations induced by 40
           R of X-rays in G_2 chromosomes of Vicia faba having
           TT-TT, TT-TB, TB-TB and TB-BB constitution (Data:
           Kihlman et al., 1978)

Constitution	Aberrations per 100 cells - control		
	Chromatid breaks	Isochromatid breaks	Chromatid exchanges
TT-TT	4.7	8.9	11.7
TT-TB	8.2	10.9	21.2
TB-TB	15.5	21.0	44.7
TB-BB	19.0	18.3	51.1

Table 3.   Analysis of break points in aberrations formed
           when TT-TB cells were irradiated with X-rays.
           Collection time 5 hours after exposure (Data:
           Kihlman et al., 1978)

Chromatid segment involved	Frequency of aberrations			
	Chromatid breaks	Chromatid exchanges	Triradial	Sum
TT	9	–	1	10
TB	24	–	3	27
TT and TT	–	5	–	5
TT and TB	–	47	–	47
TB and TB	–	48	–	48

would be the same as for the exchanges. According to the Molecular theory,
we predict that one break can give an exchange and expect the sensitivity
increase for breaks and exchanges to be the same. In their analysis of the
TT-TB experiment, the ratio of breaks 10-27 is clearly not the same as that
for exchanges 5:48 (Table 3). However, their analysis of the TB-BB
experiment shows that the ratio of breaks 12:22 is very closely the same as
that for exchanges 9:19. In addition, if we examine Table 2 in more detail
and consider the breaks and exchanges produced at 5 and 6 hour collection
time in TT-TT cells, where the lesions have to be in TT chromatids,
independent of the theory, and compare them with those in TB-TB cells, we
find that the ratio of breaks 4.7:15.5 = 1:3.3 is very closely similar to
the ratio of exchanges 11.7:44.7 = 1:3.8.

We can use the data in Table 2 more fully as follows: let us assume
that the loading of one strand of a DNA helix increases the sensitivity of
that chromatid by an amount s, then we can define the relative chromatid
sensitivities for lesion induction as $t(TT) = 1$; $t(TB) = 1 + s$; $t(BB) = 1 + 2s$.

257

If we now define $t(i)$ and $t(j)$ as the relative sensitivities of the chromatids i and j where i and j can be TT, TB or BB, then we can calculate the relative frequency of breaks and exchanges for each theory.

Classical theory predicts:

$$\text{relative frequency of breaks} = (t(i) + t(j))/2 \tag{2}$$

$$\text{relative frequency of exchanges} = ((t(i) + t(j))/2)^2 \tag{3}$$

and the ratio of breaks in TB-TB:breaks in TT-TT cells is $1 + s_c : 1$.

Exchange theory predicts:

$$\text{relative frequency of breaks} = \text{relative frequency of exchanges} = ((t(i) + t(j))/2)^2 \tag{4}$$

and the ratio of breaks in TB-TB:breaks in TT-TT cells is $(1 + s_e)^2 : 1$.

Molecular theory predicts:

$$\text{relative frequency of breaks} = \text{relative frequency of exchanges} = (t(i) + t(j))/2 \tag{5}$$

and the ratio of breaks in TB-TB:breaks in TT-TT cells is $1 + s_m : 1$.

According to Table 2, the ratio of breaks in TB-TB:breaks in TT-TT cells is $15.5:4.7 = 3.3:1$. Thus, $s_c = 2.3$, $s_e = 0.82$, $s_m = 2.3$ and we can calculate the expected relative frequencies of breaks and exchanges according to each theory for TT-TT, TT-TB, TB-TB and TB-BB cells using equations 2, 3, 4, and 5, and the relevant values of s_c, s_e, and s_m. These are shown in Table 4 and compared with the experimental values derived from

Table 4. Expected relative frequencies of chromatid breaks and exchanges on basis of different theories normalized to the relative frequencies of breaks for TT-TT and TB-TB cells

Cell	Classical		Exchange		Molecular		Experiment	
	Breaks	Exchanges	Breaks	Exchanges	Breaks	Exchanges	Breaks	Exchanges
TT-TT	1	1	1	1	1	1	1	1
TT-TB	2.15	4.62	1.98	1.98	2.15	2.15	1.74	1.81
TB-TB	3.30	10.89	3.30	3.30	3.30	3.30	3.30	3.82
TB-BB	4.45	19.80	4.97	4.97	4.45	4.45	4.04	4.36

Table 2. Figure 9 presents the data in graphical form where the actual experimental values are used and the theories are normalized to the vaues for TT-TT cells. The results in the table and figure demonstrate that no distinction can be made between the theories using the data for the breaks, but that the Classical theory can quite clearly be rejected on the basis of the exchange data, which, however, does not distinguish between the exchange and molecular theories. Figure 10 presents the experimental data from Figure 9 in a slightly different way. The frequency of exchanges is plotted against the frequency of breaks for each cell constitution. The straight line through the origin indicates that both breaks and exchanges are formed by the same type of process.

258

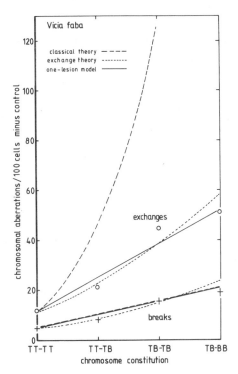

Fig. 9. A comparison of the frequencies of
chromatid breaks and exchanges induced in
four different differentially BUdR
labelled cells expected on the basis of
the Classical, Exchange and Molecular
theories and the values determined
experimentally by Kihlman et al. (1978).
The theoretical curves are normalized at
the values of breaks and exchanges found
in TT-TT cells and the value for
breaks found in TB-TB cells.

We conclude that while the results of these ingenious BUdR experiments
have been interpreted as evidence against our theory of chromosomal
aberrations in favour of the classical theory, in actual fact the majority
of the results argue strongly against the classical theory and favour the
Exchange theory or our theory without being able to discriminate between
these two theories.

CONCLUSIONS

Our general conclusion is that our theory of chromosomal aberrations
is in accordance with the unineme structure of the chromosome, provides a
molecular lesion which is known to be recombinogenic, involves known enzyme
and DNA repair processes, makes use of the repetitive DNA scattered
throughout the genome, is in line with the evidence showing DNA double
strand breaks to be the important lesions, is in agreement with the
evidence showing the target to be <7 nm in size, and has yet to be
disproved.

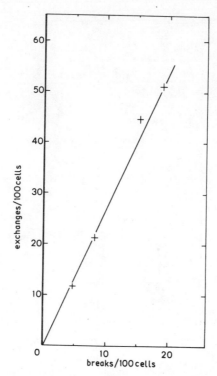

Fig. 10. A plot of the frequencies of breaks against the frequencies of exchanges measured by Kihlman et al. (1978) in four different differentially labelled cells after 40 R of X-rays. The straight line relationship between the breaks and exchanges passing through the origin indicates that both types of aberration arise from a common mechanism.

ACKNOWLEDGEMENT

This publication is contribution number 2170 of the Biology Division of the Commission of the European Communities. The work was supported by contract number BIO-E-478-NL of the Radiation Protection Programme and by the Dutch Ministries of Agriculture and Fisheries and of Welfare, Health and Culture.

REFERENCES

1. F. E. Arrighi, P. P. Saunders, G. F. Saunders, T. C. Hsu, _Experimentia_ 27:964-966 (1971).

2. C. R. Bartram, A. de Klein, A. Hagemeijer, T. van Agthoven, A. Geurts van Kessel, D. Bootsma, G. Grosveld, M. A. Ferguson-Smith, T. Davies, M. Stone, N. Heisterkamp, J. R. Stephenson, and J. Groffen, _Nature_ 306:227-280 (1983).

3. M. A. Bender, H. G. Griggs, and J. S. Bedford, _Mutat. Res._ 23:197-212 (1974).

4. W. F. Benedict, A. L. Murphree, A. Banerjee, C. A. Spina, M. C. Sparkes, and R. S. Sparkes, Science 219:973-975 (1983).

5. R. Berger, Nouv. Presse Med. 46:3121 (1973).

6. J. M. Bishop, Sci. Am. 246(3):69-78 (1982).

7. R. J. Britten and D. E. Kohne, Science 161:529-540 (1968).

8. K. E. Buckton, Int. J. Radiat. Biol. 29:475-488 (1976).

9. T. Caspersson, L. Zech, C. Johansson, and E. J. Modest, Chromosoma 30:215-227 (1970).

10. T. Caspersson, V. Hagland, B. Lindell, and L. Zech, Exp. Cell Res. 75:541-543 (1972).

11. D. G. Catcheside, D. E. Lea, and J. M. Thoday, J. Genet. 47:113-136 (1946).

12. K. H. Chadwick and H. P. Leenhouts, in: "The Molecular Theory of Radiation Biology," Springer Verlag, Heidelberg (1981).

13. K. H. Chadwick and H. P. Leenhouts, Int. J. Radiat. Biol. 33:517-529 (1978).

14. P. Cooke, M. Seabright, and M. Wheeler, Humangenetik 28:221-231 (1975).

15. S. Crews, R. Barth, L. Hood, J. Prehn, and K. Calame, Science 218:1319-1321 (1982).

16. E. H. Davidson and R. J. Britten, Q. Rev. Biol. 48:565-613 (1973).

17. A. de Klein, A. Geurts van Kessel, G. Grosveld, C. R. Bartram, A. Hagemeijer, D. Bootsma, N. K. Spurr, N. Heisterkamp, J. Groffen, and J. R. Stephenson, Nature 300:765-767 (1982).

18. M. C. Dinauer and R. V. Pierre, Lancet II:971 (1973).

19. R. F. Doolittle, M. W. Hunkapiller, L. E. Hood, S. G. Devare, K. C. Robbins, S. A. Aaronson, and H. N. Antoniades, Science 221:275-277 (1983).

20. P. H. Duesberg, Nature 304:219-226 (1983).

21. H. J. Evans and T. R. L. Bigger, Genetics 46:227-289 (1961).

22. D. Forman and J. Rowley, Nature 300:403-404 (1982).

23. D. T. Goodhead, R. P. Virsik, D. Harder, J. Thacker, R. Cox, and R. Blohm, in: "Proc. 7th Microdosimetry Symposium," J. Booz, H. G. Ebert, H. D. Hartfiel, eds., EUR 7147, CEC, Brussels (1980), pp. 1275-1285.

24. F. T. Hatch, A. J. Bodner, J. A. Mazrimas, and D. H. Moore, Chromosoma 58:155-168 (1976).

25. N. Heisterkamp, J. R. Stephenson, J. Groffen, P. F. Hansen, A. de Klein, C. R. Bartram, and G. Grosveld, Nature 306:239-242 (1983).

26. M. Holmberg and J. Jonasson, Hereditas 74:57-67 (1973).

27. R. Kavenoff and B. H. Zimm, Chromosoma 41:1-27 (1973).

28. B. A. Kihlman, H. C. Andersson, and A. T. Natarajan, in: "Chromosomes Today 6," A. de la Chapelle and M. Sorsa, eds., Elsevier, Amsterdam (1977), pp. 287-296.

29. B. A. Kihlman, A. T. Natarajan, and H. C. Andersson, Mutat. Res. 52:181-198 (1978).

30. A. G. Knudson, L. C. Strong, and D. E. Anderson, in: "Prog. in Med. Genet.," A. G. Steinberg and A. G. Bearn, eds., Grane and Stratton, New York (1973), pp. 113-158.

31. R. D. Kornberg, Science 184:868-871 (1974).

32. M. Kucerova and Z. Polivkova, Mutat. Res. 34:279-290 (1976).

33. D. E. Lea and D. G. Catcheside, J. Genet. 44:216-245 (1942).

34. M. M. Lebeau and J. D. Rowley, Nature 308:607-608 (1984).

35. W-H. Lee, A. L. Murphree and W. F. Benedict, Nature 309:458-460 (1984).

36. H. P. Leenhouts and K. H. Chadwick, Theor. App. Genet. 44:167-172 (1974).

37. C. D. Little, M. M. Nan, D. N. Carney, A. F. Gazdar and J. F. Minna, Nature 306:194-196 (1983).

38. J. McCann and B. N. Ames, Proc. Natl. Acad. Sci. USA 73:950-954 (1976).

39. A. T. Natarajan and G. Ahnstrom, Chromosoma 28:48-61 (1969).

40. A. T. Natarajan and G. Ahnstrom, Chromosoma 30:250-257 (1970).

41. A. T. Natarajan and G. Obe, Mutat. Res. 52:137-149 (1978).

42. A. T. Natarajan, G. Obe, A. A. van Zealand, F. Palitti, M. Meijers, and E. A. M. Verdegaal-Immerzeel, Mutat. Res. 69:293-305 (1980a).

43. A. T. Natarajan, B. A. Kihlman, and G. Obe, Mutat. Res. 73:307-317 (1980b).

44. A. T. Natarajan and T. S. B. Zwanenburg, Mutat. Res. 95:1-6 (1982).

45. P. Nowell, J. Finan, R. Dalla Favera, R. C. Gallo, A. ar-Rushdi, H. Romanczuk, J. R. Selden, B. S. Emanuel, G. Rovera and C. M. Croce, Nature 306:494-497 (1983).

46. P. Petit and C. Cauchie, Lancet II:94 (1973).

47. T. H. Rabbitts, P. H. Hamlyn and R. Baer, Nature 306:760-765 (1983).

48. T. Raposa, A. T. Natarajan, and I. Granberg, J. Natl. Cancer Inst. 52:1935-1938 (1974).

49. E. P. Reddy, R. K. Reynolds, E. Santos, and M. Barbacid, Nature 300:149-152 (1982).

50. M. A. Resnick, J. Theor. Biol. 59:97-106 (1976).

51. S. H. Revell, in: "Proc. Radiobiol. Symp. Liege," Butterworth, London (1955) pp. 243-253.

52. S. H. Revell, Proc. R. Soc. Ser. B. (London) 150:563-589 (1959).

53. S. H. Revell, in: "Radiation Induced Chromosome Aberrations," S. Wolff, ed., Columbia University Press, New York (1963) pp. 42-72.

54. S. H. Revell, Mutat. Res. 3:34-53 (1966).

55. J. D. Rowley, Nature 243:290-293 (1973a).

56. J. D. Rowley, Ann. Genet. 16:109-112 (1973b).

57. C. San Roman and M. Bobrow, Mutat. Res. 18:325-332 (1973).

58. J. R. K. Savage, Radiat. Bot. 15:87-140 (1975).

59. K. Sax, Proc. Natl. Acad. Sci. USA 25:225-233 (1939).

60. K. Sax, Genetics 25:41-68 (1940).

61. K. Sax, Cold Spring Harbor Symp. 9:93-103 (1941).

62. M. Seabright, Chromosoma 40:333-346 (1973).

63. R. B. Setlow, Nature 271:713-717 (1978).

64. N. Sugawara and J. W. Szostak, Proc. Natl. Acad. Sci. USA 80:5675-5679 (1983).

65. S. Sukumar, V. Notario, D. Martin-Zanca and M. Barbacid, Nature 306:658-661 (1983).

66. J. W. Szostak, T. L. Orr-Weaver, R. J. Rothstein and F. W. Stahl, Cell 33:25-35 (1983).

67. J. Thacker, R. Cox, and D. T. Goodhead, Int. J. Radiat. Biol. 38:469-472 (1980).

68. J. Thacker, D. T. Goodhead and R. E. Wilkinson, in: "Proc. 8th Microdosimetry Symp.," J. Booz and H. G. Ebert, eds., EUR 8395, CEC, Brussels (1982), pp. 587-595.

69. J. M. Thoday, J. Genet. 43:189 (1942).

70. J. M. Thoday, Brit. J. Radiol. 24:572-576, 622-628 (1951).

71. C. A. Thomas, B. A. Hamkalo, D. N. Misra, and C. S. Lee, J. Mol. Biol. 51:621-632 (1970).

72. H. Van der Berghe, J. P. Fryns, and F. Devos, Humangenetick 20:163-166 (1973).

73. H. Van Steenis, R. Tuscany, and B. Leigh, Mutat. Res. 23:223-228 (1974).

74. R. P. Virsik, R. Blohm, K. P. Hermann and D. Harder, in: "Proc. 7th Microdosimetry Symp.," J. Booz, H. G. Ebert, and H. D. Hartfiel, eds., EUR 7147, CEC, Brussels (1980) pp. 943-955.

75. R. P. Virsik, D. T. Goodhead, R. Cox, J. Thacker, C. Schafer, and D. Harder, Int. J. Radiat. Biol. 38:545-557 (1980).

76. M. D. Waterfield, G. T. Scrace, N. Whittle, P. Stroobant, A. Johnsson, A. Wasteson, B. Westermark, C-H. Heldin, J. S. Huang, and T. F. Denel, Nature 304:35-39 (1983).

77. J. D. Watson and F. H. C. Crick, Nature 171:737-738 (1953).

78. R. W. Weinberg, Sci. Amer. 249(5):102-116 (1983).

79. J. Whang-Peng, T. A. Knudsen, and E. C. Lee, J. Natl. Cancer Inst., 51:2009-2012 (1973).

80. J. S. Yoon and R. H. Richardson, Genetics 88:305-316 (1978).

81. J. J. Yunis, Science 221:227-236 (1983).

CHROMOSOME BREAK-POINTS, SOMATIC MUTATION AND ONCOGENE ACTIVATION: SOME COMMENTS

K. H. Chadwick and H. P. Leenhouts

National Institute for Public Health and Environmental
Hygiene, Bilthoven
Association Euratom-ITAL
Wageningen, The Netherlands

INTRODUCTION

In previous publications (3, 8) we have attempted to associate the DNA double strand break with the induction of malignancy by making use of the "somatic mutation" theory of malignancy. In particular, we tried to align our ideas on chromosome aberrations with the then current ideas on the nature of malignancy which suggested that the factor governing malignancy behaved as a recessive gene. This idea had been developed from cell fusion experiments between malignant and non-malignant cells where it was found that the malignant factor was suppressed in the hybrids initially, but returned eventually with the loss of chromosomes from the hybrid cell (6) (see Figure 1). These results in mouse-mouse and mouse-human hybrids which were not very chromosome stable were supported by work with human-human hybrids which were much more chromosomally stable (12). When we developed these ideas we suggested that with the further development of the analysis of malignancy, we would probably have to revise our ideas, although we were convinced that radiation induced cancer and somatic mutation were directly related. However, at that time we did not anticipate the tremendous development in the investigation of the role of oncogenes in malignancy which has occurred during the past few years. In this paper we review the ideas we developed on the basis of the cell fusion-hybrid experiments and discuss some of the more recent developments in the molecular biology of malignancy with respect to the role of chromosome aberrations in the induction of malignancy.

The Recessive Malignant Genotype

The results of the cell-fusion experiments which indicated that the factor controlling malignancy behaved as a recessive genetic character and could be suppressed by a dominant normal chromosomal factor suggested to us that a normal diploid cell could be in one of two genetic situations; it could be a diploid carrier cell already having the recessive malignant gene but being unable to express it because of the presence of the normal suppressing factors, or it could be a diploid non-carrier cell.

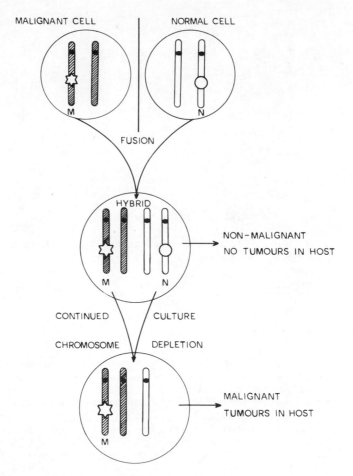

Fig. 1.   Schematic representation of the interpretation of the
          cell fusion experiments used to investigate the genetic
          character of malignancy. M represents the malignant
          factor, N the controlling suppressive factor.

In the case of the diploid carrier cell a chromosome aberration
affecting the normal suppressing factor will permit the expression of the
malignant factor and make the cell potentially malignant. This is shown
schematically in Figure 2 which also includes the possibility that a second
aberration could eliminate the malignant factor itself and render the cell
non-malignant. This scheme leads to an equation for cell transformation
per surviving cell as a function of radiation dose of:

$$T = (1 - \exp(-q(\alpha D + \beta D^2)))\ \ \exp(-s(\alpha D + \beta D^2)) \tag{1}$$

where $\alpha D + \beta D^2$ represents the dose relationship for the induction of DNA
          double strand breaks,

     q   is the probability that a double strand break removes the
          normal suppressive factor

and   s   is the probability that a double strand break mutates the
          malignant factor to block its expression.

Figure 3 demonstrates the application of this equation to the data of Borek and Hall (1973) on the transformation of hamster embryo cells by radiation.

In Figure 4 we present a scheme for the effect of radiation on a diploid non-carrier cell in which two possibilities are shown: if

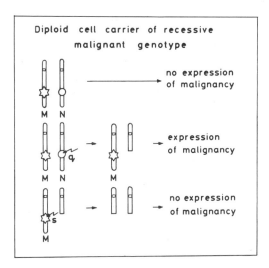

Fig. 2.   Schematic representation for the induction of cell transformation by radiation in a diploid cell which already carries the malignant factor. N represents the controlling suppressive factor, M represents the malignant factor.

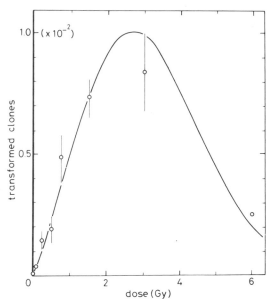

Fig. 3.   Application of equation (1) to the data of Borek and Hall (1973) for the transformation of primary cultures of hamster embryo cells induced by radiation.

radiation cannot induce the malignant factor then a diploid non-carrier
cell will never be converted by radiation alone to a malignant state; if
radiation can induce the malignant factor then one would expect two
radiation events to be necessary to convert the non-carrier cell to a
potentially malignant state. In this case, the cell transformation
equation is given by:

$$T_{d,n} = (1 - \exp(-q_m(\alpha D + \beta D^2)))\ (1-\exp(-q(\alpha D + \beta D^2)))\ \exp(-s(\alpha D + \beta D^2))\quad (2)$$

where q_m is the probability that a double strand break induces the
malignant factor.

Figure 5 compares the cell transformation equations for a diploid
carrier and non-carrier cell. The incidence for the non-carrier cell,
assuming the malignant factor can be induced by radiation would be much
lower and have different dose kinetics than that for a carrier cell.

Now, we try to consider how these proposals of carrier and non-carrier
cells appear in terms of the latest developments in the molecular biology
of malignancy.

Cell Fusion Studies Using Human Cells

The chromosomal instabilities originally encountered in mouse-mouse and
mouse-human hybrids appear to have been avoided in the human-human hybrids.
The better stability of these hybrids permits a more detailed study of the
properties of the hybrids (13). Most of the hybrids studied by Stanbridge
and his colleagues were formed by fusing the tumorigenic Hela cells with
normal diploid fibroblasts. These hybrid cells grew well in both normal
medium and in a minimal medium in which normal cells do not proliferate,
even so the hybrid cells did not induce tumours in the different immuno

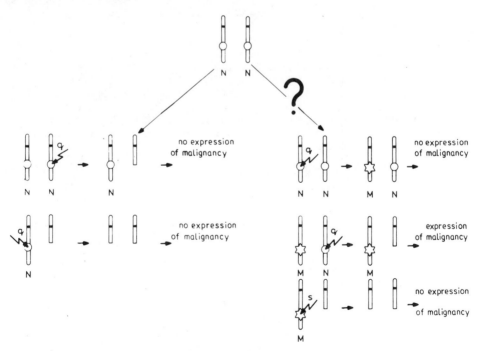

Fig. 4.   Schematic representation of the possible effects of radiation
on a diploid non-carrier cell.

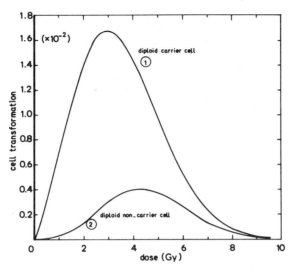

Fig. 5.   Possible theoretical dose-response relationships for
cell transformation. Curve 1 in a diploid carrier cell
(Equation 1); Curve 2 in a non-carrier cell if
radiation can induce the malignant factor (Equation 2). α
= 7.10^{-2} Gy^{-1}; β = 5.10^{-2} Gy^{-2}; q = 0.07, s = 1.5; q_m =
0.3.

suppressed mice into which they were injected. After continued growth in
culture the hybrids occasionally became tumorigenic and the conversion to
tumorigenicity was always accompanied by the loss of a few chromosomes.
Chromosome banding techniques have indicated that the loss of chromosomes
11 and 14, respectively, is associated with the reexpression of the
malignant phenotype.

Attempts to study hybrids between normal human diploid fibroblasts and
other malignant human cells have been largely frustrated because the
hybrids could not be established as a continuously growing culture. One
hybrid between a lung carcinoma cell and normal fibroblasts was established
and proved to be non-malignant. Using sarcoma cell lines, fused to normal
fibroblasts, hybrid populations have been established, but only when at
least a tetraploid complement of the sarcoma cell was present in the
hybrid. In these cases, there did not appear to be a suppression of
malignancy by the normal fibroblast chromosomes. This suggests that in
this system a gene dosage effect may be operating to both give the hybrids
the ability to continue to divide and also to make them malignant.

In an attempt to study whether malignancy was a single or multiple
genetic locus effect, Stanbridge et al. (1982) fused several different
combinations of human malignant cell lines together. The results were
interesting because when carcinoma lines were fused together the hybrids
were highly tumorigenic but when carcinoma cells were fused with sarcoma
cells or with melanoma cells the hybrids were non-tumorigenic. This led to
the conclusion that in carcinoma cells a common genetic locus governs the
expression of malignancy and complementation does not occur in hybrids
formed from malignant cells of the same somatic origin. There seem to be a
number of genes which control the expression of malignancy and there may be
one gene for each somatic type of malignant cell.

Stanbridge et al. (1982) conclude that their studies lead to a two-
step model (Figure 6) for the progression of a normal cell to a neoplastic

269

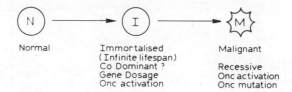

Normal   Immortalised   Malignant
(Infinite lifespan)
Co Dominant ?   Recessive
Gene Dosage   Onc activation
Onc activation   Onc mutation

Fig. 6.　A two-step model for the progression of a normal
cell to a malignant cell. This sort of model can
be derived from the cell fusion studies (13) and
from the oncogene studies (15).

one. Each step is considered to be under a separate genetic control, the
first step leads a normal cell with a limited ability to divide into a
state of unlimited proliferation and a second step converts the
proliferating non-tumorigenic cell to the tumorigenic state. Stanbridge et
al. (1982) also state that "the key difference between the transformed
(proliferating) non-tumorigenic cells and their tumorigenic segregants is
their response to growth regulatory signals in the intact animal".

The two step model is very interesting especially in view of the ideas
now arising from work with oncogenes on the progression of normal cells via
immortalization (unlimited proliferation) to malignancy.

The Typical Chromosomal Rearrangements

The use of refined chromosome banding techniques over the past 15
years has provided cytologists with the means not only to identify the
different individual chromosomes in a cell but also to study the
chromosomal complement of the malignant cell. This last aspect of cytology
has been most fruitful and it can now be concluded that very many different
cancers have typical chromosomal defects (16). The common defects are
reciprocal translocations between two chromosomes or specific band
deletions. In the reciprocal translocations one chromosome breaks at a
specific site consistently (donor chromosome) while the break point in the
second chromosome may vary (receptor chromosome). Occasionally a specific
chromosome occurs in triplicate (trisomy) in certain cancers. Recent
molecular biological techniques have identified the translocations as truly
reciprocal and Mitelman (1984) has found that the number of chromosomal
regions associated with the aberrations typical of human malignancies is
restricted.

The typical chromosomal aberrations are obviously closely associated
with the development of the specific malignancies but the question remains
as to whether they are the initiating event or only a direct consequence of
the malignancy. Table 1 presents a list of several malignancies together
with the typical chromosomal defect and where possible the oncogenes
identified with the defect or the relevant chromosomes. There now seems to
be some information which makes a consideration of the relevance of the
typical aberrations to the malignant character possible. In the first
place the aberrations found are very consistent, for instance the (9.22)
translocation is found in 95% of the cases of chronic myelogenous leukemia,
the (8.14) translocation in 100% of Burkitt's lymphoma, monosomy of
chromosome 22 in 95% of meningiomas, a deletion of chromosome 13 in 85% of
retinoblastomas. The retinoblastoma is interesting because it is a
hereditary malignancy, although it also occurs as a sporadic non-hereditary
event. In the hereditary cases all cells of the body show the deletion of
the band on chromosome 13 but in the sporadic non-hereditary cases the
deletion is only found in the tumour cells. Wilm's tumour is a similar

Table 1. A list of malignancies together with the typical chromosome aberrations and the oncogenes which have been associated with the chromosomes, though not necessarily at the break-points

Disease	Chromosome aberration	Oncogenes
− Leukemia		
Chronic myelogenous leukemia	t (9 : 22)	abl : sis
Acute non-lymphocytic leukemia		
M1	t (9 : 22)	abl : sis
M2	t (8 : 21)	myc,mos : −
M3	t (15 : 17)	fes : −
M4	inv 16	−
M4, M5	t (9 : 11)	abl : Ha-ras,ets
M1-6	del 5 q	fms
	del 7 q	−
	+ 8	myc,mos :
Chronic lymphocytic leukemia	+ 12	Ki-ras
	t (11 : 14)	Ha-ras,ets : −
Acute lymphocytic leukemia		
L1-L2	t (9 : 22)	abl : sis
L2	t (4 : 11)	: Ha-ras,ets
L3	t (8 : 14)	myc,mos : −
− Lymphomas		
Burkitt's, non-Burkitt's, large cell immunoblastic	t (8 : 14)	myc,mos : −
Folicular	t (14 : 18)	− : −
Small cell lymphocytic	+ 12	Ki-ras
	t (11 : 14)	Ha-ras,ets : −
− Carcinomas		
Neuroblastoma	del 1 p	ski,N-ras,Blym
Small cell lung	del 3 p	raf
Ovary papillary cystadeno	t (6 : 14)	myb : −
Retinoblastoma	del 13 q	−
Wilm's tumour	del 11 p	Ha-ras,ets
− Benign Solid tumours		
Mixed paratoid gland	t (3 : 8)	raf : myc,mos
Meningioma	− 22	sis

case, individuals showing a constitutional absence of the band p13 on chromosome 11 are predisposed to the aniridia Wilm's tumour syndrome, whereas in the non-hereditary cases this deletion is only found in the tumour. However, this deletion is not sufficient for the development of the tumour since only 40% of patients with the deletion and aniridia developed the tumour (16). It thus appears that the deletion predisposes a patient to neoplasia but that a second event is necessary for the malignancy to be initiated.

A recent very interesting development has been the chromosomal association of oncogenes to specific chromosomes and, in some cases, to the break-points of the typical chromosomal aberrations. C-myc oncogene is at the break-point of chromosome 8 and is translocated to chromosome 14 in Burkitt's lymphoma (Figure 7), c-abl is located on the terminal band of chromosome 9 which is broken in the (9, 22) translocation of chronic myelogenous leukemia, c-mos is associated with chromosome 8 at the band involved in the (8, 21) translocation found in some acute non-lymphocytic leukemia (ANLL), c-fes is associated with a (15,17) translocation found in another subgroup of ANLL. In some cases, the oncogenes show activation or increased transcription, in others an altered gene product is detected and in others no change in the oncogene product can be detected.

The specific aberrations and the association of oncogenes with these aberrations would appear to indicate that the chromosomal rearrangements are intimately involved in the development of malignancy but are perhaps not in themselves totally sufficient to be the only initiating event. We believe that the induction of chromosomal rearrangements probably represents the dominant role of radiation in the induction of malignancy.

Oncogenes

Retroviruses (RNA viruses) have been isolated from spontaneous animal tumours and have been shown to have in addition to the genes required for the construction of new virus particles, a gene which is not essential for the virus but which gives the virus the ability to transform a host cell to malignancy, the viral oncogene (v-onc). These viral oncogenes "are the fastest acting and most inevitable carcinogenic agent known to date" (5). These viral oncogenes appear to have been copied as a rare event from genes in the cell of the host in which the virus replicates. The cellular genes

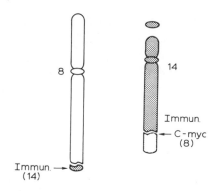

Fig. 7.   Schematic representation of the translocation
           between chromsome 8 and chromsome 14 found in
           Burkitt's lymphoma. C-myc moves from 8
           to join the broken heavy chain immunoglobin gene
           (14), part of which moves reciprocally to
           chromosome 8.

272

are called cellular oncogenes (c-onc), and some 20 of these genes have now
been identified. These cellular oncogenes are found in a wide variety of
species from Drosophila through mouse to man and have thus been very
strongly preserved through evolution. They obviously have an important
role to play in normal cellular function and the recent association of the
products of some of these genes with cell growth factors may partially
explain this importance (14, 4).

The discovery of these viral oncogenes and their cellular counter
parts led to two theories for cancer induction, the oncogene theory and the
protovirus theory. The oncogene theory proposed that all normal cells
contain unexpressed oncogenes and that these genes could be activated by
carcinogens or virus action. The protovirus theory proposed that normal
cells contain potential (proto) oncogenes which by somatic mutation and
retroviral or cellular reverse transcription could become viral or cellular
oncogenes (5, 1). The basic difference between the two theories is that
the oncogene theory implies that all cells carry genes which can cause
cancer if they are activated, while the protovirus theory suggests that the
normal cellular genes can only cause cancer after they have been altered or
mutated in someway. The oncogene theory suggests that the cellular
oncogenes should be exactly homologous to the viral oncogenes, the
protovirus theory suggests that this homology should not be perfect but the
v-onc and c-onc should be closely similar. Although it appeared at first
as if the v-onc and c-onc were exactly homologous (1) it now looks as if
there are subtle differences between the v-onc and c-onc genes (5, 15).

The study of retroviruses has revealed several oncogenes, but
interestingly, the isolation of the DNA piece from a malignant cell which
is capable of transfecting immortalized mouse cells from a non-tumorigenic
to a tumorigenic state (15) has revealed another group of oncogenes. One
of these oncogenes, from a human bladder carcinoma, defined by the gene
transfer experiments has been found to differ by only a 1 base pair
transition point mutation from the normal cellular proto-oncogene.
Furthermore, an overlap has been noted between the group of oncogenes found
from the study of retroviruses and those from the group found by gene
transfer. Indeed, the bladder carcinoma oncogene is a close relative of
the oncogene carried by the Harvey sarcoma virus derived from the rat, v-
Ha-ras. Other related ras oncogenes have been found associated with human
carcinomas of the colon, lung, bladder, and pancreas and in various
leukemias, a lymphoma, neuroblastoma, and sarcomas. This suggests that the
particular cellular proto-oncogene can be transformed to become an active
oncogene in several different tissues.

The transformation event appears to be a single step event but the
detection of this Ha-ras oncogene in the immortalized NIH 3T3 mouse cells
suggested that this event was possibly only one component of a complex
process. The use of non-immortalized cells together with the mutated Ha-
ras oncogene did not lead to tumorigenic cells even though the cellular
morphology induced by Ha-ras could be observed (7). However, when Ha-ras
was used in cooperation with another cellular oncogene, an active myc, in
the non-immortalized cells, dense foci of tumorigenic cells were found
(7). Thus, the combined effect of ras and myc converted the normal cells
to malignancy, a step which neither ras nor myc could do alone. These
results suggested an explanation of why multiple cellular oncogenes had been
found to be active in certain tumours, and they also suggested a molecular
explanation of the multiple step process of carcinogenesis.

Indeed these results indicate at least a two-step process of
immortalization and malignancy though Land et al. (1983) think that there
may be three steps as the tumours induced by cells transformed by ras + myc
stopped growing, in contrast to tumours caused by cells transformed by ras

+ large T antigen which grew to kill the host. However, recently it has been shown that normal cells can be transformed to malignancy by the enhanced transcription of the mutated Ha-ras gene from the bladder carcinoma. Enhanced transcription of the unmutated Ha-ras gene caused only immortalization, normal Ha-ras gene without enhanced transcription had no effect and strangely, the mutated Ha-ras gene without enhanced transcription also caused immortalization (11). The authors point out that the mutated Ha-ras gene does not need a cooperating gene to give malignant conversion but also point out that there are still two distinct steps, the mutation of the Ha-ras gene plus its enhanced transcription required to give the conversion.

DISCUSSION

The investigation of the molecular biology of the malignant state is proceeding at a tremendous rate and not all the information appears to lead to a simplificaction of the understanding of the origin of this disease. However, certain basic aspects new seem to be well established.

1. At least two steps, under separate genetic control, appear to be involved in the conversion of normal cells to malignancy. One step converts a normal cell to unlimited growth, i.e., it immortalizes the cell, the second step progresses the cell from a non-malignant to a malignant state (Figure 6).

2. The progression step appears to be recessive with a possible dependence on gene dosage.

3. Typical chromosome rearrangements are associated with specific neoplasia, often involve oncogene rearrangements and may act in the deregulation of oncogenes.

4. Oncogenes differ from the cellular proto-oncogenes sometimes by very small point mutations.

5. Very many human malignant cell lines and tumours demonstrate multiple c-oncogene expression (10).

The important problem for us is how does radiation influence the conversion of a normal non-malignant cell to a malignant cell? It is clear that radiation could induce the typical chromosomal rearrangements and that this could possibly act as the progression step by activating one or more oncogenes.

The question that remains uppermost in our minds is whether one single radiation event could achieve this conversion process or are other events needed to "predispose" the cell to malignancy.

At present, we do not think that an answer can be given, but we think that information on the following points would help to formulate an answer:

a. is the point mutation which makes Ha-ras so effective in progressing immortalized cells to malignancy typical of the change required in cellular proto-oncogenes to make them "progressor" oncogenes or can a gross aberration of a cellular proto-oncogene convert it to a "progressor" oncogene;

b. can a gross aberration in a cellular proto-oncogene convert it by activating its transcription into an "immortalization" oncogene;

    c. is the sequence always from normal to immortalization to malignancy or can the malignancy step occur first and remain quiescent until the immortalization event.

If the Ha-<u>ras</u> gene is really typical, we do not see how a radiation induced double strand break could lead to both the point mutation and the enhanced transcription of the gene via a chromosomal rearrangement in one event.

We return to our figure questioning the effect of radiation on a non-carrier cell (Figure 4). Although we probably have to refine our ideas on the nature of the "non-carrier" and "carrier" cell, we are still left with the question whether radiation can convert a "non-carrier" normal cell directly to the state of malignancy.

CONCLUSION

We conclude that although molecular biology has advanced the state of knowledge on the progression of a normal cell to the malignant state tremendously in the past 5 years and we can accept that a DNA double strand break giving a chromosomal rearrangement, possibly involving oncogenes, could convert a "pre-disposed" cell to become malignant, we are not yet sure that radiation in itself can convert a normal cell directly to the malignant state.

We believe that it is important for the philosophical basis of risk evaluation to be able to relate hypotheses of radiation action to the prevailing and advancing concepts of the biology of the cancer cell.

ACKNOWLEDGEMENT

This publication is contribution number 2172 of the Biology Division of the Commission of the European Communities. The work was supported by contract number BIO-E-478-NL of the Radiation Protection Programme and by the Dutch Ministries of Agriculture and Fisheries and of Welfare, Health and Culture.

REFERENCES

1. J. M. Bishop, <u>Sci. Amer.</u> 246:68-79 (1982).

2. C. Borek and E. J. Hall, <u>Nature</u> 243:450-453 (1973).

3. K. H. Chadwick and H. P. Leenhouts, <u>in</u>: "The Molecular Theory of Radiation Biology," Springer Verlag, Heidelberg (1981).

4. R. F. Doolittle, M. W. Hunkapiller, L. E. Hood, S. G. Devare, K. C. Robbins, S. A. Aaronson, and H. N. Antoniades, <u>Science</u> 221:275-277 (1983).

5. P. H. Duesberg, <u>Nature</u> 304:219-226 (1983).

6. H. Harris, <u>J. Natl. Cancer Inst</u> 48:851-864 (1972).

7. H. Land, L. F. Parada, and R. A. Weinberg, <u>Science</u> 222:771-778 (1983).

8. H. P. Leenhouts and K. H. Chadwick, <u>Int. J. Radiat. Biol.</u> 33:357-370 (1978).

9. F. Mitelman, _Nature_ 310:325-327 (1984).

10. D. J. Slamon, J. B. deKernion, I. M. Verma, and M. J. Cline, _Science_ 224:256-262 (1984).

11. D. A. Spandidos and N. M. Wilkie, _Nature_ 310:469-475 (1984).

12. E. J. Stanbridge, _Nature_ 260:17-20 (1976).

13. E. J. Stanbridge, C. J. Der, C-J. Doersen, R. Y. Nishimi, D. M. Peehl, B. E. Weissman, and J. E. Wilkinson, _Science_ 215:252-259 (1982).

14. M. D. Waterfield, G. T. Scrace, N. Whittle, P. Stroobant, A. Johnson, A. Wasterson, B. Westermark, C-H. Heldin, J. S. Huang, and T. F. Denel, _Nature_ 304:35-39 (1983).

15. R. A. Weinberg, _Scie._ _Amer._ 249:102-117 (1983).

16. J. J. Yunis, _Science_ 221:227-236 (1983).

THE YIELD OF CHROMOSOMAL ABERRATIONS AND ITS CORRELATION WITH OTHER BIOLOGICAL ENDPOINTS

H. P. Leenhouts and K. H. Chadwick

National Institute for Public Health and Environmental
Hygiene, Bilthoven
and Association Euratom-ITAL
Wageningen, The Netherlands

INTRODUCTION

We have proposed in our preceding chapter that all radiation induced chromosomal aberrations arise from one DNA double strand break by a process of chromosomal repair. In this paper we consider the yield of chromosomal aberrations as a function of dose and consider the effect of different dose rates and types of radiation on the yield. We also show that if the DNA double strand break is proposed as the crucial lesion, then mathematical correlations between different endpoints can be predicted and are found experimentally. We discuss these correlations, their implications and the evidence which suggests that the crucial lesion really is the DNA double strand break.

The Yield of Chromosomal Aberrations

Figure 1 presents a schematic diagram of how we consider DNA double strand breaks can be induced by radiation. We do not present here a detailed derivation of the coefficients "α" and "β" but would draw attention to the fact that in the complete derivation (4) these coefficients contain parameters to take into account the effects of repair and of different types of radiation.

The number (N) of DNA double strand breaks induced by a dose (D) is given by:

$$N = \alpha D + \beta D^2 \tag{1}$$

where α is the probability per cell per unit dose that both strands of the DNA helix are broken simultaneously in the passage of one ionizing particle,

and β is the probability per cell per unit dose squared that two independently induced DNA single strand breaks form a double strand break.

If c_0 is the experimental scoring efficiency for a specific type of aberration and f_c is a function of repair and is the probability that an

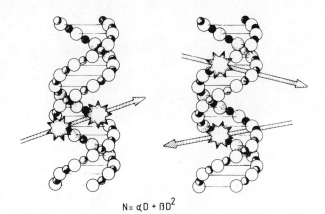

$$N = \alpha D + \beta D^2$$

Fig. 1.   Schematic representation of the induction of DNA
double strand breaks by ionizing radiation showing
the linear- quadratic dose relationship.

induced DNA double strand break leads to the formation of the specific
aberration then the yield (Y) of specific aberrations per cell is given by:

$$Y = c_0 f_c \, (\alpha D + \beta D^2), \tag{2}$$

and if $c = c_0 f_c$

$$Y = c(\alpha D + \beta D^2). \tag{3}$$

This is one form of the well-known linear-quadratic dose equation
which is known to describe accurately the yield of aberrations. This
equation is different from other derivations of the linear-quadratic equation (20) in as much as our equation refers to a specific type of molecular damage in a molecule having a well defined three dimensional structure and
well known repair properties. The association of the equation with the
molecular damage means that repair functions can be identified and their
effects predicted mathematically; it probably makes the hypothesis more
"visible", however, it also introduces serious restrictions on the hypothesis as everything must be explained within the known properties of the
molecule.

One problem we have encountered concerns the yield of DNA double
strand breaks which has often been found to be a linear function of dose
when measured immediately after radiation although within 1 hour of
radiation the yield becomes distinctly linear-quadratic (36, 11, 12). It
is not known exactly why the function changes but time and probably repair
appear to be involved. We are still convinced that the β-term is a true
"two-hit" term and speculate on the basis of certain radical scavenging
experiments (5) and our own calculations (21) that a different radical
mechanism is involved in the β-term than in the "α"-term. As shown in
Figure 2, we believe that the α-term double strand break arises from two OH
radicals formed simultaneously within 1 nm of the two DNA sugar-phosphate
strands. The β-term, on the other hand, we believe arises from one OH
radical close to one of the strands, followed by some "relaxation" of the
DNA helix at that point, which takes a little time and makes the second
undamaged strand vulnerable to attack by a different radical which is

formed up to 30 nm from the DNA and which in first instance only damages the strand without breaking it. We then propose that this double stranded lesion is recombinogenic and is converted to a break during the following repair process. In this way, we maintain a "two-hit term" which requires time and repair to be revealed.

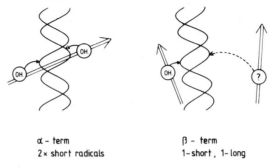

α - term
2× short radicals

β - term
1-short, 1-long

Details of β-term

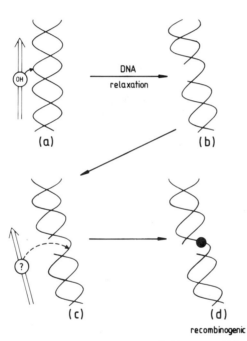

Fig. 2.   Schematic representation of the possible mechanisms involved in the induction of the "α" term (two short range OH radicals) and of the "β" term (one short range OH radical followed by helix relaxations and one long range radical followed by repair).

The Dose Rate Effect and the LET Effect

The yield equation 3 coupled with the molecular lesion permits some considerations to be made about the effect of dose rate and of different types of radiation on the yield of chromosomal aberrations.

The α-term is formed by two simultaneous events in the same track and is of course independent of time and dose rate.

The -term is formed by two independent events and the time between the two events will obviously depend on the dose rate; the lower the dose rate the more time there will be between the two events, and the more time there will be for the first single strand break to repair before the second event occurs. Thus, with decreasing dose rate the -coefficient, which carries a parameter f_1 to account for the repair of single strand breaks, will also decrease and at very low dose rates will become zero. Thus, at very low dose rates the yield of aberrations will become:

$$Y = c\alpha D \qquad (4)$$

A further decrease in the dose rate will not alter the yield equation. If it is assumed that the repair of DNA single strand breaks follows a first order process with time it can be shown (4) that

$$f_1 = (e^{-\lambda t} - 1 + \lambda t) \cdot 2/(\lambda t)^2 \qquad (5)$$

where λ is the repair rate constant for single strand breaks and the yield of aberrations can be written as

$$Y = c(\alpha D + f_1 \beta_\infty D^2) \qquad (6)$$

where β_∞ is the β found after an acute irradiation.

This expression for f_1 is similar to the expressions derived by others using a two-lesion type of model with repair of sub-lesions (28, 18, 19).

The interesting feature of the equation 5 for f_1 and its inclusion in equation 6 is that if the repair of "sub-lesions", identified here as single strand breaks, is exponential in time, than an accurate analysis of the dose rate effect can only be made if the yield curve is made using the same exposure time for each dose. A series of yield curves can be made using a series of exposure times and a full analysis according to equation 6 can be made. Lloyd et al (1984) have recently made this series of experiments for the yield of dicentrics and rings in human lymphocytes and have shown that the analysis is compatible with an equation which is equivalent to equation 6, they find a repair constant of $\lambda = 0.5$ h^{-1} (Figure 3).

Bauchinger and Schmid have also looked carefully at the dose rate effect and have shown that the dose relationship for dicentrics in human lymphocytes was linear-quadratic at both 0.5 Gy/min and at 0.017 Gy/min and that the α-term remained constant (2, 3). They also showed that the curve at 0.017 Gy/min could be derived from that found at 0.5 Gy/min by using the G(x) function of Lea (1946), a function identical to our function for f_1, and the repair rate of the sub-lesions which they had previously determined in split dose experiments (29).

Virsik and Harder (1980a) have also used split dose measurements to study the repair of sub-lesions and have shown that the repair rate was independent of dose and radiation quality for radiations of low LET.

These results support the linear-quadratic equation, indicate that the β -term is truly a two-hit term and suggest the exponential repair of the sub-lesions. They are in accordance with our theoretical proposals but do not say anything about the molecular nature of the target or the sub-lesion.

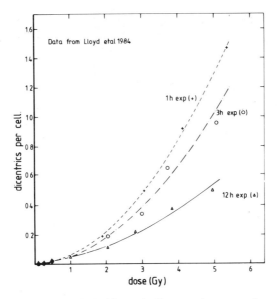

Fig. 3. The effect of different dose rates, or irradiation
times on the dose response relationship for the yield
of chromosome aberrations (data from: ref. 25).

Three groups have studied the efficiency of aberration induction as a
function of radiation quality, two groups have worked with human lymphocytes (22-24, 13-14, 26, 35) and one group has worked with different cell
cultures (37-38, 1). All the groups have found that the α-term is strongly
dependent on radiation quality and increases as the radiation becomes more
densely ionizing. Qualitatively the increase in "α" can be easily understood in terms of the three dimensional structure and dimensions of the DNA
molecule. The more densely ionizing the radiation is the more closely
together are the ionization events along a particle track and the greater
the chance that two ionization events occur close to the two strands of the
DNA helix. Quantitatively the calculation of "α" for different radiations
is rather complicated but our recent calculations using modern concepts of
radiation track structure and the dimensions of the DNA molecule suggest
that the type of dependence of "α" on radiation quality generally found
(Figure 4) is compatible with our proposal that the crucial lesion for
aberration formation is a DNA double strand break.

Correlations

In the development of our theoretical model we have not only suggested
that the DNA double strand break was the crucial lesion for chromosomal
aberrations but also that it could lead to cell lethality and to mutation
induction. An important, and testable, consequence of this suggestion is
that a direct correlation should exist between two different biological
endpoints when they are measured in the same experiment. In addition, it
should be possible to correlate the endpoint with DNA strand breakage when
they are measured by the same experiment.

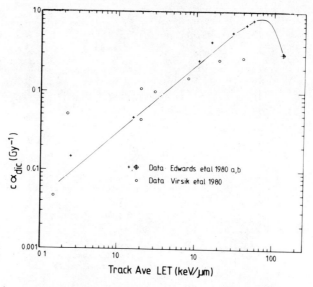

Fig. 4.   The dependence of the "α" term on the yield of
chromosomal aberrations on the radiation quality
(data from: refs. 14, 35).

Firstly, we define mathematically the expected correlations before
examining suitable data.

If the number of DNA double strand breaks is given by

$$N = \alpha D + \beta D^2 \tag{1}$$

and if p, q, and c are the probabilities that a double strand break causes
cell killing, mutation, and chromosomal aberrations, respectively, then

$$\text{Cell Survival} \qquad S = \exp(-pN) \tag{7}$$

$$\text{Mutation Frequency} \quad M = 1 - \exp(-qN) \stackrel{\sim}{=} qN \tag{8}$$

$$\text{and Aberration Yield} \qquad Y = cN \tag{9}$$

$N = \alpha D + \beta D^2$ is common to equations 7, 8, and 9 which can be combined
to eliminate N and give the following correlations:

$$\text{Cell Survival - Mutations} \qquad \ell nS = (-p/q) M \tag{10}$$

$$\text{Cell Survival - Aberration Yield} \quad \ell nS = (p/c) Y \tag{11}$$

These equations predict a linear relationship between cell survival
and mutation frequency or aberration yield.

In addition, it will be clear that if the yield of one type of
aberration (Y_1) is given by

$$Y_1 = c_1 N \tag{12}$$

and the yield of a second type of aberration Y_2 is given by

$$Y_2 = c_2 N \qquad (13)$$

then a correlation exists between Y_1 and Y_2 such that

$$Y_1 = \frac{c_1}{c_2} Y_2 \qquad (14)$$

We have previously published several correlations between two different types of aberrations and found them to be in agreement with equation 14 (4). In Figure 5 we present data on dicentrics and acentrics induced in human lymphocytes by different types of radiation. Since we first published this figure in 1981, we have been able to add data for two additional types of radiation which fall along exactly the same correlation. It should be noted that the correlation defined by equation 14 would also be expected on the basis of the exchange theory where all aberrations are assumed to arise from the same sorts of lesions via exchange. It would not be expected on the basis of the Classical theory.

If we now turn to correlations (which are unique to our theoretical model, and more especially to that) between cell survival and aberration yield predicted by equation 11, Figure 6 shows the most comprehensive set of data we have analysed so far. Dewey et al. (1970, 1971a, b) measured cell survival and aberration yield in synchronous cells exposed with and without the incorporation of the sensitizer BUdR. Dewey et al. also published correlations between survival and chromatid arm breaks although they did not have theoretical grounds for the correlation. They found a good correlation up to three breaks per cell but had counted deletions as one break, exchanges as two breaks and tri-radials as four breaks. In our analysis of their data we have counted deletions and exchanges as one break and tri-radials as two breaks. Figure 7 presents all the data in one correlation and shows a good straight-line relationship, in accordance with equation 11 up to five breaks per cell. Dewey et al. (1978) have also found a similar correlation when combined hyperthermia and X-rays were used.

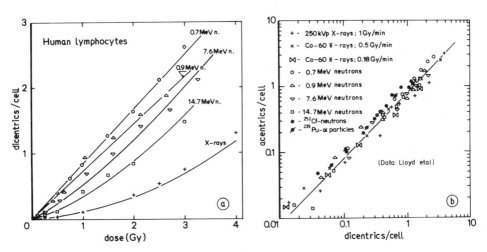

Fig. 5. The correlation between dicentrics and acentric fragments induced in human lymphocytes by different types of radiation analyzed according to equation 14 (data from: refs. 22, 23).

Figure 8 shows another correlation of the same sort, logarithm of survival versus aberrations, derived from the data of Thacker et al. (1982) (taken directly from their Figures 1 and 2) for carbon-X-rays and 250 kVp X-rays.

A consideration of the LET dependence of chromosomal aberration induction and survival has led Virsik and Harder (1980b) and Zoetelief and Barendsen (1983) to conclude that chromosomal aberrations are responsible for cell killing, even though Virsik ad Harder compared aberrations in lymphocytes and cell death in bone marrow cells and Zoetelief and Barendsen studies only dicentrics and centric rings and concluded that these were not the only aberrations which caused cell killing.

Our conclusion is not that chromosomal aberrations cause cell killing as such, but that both biological endpoints arise from the same basic type of molecular lesion, the DNA double strand break.

Two relatively recent publications throw some rather clear light on the correlation between survival and residual DNA strand breaks. The first by Weibezahn et al. (1980) measured survival and DNA strand breaks immediately and 1 hour after irradiation of Chinese hamster cells with X-rays and π-mesons. Figure 9 shows the correlation between the logarithm of

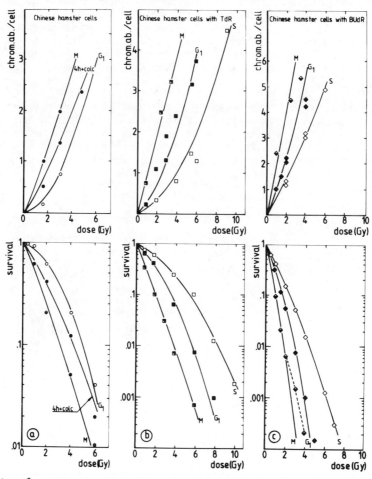

Fig. 6. The dose response relationships for survival and aberration yield in synchronized Chinese hamster cells with and without BUdR sensitized (data from: refs. 7-9).

284

survival and the residual DNA strand breaks 1 hour after irradiation. The straightline correlations are clearly in accordance with equation 7, the fact that the correaltions are not identical for both radiations can probably be explained because the cells are not quite in exactly the same situation one hour after the two types of radiation.

The second correlation is taken directly from the work of Dikomey et al. (1982) who studied survival and DNA strand breakage 1 hour after combined treatments of hyperthermia and X-rays. As the Figure 10 shows the correlation for all three different treatments is the same and is in accordance with equation 7.

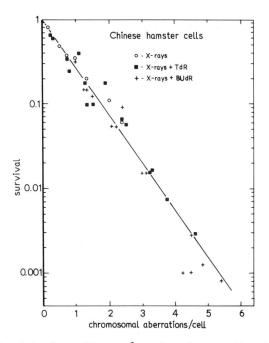

Fig. 7. The data from Figure 6 analyzed according to equation 11 showing the single straight line correlation for all the data.

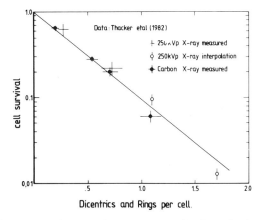

Fig. 8. Another correlation between survival and aberration yield for soft X-rays and conventional X-rays analyzed according to equation 11 (data from: ref. 32).

In our opinion, these correlations in which the molecular lesions have been measured at the same radiation doses as cell survival, demonstrate the clear and direct association between the DNA double strand breaks measured in the cells at 1 hour after irradiation and the cells' ability to continue to divide and survive.

We present one further correlation, that between survival and somatic mutation, because of its relevance to the induction of cancer. We have previously presented some examples of this correlation predicted by equation 10 (4) and show here the data of Rao and Hopwood (1982) in Figure 11. These data show the same correlation between the logarithm of survival and mutation frequency in stationary cells with and without a post damage. This result has been confirmed by the recent publication of Iliakis (1984) and a reproduction of the correlation Iliakis made is shown in Figure 12.

One set of data (15), although showing a good linear correlation between logarithm of survival and mutation, did not give the same correlation for different radiation types and was apparently in contradiction with our prediction that the correlations should be independent of the way in which the initial lesions are induced. Goodhead, et al. (1980) have suggested that at least part of this discrepancy might be explained by the fact that high LET radiation will induce several lesions in one cell by the passage of one particle track and that the lesions will not be distributed through a cell population according to Poissonian statistics. Our own recent calculations on DNA double strand break induction by different radiations support this and suggest that all of the difference between the correlations could be explained in this way.

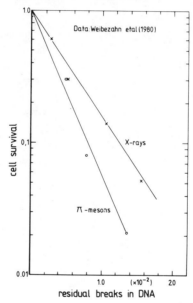

Fig. 9. The correlation between survival and residual DNA strand breaks measured 1 hour after irradiation for X-rays and π-mesons analyzed according to equation 7 (data from: ref. 36).

In the Figures 5-12 we have presented a series of direct correlations between the different endpoints survival, aberration induction and mutation frequency and in Figures 9 and 10 is shown that survival is directly correlated with DNA strand breaks at 1 hour after irradiation. Important evidence which supports our suggestion that one type of lesion is responsible for the different effects, is the work of Goodhead, et al. (16, 32) who

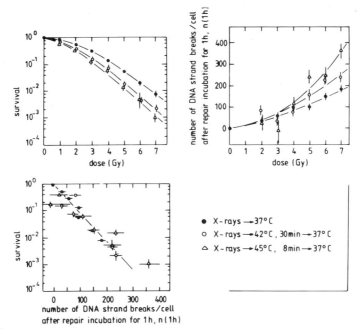

Fig. 10. The correlation between survival and residual DNA
strand breaks measured 1 hour after three different
X-ray-hyperthermia treatments analysed according to
equation 7 (redrawn from: 11).

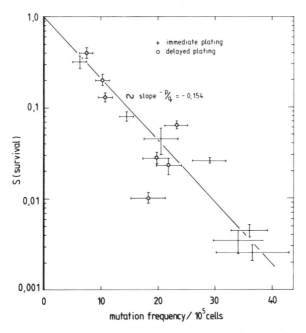

Fig. 11. The correlation between survival and mutation
frequency with and without repair of potentially
lethal damage analysed according to equation 10 (data
from: ref. 27).

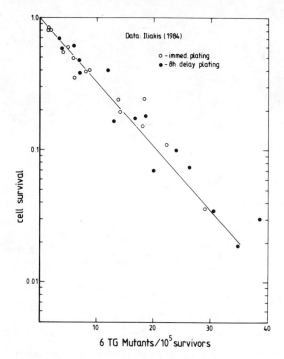

Fig. 12. The correlation between survival and mutation
frequency with and without repair of potentially
lethal damage found by Iliakis (1984) and in
accordance with equation 10.

have shown that very soft carbon X-rays are very efficient for the
induction of cell killing, aberrations and mutations and that the target
for all these effect must be smaller than 7 nm. We thus have a series of
links from the molecular lesion, the DNA double strand break, through
survival to chromosomal aberrations and mutations and although we have no
correlations between survival and cell transformation, we believe that via
the somatic mutation the DNA double strand break is a lesion which plays an
important role in the induction of cancer.

CONCLUSION

     The linear-quadratic equation for the yield of chromosomal aberrations
is derived from our proposal for the induction of DNA double strand breaks.
The dose rate effect can be explained by the repair of sublesions associated in our model with DNA single strand breaks. The LET dependence of
the yield of aberrations is compatible with the DNA double strand break as
the critical lesion.

     The series of correlations provide convincing evidence that the diffe-
rent biological endpoints all arise from the same basic type of lesion.
One correlation might arise as a pure coincidence but when a series of 9
different experiments all giving differently curved dose response relationships can be associated in one linear correlation (7, 8, 9) then the
correlation can no longer be considered as a coincidence but means that the
two correlating biological endpoints share a common origin. When we
discussed the correlations previously (4), we had no direct associations to

the molecular lesions and could only conclude from the mutation and aberration correlations that the lesion must be in the DNA molecule. We now have direct correlations which associate cell survival with the number of DNA double strand breaks measured at one hour after irradiation.

ACKNOWLEDGEMENT

This publication is contribution number 2171 of the Biology Division of the Commission of the European Communities. The work was supported by contract number BIO-E-478-NL of the Radiation Protection Programme and by the Dutch Ministries of Agriculture and Fisheries and of Welfare, Health and Culture.

REFERENCES

1. G. W. Barendsen, Int. J. Radiat. Biol. 36:49-63 (1979).

2. M. Bauchinger, E. Schmid, and J. Dresp, Int. J. Radiat. Biol. 35:229-233, (1979).

3. M. Bauchinger, E. Schmid, S. Streng, and J. Dresp, Radiat. Environ. Biophys. 22:225-230 (1983).

4. K. H. Chadwick and H. P. Leenhouts, "The Molecular Theory of Radiation Biology," Springer Verlag, Heidelberg (1981).

5. J. D. Chapman, A. P. Reuvers, S. D. Doern, C. J. Gillespie, and D. L. Dugle, in: "Proc. 5th Microdosimetry Symposium," J. Booz, H. G. Ebert, and B. G. R. Smith, eds. EUR 5452, CEC, Brussels (1976), pp. 775-793.

6. R. Cox and W. K. Masson, Int. J. Radiat. Biol. 36:149-160 (1979).

7. W. C. Dewey, S. C. Furman, and H. H. Miller, Radiat. Res. 43:561-581 (1970).

8. W. C. Dewey, L. E. Stone, H. H. Miller, and R. E. Giblak, Radiat. Res. 47:672-688 (1971a).

9. W. C. Dewey, H. H. Miller, and D. B. Leeper, Proc. Nat. Acad. Sci. USA 68:667-671 (1971b).

10. W. C. Dewey, S. A. Sapareto, and D. A. Betten, Radiat. Res. 76:48-59 (1978).

11. E. Dikomey, Int. J. Radiat. Biol. 41:603-614 (1982).

12. D. L. Dugle, C. J. Gillespie, and J. D. Chapman, Proc. Nat. Acad. Sci. USA 73:809-812 (1976).

13. A. A. Edwards, R. J. Purrott, J. S. Prosser, and D. C. Lloyd, Int. J. Radiat. Biol. 38:83-91 (1980a).

14. A. A. Edward, D. C. Lloyd, and R. J. Purrott, in: "Proc. 7th Microdosimetry Symposium," J. Booz, H. G. Ebert, and H. D. Hartfiel, eds., EUR 7147, CEC, Brussels (1980), pp. 1263-1274.

15. D. T. Goodhead, R. J. Munson, J. Thacker, and R. Cox, Int. J. Radiat. Biol. 37:135-167 (1980).

16. D. T. Goodhead, J. Thacker, and R. Cox, *Int. J. Radiat. Biol.* 36:101–114 (1979).

17. G. Iliakis, *Mutat. Res.* 126:215–225 (1984).

18. A. M. Kellerer and H. H. Rossi, *Curr. Top. Radiat. Res. Q.* 8:85–158 (1972).

19. D. E. Lea, "Actions of Radiations on Living Cells," University Press, Cambridge (1946).

20. D. E. Lea and D. G. Catcheside, *J. Genet.* 44:216–245 (1942).

21. H. P. Leenhouts and K. H. Chadwick, *in:* "Proc. 5th Microdosimetry Symposium," J. Booz, H. G. Ebert, and B. G. R. Smith, eds., EUR 5452, CEC, Brussels (1976), pp. 289–308.

22. D. C. Lloyd, R. J. Purrott, G. W. Dolphin, D. Bolton, A. A. Edwards, and M. J. Corp, *Int. J. Radiat. Biol.* 28:75–90 (1975).

23. D. C. Lloyd, R. J. Purrott, G. W. Dolphin, and A. A. Edwards, *Int. J. Radiat. Biol.* 29:169–182 (1976).

24. D. C. Lloyd, R. J. Purrott, E. J. Reeder, A. A. Edwards, and G. W. Dolphin, *Int. J. Radiat. Biol.* 34:177–186 (1978).

25. D. C. Lloyd, A. A. Edwards, J. S. Prosser, and M. J. Corp, *Radiat. Environ. Biophys.* 23:179–190 (1984).

26. R. J. Purrott, A. A. Edwards, D. C. Lloyd, and J. W. Stather, *Int. J. Radiat. Biol.* 38:277–284 (1980).

27. B. S. Rao and L. E. Hopwood, *Int. J. Radiat. Biol.* 42:501–508 (1982).

28. W. C. Roesch, *in:* "Proc. 3rd Symposium Neutron Dosimetry in Biology and Medicine," G. Burger and H. G. Ebert, eds., CEC, Luxembourg (1982), pp. 1–27.

29. E. Schmid, M. Bauchinger, and W. Mergenthaler, *Int. J. Radiat. Biol.* 30:339–346 (1976).

30. J. Thacker, A. Stretch, and M. A. Stephens, *Mutat. Res.* 42:313–326 (1977).

31. J. Thacker, A. Stretch, and M. A. Stephens, *Int. J. Radiat. Biol.* 36:137–148 (1979).

32. J. Thacker, D. T. Goodhead, and R. E. Wilkinson, *in:* "Proc. 8th Microdosimetry Symposium," J. Booz and H. G. Ebert, eds., EUR 8395, CEC, Brussels (1982), pp. 587–595.

33. R. P. Virsik and D. Harder, *Radiat. Envirn. Biophys.* 18:221–238 (1980a).

34. R. P. Virsik and D. Harder, *Radiat. Envirn. Biophys.* 18:73–77 (1980b).

35. R. B. Virsik, R. Blohm, K-P Hermann, and D. Harder, *in*" Proc. 7th Microdosimetry Symposium," J. Booz, H. G. Ebert, and H. D. Hartfiel, eds., EUR 7147, CEC, Brussels (1980), pp. 943–955.

36. K. F. Weibezahn, C. Sexauer, and T. Coquerelle, <u>Int. J. Radiat. Biol.</u> 38:365-371 (1980).

37. J. Zoetelief and G. W. Barendsen, <u>in</u>: "Proc. 8th Microdosimetry Symposium," J. Booz, H. G. Ebert, and H. D. Hartfiel, eds., EUR 7147, CEC, Brussels (1980), pp. 883-898.

38. J. Zoetelief and G. W. Barendsen, <u>Int. J. Radiat. Biol.</u> 43:349-362 (1983).

X-RAY-INDUCED DNA DOUBLE STRAND BREAKS IN POLYNUCLEOSOMES

F. Barone*, M. Belli*, E. Rongoni*, O. Sapora**,
and M. A. Tabocchini*

*Laboratorio di Fisica and **Laboratorio di Tossicologia
Comparata ed Ecotossicologia
Istituto Superiore di Sanita
Rome, Italy

INTRODUCTION

Most of the studies on DNA damage induced by ionizing radiations are based on the assumption that lesions are randomly distributed along the cellular DNA. However, Roti Roti et al. reported that the efficiency of gamma radiation in producing DNA thymine damage (tγ) depends on the amount of proteins associated with DNA (1). Since chromatin structure is not uniform in the genome and changes during replication and transcription, it seems reasonable to assume that different DNA regions may have different radiosensitivity. In fact, a non-random distribution in DNA damage was recently found by some authors. After gamma irradiation, Chiu et al. (2) observed that both single strand breaks (ssb) production and repair were greater in actively transcribing genes than in total nuclear DNA. Warters and Childers (3) found that the newly replicated DNA was hypersensitive to the induction of tγ-type damage. These findings have been related to the different accessibilities of DNA regions to diffusible radicals and repair enzymes, and point out the importance of the association of DNA with the protein component of chromatin.

The elementary units of chromatin are nucleosomes, consisting in "core particles", where the DNA is wrapped around a histone octamer, inserted between "linker" regions, where DNA is associated primarily with histone H1, and is more susceptible to nuclease action (4). It seems likely that nucleosomal organization itself could involve a differential radiosensitivity in "core" and "linker" DNA.

In this paper we describe our studies on the distribution of DNA double strand breaks (dsb) obtained analyzing the X-ray-induced fragmentation of isolated hen erythrocyte nucleosomes and their oligomers, as well as the DNA extracted from them.

MATERIALS AND METHODS

All the extraction procedures were carried out at 4°C unless otherwise specified.

Five ml of hen erythrocytes were lysed with 0.5% (v/v) NONIDET P40 in buffer A (110 mM KCl, 30mM NaCl, 0.4 mM PMSF, 0.2 mM $MgCl_2$, 10 mM tris-HCl, pH(7.4). Nuclei were centrifuged and resuspended in the same buffer containing 1 mM $CaCl_2$ to give a final DNA concentration of 2 mg/ml and then digested with 30 U/ml of micrococcal nuclease (Worthington) for 10 min. at $37^{O}C$. The reaction was stopped chilling the sample and adding EDTA to 0.25 mM final concentration. The digested chromatin was released from nuclei after an overnight dialysis against buffer B (40 mM KCl, 0.2 mM EDTA, 0.4 mM PMSF, 10 mM tris-HCl, pH 7.4), with gentle mixing to avoid nuclei aggregation. Soluble chromatin was centrifuged to remove nuclear debris and then layered on top of 5-30% linear sucrose gradients which were centrifuged for 16 hr. at 26,000 rpm 4 degrees in a SW28 rotor. At the end of the run the gradients were fractionated; the first three peaks, corresponding to mono-, di-, and trinucleosomes, respectively, were separated and further purified by a second sucrose gradient centrifugation.

The samples were then dialysed against buffer B without PMSF and their concentration was adjusted to obtained a DNA concentration of about 0.15 mg/ml.

DNA was extracted from irradiated and unirradiated samples by digestion with RNase T1 and proteinase K at $37^{O}C$ in the presence of 2M NaCl and 2% Sarkosyl. Extracts were then treated with phenol and chloroform, and DNA was precipitated adding two volumes of ethanol. The suspension was centrifuged and the precipitate dissolved in the same buffer and at the same concentration as reported for polynucleosomes. Assays with Hoechst 2495 fluorescent dye were carried out to detect possible protein contamination.

The samples were irradiated using a Picker X-ray apparatus (230 kVp, 15 mA) delivering a dose rate of 1.65 kGy/hr. After irradiation, 0.2 ml samples were layered on top of 5-30% linear sucrose gradients and centrifuged in a SW41 rotor at $4^{O}C$ for 17 hr. at 31,000 rpm for polynucleosomes or for 27 hr. at 40,000 rpm for extracted DNA. The optical density profiles of the gradients were recorded at 254 nm and converted into digital form, to normalize the area under the profile, so that comparison of the results was made independent of possible differences among sample concentrations.

RESULTS AND DISCUSSION

In the attempt to investigate the initial DNA damage distribution, we decided to study the effect of X-rays on isolated polynucleosomes rather than on intact cells, in order to avoid difficulties in the understanding the experimental results, due to cellular metabolic processes and extraction artifacts. Another advantage of this approach is the good characterization of the system used, while a disadvantage is the relatively high doses required to break up such small targets (about 1-10 kGy).

The procedure we used for polynucleosome preparation gave a good yield of mono-, di-, and trinucleosomes, with a satisfactory separation of the corresponding peaks (Figure 1). At the same time, the digestion with micrococcal nuclease, at the conditions we used, did not introduced undesired nicks in the DNA strands, as shown by polyacrilamide gel electrophoresis in alkaline conditions.

In Figure 2 the results, obtained irradiating mono-, di-, and trinucleosomes with increasing doses of X-rays, are shown. The di- and trinucleosome sedimentation profiles exhibit a discrete distribution, with the production of the lower oligomers, which increases with the dose

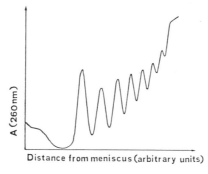

Fig. 1.   Sedimentation profile of soluble chromatin
          obtained by nuclei digestion with micrococcal
          nuclease.

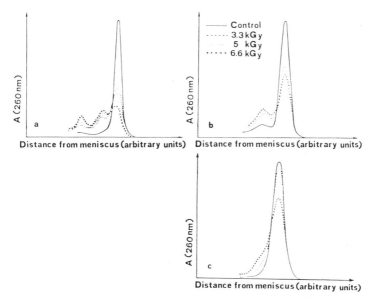

Fig. 2.   Sedimentation profiles of polynucleosomes irradiated at
          several doses: (a) trinucleosomes; (b) dinucleosomes;
          (c) mononucleosomes.

(Figure 2a, b). On the contrary, a qualitatively different pattern can be
observed when mononucleosomes are irradiated (Figure 2c). No other peaks
appear after irradiation in the dose range used, and only a limited
broadening is produced in the low molecular part of the sedimentation
patterns.

     The results point out that polynucleosome fragmentation is specific
and occurs preferentially in the linker regions. Since this fragmentation
is related to DNA double strand breaks (dsb), the question to be raised is
whether the dsb are mainly located in the DNA linker regions, or they are
randomly distributed but partially hidden in the core region. In this
case, the histone octamer can provide the structural support to hold the
DNA fragments together.

     To clarify this point, we investigated the dsb distribution in DNA
extracted from the irradiated trinucleosomes (Figure 3a). Similarly, to
what found for trinucleosomes, the sedimentation pattern indicates a

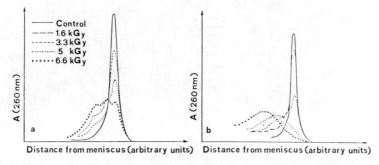

Fig. 3.   Sedimentation profiles of: (a) DNA extracted from
irradiated trinucleosomes; (b) DNA irradiated after
isolation from unirradiated trinucleosomes.

specific fragmentation.   This cannot be ascribed to the presence of
residual proteins, since assay with Hoechst 24495 dye indicated that
DNA- bound proteins were less than 10% of the original amount.   These
findings strongly suggest that dsb preferentially occur in the linker
regions.   On the other hand, when we irradiated the DNA extracted from
unirradiated trimers, we obtained a completely different pattern,
characterized by a decrease of the original peak along with the appearance
of a broad distribution which moved towards lower molecular weights as the
dose increased (Figure 3b).   This kind of distribution is the one expected
for randomly produced dsb in DNA molecules of about the same size.   Similar
results have been obtained for homogeneous DNA samples, such as phage DNA,
irradiated with gamma rays (5).   Comparing the results reported in Figures
3a and b, it appears that DNA radiosensitivity is greatly affected by
chromatin organization.   In fact, only a very limited (if any) amount of
fragments with a size smaller than monomer DNA was found in DNA extracted
from irradiated polynucleosomes.   This, together with fragmentation
specificity, indicates that core regions are more resistant than linker
regions and isolated DNA.

In conclusion, these results indicate that, in our experimental
system, DNA dsb introduced by X-rays are not randomly distributed and that
interaction with histones makes core DNA more resistant against radiation.

REFERENCES

1. J. L. Roti Roti, G. S. Stein, and P. A. Cerutti, Biochemistry 13:1900-
    1905 (1974).

2. S. M. Chiu, N. L. Oleinick, L. R. Friedman, and P. J. Stambrook,
    Biochim. Biophys. Acta 699:15-21 (1982).

3. R. L. Warters and T. J. Childers, Radiat. Res. 90:564-574 (1982).

4. K. E. Van Holde and W. O. Weischet, in: "The Cell Nucleus-Chromatin,
    Vol. IV," Academic Press, New York, pp. 75-105 (1978).

5. G. P. Van der Schans and J. B. Aten, Anal. Biochem. 32:14-30 (1969).

CHEMICAL INHIBITION OF THE REPAIR OF DNA SINGLE STRAND BREAKS PRODUCED BY X-IRRADIATION OR HYDROGEN PEROXIDE IN CULTURED MAMMALIAN CELLS

O. Cantoni and F. Cattabeni

Istituto di Farmacologia e Farmacognosia
Universita degli Studi di Urbino
Chiara, 27
61019 Urbino, Italy

ABSTRACT

The effect of various metal compounds, formaldehyde and adriamycin on the rejoining of X-rays induced DNA single strand breaks was examined using the alkaline elution technique. Of the compounds tested, chromate, mercury (II) and formaldehyde decreased the ability of cells to rejoin DNA strand breaks. The inhibition of DNA repair could be demonstrated also using another system where strand breaks were produced by exposing cells for 1 hr. to 30 μM H_2O_2, at ice temperature.

$NiCl_2$, $CoCl_2$, $Pb(C_2H_3O_2)_2$, $Cr(C_2H_3O_2)_3$, $CdCl_2$ and adriamycin were not effective in inhibiting strand break rejoining.

The possible biological significance of DNA repair inhibition is discussed.

INTRODUCTION

A large body of evidence suggests that the majority of known carcinogens have significant actions involving DNA (1). Such interactions may be closely related to cytotoxicity or to the progression of a normal cell to a cancer cell. The interactions of a carcinogen with DNA result in the formation of different classes of DNA lesions such as single and double strand breaks, alkali labile sites (base free sites or phosphotriesters), interstrand crosslinks or DNA-protein crosslinks. During recent years several specific inhibitors of the repair of these lesions have been found which have increased the understanding of the enzymatic steps involved in the repair of DNA damage (2, 3). In regard to biological consequences, it is not easy to visualize if and how repair inhibition could modify cellular response to the insult of DNA damaging agents. However, advances have been made along several different lines (see Discussion) which actually or potentially permit to postulate that repair inhibitors might affect cytotoxicity, mutagenicity and transforming ability of DNA damaging agents.

The aim of this study was to assess if various metal compounds, formaldehyde or adriamycin could interfere with repair of DNA single strand breaks produced by X-irradiation or hydrogen peroxide.

MATERIALS AND METHODS

Chinese Hamster Ovary (CHO) cells were maintained in McCoy's 5a medium supplemented with 10% fetal bovine serum (FBS). All experiments were carried out with asynchronous cultures in the logarithmic growth phase with a generation time of 14-16 hr.

Cells were irradiated or exposed to H_2O_2 for 1 hr. at ice temperature and then incubated in a salts/glucose medium that either did or did not contain repair inhibitors. Single strand breaks were assayed by the alkaline elution technique as previously described (4, 5). Proteinase K was used only in the case of $CaCrO_4$, formaldehyde and adriamycin.

DNA breakage has been expressed as strand scission factor (SSF) that was calculated from the alkaline elution patterns by the following relationship: SSF = - log A/B where A = amount of DNA retained in the sixth fraction of the treated sample and B = DNA retained in the sixth fraction of the untreated sample.

RESULTS

The rejoining of strand breaks produced by X-rays (400 rads) is a rapid process involving at least two kinetically distinct phases. A fast process with a half-life of 3-5 min. and a slow process of 60 or more min. (Figure 1A). Also H_2O_2 (30 M for 1 hr. on ice) induced strand breaks are rapidly repaired (Figure 1B). The fast process is similar to that occurring during the repair of X-rays induced DNA damage. The slow process differs in that, unlike X-rays, H_2O_2 generates breaks that are quantitatively resealed at the end of the 1 hr. repair time. The toxicity of the two agents is markedly different as indicated by the fact that a

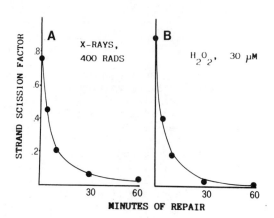

Fig. 1. The resealing rate of DNA single strand breaks produced by X-rays or hydrogen peroxide. CHO cells were irradiated with 400 rads (A) or were treated with 30 M H_2O_2 for 1 hr. on ice (B). Strand breaks were measured by the alkaline elution technique at various time periods of incubation in a salts/glucose medium, at 21^OC. DNA breakage is expressed as strand scission factor that was calculated from the elution pattern, as detailed in Methods section.

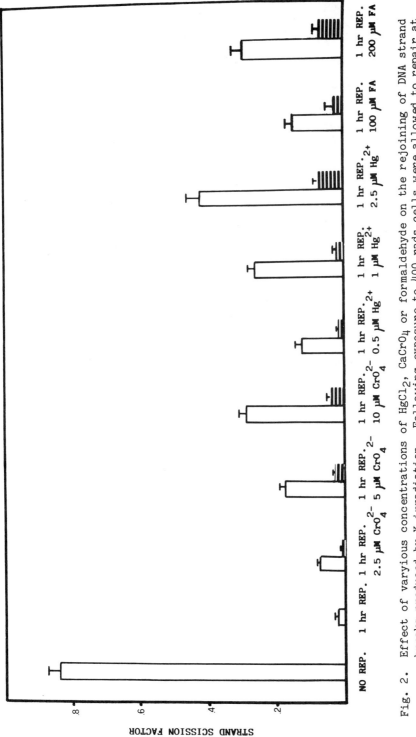

Fig. 2. Effect of varyious concentrations of HgCl$_2$, CaCrO$_4$ or formaldehyde on the rejoining of DNA strand breaks produced by X-irradiation. Following exposure to 400 rads cells were allowed to repair at 21°C for 60 min. in the presence of absence of HgCl$_2$, CaCrO$_4$ or formaldehyde. The same treatments were performed in unirradiated cells. DNA strand breaks were assayed by the alkaline elution technique and were expressed as strand scission factor.

much higher level of DNA damage is required by H_2O_2, as compared to X-rays, to produce an equivalent level of cell killing. For example, a concentration of H_2O_2 (30 µM) generating a number of DNA breaks equivalent to that produced by 400 rads (50% cell killing) is not toxic and concentrations of H_2O_2 as high as 900 M are required to achieve a 50% decrease in cloning efficiency (6).

The ability of cells to rejoin strand breaks generated by X-rays or H_2O_2 was measured after 1 hr. repair in the absence or presence of various compounds. Figure 2 shows that $HgCl_2$, $CaCrO_4$ and formaldehyde produce a concentration dependent inhibition of the repair of radiation damage at concentrations producing minimal toxicity (not shown). Additionally, measurement of DNA damage in non-irradiated cells indicates that the presence of these agents has little or no effect on this initial yield (Figure 2). A similar degree of repair inhibition can be obtained if the initial damage is produced by exposing cells to 30 M H_2O_2 for 1 hr. at ice temperature (Table 1). Several metal compounds such as $NiCl_2$ (100 µM), $CoCl_2$ (50 µM), $Pb(C_2H_3O_2)_2$ (100 µM), $Cr(C_2H_3O_2)_3$ (250 µM), and $CdCl_2$ (100 µM) do not inhibit the repair of radiation damage (Table 2). The anticancer drug adriamycin was also tested for its ability to inhibit repair. However, a similar yield of DNA breaks is observed in irradiated or non-irradiated cells after 1 hr. incubation in 0.5-2 µM adriamycin (Figure 3).

DISCUSSION

In previous work we have found that addition of non-cytotoxic, non-DNA-damaging concentrations of $HgCl_2$ to cells following treatment with X-rays greatly inhibited the repair of DNA strand breaks (5). These

Table 1. Effect of $HgCl_2$, $CaCrO_4$ and formaldehyde on the rejoining of DNA strand produced by hydrogen peroxide *

Compound	Concentration (uM)	SSF[1]	SSF[2]
none	–	0.003	–
$HgCl_2$	0.5	0.132	0.012
	1	0.281	0.026
	2.5	0.440	0.080
$CaCrO_4$	2.5	0.081	0.011
	5	0.183	0.034
	10	0.294	0.052
Formaldehyde	100	0.183	0.032
	200	0.295	0.081

SSF[1] = cells were exposed for 1 hr to 30 uM H_2O_2 at ice temperature and then allowed to repair in the absence or presence of repair inhibitors.

SSF[2] = Cells were treated with $HgCl_2$, $CaCrO_4$ or formaldehyde without previous exposure to H_2O_2.

* DNA strand breaks were assayed by alkaline elution and SSF was calculated as detailed in the Methods section.

300

Table 2. Effect of various metal compounds on the rejoining of DNA strand breaks produced by X-irradiation *

Metal compound	Concentration (uM)	SSF[1]	SSF[2]
none	–	0.021	–
NiCl$_2$	100	0.023	0.003
CoCl$_2$	50	0.020	0.010
Pb(C$_2$H$_3$O$_2$)$_2$	100	0.026	0.007
Cr(C$_2$H$_3$O$_2$)$_3$	250	0.018	0.009
CdCl$_2$	100	0.021	0.015

SSF[1] = cells were irradiated with 400 rads and then allowed to repair in the absence or presence of metal compound.

SSF[2] = unirradiated cells were treated for 1 hr.

* DNA strand breaks were assayed by alkaline elution and SSF was calculated as detailed in the Methods section.

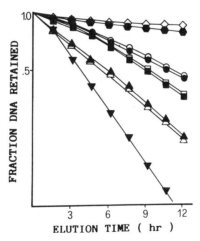

Fig. 3. Effect of varying concentrations of adriamycin on the rejoining of DNA strand breaks induced by X-rays. Cells were treated with 400 rads and their DNA was analyzed by the alkaline elution technique immediately following irradiation (▼—▼) or after incubation of the cultures at 21° for an additional 60 min. in a salts/glucose medium in the absence (◇—◇) or presence of 0.5 (●—●), 1 (■—■) and 2 µM adriamycin (▲—▲). Unirradiated cells were also exposed to 0 (◇—◇), 0.5 (○—○), 1 (□—□) and 2 µM adriamycin (⬠—⬠).

experiments were made on CHO cells repairing in a medium (McCoy's 5a) containing 10% FBS, at a temperature of 37°C. In the current study, we have used a system involving a postirradiation incubation in a salts/glucose medium at 21°C. Under these conditions, repair was efficient and more reproducible results could be obtained. In fact, as we have previously shown, different amounts and/or different batches of serum were able to affect significantly the cyto- and geno-toxic actions of metal ions such as Ni^{2+} (7) Hg^{2+} and CrO_4^{2-} (8). Of the metal compounds tested, $HgCl_2$ and $CaCrO_4$ appeared to decrease the ability of cells to reseal DNA breaks whereas other metals such as $NiCl_2$, $CoCl_2$, $Pb(C_2H_3O_2)_2$, $Cr(C_2H_3O_2)_3$ and $CdCl_2$ did not display any inhibitory effect of the repair process.

Formaldehyde, in agreement with a previously published report (9), was an inhibitor of DNA repair. These results do not allow mechanistic speculations but studies in progress suggest that the enzyme DNA ligase could be the target in the case of $CaCrO_4$ and formaldehyde and DNA polymerases in the case of $HgCl_2$ (Unpublished). These conclusions were derived from studies attempting to correlate inhibition of DNA repair with other biological effects such as DNA synthesis, DNA chain elongation, cell survival and the effect on ultraviolet light induced unscheduled DNA synthesis. However, these experiments did not directly demonstrate inhibition of DNA repair enzymes and, therefore, the possibility that inhibition of the repair process occurs by different mechanism(s) cannot be ruled out.

It has been shown that adriamycin may act as an inhibitor of DNA repair synthesis induced by nitrogen mustard, ultraviolet radiation and methyl-methane-sulphonate (10, 11). Tanaka and Youshida (12) have reported that this anticancer drug directly inhibits alpha and beta polymrases (12) and, therefore, one should expect that postirradiation incubation in the presence of adriamycin will result in the accumulation of strand breaks. Unexpectedly, adriamycin did not affect the rejoining of DNA strand breaks. Both alpha and beta polymerases are thought to be involved in the repair of radiation damage (3); however, only 3-5 nucleotides are excised by the short patch repair activated by X-rays (13) and the enzymes, though inhibited, may still be able to polymerize such a limited number of nucleotides. This could explain the lack of effect of adriamycin in this study.

The repair inhibitory action of chromate, mercury (II), and formaldehyde was also demonstrated using another system where strand breaks were produced by exposing cells to 30 µM H_2O_2 for 1 hr. on ice. This concentration of H_2O_2 is far below the minimum cytotoxic level (on the contrary the dose of X-rays used, 400 rads, produced 50% cell killing) and, therefore, the effect of non-toxic concentrations of DNA repair inhibitors can be assessed with less or no reasons to suspect that inhibition of DNA repair represents a part of an overall inhibition of cellular metabolism. Thus, H_2O_2 induced DNA strand breaks represent a suitable system for estimating the ability of given compound to act on DNA homeostasis by inhibiting repair processes.

The biological significance of these effects on DNA repair is uncertain. In theory, inhibition of DNA repair could amplify the toxicity of DNA damaging agents. Previous work from other laboratories has indicated that nitrosoureas with strong carbamoylating activity are inhibitors of DNA repair (14). The authors suggested that the cytocidal effect of these agents, generally attributed to their alkylating activity was potentiated through an inhibition of the repair of damaged DNA. In other studies, inhibitors such as hydroxyurea, 1-β-arabinofuranosylcytosine, diamide (13) and 3-aminobenzamide (6, 15), acting at different biochemical steps of the repair of radiation damage, increased cellular radiosensitivity. In general, data from the literature support the idea that inhibitors of DNA repair might potentiate cytotoxicity produced by DNA damaging agents. This is not surprising if we assume that inhibition of repair, during the time when fixation of the damage occurs, should allow higher proportion of potentially lethal lesions to progress to lethal lesions.

However, inhibition of DNA repair can be of other biological significance rather than be merely relevant to cytotoxicity. Since unfaithful repair of DNA has been highlighted as a critical event in the oncogenic transformation, it is a fair (as yet untested) assumption that inhibitors of DNA repair will decrease the effective time available for repair and, in turn, this could result in the fixation of premutational damage in the DNA genome, as a result of replication. Additionally, a feature common to different classes of cocarcinogens is that of being inhibitors of DNA repair (16) and, therefore, repair inhibition could be related at least in part, to the process of cocarcinogenesis. Our results, as far as they go, support this idea. In fact, formaldehyde has been implicated as a cocarcinogen (17) and, though no definitive information indicates that chromate and mercury (II) act as cocarcinogens, there are two reports demonstrating that they potentiate the mutagenicity of other carcinogens (18, 19).

In conclusion, further studies are necessary to understand the role that inhibitors of DNA repair play in carcinogenesis. Future work will be directed toward the identification of agents acting on DNA homeostasis by inhibiting DNA repair.

REFERENCES

1. M. J. Waring, Ann. Rev. Biochem. 50:159 (1981).

2. C. S. Downes, A. R. S. Collins, and R. T. Johnson, Mutat. Res. 112:75 (1983).

3. R. M. Miller and D. N. Chinault, J. Biol. Chem. 257:10204 (1982).

4. K. W. Kohn, R. A. G. Ewig, L. C. Erickson, and L. A. Zwelling, in: "DNA Repair - A Laboratory Manual of Research Procedures," E. Friedberg and P. C. Hanawalt, eds., Vol. 1, Part B (1981) pp. 378.

5. O. Cantoni and M. Costa, Molecular Pharmacol. 24:84 (1983).

6. O. Cantoni, D. Murray, and R. Meyn, Biochem. Biophys. Acta. In press.

7. M. P. Abbracchio, R. M. Evans, J. D. Heck, O. Cantoni, and M. Costa, Biol. trace El. Res. 4:289 (1982).

8. O. Cantoni, P. Sestiei and F. Cattabeni, Bull. Environ. Cont. Tox. In Press.

9. R. C. Grafstrom, A. J. Fornace, H. Autrup, J. F. Lachner, and C. Harris, Science 220:216 (1983).

10. U. Ringborg and B. Lambert, in: "DNA Repair Late Effects," H. Altmann, H. Riklis, and H. Slor (1980), pp. 311.

11. R. Lewensohn and U. Ringborg, Cancer Letters 18:305 (1983).

12. M. Tanaka and S. Yoshida, Biochem. 87:911 (1980).

13. J. F. Ward, E. I. Joner, and W. F. Blakely, Cancer Res. 44:59 (1984).

14. H. E. Kann, K. W. Kohn, and J. M. Lyles, Cancer Res. 34:398 (1974).

15. L. A. Zwelling, D. Kerrigan, and Y. Pommier, Biochem. Biophys. Res. Comm. 104:897 (1982).

16. D. Gaudin, R. S. Gregg, and K. L. Yelding, Biochem. Res. Comm. 45:630 (1971).

17. J. A. Swenberg, C. S. Barrow, C. J. Boreiko, H. Heck, R. J. Levine, K. T. Morgan, and T. B. Starr, Carcinogenesis 4:945 (1983).

18. J. M. LaVelle and C. M. Witmer, Mutat. Res. 106:297 (1982).

CONJUGATED DIENES AND TBA REACTIVE MATERIAL AS COMPONENTS OF CHROMOSOME

BREAKAGE FACTORS

S. H. Khan and I. Emerit

Laboratory of Experimental Cytogenetics
Institut Biomedical des Cordeliers
Universite Pierre et Marie Curies and CNRS
15, rue de l'Ecole de Medecine
Paris, France

ABSTRACT

Clastogenic components have been described as so-called chromosome breakage factors or "clastogenic factors" (CF) as an indirect effect of ionizing radiation. They have been also observed in the hereditary breakage syndromes Ataxia telangiectasia and Bloom's syndrome, in chronic inflammatory diseases and in supernatants of cell cultures exposed to the tumor promoter phorbol-myristate-acetate (PMA) or to a superoxide generating xanthine-xanthine oxidase system. The formation and action mechanisms of CF are intimely linked to the generation of superoxide anion radicals, since superoxide dismutase can prevent their formation and their chromosome damaging effect. However, the observation that the clastogenic material is transferable from one culture system to the other cannot be understood by short-lived free radicals. Oxygen radicals and other oxidants appear to be toxic in large part because they initiate the chain reaction of lipid peroxidation in membranes. Oxidative damage to membranes may be at the origin of the clastogenic material called CF by formation of lipid hydroperoxides and fragmentation products. According to this hypothesis, we have examined the supernatants of lymphocyte cultures for the presence of lipid peroxidation products. These cell cultures had been exposed to PMA or a xanthine-xanthine oxidase reaction which represent two in vitro model systems: The PMA induced CF may serve as a model for CF in chronic inflammatory diseases, and the induction of CF by xanthine-xanthine oxidase reaction may be a model for the oxidative damage observed in the phenomenon of ischemia/reperfusion injury.

INTRODUCTION

Clastogenic components have been described as so-called chromosome "breakage factors" or "clastogenic factors" as an indirect effect of radiation (11, for review). They have been also observed in the cancer-prone hereditary breakage syndromes ataxia telangiectasia (23) and Bloom's syndrome (6) and in various chronic inflammatory diseases with autoimmune reactions (for review see Emerit 1982 and 1983). In all these conditions, the clastogenic factors (CF) have been isolated from serum or supernatants of lymphocyte or fibroblast cultures. Their molecular weight is less than 10,000 daltons, and their formation and action mechanism is intimely linked to the generation of superoxide anion radicals, as superoxide dismutase has been found protective both against the production of CF and their chromosome damaging effect.

Recently, we have shown that lymphocytes exposed in culture to the tumor promoter phorbol-myristate-acetate (PMA) produce a CF which seems to be the consequence of the capacity of this phorbol ester to stimulate a respiratory burst in competent cells. It's molecular weight is also less than 10,000 daltons and its production and clastogenic action can be prevented by superoxide dismutase (8, 9). Since generation of superoxide anion radicals in the culture medium of lymphocyte cultures by the xanthine plus xanthine oxidase reaction results in chromosome damage and an increase in sister chromatid exchanges (7), we wondered whether the supernatant of these cultures also contained a CF. The cytogenetic analysis of the test cultures exposed to these supernatants indeed confirmed the presence of transferable clastogenic material, i.e., formation of CF (10).

In the present work we used both experimental systems to produce CF to study and compare their biochemical nature. The PMA induced CF may serve as a model for CF in chronic inflammatory diseases, since the respiratory burst of PMA is comparable to that of phagocytosing inflammatory cells. On the other hand, induction of a CF by the xanthine plus xanthine oxidase reaction may be a model for the oxidative damage observed in the phenomenon of ischemia/reperfusion injury (21). This phenomenon involves the reaction of xanthine oxidase, hypoxanthine and molecular oxygen to produce a burst of oxygen radicals with reperfusion after myocardial, cerebral, intestinal or renal ischemia (1, 12, 15, 18). In a number of conditions, in which low oxygen tension, proteolysis and calcium seem to play a role, there is conversion of xanthine dehydrogenase to xanthine oxidase.

In both the aforementioned model systems, oxygen radicals appear to be toxic because they initiate the chain reaction of lipid peroxidation in membranes. It is well known that oxidative damage to membranes after a low dose of ionizing radiation results in the generation of lipid peroxides (19). Interaction with oxidizing lipids may inactive transforming DNA (20) and radiomimetic effects of peroxidizing lipids on nucleic acids and their bases have been observed (22). Oxidative damage to membranes may also lead to activation of phospholipase A_2 and stimulation of the arachidonic acid cascade. Chromosomal breakage by the tumor promoter phorbol-myristate-acetate (PMA) could be prevented not only by antioxidants but also by inhibitors of arachidonic acid (AA) metabolism indicating that enzymatic oxidation of AA via the cyclo- and lipo-oxygenase pathways leads to the formation of clastogenic material (9). PMA and other membrane active agents may induce "membrane-mediated" chromosomal damage by this mechanism (2, 3).

According to the working hypothesis, that lipid peroxidation products could be involved in the clastogenic effect, we have looked for and compared the formation of these products in the supernatants of X-XO and PMA treated cultures at different time intervals of their incubation period.

Venous blood was collected from normal volunteers. Each culture flask contained 5 ml of tissue culture medium 199 without phenol red (Flow Lab., Paris), 1.5 ml heat-inactivated human AB serum and 2.5×10^6 isolated lymphocytes. The lymphocytes were prepared by differential centrifugation of heparinized blood on Isopaque-Ficoll (Nyegaard, Oslo) and were essentially free of neutrophils and erythrocytes but contaminated with

306

monocytes and platelets. The cell cultures were stimulated to divide with phytohemagglutinin P (PHA) (Difco Lab., Detroit). At hour 0 of the cultivation period, hypoxanthine (X) and xanthine oxidase (XO) were added to the culture medium to a final concentration of 7 and 10 µg/ml, respectively. Both chemicals were purchased from Boehringer, Mannheim. PMA (CCR Inc., Eden Prairie, MI) was dissolved in spectral grade acetone at a final concentration of 100 ng/ml. In control cell cultures equal amount of acetone was added. At these concentrations, no influence on cell cultures was observed by previous cytogenetic analysis.

After various cultivation times, lymphocyte culture media were centrifuged at 3500 rpm for 10 min. and the supernatants were collected for the measurement of conjugated dienes and TBA reactive material. Both assays were performed as follows.

Conjugated Dienes

0.5 ml each in duplicate of the collected supernatants were acidified to pH 3.5 with N HCl and extracted with ethylacetate. The ethylacetate was evaporated in a rotary evaporator and the residue was dissolved in 5 ml of cyclohexane (UV spectroscopy grade, Fluka). Absorbance of the duplicate samples against a cyclohexane blank was measured twice at 233 nm with a Varian spectrophotometer Series 634. Difference in absorbance of extracts of X-XO and PMA treated, and their control supernatants was recorded; formation of conjugated dienes in the X-XO and PMA treated samples was expressed in terms of percentage increase in absorbance.

TBA Reactive Material

0.5 ml each in duplicate of the collected supernatants were acidified by addition of 3.5 ml N/12 H_2SO_4 (Sigma Chem. Comp., Paris). Then 1.0 ml of thiobarbituric acid (TBA) (Sigma) reagent was added and the samples heated to 95° for 60 minutes in a water bath. TBA reagent was prepared by mixing 0.67% TBA in 0.1 N NaOH-glacial acetic acid (1/1, V/V Prolabo, Paris) just before use. After cooling with tap water, 5.0 ml of n-butanol (Sigma) were added, and the mixture was shaken vigorously. After centrifugation at 4000 rpm for 15 min., the fluorescence of the n-butanol layer was measured at 515 nm excition and 552 nm emission wavelength with a Kontron spectrofluorimeter SFM M 23/B. Tetraethoxypropan (Fluka) which linearly converts to malondialdehyde (MDA), was used as a standard. The fluorescence intensity of a standard solution obtained by reacting 1 ml of 10^{-6} M tetraethoxypropan with TBA was defined at 100%. The data is expressed as % increase in fluorescence intensity relative to medium from untreated control cultures.

The results obtained with both assays are given in Table 1. As shown, the presence of lipid peroxidation products could be demonstrated for both experimental systems and with both assays:

o If the absorbance at 233 nm (conjugated dienes) is compared between treated and control supernatants, an increase was found in both X-XO and PMA treated cultures. This increase was already detectable 1 hr. after exposure of the cells to X-XO or PMA. In X-XO treated cultures, the values increased during the first 12 hrs. and then decreased during the following hours of cultivation which lasted until 72 hrs. For PMA treated cultures, the values were almost constant during the first 24 hrs. with slight increase during the subsequent 48 hrs. Apart from the difference in time dependency in both the experimental systems, the values were higher for X-XO than for PMA treated cultures.

Table 1. Results of both assays measuring lipid peroxidation in the
supernatants of X-XO or PMA treated cultures in comparison to
controls. The figure represent percent increases in absorbance
(conjugated dienes) or fluorescence (MDA) between treated and
control samples. In brackets are the number of independent
experiments.

Incubation time(hrs)	% increase in absorbance at 233nm		% increase in TBA reactive material	
	X-XO	PMA	X-XO	PMA
1	4.7 $\pm$ 2.1 (3)	3.3 $\pm$ 2.2 (3)	— (5)	6.7 $\pm$ 6.1 (3)
3	7.0 $\pm$ 0.9 (4)	2.9 $\pm$ 3.3(5)	— (5)	10.5 $\pm$ 2.4(5)
6	8.9 $\pm$ 1.6 (3)	2.8 $\pm$ 1.6(5)	— (4)	8.8 $\pm$ 3.4 (5)
12	11.3 $\pm$ 4.0 (5)	2.6 $\pm$ 1.8(5)	— (5)	8.7 $\pm$ 3.4 (5)
18	3.8 $\pm$ 1.5 (2)	3.9 $\pm$ 2.2(5)	2.7 $\pm$ 3.5(4)	5.9 $\pm$ 3.9 (5)
24	7.2 $\pm$ 5.4 (4)	3.1 $\pm$ 1.9(5)	10.3 $\pm$ 1.7(6)	6.8 $\pm$ 1.8(5)
48	6.2 $\pm$ 5.8 (4)	4.1 $\pm$ 2.4(5)	9.4 $\pm$ 3.6(8)	7.2 $\pm$ 1.4(5)
72	5.9 $\pm$ 4.4 (7)	5.1 $\pm$ 0.8(5)	9.1 $\pm$ 6.4(9)	6.2 $\pm$ 1.7(5)

o The TBA assay showed even more striking differences for both
experimental systems. The values were consistently negative during the
first 12 hrs. in the X-XO treated cell cultures, slightly positive at 18
hrs. and considerably increased at 24-72 hrs. On the contrary, positive
values were found during the initial hours in PMA treated cell cultures
and persisted until 72 hrs.

Previous cytogenetic analysis had shown that the supernatants from X-
XO treated cell cultures contained clastogenic material only after a delay
of about 15 hrs. (11% mitoses with chromosome aberrations compared to 4.5%
in control). There was further increase in the clastogenic activity of the
supernatants after 21 hrs. (18%) and 24 hrs. (23.6%). The activity
remained unchanged for supernatants collected after 48 and 72 hrs. (22 and
23%, respectively) (10). In PMA treated cultures, cytogenetic analysis had
shown a slight increase in clastogenic activity after incubation of
lymphocytes during 3 hours (mean of 3 experiments 9.3% abnormal mitoses,
acetone treated controls 2.0%). Significantly increased clastogenic
activity was observed in the supernatants after 24 hours (18.0%).
Comparative studies of media collected at 24, 48, and 72 hours consistently
showed higher values at 48 and 72 hrs. than at 24 hrs. Thus, whereas a
time correlation between lipid peroxidation products and clastogenic
activity could be observed in the X-XO system for TBA reactive material at
24 hrs. of incubation, such a correlation is yet to be explained in PMA
treated cultures in which different cell types play different roles with
respect to the lipid peroxidation.

The process of lipid peroxidation starts with the formation of
conjugated dienes by rearrangement of double bonds in polyunsaturated fatty
acids of membrane lipids. It is followed by the formation of
hydroperoxides, carbonyl, and hydrocarbon products. According to this
scheme, the assay for conjugated dienes would measure an early event in the
process, while the TBA reaction would measure decomposition products, most

likely MDA. However, we have to keep in mind that the exact mechanisms of these reaction are not clearly elucidated (25) and these lipid peroxidation products have to be studied in more detail by HPLC analysis.

As far as the role of oxygen derived free radicals is concernd, the prevailing view is that the $OH^\cdot$ radical is the most important form of active oxygen for the initiation of lipid peroxidation. In the case of X-XO treated cell cultures, $OH^\cdot$ radical may be formed in an iron catalysed Haber-Weiss reaction, by the interaction of O_2^- and H_2O_2. While O_2^- is produced as a byproduct of oxidation of xanthine to uric acid, H_2O_2 is formed by the rapid spontaneous dismutation of superoxide. In this system oxygen free radicals are produced by chemical means in the extracellular environment.

In PMA treated cultures the source of oxygen free radical is cellular. The PMA effect is analogous to the phagocytic process in PMN which produce superoxide and hydrogen peroxide (16, 13). Monocytes also display increased O_2^- production and stimulated cells manifest enhanced cytotoxic efficacy (13). Platelets aggregate upon PMA treatment and release serotonin and other pharmacological mediators (24), 26). Monocytes and platelets are contaminating our lymphocyte cultures, and we had already reported that CF consisted of clastogenic material produced by the different types of cells (9). Lymphocytes produce little or no O_2^-, but on stimulation by PHA release cell bound arachidonic acid (AA) in the medium (17). This AA would be then available for co-oxidation in the culture medium. Furthermore, it is known that PMA stimulates the arachidonic acid cascade by the activation of phospholipase A_2. This leads to the formation of the metabolites of AA via the cyclo- and lipooxygenase pathways. Among these metabolites, prostaglandin endoperoxides such as PGG_2 and PGH_2 are TBA positive, and during the enzymatic conversion of these endoperoxides to prostacyclin and thromboxanes, a significant amount of MDA is produced concomitantly with HHT and HHD (14). It has been also found that hydroperoxides such as 5 HPETE which are produced from AA via the lipoxygenase pathway have conjugated diene structure. Since stimulation of the AA cascade is an immediate response of cells after exposure to PMA, it is not astonishing that both assays in our present work are positive already after 1 hr. incubation. The interaction of cellular O_2^- production and initiation of the AA cascade by PMA make this system more complex than the X-XO system.

In conclusion, if our work confirms the process of lipid peroxidation in both CF producing culture systems, more detailed analysis of the products and of their individual clastogenic properties have to be undertaken. The identification of these products may be important with respect to certain human disease processes in which the importance of oxygen free radicals has been underlined in the last decade. Production of CF in vitro by X-XO and by PMA may be helpful as models for the study of ischemia/reperfusion injury, and chronic inflammatory diseases, respectively.

REFERENCES

1. G. B. Bulkley, The role of oxygen free radicals in human disease processes, Surgery 94:407-419 (1983).

2. P. Cerutti, Prooxidant states and promotion, Science (1984), 227:375-381 (1986).

3. P. Cerutti, I. Emerit, and P. Amstad, Membrane-mediated chromosomal damage, in: "Genes and Proteins in Oncogenesis," I. Weinstein and H. Vogel, eds., Academic Press, New York (1983), pp. 55-69.

4. I. Emerit, Chromosome breakage factors: origin and possible significance, Progress in Mutat. Res. 4:61-72 (1982).

5. I. Emerit, Properties and action mechanism of clastogenic factors, Lymphokines 8:413-424 (1983).

6. I. Emerit and P. Cerutti, Clastogenic activity from Bloom's Syndrome fibroblast cultures, Proc. Natl. Acad. Sci. 78:1868-1872 (1981).

7. I. Emerit, M. Keck, A. Levy, J. Feingold, and A. M. Michelson, Activated oxygen species at the origin of chromosome breakage and sister chromatid exchanges, Mutat. Res. 103:165-172 (1980).

8. I. Emerit and P. Cerutti, Tumor promoter phorbol-12-myristate-13-acetate induces a clastogenic factor in human lymphocytes, Proc. Natl. Acad. 79:7509-7513 (1982).

9. I. Emerit and P. Cerutti, Clastogenic action of phorbol-12-myristate-13-acetate in mixed human leukocyte cultures, Carcinogenesis 4:1313-1316 (1983).

10. I. Emerit, S. H. Khan, and P. Cerutti, Superoxide treatment of lymphocyte cultures induces the formation of transferable clastogenic material, J. Free Radicals Biol. Med., 1:51-57 (1985).

11. G. B. Faguet, S. M. Reichard, and D. A. Welter, Radiation-induced clastogenic plasma factors, Cancer Genet. Cytogent. 12:73-83 (1984).

12. T. J. Gardner, J. R. Steward, A. S. Casale, J. M. Downey, and D. E. Chambers, Reduction of myocardial ischemic injury with oxygen-derived free radical scavengers, Surgery 94:423-427 (1983).

13. B. D. Goldstein, G. Witz, M. Amoruso, D. S. Stone, and W. Troll, Stimulation of human polymorphonuclear leukocyte superoxide anion radical production by tumor promoters, Cancer Lett. 11:257-262 (1981).

14. O. Hayashi and T. Shimizu, Metabolic and functional significance of prostaglandins in lipid peroxide research, in: "Lipid peroxides in Biology and Medicine," K. Yagi, ed., Academic Press, New York, (1982), pp. 41-53.

15. H. A. Kontos, E. P. Wei, C. W. Christman, J. E. Levasseur, J. T. Povlishock, and E. F. Ellis, Free radicals in cerebral vascular responses. Physiologist 26:165-169 (1983).

16. R. I. Lehrer and L. Cohen, Receptor-mediated regulation of superoxide production in human neutrophils stimulated by phorbol myristate acetate, J. Clin. Invest. 68:1314-1320 (1981).

17. C. W. Parker, J. P. Kelly, S. F. Falkenhein, and M. G. Huber, Release of arachidonic acid from human lymphocytes in response to mitogenic lectins, J. Exp. Med. 149:1487-1503 (1979).

18. D. A. Parks, G. B. Bulkley, and D. N. Granger, Role of oxygen derived free radicals in digestive tract disease, Surgery 94:415-422 (1983).

19. A. Petkau, Radiation carcinogenesis from a membrane perspective, Acta Physiol. Scand. Suppl. 492:81-99 (1980).

20. D. B. Pietronigro, W. B. Jones, K. Kalty, and H. B. Demopoulos, Interaction of DNA and liposomes as a model for membrane-mediated DNA damage, Nature 267:78-79 (1977).

21. R. S. Roy and J. M. McCord, Superoxide and ischemia: conversion of xanthine dehydrogenase in xanthine oxidase, in: "Proc. Third International Conference on Superoxide and Superoxide Dismutase," R. Greenwald and G. Cohen, eds., Elsevier North Holland Biomedical Press (1983), pp. 145-153.

22. K. M. Schaich and D. C. Borg, Radiomimetic effects of peroxidizing lipids in nucleic acids and their bases, in: "Proc. Third International Conference on Oxygen Radicals in Chemistry and Biology," Munchen (1983).

23. M. Shaham, Y. Becker, and M. Cohen, A Diffusable clastogenic factor in ataxia telangiectasis Cytogent. Cell Gent. 27:155-161 (1980).

24. J. G. White, G. H. R. Rao, and R. D. Estensen, Investigation of the release reaction in platelets exposed to phorbol myristate acetate, Am. J. Pathol. 75:301-314 (1974).

25. K. Yagi, Assay for serum lipid peroxide level and its clinical significance, in: "Lipid peroxides in Biology and Medicine," K. Yagi, ed., Academic Press, New York (1982).

26. M. B. Zucker, W. Troll, and S. Belman, The tumor promoter phorbol ester (12-0-tetradecanoyl-phorbol-13-acetate), a potent aggregating agent for blood platelets, J. Cell Biol. 60:325-336 (1974).

CONVERSION OF COVALENTLY CLOSED CIRCULAR DNA INTO CIRCULAR AND LINEAR DNA
BY IONIZING RADIATION IN THE PRESENCE AND ABSENCE OF DNA-BINDING OR
INTERCALATING DRUGS

P. Ohneseit and W. Kohnlein

Institute for Radiation Biology
University of Munster
Germany

INTRODUCTION

It is generally accepted that hydroxyl radicals produced by the action
of ionizing radiation in dilute aqueous solutions are predominantly
responsible for the induction of strand breaks in DNA. It is also known
that Tris buffer and citrate buffer can act as OH-scavengers.
Nevertheless, Tris is still used as a solvent for DNA in irradiation
experiments, even very recently, as can be seen from the work of McCormack
et al. and Belli, reported during this meeting. We therefore considered it
appropriate to study the OH-scavenging capacity of different buffers by
measuring the DNA strand break production after ionizing radiation,
starting with Tris buffer and phosphate buffer. Furthermore, we wanted to
know whether drugs, known to interact with the DNA molecule, affect the
radiation induced degradation and whether there is any correlation to the
binding properties. Such knowledge might be important for the formulation
of safety standards.

In a recent work Cobreros et al. (1982) found sensitization and
protection as well using calf thymus DNA in 0.01 M NaCl and various drugs,
employing analytical ultracentrifugation. However, no correlation was
found between the modifying character of the added drugs and the different
binding mechanisms to DNA. We have, therefore, extended such
investigations and irradiated DNA in the presence and absence of the
intercalating drugs ethidium bromide, neocarzinostatin, and daunomycin as
well as chloroquine which probably also binds to DNA by intercalation.
Furthermore, we added chromomycin A_3 and mitomycin C, the last one known to
bind covalently to DNA. We used covalently closed circular (ccc) DNA and
analyzed strand break production by agarose gel electrophoresis.

Compared to analytical or preparative ultracentrifugation studies the
advantage of this system is the high sensitivity in the low dose range, the
option to run many samples simultaneously, and the much easier method to
reduce experimental data to numbers of strand breaks.

MATERIALS AND METHODS

DNA-Preparation

These experiments were performed using covalently closed circular DNA of Col E1 plasmids from E. coli JC 411[thy-]. Plasmid amplification was induced by treatment of the E. coli-cultures with chloramphenicol in the presence of ^{3}H-thymidine. Cleared lysates were prepared following the procedure described by Clewell and Helinski (1969). Isolation of cccDNA from cleared lysates was performed according to Colman et al. (1978) using hydroxylapatite chromatography. Final DNA-preparation consisted of up to 90% supercoiled DNA.

Assay for DNA-Degradation

Supercoiled (form I) DNA is converted to relaxed circular DNA (form II) by a single-strand break; a double-strand break converts either of these forms to a linear molecule (form III). According to their different retardation coefficients these three topological forms can be separated by agarose gel electrophoresis. Quantitation of strand breakage was based on the assumption that breaks are induced at random and that the fraction of unbroken cccDNA molecules therefore followed Poisson statistics. When the fraction of unbroken supercircles in the untreated control has been normalized to 1.0 the number of breaks $(n_1 + n_2)$ per plasmid DNA molecule in a treated sample is given by $(n_1 + n_2) = -\ln F_I$, where F_I is the fraction of unbroken supercoils in that particular sample. The number of double-strand breaks (n_2) can be obtained from the fraction of linear molecules of full size using the first term of a Poisson distribution $F = n_2 \times e^{-n_2}$ (Povirk, et al., 1977). DNA samples were analyzed on horizontal agarose gels (1%).

Irradiation

DNA solutions (12 g/ml final) were irradiated in air using a 150 KeV X-ray tube with an additional Al-filter of 0.76 mm; the dose rate was 10 Gy/min as measured by Fricke dosimetry.

Drugs

The influence of the following drugs on DNA strand breakage upon irradiation was studied in 50 mM phosphate buffer: ethidium bromide (Calbiochem-Behring), neocarzinostatin (Kayaku Antibiotics), daunomycin and chloroquine (Serva), chromomycin A_3 and mitomycin C (Sigma).

Yields

G-values were calculated according to the equation given by Blok and Loman (1973): $G = (100/r \times D_{37})N_0$, where N_0 is the DNA concentration expressed as numbers of molecules per ml and r is the number of eV per gram per Gy (6.24×10^{15}).

RESULTS AND DISCUSSION

Role of Buffers on Strand Breakage

The increase of linear DNA molecules of full length was very remote indicating that under the conditions used no double-strand breaks were produced ($n_2 = 0$). Thus, the fraction of remaining supercoiled DNA molecules yields directly the number of single-strand breaks (n_1). As can be seen in Figure 1, the number of strand breaks increased linearly with dose and was larger by a factor of 40 for DNA dissolved in phosphate buffer as compared to DNA in Tris buffer. This is in good agreement with the finding that OH-radicals are mainly responsible for strand break production

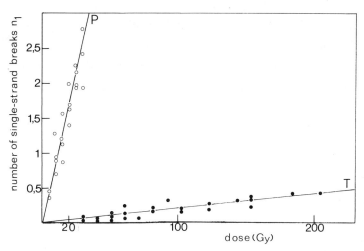

Fig. 1.   Production of single-strand breaks in Col E1 DNA, as
           determined from conversion of supercoils into linear
           and relaxed molecules after ionizing radiation in 50 mM
           phosphate buffer (○) or 50 mM Tris buffer (●).
           Radiation dose given in Gray. The G-values for ssb are
           4.7×10^{-3} and 0.12×10^{-3} in phosphate buffer and Tris
           buffer, respectively.

and with the high scavenging capacity of Tris ions for OH-radicals. Achey
et al. (1974) also reported a high protection efficiency of 50 mM Tris and
found that DNA is about 35 times more susceptible to strand break
production in phosphate than in Tris buffer. From the linear dose effect
curves D_{37} and G-values were deduced (see Table 1).

Effects of Drugs on the Radiation Sensitivity of DNA

These experiments were done in 50 mM phosphate buffer where no
additional scavenging of OH-radicals was observed and the highest yield of
single-strand breaks was found.

Ethidium Bromide   In the presence of one molecule ethidium bromide
(EB) per two base pairs no change in strand break production was observed
(Figure 2). At that concentration about 70% of EB is bound as can be
calculated from the known binding constant of 6.6×10^6 M^{-1} (Le Pecq and
Paoletti, 1967). The intercalating drug (Di Marco et al., 1975), does,
however, change the yield of single-strand breaks in DNA upon irradiation.
At a concentration of one drug molecule per 3 base pairs the yield of
strand breaks was reduced by a factor of 3.2 as compared to the drug free
control (Figure 2). Increasing the drug concentration caused further
reduction of strand breakage. At the used concentrations most of the drug
molecules can be considered as free and, therefore, the observed protection
effect must result from a high OH-radical scavenging capacity while the drug
binding process has no influence on the radiation sensitivity. This
finding is in contradiction to the results of Cobreros et al. who found at
a concentration of one drug molecule per 4 base pairs an increase of
sensitivity by a factor of four when the DNA was irradiated with 100 Gy in
0.01 M NaCl.

Chloroquine   The influence of the antimalaria drug chloroquine
(Yielding et al., 1971) was investigated at a concentration of 5 drug
molecules per base pair. At equal radiation doses, chloroquine treated DNA

Table 1. G-values for X-ray induced strand breakage in Col E1 DNA and protection factors for various drugs at the indicated drug to base pair ratios.*

Buffer or drug	MW	Conc. M	Drug/base pair	G-values for ssb	Protection factor
phosphate		$50 \cdot 10^{-3}$		$4.7 \cdot 10^{-3}$	1
Tris		$50 \cdot 10^{-3}$		$0.12 \cdot 10^{-3}$	40
EB	394	$1 \cdot 10^{-5}$	1 : 2	$4.7 \cdot 10^{-3}$	1
daunomycin-HCl	564	$6.3 \cdot 10^{-6}$	1 : 3	$1.5 \cdot 10^{-3}$	3.2
chloroquine-diphosphate	519	$1 \cdot 10^{-4}$	5 : 1	$2.3 \cdot 10^{-3}$	2.0
		$3 \cdot 10^{-4}$	16 : 1	$1.7 \cdot 10^{-3}$	2.8
chromomycin	1183	$7.2 \cdot 10^{-5}$	4 : 1		
with Mg^{++}				$1.3 \cdot 10^{-3}$	3.6
without Mg^{++}				$0.8 \cdot 10^{-3}$	5.9
mitomycin	334	$1.2 \cdot 10^{-4}$	7 : 1	$4.1 \cdot 10^{-3}$	1.1
		$2.4 \cdot 10^{-4}$	13 : 1	$3.8 \cdot 10^{-3}$	1.3
		$3.6 \cdot 10^{-4}$	19 : 1	$2.6 \cdot 10^{-3}$	1.8
NCS	10 000	$5 \cdot 10^{-7}$	1 : 38	$1 \cdot 10^{-3}$	4.7

*In the presence of drug DNA (12 µg/ml = $1.9 \cdot 10^{-5}$M base pairs) was irradiated in 50 mM phosphate buffer.

is less degraded (factor 2) than untreated DNA (Figure 2). At comparable conditions the protection effect was much higher for daunomycin than for chloroquine, indicating that chloroquine has a lower capacity for scavenging OH-radicals.

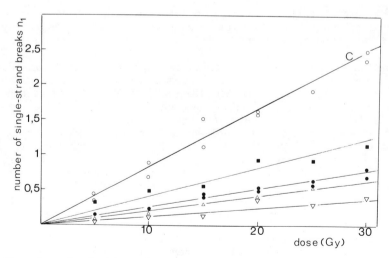

Fig. 2. Production of single-strand breaks in Col E1 DNA by ionizing radiation (5-30 Gy) in 50 mM phosphate buffer alone (C) and in the presence of the following drugs: ethidium bromide (1 x 10^{-5}) O, chloroquine (0.1 x 10^{-3})■, daunomycin (6.3 x 10^{-6})●, chromomycin (7.2 x 10^{-5}) with Mg^{++}△, without Mg^{++}▽.

Chromomycin A$_3$ This antitumor antibiotic interacts with DNA in the presence of Mg^{++} (Kersten et al., 1966). Using the association constant of 6 x 10^4 M^{-1} given by Nayak et al. (1975), we calculated for a drug concentration of 7.2 x 10^{-5} M and 1 x 10^{-5} M MgCl$_2$ that only 4% of the drug molecules are bound to DNA. Under these conditions, the observed protection factor was 3.6 (Figure 2). An even higher reduction of single-strand breaks was found at the same drug concentration in the absence of Mg^{++}. It was, therefore, concluded that the protection is not due to a shielding of DNA by the bound drug molecules but rather due to a competition between free chromomycin A$_3$ and DNA for OH-radicals. Again, these results are in disagreement to the observation of Coberos et al. (1982).

Mitomycin C   The antibiotic mitomycin C binds covalently to DNA and induces interstrand crosslinks (Iyer & Szybalski, 1963). When mixtures of mitomycin C and DNA were irradiated, the strand break production was also reduced. However, rather high drug concentrations were necessary. At 7 drug molecules per base pair the production of strand breaks was reduced by only 12%. A further reduction was seen at even higher drug concentrations (see Figure 3 and Table 1). In our investigations mitomycin C has the lowest scavenging capacity for OH-radicals compared to the other drugs on a molar basis. This is in contradiction to the results of Cobreros et al. who reported the highest protection effect for mitomycin C. Even at a ratio of one drug molecule per base pair they found a protection factor of 5.

Neocarzinostatin   This antitumor protein was included because of its interesting interaction mechanism with DNA (Povirk & Goldberg, 1980, Jung, Napier, et al., 1980). Since DNA strand breaks are produced by NCS (Beerman & Goldberg, 1974) and by ionizing radiation, it was expected that a combination of both agents would at least have an additive and possibly even a synergistic effect. It was, however, observed that neocarzinostatin reduces the radiosensitivity by a factor of about 5 if present at a concentration of only one drug molecule per 38 base pairs (Figure 3). This is the highest protection efficiency we have observed so far. One has,

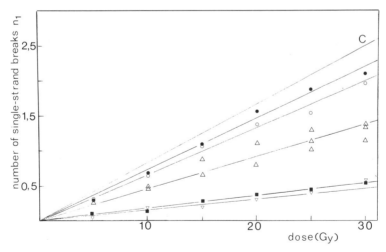

Fig. 3.   Production of single-strand breaks in Col E1 DNA by ionizing radiation (5-30 Gy) in 50 mM phosphate buffer alone (C) and in the presence of the following drugs: mitomycin (1.2 x 10^{-4}M)●, (2.4 x 10^{-4}M)○, (3.6 x 10^{-7}M)△, neocarizinostatin (5 x 10^{-7}M)■, chromophore free NCS (5 x 10^{-7}M)▽.

however, to consider the large molecular weight of NCS; even so, the scavenging capacity of NCS for radiation induced OH-radicals is remarkable.

CONCLUSIONS

DNA strand breakage was found to be very sensitive to the buffer system in which the DNA was irradiated. Buffers acting as scavengers for OH-radicals strongly reduce the yield of strand breaks. In phosphate buffer where no OH-radicals are scavenged a yield of 4.7×10^{-3} was found. In Tris buffer the corresponding value was only 0.12×10^{-3}. Compared to the G-value for OH-radicals ($G_{OH} = 2.7$), the yield for single-strand breaks is very low. In phosphate buffer one out of 600 OH-radicals finally leads to a single-strand break. A similar reduction in radiation products was observed by Kohnlein and Merwitz (1983) studying the demethylation of DNA in citrate buffer which is also known to be an OH-radical scavenger.

In the presence of neocarzinostatin, daunomycin, chloroquine, mitomycin C, and chromomycin A_3 generally a reduction of single-strand breaks was found which was more pronounced at higher drug concentrations. In Table 1 the reduction factors are compiled together with drug concentration and drug to base pair ratio. Ethidium bromide did not change the radiosensitivity of Col E1 DNA. Our finding is partly in contradiction to the results of Cobreros et al. (1982) who observed a strong sensitization effect with daunomycin and chromomycin A_3. They used irradiation doses up to 500 Gy and 0.01 M NaCl as DNA solvent. Our results obtained in a much lower dose range can be best explained assuming that the used drugs can act as scavengers for OH-radicals thus exerting an antagonistic effect.

The interaction mechanisms of the drugs with DNA (intercalation for chloroquine, daunomycin, and neocarzinostatin and binding for mitomycin C and chromomycin A_3) has apparently no influence on the protection effect.

Although the investigated drugs reduce the effect of ionizing radiation, they still retain their cytotoxic and carcinogenic potentials. Our findings will not yield new hints for the formulation of safety standards. They might, however, contribute to a better understanding of combined treatment of tumors with radiation and cytotoxic chemicals.

REFERENCES

1. P. M. Achey, H. Z. Duryea, and G. S. Michaels, Rad. Res. 58:83 (1974).

2. T. A. Beerman and I. H. Goldberg, Biochem. Biophys. Res. Commun. 59:1254 (1974).

3. J. Blok and H. Loman, Curr. Top. Radiat. Res. 34:468 (1973).

4. G. Cobreros, M. C. Lopez Zumel, and P. Usobiaga, Rad. Res. 92:255 (1982).

5. A. Colman, M. J. Byers, S. B. Primrose, and A. Lyons, Eur. J. Biochem. 91:303 (1978).

6. D. B. Clewell and D. R. Helinski, Proc. Nat. Acad. Sci. USA 62:1159 (1969).

7. A. Di Marco and F. Arcamone, Drug Res. 25:368 (1975).

8. V. N. Iyer and W. Szybalski, Proc. Nat. Acad. Sci. USA 50:355 (1963).

9. G. Jung, R. S. Lewis, and W. Kohnlein, Biochem. Biophys. Acta 608:147 (1980).

10. W. Kersten, H. Kersten and W. Szybalski, Biochemistry 5:236 (1966).

11. W. Kohnlein and O. Merwitz, in: "18th Annual Meeting European Society for Radiation Biology, Book of Abstracts," 171 (1984).

12. J.-B. Le Pecq and C. Paoletti, J. Mol. Biol. 27:87 (1967).

13. M. A. Napier, L. S. Kappen and I. H. Goldberg, Biochemistry 19:1767 (1980).

14. R. Nayak, M. Sirsi, and S. K. Podder, Biochim. Biophys. Acta 378:195 (1975).

15. L. F. Povirk, W. Wubker, W. Kohnlein, and F. Hutchinson, Nuc. Acids Res. 4:3573 (1977).

16. L. F. Povirk and I. H. Goldberg, Biochemistry 19:4773 (1980).

17. K. L. Yielding, L. W. Blodgett, H. Sternglanz, and D. Gaudin, in: "Progress in Mol. & Subcell. Biol., Vol. 2," F. E. Hahn et al., eds., Springer-Verlag, Berlin, Heidelberg, New York (1971), pp. 69-90.

HOW SOON AFTER IRRADIATION DO CHROMOSOME ABERRATIONS FORM AND BECOME
IRREVERSIBLE: A DIRECT ANALYSIS BY MEANS OF THE PREMATURE CHROMOSOME
CONDENSATION TECHNIQUE

G. E. Pantelias, J. K. Wiencke and V. Afzal

Laboratory of Radiobiology and Environmental Health
University of California
San Francisco, CA 94143

ABSTRACT

     Radiation-induced chromosome breaks and rearrangements may play a
crucial role in both mutagenesis and carcinogenesis. Yet, because radiation induces far more initial chromosome breaks than are observed as aberrations at metaphase, it has not been possible to examine the kinetics of
primary breakage and rejoining in lymphocytes. A simple method for cell
fusion and premature condensation induction is used to study primary
chromosome breakage, rejoining and formation of irreversible chromosome
rearrangements (e.g., rings, dicentrics) in G_0 human lymphocytes. The
dose-response relations for chromosome fragments analyzed immediately or 1,
2 or 24 h after exposure were found to be linear. Chromosome fragment
rejoining and ring formation were completed about 6 h after irradiation.
With the use of C-banded chromosome preparations, it could be seen that
dicentric chromosomes were also formed in the G_0 lymphocytes during the
chromosome fragment rejoining process. Regardless of dose and post-irradiation time, rings were found to follow a Poisson distribution, whereas
chromosome fragments were overdispersed.

INTRODUCTION

     Most human cancers are associated with chromosomal rearrangements
believed to be the result of somatic mutations in cells whose karyotypes
were originally normal. Ionizing radiations are potent inducers of chromosome aberrations in human cells. Since chromosome breaks and rearrangements may play a crucial role in both mutagenesis and carcinogenesis,
analysis of dose-effect and rejoining kinetics of radiation-induced chromosome fragments may provide not only evidence of radiation injury and
repair, but also a biophysical basis for the mathematical models required
in risk assessment, especially in the case of low doses.

     Improvements in the techniques of cell culture and, particularly, the
development of procedure to stimulate peripheral blood lymphocytes have
facilitated considerably the study of various kinds of aberrations, their
distribution among the cells, and their recovery kinetics. It is widely
accepted today that the radiation-induced chromosome aberrations result
from interaction or accumulation of primary lesions (1, 2). Moreover, it
is assumed that one-track (single ionizing particle) and two-track actions

(two independent ionizing particles) play a role in the production of radiation lesions. These assumptions result in a linear quadratic relation for radiation injury, i.e., observed effect = $\alpha D + \beta D^2$, where α is proportional to the probability per unit dose per cell that two lesions are induced by the same particle, and β is related to the probability that they are induced by different particles. On the contrary, Luchnik (3) claims that the parameters 2 and β have no biophysical or cytogenetic significance. He concludes that the linear quadratic relation should be considered as empirical and cannot be regarded as a relation describing the mechanism of chromosomal aberration production. A similar conclusion has been reached by Goodhead (4). He claims that lesions are determined directly by the energy deposited within single tracks. As a result, the one-track action should be dominant for all conventional radiations and the dose-response relationship fitted by the linear-quadratic model could be explained by introducing a saturable repair system for the lesions.

Attempts to test the validity of the various hypotheses and models of chromosome aberration formation in lymphocyte cultures have been hampered by some inherent limitations of the system. Mainly because there is a period of time between irradiation and cell division, during which chromosomes cannot be examined, the relation between the initial events induced by radiation and the cytologically visible chromosome aberrations cannot be established directly. Furthermore, because of repair of damage and delay in cell progression of the damaged cells, conclusions based on the aberration frequencies observed in cells in metaphase may not be valid for primary breaks induced by radiation.

The direct visualization of chromosome aberrations in interphase cells has now been made possible by techniques based on the phenomenon of premature chromosome condensation (PCC) (5). In this report, the PCC technique is applied to study the kinetics of radiation-induced primary chromosome breaks and the formation of irreversible chromosome rearrangements such as rings and dicentrics in unstimulated G_0 human lymphocytes. Moreover, the distribution of chromosome fragments and rings among the cells is analyzed with respect to the Poisson distribution.

MATERIALS AND METHODS

The procedures for polyethylene glycol (PEG)-mediated cell fusion and PCC induction have been described previously (6).

To identify the centromeric regions of the lymphyocyte prematurely condensed chromosomes (PCCs), air-dried chromosome preparations were C-banded (7).

Whole human blood or isolated lymphocytes were irradiated at room temperature with a Philip's RT250 X-ray machine (250 kVp; HVL = 1.1 mmCu; 115 rad/min). When the chromosome damage was to be estimated immediately after irradiation, the lymphocytes were mixed with mitotic CHO cells, chilled at $0^{\circ}C$, and then irradiated at this temperature. Immediately after irradiation, the cell mixture was treated with PEG for cell fusion ad PCC induction.

The prepared slides were randomly coded, and for each dose and post-irradiation time, the PCCs of at least 100 lymphocytes were analyzed for chromosome aberrations. The chromosome damage was quantified either as the number of rings per cell or, for fragments, as the number of chromosome pieces in excess of 46.

The distribution of rings and fragments among the cells were analyzed
with respect to the Poisson distribution by the method of Papworth (8).
The variance and the mean of the observed distributions are compared in
order to determine whether they are significantly different. In this test,
the quantity µ defined by equation (i) approximates to a unit normal deviate.

$$\mu = \frac{d - (N - 1)}{\sqrt{v\ ard}}$$

Where d is a coefficient of dispersion defined by equation (ii)

$$d = \frac{(N - 1)\sigma^2}{y} \qquad \sigma^2$$

and Var d = 2(N - 1 (1 - 1/NY) where N, Y, and σ^2 are the total number of
cells analyzed, the mean number of chromatid aberrations per cell, and an
estimate of the population variance, respectively.

For a Poisson distribution, the variance equals the mean and so the
quantity µ equals zero. A positive value of   indicates over-dispersion,
i.e., cells with higher and lower aberrations frequencies are more numerous
than in a Poisson distribution. On the contrary, a negative value of
indicates underdispersion, i.e., cells with aberration frequencies close to
the mean are more numerous than in a Poisson distribution. If the absolute
value of   is smaller than 1.96, then the underlying distribution is
Poissonian with a 95 percent level of significance.

RESULTS

Dose-response curves for chromosome fragments obtained immediately or
1, 2, or 24 h after exposure to various X-ray doses were found to be linear
(Figure 1). The rapid rejoining of chromosome fragments that takes place
in the first 3 h after exposure was not correlated with a simultaneous
increase in the yield of rings (Figure 2). Moreover, it was observed that
after 6 h there was no further chromosome fragment rejoining or ring
formation.

To determine whether dicentric chromosomes were formed in the
irradiated lymphocytes during the process of chromosome fragment rejoining,
the chromosomes were C-banded. Unirradiated lymphocyte PCCs exhibit one
centromeric region per chromosome, whereas immediately after 645 rad of X-
rays, acentric fragments were the predominant chromosome aberrations.
However, when the C-banding technique was applied to chromosome spreads
prepared 6 h after exposure, acentric fragments were infrequent but centric
rings and dicentric chromosomes could be seen.

The data for the distribution of lymphocyte chromosome fragments
and rings among the cells immediately after whole blood irradiation (Tables 1
and 2), or at various times after exposure (Table 3 and 4), show that,
regardless of the dose administered and post-irradiation time, rings
followed a Poisson distribution whereas the chromosome fragments were
overdispersed.

DISCUSSION

The linearity of the dose-response curve for chromosome fragments
obtained immediately after irradiation (Figure 1) suggests that chromosome
fragments are determined directly by the energy deposited. If interactions

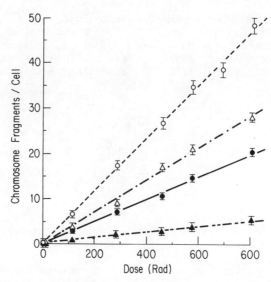

Fig. 1.   Yield of chromosome fragments per cell in human peripheral blood
lymphocytes exposed _in vitro_ to X-ray doses up to 805 rads. The
yield of excess chromosome fragments per cell (Y) is fitted by
the linear regression equation, $Y = \alpha + \beta D$. Immediately after
exposure (O), $\alpha = 0.040$, $\beta = 0.059$, and S.E. (β) = 0.0009. One
hour after exposure (X), $\alpha = 0.054$, $\beta = 0.035$, and S.E. (β) =
0.0006. Two hours after exposure (●), $\alpha = 0.092$, $\beta = 0.025$, and
S.E. (β) = 0.0005. Twenty-four hours after exposure (▲), $\alpha =$
0.408, $\beta = 0.006$, and S.E. (β) = 0.0003. Bars represent standard
deviations calculated from two to three independent experiments.
(Data taken from Pantelias and Maillie, 1984.)

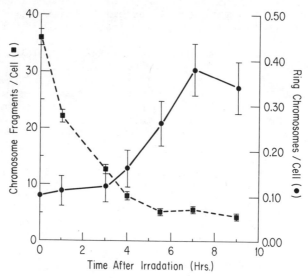

Fig. 2.   Yield of chromosome fragments (■) and ring chromosomes (●) per

cell in human peripheral blood lymphocytes exposed _in vitro_ to
645 rads of X-rays and analyzed at various times after exposure.
(Data taken from Panelias and Maillie, 1984.)

Table 1. Distribution of excess fragments among the cells immediately after X-ray irradiation for doses up to 500 rads - values of Y, σ^2, and μ

Dose (rad)	Cells scored	Excess fragments scored	0	1	2	3	4	5	6	7	8	9	10	11	12	13	14	15	16	17	18	19	20	21	22	23	Y	σ^2	u
5	120	47	93	21	1	3	0	0	1	0	0	1															.39	1.25	17.20
25	110	108	53	27	21	3	2	3	0	1																	.98	1.7	5.45
100	100	296	15	21	10	15	19	7	4	3	2	2	2															2.96	5.80	6.78
250	100	631	0	4	5	11	15	8	18	7	6	8	8	2	3	2	2	1									6.31	10.33	4.50
500	100	1209	0	0	0	1	3	1	5	10	5	6	14	6	7	3	7	5	5	7	6	3	2	1	1	2	12.09	21.90	5.96

Table 2. Distribution of rings among the cells immediately after X-ray irradiation for doses up to 500 rads. Values of Y, σ^2, and μ

| Dose (rad) | Cells scored | Rings | Distribution | | | | | |
			0	1	2	Y	σ^2	u
100	254	26	229	24	1	0.10	0.10	0
250	160	19	141	19	0	0.119	0.105	−1.08
500	177	25	153	23	1	0.14	0.116	−1.67

of two primary lesions are subsequently expressed as fragments, then these primary lesions should result from one-tract actions. Moreover, from the linearity of the dose-response curves obtained at 1, 2, and 24 h after exposure, it can be inferred that at each dose a fixed percentage of the initially induced chromosome fragments undergo rejoining. This conclusion contradicts the hypothesis of dose-dependent differential repair that has been used to explain the low-LET dose-response curves obtained by conventional cytogenetic techniques (4). Indeed, these data on radiation-induced primary chromosome fragments show that repair does not affect the linearity of the dose-response curve.

The yield of rings at 24 h after irradiation has been shown to fit a linear quadratic equation (9). Preliminary results using the C-banding technique suggest that the kinetics of dicentric chromosome formation follows a pattern similar to that of ring formation. Therefore, it can be concluded that the linear quadratic model, which fits most of the experimental results for dicentrics and rings obtained by conventional metaphase cytogenetic techniques, also fits the data obtained from interphase cells.

The relation of chromosome fragment rejoining and ring formation shown in Figure 2 suggests that most of the rejoining and ring formation takes place during the first 6 h after exposure. Similar estimates of the rejoining time have been reported in conventional cytogenetic dose-fractionation experiments designed to measure chromosome repair in human lymphocytes. The repair time after a dose of 100 rads of X-rays was found to be approximately 4 to 5 h (10). It is worth noting that while chromosome fragments are capable of restituting, exchanges (e.g. rings, dicentrics) once formed are permanent. Ring and dicentric chromosomes in lymphocyte PCCs could provide, therefore, confirmatory evidence of an

Table 3. Distribution of excess fragments among the cells after a 500 rad X-ray irradiation at varying post-irradiation times up to 48 hours – values of Y, σ^2, and μ

Time (hr)	Cells scored	Excess frag-ments scored	0	1	2	3	4	5	6	7	8	9	10	11	12	13	14	15	16	17	18	19	20	21	22	23	24	25	26	27	28	29	Y	σ^2	u
0	100	1180	0	0	2	2	3	1	0	6	13	2	5	7	22	4	13	0	4	4	6	2	1	0	3								11.80	18.98	4.28
3	100	1074	1	1	8	1	6	2	7	10	4	4	2	11	3	6	5	5	7	0	3	2	3	2	2	0	0	0	0	0	0	2	10.74	36.27	16.73
8	100	650	0	2	11	9	11	9	16	6	10	4	6	5	5	2	0	0	0	0	0	1											6.5	12.05	6.04
24	113	582	6	6	18	9	23	7	9	8	7	8	4	1	2	1	0	1	2	1													5.15	13.09	11.55
48	100	564	10	11	11	9	15	2	10	5	5	3	1	1	7	1	2	0	4	0	1	0	0	1	0	1							5.64	25.34	24.6

Table 4. Distribution of rings among the cells after a 500 rad X-ray irradiation at varying post-irradiation times up to 48 hours. Values of Y, σ^2, and μ

Time (hr)	Cells scored	Rings	Distribution					Y	σ^2	u
			0	1	2	3	4			
0	185	25	162	21	2			.135	.138	0.218
3	165	46	119	40	3			.280	.236	-1.44
8	156	60	96	40	10			.380	.356	-0.56
24	166	81	100	52	13	1		.49	.44	-0.90
48	169	87	100	54	13	1	1	.51	.51	0

exposure, especially when blood samples are analyzed a long time after radiation.

With respect to the frequency distribution of rings and chromosome fragments among the cells, it was found that rings follow a Poisson distribution, i.e., are randomly distributed. Chromosome fragments, however, do not follow a Poisson distribution, which is in agreement with previously reported results for acentric chromosome fragments in lymphocytes analyzed at metaphase (11). A conclusion regarding the distribution of primary lesions may then be drawn from these results. Indeed, since very few rings and presumably dicentrics are expected to be formed immediately after irradiation, the distribution of fragments should follow very closely the distribution of primary lesions. Consequently, the primary lesions themselves should be significantly overdispersed.

Finally, data in Table 3 show that about 20 percent of the cells analyzed at 8, 24, and 48 h post-irradiation time still had nine or more excess fragments per cell. Therefore, it may be concluded that this percentage represents a lymphocyte subpopulation which shows slow repair.

ACKNOWLEDGEMENTS

This work was supported by Department of Energy Contract No. DE-AM03-76-SF01012.

REFERENCES

1. A. M. Kellerer and H. H. Rossi, The theory of dual radiation action, Curr. Top. Rad. Res. 8:85-158 (1972).

2. K. H. Chadwick and H. P. Leenhouts, A molecular theory of cell survival, Phys. Med. Biol. 18:78-87 (1973).

3. N. V. Luchnik, Do one-hit chromosome exchanges exist?, Rad. Environ. Biophys. 12:197-204 (1975).

4. D. T. Goodhead, Models of radiation inactivation and mutagenesis, in: "Radiation Biology in Cancer Research," R. E. Meyn and H. R. Withers, eds., Raven Press, New York (1980), pp. 231-247.

5. R. T. Johnson and P. N. Rao, Mammalian cell fusion: induction of premature chromosome condensation in interphase nuclei, Nature 226:717-722 (1970).

6. G. E. Pantelias and H. D. Maillie, A simple method for premature chromosome condensation induction in primary human and rodent cells using polyethylene glycol, Somat. Cell Genet. 9:533-547 (1983).

7. A. T. Sumner, A simple technique for demonstrating centromeric heterochromatin, Exp. Cell Res. 75:304-306 (1972).

8. J. R. K. Savage, Sites of radiation induced chromosome exchanges, Curr. Top. Radiat. Res. Qtly. 6:129-194 (1970).

9. G. E. Pantelias and H. D. Maillie, Direct analysis of radiation-induced chromosome fragments and rings in unstimulated human peripheral blood lymphocytes by means of the premature chromosome condensation technique, Mutat. Res. (1984), in press.

10. S. Wolff, The repair of X-ray-induced chromosome aberrations in stimulated and unstimulated human lymphocytes, Mutat. Res. 15:435-444 (1972).

11. R. P. Virsik and D. Harder, Analysis of radiation-induced acentric fragments in human G_0 lymphocytes, Radiat. Environ. Biophys 19:29-40 (1981).

PRODUCTION BY RADIATION OF DNA DOUBLE STRAND BREAKS IN THREE MAMMALIAN

CELL LINES AND THEIR REPAIR IN FOETAL HUMAN FIBROBLASTS

O. Sapora*, A. Maggi*, and M. Quintiliani+

*Laboratorio di Tossicologia Comparata ed Ecotossicologia
 Istituto Superiore di Sanita
 Roma
+Istituto Tecnologie Biomediche, (CNR)
 Roma, Italia

INTRODUCTION

When first techniques became available to measure radiation induced DNA double strand breaks (DSB) (1), it was postulated that such lesions could not be repaired by living cells and were, therefore, responsible for cell death (2, 3). It was later realized that DSB were instead extensively repaired both in bacterial (4) and mammalian cells (5). Nevertheless, the assumption the DSB could be involved in the mechanism of radiation induced cell death, was not dismissed but transferred to unrepaired DSB (6). Unfortunately, the possibility of directly checking this hypothesis is severely hampered by technical reasons. Even with the more recent methodologies, radiation doses necessary to obtain significant measurement of DSB are far beyond the range of cell survival, particularly when sedimentation techniques are used. A second drawback is due to the difficulties of handling large DNA molecules attached to nuclear proteins and to isolate DNA without degrading it too much. On the other hand, it should be taken into account that, even if we were able to isolate intact chromosomal DNA of mammalian cells, no analytical techniques are actually available to deal with it.

In addition to ionizing radiation, DSB can be produced by other agents such as UV light and various drugs. In these cases a mechanism operating through repair enzymes attempting to repair DNA damage can be mainly involved (7, 8). Such a mechanism on the other hand, is believed to contribute also to DSB production by ionizing radiation (9, 10).

In this paper an experimental technique set up in our laboratory has been applied to investigate the production of DSB in three different mammalian cell lines and the repair of such damage in a primary line of human foetal fibroblast.

331

MATERIALS AND METHODS

Cell Lines and Culture Conditions

Two cell lines growing in monolayer in F14 medium supplemented with
neomicine (5 mgr/ml), NaHCO3 (2 gr/lt) and 10% foetal calf serum, were
used: namely, the Chinese hamster lung cells, V79, a well known
established line, and the human foetal lung fibroblast primary line HF19,
with doubling times of 12 and 30 hours, respectively. The third line was
the K562, established by Lozzio and Lozzio (11) from a patient with chronic
myeloid leukemia in acute phase. K562 cells were grown in suspension, in
RPMI 1642 medium supplemented with 10% foetal calf serum, streptomycin
and penicillin (50 mU/ml) and NaHCO3 (2 gr/lt), with a doubling time of 24
hours.

Irradiation

X-irradiation was carried out with a Siemens therapy unit operating at
200 KV, 15 mA with 0.2 mm copper filter at dose rates of 1.2 Gy/min and 18
Gy/min for cell survival and DSB experiments, respectively.

Cell Survival

V79 and HF19 cells were irradiated attached to tissue culture flask
surface, in growing medium, in air and at room temperature. Immediately
after irradiation cells were trypsinized, counted, diluted, and plated at
appropriate concentrations. After 8 days of incubation at $37^{O}C$, the
survival was calculated by scoring the number of visible clones. The
survival of K562 cells growing in suspension was measured using the method
of Kramer et al. (12), which measures the ability of small numbers of cells
to initiate microscopic cultures in wells of a microtiter plate.

DSB Measurement

5×10^{4} cells into 3 cm diameter plastic tissue culture plates were
labelled overnight with ^{3}H-thymidine (3.66×10^{4} Bq/ml). After 16 hours
incubation cold thymidine (final concentration 0.1 mg/ml) was added to each
sample for 30 minutes. The medium was then removed, the cells washed twice
with fresh medium and incubated for two more hours. The irradiations were
carried out at $0^{O}C$ to prevent DNA repair during irradiation.

For repair experiments the cells, after irradiation, were incubated in
fresh medium at $37^{O}C$ for different lengths of time. Experiments in the
presence of aphidicolin were carried out by incubating the cells in growing
medium containing 10 microgr./ml of the inhibitor for 60 minutes prior to
irradiation. The same medium was then maintained during repair incubation.

Cells were detached from the plastic surface using a rubber scraper
and resuspended in 0.5 ml of cold TEN (Tris-HCl 0.05 M, EDTA 0.01 M, NaCl
0.01 M pH 8.5) buffer. 0.27 ml of suspension was added into an Eppendorf 1
ml minicentrifuge tube with 0.015 ml of 10% Sarkosyl and incubated at $65^{O}C$
for 30 minutes. At the end of treatment 0.015 ml of proteinase K (10
mgr/ml) were added and the tubes incubated overnight at 37° in a device
rotating at 0.5 rpm. Then 0.2 ml of 5 M NaCl were added and the tubes kept
at $37^{O}C$ for one more hour followed by the addition of 0.4 ml of TEN buffer.
The resulting DNA solution was pumped out through the cutted bottom of each
minitube at 0.3 ml/min and layered on the top of 10 ml neutral 5-20%
sucrose gradient (0.02 M Tris-HCl, 1 M NaCl, 0.01 M EDTA, 0.1% Sarkosyl, pH
8.5) resting on 0.5 ml of 40% sucrose at the bottom of the centrifuge tube.
Gradients were centrifuged in a L8-80 Beckman Ultracentrifuge, using a SW
41 rotor at 5000 rpm for 65-70 hours and then fractionated in 30-32

fractions, collected into miniscintillation vials and counted in a L9000 Beckman scintillation counter.

DSB Calculation

Gradient profiles were analyzed using a modification (13) of an expression derived by Litwin (14) which assumes that DNA of unit length undergoes scission at random positions on the DNA strand. This method is more reliable than many of the others used to analyze sedimentation data. Molecular weights were standardized using T2 phage DNA whose molecular weight is 1.1×10^{8} daltons.

RESULTS

Figure 1 shows the survival (A) and the dose-effect curves for DSB production (B) relative to cell lines used in the experiments. V79 cells are the most resistant to lethal effect of radiation and exhibit a large initial shoulder in their survival curve, while the other two lines exhibit little or no shoulder and steeper slopes. The D 10%, i.e., the radiation dose necessary to reduce survival to 10%, are 1.7, 2.7, and 5.7 Gy for K562, HF19 and V79, respectively. On the contrary, the dose effect relation for DSB production appears to be the same for the three cell lines; and, in the dose range used in the present experiments, it is linear with a yield of 0.07 DSB/Gy/10^{10} daltons. A representative example of sedimentation profiles at different radiation doses is shown in Figure 2 for HF19 cells.

HF19 cells have been used to study the time course of repair. Sedimentation profiles obtained after irradiation with 90 (A) and 360 Gy (B) are shown in Figure 3. In our experimental conditions, the lowest dose for detecting significant differences in sedimentation profiles, with respect to unirradiated cells, is 15 Gy, however, such high doses as those indicated above were used in order to obtain clear differences between various experimental samples. During the first 60 minutes of incubation in complete medium, cells irradiated with 90 Gy are able to repair approximately 70% out of 6-7 DSB, while those irradiated with 360 Gy repaired 50% out of the 25 DSB produced. In the following 60 minutes the

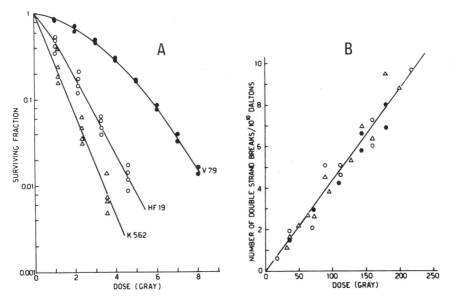

Fig. 1. X-ray survival curves (panel A) and number of DSB as a function of X-ray dose (panel B) for K562 ($\triangle$), HF19 ($\bigcirc$), and V79 cells ($\bullet$).

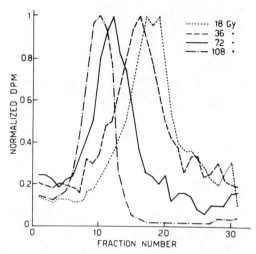

Fig. 2.   Sedimentation profiles of DNA extracted from HF19
           cells as a function of absorbed dose. The double
           stranded DNA was centrifuged for 65 hours at 5000
           rpm.

rate of repair decreases so that only a further amount of 5-10% is repaired
after 90 Gy. In cells irradiated with 360 Gy, during the 180 minutes
following the first hour of repair incubation, the damage decreases from 50
to 35-40%. The relative kinetic curves are shown in Figure 5.

Aphidicolin, a specific inhibitor of alpha polymerases, was used in
the attempt to clarify the role of polymerases in DSB repair, the specific
alfa polymerases inhibitor, aphidicolin, was used. The results obtained
are reported in Figures 4 and 5. As shown in the figures, aphidicolin does
not affect the repair of DSB produced by 90 Gy of X-rays, while the repair
of breaks produced by 360 Gy appears to proceed normally for 30-60 min and
then is completely inhibited.

DISCUSSION

The experimental technique used to evaluate DSB allows to handle high
molecular weight DNA (5-7 x 10^9 daltons) without any preconditioning
treatment (2, 5). It compares to the technique used by Pohlit et al. (15,
6), that is slightly more complicated and gives somewhat better
experimental results. These authors can in fact handle DNA of more than
10^{10} daltons and detect damage at radiation doses of about 10 Gy. The
yield of DSB they obtain is not very far from that obtained in the present
experiments. It can be noted that our data are the first showing that
three cell lines, with different sensitivity towards lethal effects of
radiation, show that same sensitivity with respect to DSB production. This
finding is consistent with the assumption that it is not the initial number
of DSB produced by radiation that can be responsible for the lethal effect,
but, eventually, the number of non-repaired DSB.

Previous data on cell lines used in our experiments only concern V79
cells and primary human fibroblasts (16, 17). Due to differences in the
experimental techniques, it is not possible to make direct comparisons in
the respective yields, while the linear relationship of breaks production
versus radiation dose has been confirmed.

No previous data have been reported on K562 cells.

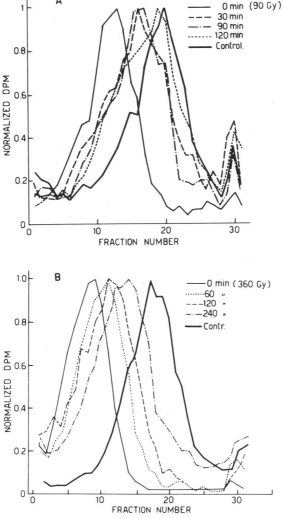

Fig. 3. Sedimentation profiles of double stranded DNA from
HF19 cells irradiated with 90 (A) or 360 GY (B) of
X-ray and incubated for different times at 37°C in
complete medium.

With regard to DSB repair in HF19 cells, our data show that
the majority of the breaks are rapidly repaired both at 90 and at 360 Gy.
Similar results were obtained by Woods (17) on primary human fibroblasts,
HF15, using the neutral elution technique. Both series of data indicate a
$T_{1/2}$, time required to repair 50% of the damage, of about 30 minutes after
radiation doses of 90-100 Gy.

The repair process does not appear to be as fast as in our cells, in
Ascites tumor cells. The data reported by Pohlit and Blocher (6) show, in
fact, that in these cells the $T_{1/2}$ is of about 120 minutes. The existence
of different repair capabilities in different cell lines is suggested by
these findings.

The effect of aphidicolin on DSB repair seems to indicate the
existence of different repair pathways according to radiation dose, that is
to say according to the level of damage. Data in Figure 5 show a late
inhibition of the repair process suggesting that from that point onward a

335

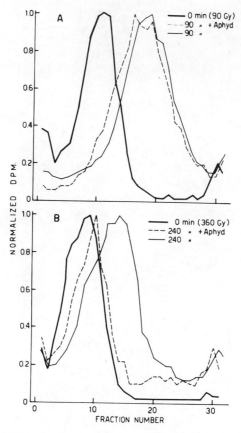

Fig. 4. Sedimentation profiles of double stranded DNA from HF19 cells irradiated with 90 (A) or 360 (B) Gy of X-ray in the presence or not of 10 microgr/ml of Aphidicolin.

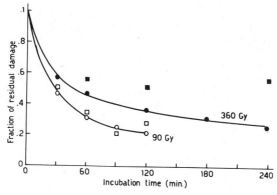

Fig. 5. Fraction of residual damage versus incubation time in HF19 cells irradiated with 90 (open symbols) or 360 Gy (closed symbols) of X-ray. Experiments carried out in the presence (□, ■) or in the absence (○, ●) of 10 microgr/ml of Aphidicolin.

mechanism depending on alfa polymerases activity takes over, while the initial component at high radiation dose, and the whole process at the low one, are not inhibited, as they would depend on non alfa polymerases activity, possibly on beta polymerase. This finding is consistent with the assumption that beta polymerase is a constitutive enzyme, always present in cells at nearly constant concentration, while alfa polymerases are to some extent inducible and fluctuating in their concentration (18).

The present state of research does not allow to go much further than to propose what stated above as a working hypothesis to be confirmed by further experimental research.

ACKNOWLEDGEMENTS

Work partially supported by the Special Project "Oncologia" of the CNR.

REFERENCES

1. H. S. Kaplan, Proc. Natl. Acad. Sci. USA 55:1442-1446 (1966).

2. D. L. Dugle, C. J. Gillespie, and J. D. Chapman, Proc. Natl. Acad. Sci. USA 73:809-812 (1976).

3. K. H. Chadwick and H. P. Leenhouts, "Molecular Theory of Radiation Biology," Springer-Verlag, Berlin, Heidelberg, New York (1981).

4. F. Krasin and F. Hutchinson, J. Mol. Biol. 116:81-98 (1977).

5. A. Cole, F. Shonka, P. Corry, and W. G. Cooper, in: "Molecular Mechanisms for Repair of DNA, Part B," P. C. Hanawalt and R. B. Setlow, eds., Plenum Press, New York (1975), pp. 665-676.

6. D. Blocher and W. Pohlit, Int. J. Radiat. Biol. 42:329-338 (1982).

7. F. Krasin and F. Hutchinson, Biophys. J. 24:645-656 (1978).

8. L. F. Povirk, W. Wubker, W. Kohnlein, and F. Hutchinson, Nucleic Ac. Res. 4:3573-3582 (1977).

9. T. Bonura, K. C. Smith, and H. S. Kaplan, Proc. Natl. Acad. Sci. USA 72:4265-4269 (1975).

10. G. Ahnstrom and P. E. Bryant, Int. J. Radiat. Biol. 41:671-676 (1982).

11. C. B. Lozzio and B. B. Lozzio, Blood 45:321-334 (1975).

12. K. H. Kraemer, L. W. Haywood, and J. K. Buchanan, Mutat. Res. 72:285-294 (1980).

13. R. A. Fox, Int. J. Radiat. Biol. 30:67-75 (1976).

14. S. J. Litwin, J. Appl. Prob. 6:275-284 (1969).

15. D. Blocher, Int. J. Radiat. Biol. 42:317-328 (1982).

16. M. D. Bradley and K. W. Kohn, Nucleic Ac. Res. 7:793-799 (1979).

17. W. G. Woods, Biochim. Biophys. Acta 655:342-348 (1981).

18. U. Bertazzoni, M. Stefanini, G. Pedrali-Noy, F. Nuzzo, and A. Falaschi, Nucleic Ac. Res. 4:141-148 (1977).

THE ROLE OF ONCOGENES IN MULTISTAGE CARCINOGENESIS

K. Brown, M. Quintanilla, M. Ramsden, and A. Balmain

Beatson Institute for Cancer Research
Garscube Estate
Switchback Road
Glasgow G61 BD
Scotland

INTRODUCTION

The existence of specific genes which could transform normal cells into tumour cells was first demonstrated in studies of retroviruses isolated from avian or rodent tumours (1). The prototype oncogene is the src gene of the avian Rous Sarcoma virus. This virus induces tumours with a short latent period in chickens and it has been demonstrated using temperature sensitive mutants that the src gene has to be expressed in order that transformation should occur (2). Over twenty additional oncogenes have subsequently been discovered in different retrovirus isolates. The products of these oncogenes can be classified into several categories according to their cellular localization or biochemical function as tyrosine kinases (src family) or GTP-binding proteins (ras family). The biological role of these products in cellular transformation is unknown, and the only oncogenes to which a function has been ascribed are those related to growth factors (sis gene) or growth factor receptors (erb B gene). Some oncogenes, for example those belonging to the ras family or the myc gene, have been isolated on several occasions in entirely independent viruses, suggesting that they play a very important role in tumour induction.

At the time when these experiments were carried out, no retrovirus had been implicated in any form of human cancer, and questions were raised about the role of viral oncogenes in the induction of "real" tumours. The first indication that oncogenes might be important in human tumour development came from the discovery that these viral genes were in fact present in the genomes of all normal cells and had been transduced or picked up by the viruses during evolution (3). This raised the possibility that these cellular "proto-oncogenes" could have an important role in the growth and/or differentiation of normal cells since they were extremely highly conserved during evolution and could be found in such diverse organisms as yeast, Drosophila, and man (4). Subsequently, evidence began to accumulate showing that the "normal" functions of proto-oncogenes could be subverted by a variety of mechanisms in tumour cells. Mechanisms which have been implicated in the activation of proto-oncogenes to an oncogenic form include (a) the induction of point mutations which alter the amino acid sequence of the gene product (5), (b) chromosomal translocations which result in the disruption of the transcriptional control mechanisms regulating the level or timing of proto-oncogene expression (6, 7), or even the generation of new fusion proteins between the products of the proto-oncogene and other cellular genes (8), (c) gene amplification associated with substantially increased levels of proto-oncogene expression (9), (d) the insertion of new promoter elements, also leading to enhanced expression or altered mRNA transcripts (10).

The ras Family

The genes which have been most frequently found in an activated form in human tumours belong to the ras family. This family comprises three known members called Harvey-, Kirsten- and N-ras. The first two were originally identified as components of the murine Harvey (H)- or Kirsten (K)- sarcoma viruses while the N-ras gene has not previously been found in any retrovirus. About 10-20% of randomly selected human tumours have activated forms of one of the ras genes. Activation in this case is defined as the capacity of DNA isolated from the tumours to transform NIH/3T3 in transfection assays. These cells have the ability to take up and express exogenously added DNA and can be particularly efficiently transformed by ras genes, but also by other, unrelated oncogenes (11-13). The acquisition of transforming properties is associated with point mutations in one of two regions of the ras genes located around codons 12 and 61.

A detailed comparison of the particular ras gene which is activated in tumours of diverse histological classification leads to the emergence of a distinct pattern (Table 1). The H-ras gene is mutated predominantly in tumours of epithelial origin, the only reported exceptions to this being two melanomas (14, 15) and virus-induced myeloid leukaemic cell line (16). On the other hand, while the N-ras gene is activated in a broad spectrum of tumour cell types including carcinomas and fibrosarcomas, it is the most frequently mutated member of the family in tumours of the haematopoietic lineage. No obvious tissue preference can be seen in the activation pattern of the Kiras gene. The activation of a particular gene in a specific cell type may indicate that this gene has a special biological function which is exclusive to the target cell, or may reflect some tissue-specific aspect of the structure or transcription of the gene which renders it more susceptible to mutation.

The main questions which arise from these observations include the following: (a) Is the activation of a ras gene a necessary or even sufficient event for tumour induction, or simply a consequence of the higher growth rate or aberrant control mechanisms in many tumours? (b) Does the mutation occur at an early or late stage of carcinogenesis and how do the biological consequences of activation relate to the multistep nature of tumour development? (c) What is the molecular basis for the preferential activation of particular members of the ras gene family in tumours of specific cell types?

The Use of Animal Model Systems

Answers to the questions raised above are obviously very difficult to obtain using human tumour material. The genetic variation in humans and the unknown etiology of the vast majority of human tumours make the question of ras gene involvement in human cancer very difficult to unravel. For this reason, a number of laboratories including our own have turned to animal model systems where tumours of defined histological type can be reproducibly induced by treatment with carcinogen agents. The particular model system we have chosen to study is based on the induction of mouse

Table 1. Activated ras genes in human tumours and tumour-derived cell lines[1]

Tumour type	Isolate number[2]		ras gene activated[3]	Reference No.
CARCINOMA:				
Bladder	EJ/T24	(C)	H	44
				45
				46
	J82	(C)	H	44
	JBT44	(T)	H	29
	A1698	(C)	K	47
Renal Pelvic	JPT26	(H)	H	29
Lung	Hs242	(C)	H	48
	Lx-1	(C)	K	44
				49
	A427	(C)	K	47
	Calu-1	(C)	K	50,51
	SK-LU-1	(C)	K	51
	A2182	(C)	K	47
	PR310	(C)	K	53
	A549	(C)	K	49
	PR371	(C)	K	53
	Lu65	(C)	K	54
	1615	(T)	K	47
	LC-10	(T)	K	28
	SW1271	(C)	N	55
Colon	SW480	(C)	K	49
	Adenocarc.	(T)	K	49
	SK-CO-1	(C)	K	52
	A2233	(C)	K	47
Pancreas	A1165	(C)	K	56
	1189	(T)	K	47
Liver	HEP G2	(C)	N	57
	2193	(T)	N	57
Gall Bladder	A1604	(C)	K	47
Ovary	OVCA-1	(C)	K	58
Teratocarcinoma	PA1	(C)	N	56

(continued)

skin papillomas and carcinomas by sequential treatment with initiators and promoters of carcinogenesis (17).

Initiation of carcinogenesis is accomplished by treatment of the mice with a low dose of the carcinogen dimethylbenzanthracene (DMBA). This gives rise to a population of putative "initiated" cells which, in the absence of further treatment, can remain dormant within the skin for periods of up to one year (18). If, however, the mice are treated 2-3 times weekly with a tumour promoter (12-0-tetradecanoyl-phorbol-13-acetate (TPA)) they develop multiple benign papillomas within 6-10 weeks. A small proportion of these tumours subsequently undergo a further change and begin to grow as invasive carcinomas (19). An additional feature of this model is that many of the characteristics of carcinogenesis in vivo can also be reproduced, at least at the morphological level, using epidermal cells cultured in vitro. The work of Yuspa and Fusenig and their colleagues has

Table 1 Continued

Tumour Type	Isolate number[2]		ras gene activated[3]	Reference No.
CARCINOMA:				
Mammary	HS578T	(C)	H	59
SARCOMA:				
Fibrosarcoma	HT1080	(C)	N	60
Rhabdomyosarcoma	RD	(C)	N	60
	1085	(T)	K	47
MELANOMA	SK2	(C)	H	15
	SK-MEL-146	(C)	H	14
	SK-MEL-93	(C)	N	14
	SK-MEL-119	(C)	N	14
	SK-MEL-147	(C)	N	14
NEUROBLASTOMA	SK-N-SH	(C)	N	51,52
LEUKAEMIA:				
Acute lymphocytic				
(immature T cell)	RPMI8402	(C)	N	61
(intermediate T cell)	T-ALL-1	(C)	N	61
"	p12	(C)	N	61
"	CCRF-CEM	(C)	K	62
"	MOLT-3	(C)	N	62
"	MOLT-4	(C)	N	62
Chronic myelocytic	PAC	(C)	N	63
Acute myelocytic	Marrow cells	(T)	N	64
Promyelocytic	HL60	(C)	N	63
LYMPHOMA:				
Burkitts	AWRamos	(C)	N	63

1. Table only shows examples published before 31.12.84.
2. (C) denotes tumour-derived cell line, (T) denotes primary tumour material used as source of transforming DNA.
3. H: c-H-ras1 gene, K: c-K-ras[2] gene, N: N-ras gene.

shown that normal epidermal cells can be treated in vitro with carcinogens and give rise to cells which are initiated but non-tumorigenic (20) or to fully transformed keratinocytes which give rise to carcinomas upon inoculation into nude mice (20, 21). Whether the putative initiated cells isolated by these procedure are the same as those which give rise to tumours in animals is an important question which has not yet been resolved, but this system obviously offers an ideal opportunity to study the molecular basis of the sequence of events which occur during carcinogenesis both in vivo and in vitro.

Our initial experiments used the NIH/3T3 transfection assay to test whether a particular oncogene was activated in skin tumours induced by initiation with DMBA and promotion with TPA. The results summarized in Table 2 show that 4 of 6 carcinomas tested were positive in the transfection assay. In each case, Southern blotting showed the activated gene to be the H-ras gene (22). A further series of experiments was carried out to determine whether the activation was an early or late event. Of eight papillomas tested, seven were positive in the transfection assay; again the activated gene in each case was the H-ras gene (23). In this system, therefore, the activation of the gene obviously is a relatively early event, and may even take place at the initiation phase of carcinogenesis.

Table 2 also shows the results obtained using other animal model system where activation of oncogenes has been investigated. Sukumar et al. (24) had previously demonstrated consistent activation of the H-ras gene in nine rat mammary carcinomas induced by a single treatment with nitrosomethylurea (NMU). More recently, Zarbl et al. extended these observations to show that 49 carcinomas had the same gene activated, and in addition that the mutation in each case was a G-A transition at codon 12 (25). In an interesting series of experiments, Guerrero et al. have shown that the particular oncogene activated in mouse thymomas depends on the carcinogenic agent used. Thymomas induced by treatment with NMU had an activated N-ras-gene, whereas in those produced as a result of radiation treatment, K-ras was the only transforming gene detected (26, 27). These results could suggest a direct interaction between the carcinogenic agent used and the particular ras gene activated, although other interpretations, for example, that different cell populations are being transformed by the different agents, cannot be excluded.

A number of general observations can be made from the comparison shown in Table 2. The first is that the proportion of tumours with activated ras genes 50-90%) is considerably higher in animal model systems than in

Table 2. Activation of ras genes in animal model systems[1]

TUMOUR	CARCINOGEN	No. POSITIVE/No. TESTED	GENE	REF.
Skin Carcinoma	DMBA/TPA	4/6	H-ras	22
Skin Papilloma	DMBA/TPA	7/8	H-ras	23
Mammary Carcinoma	NMU	48/58	H-ras	25
Thymoma	NMU	5/6	N-ras	26
Thymoma	γ-Rays	4/7	K-ras	27
Fibrosarcoma	MCA	2/4	K-ras	36

1. Abbreviations used : DMBA:dimethylbenzanthracene; NMU: nitrosomethylurea; MCA:methylcholanthrene.

randomly selected human tumours (8, 29). This probably reflects the fact that the etiology of human tumours is highly variable, and only some of the routes to tumorigenesis involve activation of these genes. One might expect much more consistent results in animal systems where the particular carcinogen used, the dose level and route of administration can all be controlled. Secondly, there is a highly reproducible activation of a specific gene in each experimental system used. The skin and mammary gland systems, both of which give rise to epithelial neoplasms, demonstrate consistent activation of the Harvey-ras gene. On the other hand, fibrosarcomas induced with methylcholanthrene appear to have an activated Kirsten-ras gene, while the thymomas have either Kirsten- or N-ras activation depending on the carcinogen used. The differential activation pattern seen in those systems is reminiscent of the situation discussed above with regard to oncogenes activated in human tumours, and thus strengthens the prospects of obtaining valuable insights into the molecular mechanisms involved in human cancer by studying these animal models.

What is the Basis of Tissue-specific Ras Gene Activation?

The finding that only the H-ras gene is reproducibly activated in chemically-induced skin tumours suggests either that this gene is particularly susceptible to mutation in epidermal cells or that perturbation specifically of H-ras gene function is very important in skin tumorigenesis. Analysis of the transcription of the H-ras gene in different mouse tissues (30, 31; M.R. and A. B., unpublished results) shows that the level of expression of this gene is not noticeably higher in epidermal cells than in other tissue types. There is, therefore, no obvious correlation between transcription level and mutational activation of the gene.

Another possibility is that there might be some aspect of the chromatin structure surrounding the H-ras gene which predisposes this particular site to the mutational effects of carcinogens. Numerous studies have implicated DNA methylation--notably the presence or absence of 5-methylcytosine residues--in the control of chromatin structure and gene expression (32-34). We, therefore, investigated the methylation state of the mouse H-ras gene in different cell types and at different stages of tumour progression in skin to determine whether there is any correlation between the activation of the gene and its methylation pattern. A comparison was carried out by digesting DNA isolated from normal mouse epidermis, brain, erythroleukaemic cells, neuroblastoma and NIH/3T3 cells with the restriction endonucleases MspI and HpaII. The results showed that the methylation status of the c-H-ras locus varies markedly in different tissue types, ranging between the highly methylated state in NIH/3T3 fibroblasts and a largely unmethylated form in epidermis, with intermediate levels in brain and hematopoietic cell lineages (35). The comparison between fibroblastic cells and epidermis is particularly interesting. The c-H-ras gene is undermethylated and capable of frequent activation in epidermis, but is highly methylated in fibroblastic cells where carcinogen-induced transformation is associated with c-K-ras activation (36, 37). It is plausible that in fibroblast or other cell types, c-H-ras activation may not occur since in addition to mutational events, demethylation steps are required to allow the effective expression of the c-H-ras transforming ability. It is also possible that demethylation of c-H-ras in epidermal DNA renders the gene more easily accessible to carcinogenic agents. This effect may be mediated by differential protein binding to c-H-ras in different cell types in association with the DNA methylation levels. Obviously, the elucidation of such possibilities require much greater insight into the role of c-H-ras plays in the cell, the mechanisms by which expression of the gene is regulated and also the mechanism of activation by carcinogen treatment.

Mechanism of Ras Gene Activation in Chemical Carcinogenesis

In all cases so far examined in detail, ras gene activation is achieved by point mutation within the coding region. This has been shown by cloning and sequencing of the normal and transforming alleles of the gene. Point mutations have been found in ras genes activated in human tumours and also in animal tumours induced by chemical treatment (5). In a detailed study by Zarbl et al., 49 rat mammary carcinomas which arose after treatment with nitrosomethylurea (NMU) has H-ras genes which were activated by the same G-A transition at the 12th codon, resulting in the replacement of glycine with glutamic acid in the P21 protein product (25). This particular mutation happens to be that predicted on the basis of direct interaction between NMU and cellular DNA, which, as a result of alkylation of deoxyguanosine residues, leads to mispairing during replication and transition mutations (38). Zarbl et al. consequently suggested that the oncogene activation may be directly linked to the interaction of NMU with the DNA.

What appears to be a more heterogeneous pattern is emerging from our studies on mouse skin tumours initiated by treatment with dimethylbenzanthracene (DMBA) and promoted with 12-0-tetradecanoyl-phorbol-13-acetate (TPA). Analysis of the P21 proteins encoded by the activated Harvey-ras genes of these tumours has identified at least 3 different forms of P21 which presumably arise by different mutations (M. Quintanilla & A. Balmain, unpublished results). This shows that the genetic changes which take place in tumours initiated by DMBA are not always identical, although it remains possible that all of the mutations are nevertheless caused by direct interaction between the carcinogen and the cellular H-ras gene. More recent sequence analysis on these tumours has shown that the majority of the mutations have taken place at codon 61 of the H-ras gene, although some tumours have mutations in codon 12. The data are consistent with the ability of DMBA to form bulky adducts with deoxyadenosine or deoxyguanosine residues, leading to the induction of several distinct point mutations (39, 40).

Ras Gene Mutations May Be the Initiation Event in Skin Carcinogenesis

We have previously shown that mutated ras genes are present in a high percentage of premalignant skin papillomas (23). This demonstrated that mutation could take place at an early stage of carcinogenesis and raised the possibility that initiation might involve direct mutation of the H-ras gene by the carcinogen used. The initiation of carcinogenesis is thought to be a mutational event, although estimates of the target size for such mutations vary widely (41, 42). The demonstration that ras gene mutations in tumours induced by chemical carcinogens are not located randomly on the genes but are situated preferentially at codon 12, in the case of mammary carcinoma induced by MNU (25), or codon 61 in the case of DMBA (25, 65) however suggests that the mutations may be caused by direct interaction with the carcinogen. It seems unlikely that selection of highly transforming mutant alleles is the cause of the specificity, since a variety of different mutations at both codons can induce transforming activity. On both the skin and mammary gland carcinogenesis systems, initiation is accomplished by a single treatment with the carcinogen. Both systems also require the use of a promoter to amplify the effect of the initial change and lead to tumour formation. In skin this is accomplished by repeated treatment with the promoter TPA, whereas mammary gland promotion is probably carried out by endogenous hormone production (24, 25). The carcinogen specificity, together with the fact that only a single treatment is carried out at the initiation phase of carcinogenesis therefore suggests that mutation takes place concomitantly with initiation. Obviously, this suggestion can only be confirmed by a much more complete analysis of mutations in tumours induced by different carcinogens within the same experimental system. Such studies are presently in progress in this laboratory.

Definitive proof of the involvement of a specific mutated gene in carcinogenesis will only be obtained by introducing the modified gene into primary cells and demonstrating that a direct consequence is tumour induction. We have recently performed some experiments along these lines which show that a mutated form of the H-ras gene can initiate mouse skin carcinogenesis in vivo in a manner very similar to that obtained using chemical initiators (66). These experiments lend strong support to the hypothesis that initiation by chemicals involves mutation of the same gene.

The impression should not be given, however, that ras gene mutation is necessarily the initiation event or even an early event in the development of all experimental or human cancers. It has, for example, been observed that cell lines derived from only one of five metastatic deposits of malignant melanoma in a single patient have activated ras oncogenes (14). This, together with the activation of Kirsten-ras in a T-cell lymphoma during passage in culture (16) may constitute examples of systems in which ras gene activation is a late event which might nevertheless contribute to the evolution of variant cell populations within a developing tumour. It is perhaps not so surprising in view of the multifaceted nature of tumour development that different experimental systems can give different results. The primary biological features which characterize the neoplastic phenotype--immortalization, anchorage-independent growth and metastatic capacity--are also highly independent and variable in different individual tumours (43) and it would, therefore, be naive to expect complete consistency in the chronological order of molecular events leading to neoplasia. As is often the case in biology, cells, in particular tumour cells, may turn out to have a surprisingly broad capacity to reach the same endpoint by a variety of different routes.

ACKNOWLEDGEMENTS

The Beatson Institute is supported by the Cancer Research Campaign of Great Britain. K. B. is the recipient of a Training Fellowship from the Medical Research Council. M. Q. is supported by an EMBO long term fellowship and by a grant from Imperial Chemical Industries PLC.

REFERENCES

1. J. M. Bishop, Cellular oncogenes and retroviruses, Ann. Rev. Biochem. 52:301-354 (1983).

2. R. L. Erikson, A. F. Purchio, E. Erikson, M. S. Collett, and J. S. Brugge, Molecular events in cells transformed by Rous sarcoma virus, J. Cell Biol. 87:319-325 (1980).

3. J. M. Bishop, Enemies within: The genesis of retrovirus oncogenes, Cell 23:5-6 (1981).

4. J. M. Bishop and H. E. Varmus, Functions and origins of retroviral transforming genes, in: "Molecular Biology of Tumour-Viruses," R. Weiss et al., eds., Cold Spring Harbor Laboratory, Cold Spring Harbor, New York (1982), pp. 999-1108.

5. A. Balmain, Transforming ras oncogenes and multistage carcinogenesis, Brit. J. Cancer 51:1-7 (1985).

6. G. Klein and E. Klein, Oncogene activation and tumour progress, Carcinogenesis 5:429-435 (1984).

7. J. D. Rowley, Human oncogene locations and chromosome aberrations, Nature 301:290-291 (1983).

8. J. Groffen, J. R. Stephenson, N. Heisterkamp, A. de Klein, C. R. Bartram, and G. Grosveld, Philadelphia chromosomal breakpoints are clustered within a limited region, bcr, on chromosome 22, Cell 36:93-99 (1984).

9. K. Alitalo, Amplification of cellular oncogenes in cancer cells, Trends Biochem. Sciences 10:194-197 (1985).

10. B. G. Neel, W. S. Hayward, H. L. Robinson, J. Fang, and S. M. Astrin, Avian leukosis virus-induced tumours have common proviral integration sites and synthesize discrete new RNAs: Oncogenesis by promoter insertion, Cell 23:323-334 (1981).

11. C. S. Cooper, M. Park, D. G. Blair, M. A. Tainsky, K. Huebner, C. M. Croce, and G. F. Vande Woude, Molecular cloning of a new transforming gene from a chemically transformed human cell line, Nature 311:29-33 (1984).

12. A. L. Schechter, D. F. Stern, L. Vaidyanathan, S. J. Decker, J. A. Drebin, M. I. Greene, and R. A. Weinberg, The neu oncogene: An erb-B-related gene encoding a 185,000-Mr tumour antigen, Nature 312:513 (1984).

13. A. Diamond, G. M. Cooper, J. Ritz, and M. A. Lane, Identification and molecular cloning of the human Blym Transforming gene activated in Burkitt's lymphoma, Nature 305:112-116 (1983).

14. A. P. Albino, R. Le Strange, A. I. Oliff, M. E. Furth, and L. J. Old, Transforming ras genes from human melanoma: A manifestation of tumour heterogeneity?, Nature 308:69-72 (1984).

15. T. Sekiya, M. Fushimi, H. Hori, S. Hirohashi, S. Nishimura, and T. Sugimura, Molecular cloning and the total nucleotide sequence of the human c-Ha-ras-1 gene activated in a melanoma from a Japanese patient, Proc. Natl. Acad. Sci. USA 81:4771-4775 (1984).

16. K. H. Vousden and C. J. Marshall, Three different activated ras genes in mouse tumours; evidence for oncogene activation during progression of a mouse lymphoma EMBO J. 3:913-917 (1984).

17. R. K. Boutwell, The function and mechanism of promoters of carcinogenesis, CRC Crit. Rev. Toxicol. 2:419-431 (1974).

18. B. L. Van Duuren, A. Sivak, C. Katz, I. Seidman, and S. Melchionne, The effect of aging and interval between primary and secondary treatment in two-stage carcinogenesis in mouse skin, Cancer Res. 35:502-505 (1975).

19. F. J. Burns, M. Vanderlaan, E. Snyder, and R. E. Albert, Induction and progression kinetics of mouse skin papillomas, in: "Carcinogenesis, Vol. 2," T. J. Slaga, A. Sivak, R. K. Boutwell, eds., Raven Press, New York (1978), pg. 91.

20. H. Hennings, O. Michael, C. Cheng, P. Steinert, K. Holbrook, and S. H. Yuspa, Calcium regulation of growth and differentiation of mouse epidermal cells in culture, Cell 19:245-254 (1980).

21. N. E. Fusenig, D. Breitkreug, R. T. Dzarlieva, P. Boukamp, A. Bohnert and W. Tilgen, Growth and differentiation characteristics of transformed keratinocytes from mouse and human skin in vitro and in vivo, J. Invest. Dermatol. 81:168s-175s (1983).

22. A. Balmain and I. B. Pragnell, Mouse skin carcinomas induced in vivo by chemical carcinogens have a transforming Harvey-ras oncogene, Nature 303:72-74 (1983).

23. A. Balmain, M. Ramsden, G. T. Bowden, and J. Smith, Activation of the mouse cellular Harvey-ras gene in chemically induced benign skin papillomas, Nature 307:658-660 (1984).

24. S. Sukumar, V. Notario, D. Martin-Zanca, and M. Barbacid, Induction of mammary carcinomas in rats by nitroso-methylurea involves malignant activation of H-ras-1 locus by single point mutations, Nature 306:658-661 (1983).

25. H. Zarbl, S. Sukumar, A. V. Arthur, D. Martin-Zanca, and M. Barbacid, Direct mutagenesis of Ha-ras-1 oncogenes by N-nitroso-N-methylurea during initiation of mammary carcinogenesis in rats, Nature 315:382-386 (1985).

26. I. Guerrero, P. Calzada, A. Mayer, and A. Pellicer, A molecular approach to leukemogenesis: Mouse lymphomas contain an activated c-ras oncogene, Proc. Natl. Acad. Sci. USA 81:202-205 (1984).

27. I. Guerrero, A. Villasante, V. Corces, and A. Pellicer, Activation of a c-K-ras oncogene by somatic mutation in mouse lymphomas induced by gamma radiation, Science 225:159-162 (1984).

28. E. Santos, D. Martin-Zanca, E. P. Reddy, M. A. Pierotti, G. Della Posta, and M. Barbacid, Malignant activation of a K-ras oncogene in lung carcinoma but not in normal tissue of the same patient, Science 223:661-664 (1984).

29. J. Fujita, O. Yoshida, Y. Yuasa, J. S. Rhim, M. Hatanaka, and S. A. Aaronson, Ha-ras oncogenes are activated by somatic alteration in human urinary tract tumours, Nature 309:464-466 (1984).

30. R. Muller, J. M. Tremblay, E. D. Adamson, and I. M. Verma, Tissue and cell type specific expression of two human c-onc genes, Nature 304:454-456 (1983).

31. R. Muller, D. J. Shamon, J. M. Tremblay, M. J. Cline, and I. M. Verma. Differential expression of cellular oncogenes during pre- and post-natal development of the mouse, Nature 299:640-644 (1982).

32. A. D. Riggs and P. A. Jones, 5-Methylcytosine, gene regulation and cancer, Adv. Cancer Res. 40:1 (1983).

33. G. Felsenfeld and J. McGhee, Methylation and gene control, Nature 296:602-603 (1982).

34. A. Razin and A. D. Riggs, DNA methylation and gene function, Science 210:604-610 (1980).

35. M. Ramsden, G. Cole, J. Smith, and A. Balmain, Differential methylation of the c-H-ras gene in normal mouse cells and during skin tumor progression, EMBO J. 4:1449-1454 (1985).

36. A. Eva and S. A. Aaronson, Frequent activation of c-kis as a transforming gene in fibrosarcomas induced by methylcholanthrene, Science 220:955-956 (1983).

37. L. F. Parada and R. A. Weinberg, Presence of a Kirsten murine sarcoma virus ras oncogene in cells transformed by 3-methylcholanthrene, Mol. Cell. Biol. 3:2298-2301 (1983).

38. G. P. Margison and P. J. O'Connor, Nucleic acid modifications by N-nitroso compounds, in: "Chemical Carcinogens and DNA, Vol. 1," Grover, ed., CRC Press, Florida (1978).

39. B. Singer and J. T. Kusmierek, Chemical mutagenesis, Ann. Rev. Biochem. 51:655-693 (1982).

40. A. Dipple, J. T. Sawicki, R. C. Moschel, and A. H. Bigger, 7,12-Dimethylbenz(a)anthracene-DNA interactions in mouse embryo cell cultures and mouse skins, in: "Extrahepatic Drug Metabolism and Chemical Carcinogenesis," J. Rydstrom, J. Montelins, and Bengtsson, eds., Elsevier Science Publishers, B.V., Amsterdam (1983) pp. 439-448.

41. J. Doniger, R. S. Day, and J. A. DiPaolo, Quantitative assessment of the role of O^6-methylguanine in the initiation of carcinogenesis by methylating agents, Proc. Natl. Acad. Sci. USA 82:421-425 (1985).

42. J. Cairns, The origin of human cancers, Nature 289:353-357 (1981).

43. L. Foulds, "Neoplastic Development, Vol. 1," Academic Press, London (1969).

44. C. J. Der, T. G. Krontiris, and G. M. Cooper, Transforming genes of human bladder and lung carcinoma cell lines are homologous to the ras genes of Harvey and Kirsten sarcoma viruses, Proc. Natl. Acad. Sci. USA 79:3637-3640 (1982).

45. E. Santos, S. R. Tronick, S. A. Aaronson, S. Pulciani, and M. Barbacid, T24 human bladder carcinoma oncogene is an activated form of the normal human homologue of BALB- and Harvey- MSV transforming genes, Nature 298:343-347 (1982).

46. L. F. Parada, C. J. Tabin, C. Shih, and R. A. Weinberg, Human EJ bladder carcinoma oncogene is homologue of Harvey sarcoma virus ras gene, Nature 297:474-478 (1982).

47. S. Pulciani, E. Santos, A. V. Lauver, L. K. Long, S. A. Aaronson, and M. Barbacid, Oncogenes in solid human tumours, Nature 300:539-542 (1982).

48. Y. Yuasa, S. K. Srivastava, C. Y. Dunn, J. S. Rhim, E. P. Reddy, and S. A. Aaronson, Acquisition of transforming properties by alternative point mutations within c-bas/has human proto-oncogene, Nature 303:775-779 (1983).

49. M. S. McCoy, J. J. Toole, J. M. Cunningham, E. H. Chang, D. R. Lowy, and R. A. Weinberg, Characterization of a human colon/lung carcinoma oncogene, Nature 302:79-81 (1983).

50. K. Shimizu, D. Birnbaum, M. A. Ruley, O. Fasano, Y. Suard, L. Edlund, E. Taparowsky, M. Goldfarb, and M. Wigler, Structure of the Ki-ras gene of the human lung carcinoma cell line Calu-1, Nature 304:497-500 (1983).

51. K. Shimizu, M. Goldfarb, Y. Suard, M. Perucho, Y. Li, T. Kamata, J. Feramisco, E. Stavnezer, J. Fogh, and M. H. Wigler, Three human transforming genes are related to the viral ras oncogenes, Proc. Natl. Acad. Sci. USA 80:2112-2116 (1983).

52. K. Shimizu, M. Goldfarb, M. Perucho, and M. Wigler, Isolation and preliminary characterization of the transforming gene of a human neuroblastoma cell line, Proc. Natl. Acad. Sci. USA 80:383-387 (1983).

53. H. Nakano, F. Yamamoto, C. Neville, D. Evans, T. Mizuno, and M. Perucho, Isolation of transforming sequences of two human lung carcinomas: Structural and functional analysis of the activated c-K-ras oncogenes, Proc. Natl. Acad. Sci. USA 81:71-75 (1984).

54. Y. Taya, K. Hosogai, S. Hirohashi, Y. Shimosato, R. Tsuchiya, N. Tsuchida, M. Fushimi, T. Sekiya, and S. Nishimura, A novel combination of K-ras and myc amplification accompanied by point mutational activation of K-ras in a human lung cancer, EMBO J. 3:2943-2946 (1984).

55. Y. Yuasa, R. A. Gol, A. Chang, I. M. Chiu, E. P. Reddy, S. R. Tronick, and S. A. Aaronson, Mechanism of activation of an N-ras oncogene of SW-1271 human lung carcinoma cells, Proc. Natl. Acad. Sci. USA 8L:3670-3674 (1984).

56. C. S. Cooper, D. G. Blair, M. K. Oskarsson, M. A. Tainsky, L. A. Eader, and G. F. Vande Woude, Characterization of human transforming genes from chemically transformed teratocarcinoma and pancreatic carcinoma cell lines, Cancer Res. 44:1-10 (1984).

57. V. Notario, S. Sukumar, E. Santos, and M. Barbacid, A common mechanism for the malignant activation of ras oncogenes in human neoplasia and in chemically induced animal tumours, in: "Cancer Cells 2/Oncogenes and Viral Genes," G. F. Vande Woude, A. J. Levine, W. C. Topp, and J. D. Watson, eds., Cold Spring Harbor Laboratory, Cold Spring Harbor, New York (1984).

58. L. A. Feig, R. C. Bast, R. C. Knapp, and G. M. Cooper, Somatic activation of ras^k gene in a human ovarian carcinoma, Science 223:698-701 (1984).

59. M. H. Kraus, Y. Yuasa, and S. A. Aaronson, A position 12-activated H-ras oncogene in all HS578T mammary carcinosarcoma cells but not normal mammary cells of the same patient, Proc. Natl. Acad. Sci. USA 81:5384-5388 (1984).

60. A. Hall, C. J. Marshall, N. K. Spurr, and R. A. Weiss, Identification of transforming gene in two human sarcoma cell lines as a new member of the ras gene family located on chromosome 1, Nature 303:396-400 (1983).

61. M. Souyri and E. Fleissner, Identification by transfection of transforming sequences in DNA of human T-cell leukemia, Proc. Natl. Acad. Sci. USA 80:6676-6679 (1983).

62. A. Eva, S. R. Tronick, R. A. Gol, J. H. Pierce, and S. A. Aaronson, Transforming genes of human hematopoietic tumors: frequent detection of ras-related oncogenes whose activation appears to be independent of tumor phenotype, Proc. Natl. Acad. Sci. USA 80:4926-4930, (1983).

63. M. J. Murray, J. M. Cunningham, L. F. Parada, F. Dautry, P. Lebowitz, and R. A. Weinberg, The HL-60 transforming sequence: A _ras_ oncogene co-existing with altered _myc_ genes in hematopoietic tumours, _Cell_ 33:749-757 (1983).

64. C. Gambke, E. Signer, and C. Moroni, Activation of N-_ras_ gene in bone marrow cells from a patient with acute myeloblastic leukaemia, _Nature_ 307:476-478 (1984).

65. M. Quintanilla, K. Brown, M. Ramsden and A. Balmain, Carcinogen-specific mutation and amplification of Ha-ras during mouse skin carcinogenesis, _Nature_ 322:78-80 (1986).

66. K. Brown, M. Quintanilla, M. Ramsden, I. B. Kerr, S. Young and A. Balmain, V-ras Genes from Harvey and BALB Murine Sarcoma Viruses can act as Initiators of Two-Stage Mouse Skin Carcinogenesis, _Cell_ 46; 447-456 (1986).

A REGULATORY SEQUENCE OF SIMIAN VIRUS 40 IS INACTIVATED BY UV-INDUCED DAMAGE

T. C. Brown and P. A. Cerutti

Department of Carcinogenesis
Swiss Institute for Experimental Cancer Research
CH-1066 Epalinges/Lausanne
Switzerland

Damage in the DNA of eurocaryotic cells can modulate gene expression by several independent mechanisms. Lesions can block RNA synthesis by posing obstacles to RNA polymerase II. In general, bulky lesions are effective (1, 2), if temporary (3), blocks to transcription while damage introduced by alkylating agents is less potent (4). Damage can also affect gene expression by altering the pattern of methylated cytosine residues in DNA, either by inhibiting the activity of eucaryotic maintenance methyl transferase (5) or because DNA synthesized during excision repair is incompletely methylated (6). The ability of damage to alter methylation patterns may lead to heritable changes in gene expression (7). Chromosomal proteins close to the sites of damage in DNA (8) may be modified by the addition of poly ADP-ribose (9). Such modification may change the conformation of the chromatin in a way that alters gene expression (10). Finally, damage may block protein-DNA interactions required for transcription by distorting the DNA sequences that ordinarily serve as protein binding sites (11-13).

The latter possibility, that damage in DNA disrupts transcriptional control, has received little attention. Transcriptional control sequences comprise a very small part of the total DNA found in a cell or a virus, and damage within regulatory sequences in general is not readily discernable because it does not produce a distinct change in phenotype. Very high doses of radiation or chemical carcinogens are required to modify a large proportion of such sequences in a target population. Thus, although lesions have been shown in several case to disrupt specific protein-DNA interactions (11-13), the critical question is whether the levels of damage that inactivate or transform cells exert any effect on transcriptional control.

We have examined the effects of damage in the transcriptional control sequences of Simian Virus 40 by constructing viral DNA molecules with UV-induced damage located exclusively within a 302 base-pair (bp) region of the genome that governs the expression of viral genes (14). We reasoned that the survival of transfected viral DNA would be hypersensitive to lesions within this region if the disruption of the regulatory functions specified by this sequence played an important role in the toxicity of DNA damage. In contrast, no hypersensitivity would be expected if damage in this region inactivated DNA solely by inhibiting DNA replication, since lesions would block replication to the same extent regardless of their location.

Our strategy for constructing SV40 DNA molecules exploits the presence of two unique restriction sites, Bg1I and KpnI, within the control region (15) (Figure 1). Cleavage of SV40 DNA with these two enzymes produces a large (4941 bp) fragment containing the protein-coding regions of the viral genome and a 302 bp fragment that contains the promoter and enhancer sequences required for transcriptional of the early (16-18) and late (19) viral genes, and a part of the origin of viral DNA replication (20). We exposed purified SV40 DNA to 700-2100 $J.m^{-2}$ of UV (254 nm principal wavelength) and used a chromatographic procedure (21) to determine the amount of damage introduced by irradiation. For each dose of UV, the same fraction of thymine was converted to thymine-thymine dimers in both the large and small fragments. We digested UV-damaged and undamaged SV40 DNA with Bg1I and KpnI and isolated the two resulting fragments. For each series of genomes to be constructed, an aliquot of the large undamaged fragment was ligated to either a damaged or undamaged small fragment. Separation of the ligation products by electrophoresis in agarose allowed purification of complete circular viral genomes that contained either no damage, or defined amounts of damage within the transcriptional control region.

SV40 DNA with various amounts of damage either randomly distributed over the entire genome or confined to within the 302 bp control region was used to transfect host CV-1 cells. The survival of damaged DNA was expressed as plaque-forming units per picogram of transfected DNA, compared to undamaged controls. Results of three independent experiments, each carried out with a different preparation of viral DNA, indicate that lesions within the 302 bp control region are 3.22 $\pm$ 0.11 -fold more effective in inactivating viral DNA than is the same amount of damage randomly distributed in the viral genome. Thus, damage within the transcriptional control region, which represents only 5.8% of the viral genome (15), accounts for 19% of the overall inactivation of the viral DNA.

Some of the damage introduced into the transfected DNA is undoubtedly excised by the repair mechanisms of the host CV-1 cells. Our results indicate that SV40 DNA is inactivated by the introduction of 32 pyrimidine dimers if the damage is randomly distributed, or by 9-10 dimers if the damage is contained in the transcriptional control region (14). Excision

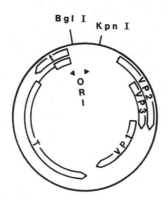

Fig. 1.   Map of the SV40 genome showing genetic
functions and the restriction sites used
to generate the fragment of interest in
this study.

repair in human cells, which is about as efficient as that in simian CV-1 cells (22) reverses 85-90% of the lethal effect of UV-induced damage in SV40 (23). If we make the conservative estimate that 80% of the UV-induced pyrimidine dimers are excised from SV40 by the host CV-1 cells then the viral DNA is inactivated by 6-7 persistent, randomly distributed lesions or by 2 persistent lesions within the control region.

The 302 bp control region contains sequences that govern the transcription of the viral early (16-18) and late (19) genes, and also contains part of the origin of viral DNA replication (20). From our results, it is likely that at least one of these three functions is extremely sensitive to disruption by the presence of UV-induced DNA damage. We postulate that the hypersensitivity of this region to lesions is due to an inactivation of transcription of the early genes. Blocking the expression of early genes would inactivate the virus by preventing the synthesis of the large T antigen, a viral early gene product whose presence is essential to the initiation of viral DNA replication (24, 25). In contrast, disruption of viral late gene expression is probable not a critical event because these genes are required only after several rounds of viral DNA replication have taken place, and their expression can therefore originate from undamaged progeny viral genomes. It remains possible that damage at the origin of DNA replication inactivates the virus by preventing the initiation of the first replication event. The hypersensitive region, however, contains less than half of the "core origin" sequences found to be the most important for viral DNA replication (26) and preliminary results with a larger KpnI-TaqI fragment indicate that the rest of the core origin does not represent a hypersensitive site. UV-induced damage is mutagenic (27), and some mutations within the hypersensitive region inactivate the virus (28). Mutation is, however, a relatively rare event even in heavily irradiated virus and would not be expected to account for a major part of lethality. We suspect, therefore, that the viral DNA is critically sensitive to damage in the transcriptional control region because the lesions alter the structure of certain DNA sequences in a way that disrupts the protein-DNA interactions required for the efficient transcription of the viral early genes.

Our results with the SV40 control region may underestimate the sensitivity of cellular transcriptional control sequences because the promoter and enhancer elements of the SV40 early genes, and to some extent the late genes, are functionally diploid. That is, early gene transcriptional is under the control of two blocs of DNA sequences one of which (72 bp) is present in two copies and one (21 bp) in three copies (15). A single copy of the 72 bp repeat (16-18, 25), and two of the three 21 bp repeats (25) suffice to promote early gene expression, and a single copy of the 72 bp repeat renders the virus viable (29-31). Some cellular transcriptional promoters contain repeated elements (32-35) that may, like those of SV40, represent multiple independent sequences that would retain part of their activity despite the introduction of a limited amount of damage. Functionally haploid promoters, however, may be extremely sensitive to the presence of a small number of lesions.

We conclude that the transcriptional control region of SV40 is prone to inactivation by low levels of DNA damage, and that the modulation of gene expression by lesions in this region makes a measurable contribution to the lethal effect of damage in the viral genome. In the experiments described here the measured endpoint of disrupted gene expression is inactivation of the viral DNA. This is true, however, only because the inactivated gene is essential to the survival of the virus. Changes in gene expression caused by modification of the promoters of nonessential genes in damaged eucaryotic cells could lead, in some cases, to subtle alterations in the state of differentiation of the cell, either by inactivation of some genes or by activating genes through inactivation of their repressors. Certain combinations of gene modulation could contribute to the development of oncogenic transformation.

NOTE ADDED IN PROOF: Since submission of this manuscript, we have completed experiments showing that viral sensitivity to damage in the BglI-KpnI regulatory regions is almost completely abolished in cos-1 cells. Constitutive production of viral early gene products in these cells complements the inability of irradiated virus to express early genes, but cos-1 cells are unable to provide damaged virus with a functional, cis-acting replication origin. Accordingly, our results identify gene expression rather than the initiation of DNA replication as the major target for lethal damage in the regulatory region of the SV40 genome.

REFERENCES

1. W. Saurbier and K. Hercules, Ann. Rev. Gen. 12:329-364 (1978).

2. P. B. Hackett, H. E. Varmus, and J. M. Bishop, Virology 112:752-756 (1981).

3. L. V. Mayne and A. R. Lehmann, Cancer Res. 42:1473-1478 (1982).

4. B. Singer and J. T. Kusmierek, Ann. Rev. Biochem. 52:665-693 (1982).

5. V. L. Wilson and P. A. Jones, Cell 32:239-246 (1983).

6. M. B. Kastan, B. J. Gowans, and M. W. Lieberman, Cell 30:509-516 (1982).

7. R. Holliday, Br. J. Cancer 40:513-522 (1979).

8. N. Malik, M. Miwa, T. Sugimura, P. Thaves, and M. E. Smulson, Proc. Natl. Acad. Sci. USA 80:2554-2558 (1983).

9. S. Shall, in: "ADP-ribosylation Reactions," O. Hayaishi and K. Ueda, Academic Press, New York (1982), pp. 478-520.

10. G. G. Poirier, G. de Murcia, J. Jongstra-Bilen, C. Niedergang, and P. Mandel, Proc. Natl. Acad. Sci. USA 79:3423-3427 (1982).

11. U. Sienbenlist, R. B. Simpson, and W. Gilbert, Cell 20:269-281 (1980).

12. M. Ptashne, A. Jeffrey, A. D. Johnson, R. Maurer, B. J. Meyer, C. O. Pabo, T. M. Roberts, and R. T. Sauer, Cell 19:1-11 (1980).

13. J. E. Cleaver, J. Mol. Biol. 170:305-317 (1983).

14. T. C. Brown and P. A. Cerutti, EMBO J. 5:197-203 (1986).

15. in: "DNA Tumor Viruses, 2nd Ed.," J. Tooze, ed., Cold Spring Harbor Laboratory, Cold Spring Harbor, New York (1980), pp. 799-829.

16. C. Benoist and P. Chambon, Nature 290:310-315 (1981).

17. D. J. Mathis and P. Chambon, Nature 290:304-310 (1981).

18. M. Fromm and P. Berg, J. Mol. Appl. Gen. 1:457-481 (1982).

19. S. W. Hartzell, B. J. Byrne, and K. N. Subramanian, <u>Proc. Natl. Acad. Sci. USA</u> 81:23-27 (1984).

20. R. T. Hay and M. L. DePamphilis, <u>Cell</u> 28:767-779 (1982).

21. H. J. Niggli and P. A. Cerutti, <u>Biochemistry</u> 22:1390-1395 (1983).

22. J. I. Williams and J. E. Cleaver, <u>Biophysical J.</u> 22:265-279 (1978).

23. P. J. Abrahams and A. J. Van der Eb, <u>Mut. Res.</u> 35:13-22 (1976).

24. P. Tegtmeyer, <u>J. Virol.</u> 15:613-618 (1975).

25. R. M. Meyers, D. C. Rio, A. K. Robbins, and R. Tjian, <u>Cell</u> 25:373-384 (1981).

26. D. J. Bergsma, D. M. Olive, S. W. Hartzell, and K. N. Subramanian, <u>Proc. Natl. Acad. Sci. USA</u> 79:381-385 (1982).

27. F. Bourre and A. Sarasin, <u>Nature</u> 305:68-70 (1983).

28. D. Di Maio and D. J. Nathans, <u>J. Mol. Biol.</u> 140:129-142 (1980).

29. T. E. Shenk, J. Carbon, and P. Berg, <u>J. Virol.</u> 18:664-671 (1976).

30. A. Barkan and J. E. Merz, <u>J. Virol.</u> 37:730-737 (1980).

31. H. Van Heuverswyn and W. Fiers, <u>Eur. J. Biochem.</u> 100:51-60 (1979).

32. M. Karin, A. Haslinger, H. Holtgreve, R. I. Richards, P. Krauter, H. M. Westphal and M. Beato, <u>Nature</u> 308:513-519 (1984).

33. R. Renkowitz, G. Schutz, D. Von der Ahe, and M. Beato, <u>Cell</u> 37:503-510 (1984).

34. T. F. Donahue, R. S. Daves, G. Lucchini, and G. R. Fink, <u>Cell</u> 36:89-98 (1983).

35. L. Guarente, B. Lalonde, P. Gifford and E. Alani, <u>Cell</u> 36:503-511 (1984).

MECHANISMS OF SPONTANEOUS MUTAGENESIS: IMPLICATIONS FOR SPONTANEOUS

CARCINOGENESIS

Kendric C. Smith and Neil J. Sargentini

Department of Radiology
Stanford University School of Medicine
Stanford, CA 94305

INTRODUCTION

Spontaneous mutations have been defined as mutations that arise by mechanisms that have yet to be identified. While we will discuss the major hypotheses for spontaneous mutagenesis, our main objective is to discuss the roles of DNA damage (especially that caused by normal metabolic reactions) and of DNA repair genes in spontaneous mutagenesis, and the possible relevance of this information to our understanding of spontaneous carcinogenesis.

We have recently published a review on the roles of DNA repair, replication and recombination in spontaneous mutagenesis (1). In the present report, we will only present a brief overview of these topics. Other reviews on spontaneous mutagenesis have appeared (2-8).

WHAT KINDS OF MUTATIONS OCCUR SPONTANEOUSLY?

In a study performed to quantitate the general classes of mutations that occur spontaneously, Hartman et al. (9) classified 83 spontaneous histidine auxotrophs of Salmonella typhimurium and found that 53% were caused by base substitution (either transitions or transversions), 11% were caused by frameshifts (i.e., insertions or deletions of one or a few base pairs), 23% were caused by deletions (i.e., deletions of more than a few base pairs), and 13% were apparently (1) caused by insertions (i.e., insertions of large DNA elements). Since studies of this sort only detect mutations that inactivate a gene product, one can presume that many missense mutations are overlooked in such studies because they have little or no effect on the measured phenotype (i.e., they are silent mutations). Thus, the listed proportion for base substitution mutations is most likely an underestimate, while those listed for the other classes of mutations are most likely overestimates. Therefore, base substitution appears to be the most common form of spontaneous mutation in bacteria. A similar conclusion can also be made for yeast (reviewed in reference 1).

REPLICATION ERRORS

    Although the processes of replication, recombination, and repair tend
to overlap, this section on the role of replication errors in spontaneous
mutagenesis is meant to focus only on the DNA replication that is part of
the normal process of cell division. Therefore, damage in a DNA template
must not block DNA replication, i.e., it must be miscoding damage rather
than noncoding damage. Mechanisms proposed for mutagenesis under these
conditions include: (1) base tautomerization, (2) miscoding DNA damage,
(3) polymerase errors, and (4) mutators, antimutators and mismatch repair.

    <u>Base Tautomerization</u> Based on their model for the structure of DNA,
Watson and Crick (10) proposed that transition mutagenesis (A$\longleftrightarrow$G, or C$\longleftrightarrow$
T) may be due to the formation of base tautomers by proton migration.
Similarly, Topal and Fresco (11) used tautomerization and base rotation to
explain transversion mutagenesis (A or G $\longleftrightarrow$ C or T). The essence of this
model is that, at the moment of replication, a base in the DNA template
develops an inappropriate coding property that leads to the incorporation
of an incorrect base in the nascent DNA. Theoretically, base
tautomerization could explain most of the spontaneous mutagenesis that is
due to base-substitution, however, such a model is inconsistent with the
data for the genetic control of spontaneous mutagenesis, which will be
discussed below (i.e., the role of DNA repair).

    <u>Miscoding Base Damage</u> Modified bases may code differently than
unmodified bases. For example, deaminated 5-methylcytosine (i.e., thymine)
codes for adenine, and thus will cause a GC $\longleftrightarrow$ AT transition. Since there
is a good correlation between the occurrence of 5-methylcytosine in the
<u>lacI</u> gene and the occurrence of mutation hotspots (12), this suggests that
5-methylcytosine deamination plays a role in spontaneous mutagenesis.
Other examples of this type of mutagenesis have been reviewed (1, 8).

    <u>Polymerase Errors</u> Loeb and Kunkel (6) have reviewed abundant data
showing that DNA polymerases occasionally incorporate incorrect bases. The
polymerase error rate is affected by the base sequence of the template, the
nature of the misincorporated base, and the nature and source of the DNA
polymerase (6). The polymerase error rate is also affected by
perturbations in the relative sizes of the pools of nucleoside
triphosphates (reviewed in reference 13), and of divalent cations such as
Mg^{++} and Mn^{++} (e.g., 14).

    While the base sequence of the template clearly has an effect on
misincorporation, i.e., base-substitution errors (e.g., 15), it seems also
to be an important factor in small and large addition/deletion mutations.
In a model for misalignment mutagenesis, Streisinger et al. (16) described
how the occurrences of short, redundant base sequences in DNA were
correlated with the sites of frameshift mutations and of mutations
involving large additions or deletions of DNA. In a related fashion,
Ripley (17) and Ripley and Glickman (18) have correlated the occurrence of
DNA palindromes with the occurrence of certain frameshift and deletion
mutations that are not easily explained by the Streisinger model. Such
models of misalignment mutagenesis, and data to support them, have recently
been reviewed by Drake et al. (8). These models seem valid because of the
good correlation between their predictions and the occurrence of
spontaneous addition/deletion mutations at certain chromosomal sites.

    <u>Mutators, Antimutators,</u> and <u>Mismatch Repair</u> The mutator
and antimutator mutations to be discussed in this section were selected
because they are known to affect the normal replication process, or because
they do not sensitize cells to killing by DNA damage, or because their
mutator effect is independent of the <u>recA</u> gene, i.e., the gene that

controls most mutagenesis after DNA damage induction (reviewed in reference 19). Mismatch repair is generally regarded as a postreplication proof-reading process (20), rather than a repair process for DNA damage.

The isolation and characterization of mutator mutants in such organisms as bacteriophage, bacteria, fungi, Drosophila, and Maize (reviewed in references 5, 21) have been valuable in understanding how spontaneous mutations can occur, but have been much less informative as to how spontaneous mutations do occur. Answers to the latter question come directly from the study and understanding of antimutator mutants. However, only a few antimutator mutants have been found.

Mutations affecting the DNA polymerase of phage T4 result in enhanced transition (22) and transversion (23) mutations. Antimutator phage T4 DNA polymerase mutants have also been described (24, 25). Muzyczka et al. (26) concluded that spontaneous mutagenesis in phage T4 is the result of the antagonistic interaction of the polymerase function (to make replication errors) and the 3'-5' exonuclease function (to correct replication errors).

The possible role in spontaneous mutagenesis of the dnaE mutants of Escherichia coli, which have altered DNA replication polymerases, is probably related to the fidelity of DNA replication. One might consider that the dnaE and lig (DNA ligase) mutants may enhance spontaneous mutagenesis by blocking the replication fork or the resealing of DNA strand breaks, respectively. Both of these actions appear to result in the induction of the SOS phenomenon (reviewed in reference 27), which can lead to enhanced spontaneous mutagenesis, as evidenced by data for the tif (28) and dnaB (29) strains. However, the mutator phenotype of such mutants is recA independent in each case that has been tested, and this recA-independent phenotype has generally been used as a means of defining a replication-error involvement (e.g., 5).

The availability of substrates for DNA synthesis may indirectly affect spontaneous mutagenesis. The purB (purine auxotrophy) mutant (30) would seem to exhibit its antimutator effect by increasing the fidelity of DNA replication via changes in the relative pool sizes of DNA precursors (reviewed in reference 13). DNA precursor pool sizes are also relevant to the regulation of the mutD (31) and tif (32) mutator effects, which suggest that altered deoxynucleoside triphosphate selection can be an important mechanism of spontaneous mutagenesis.

After an incorrect nucleotide has been incorporated into DNA, the cell still can use mismatch repair to correct the error. The mutS, mutH, mutL, and uvrD mutations and the dam mutation are known to affect mismatch repair (33). These mutators are thought to reduce DNA fidelity through a reduction in "proof-reading" function.

Mutator cell lines have also been described in fungi, Drosophila (reviewed in reference 1), and mammalian cells. Meuth et al. (34) described three thymidine auxotrophic lines of Chinese hamster ovary cells that exhibit enhanced spontaneous reversion to thymidine prototrophy, and enhanced spontaneous frequencies of 6-thioguanine and ouabain resistance. Weinberg et al. (35) described three lines of murine T-lymphosarcoma cells that show altered deoxynucleoside triphosphate pools, and enhanced frequencies of spontaneous dexamethasone and 6-thioguanine resistance. Both groups of workers concluded that abnormal deoxycytidine triphosphate pools are responsible for the enhanced rates of spontaneous mutagenesis that they observed.

RECOMBINATION ERRORS

Evidence for a role of genetic recombination in spontaneous mutagenesis has come from an analysis of the meiotic effect in yeast (reviewed in reference 2). That is, certain spontaneous addition/deletion type reversions are much enhanced during meiosis relative to mitosis (36, 37). Because of the strong correlation between addition/deletion reversions and outside marker exchange during meiosis, it was concluded that the reversions were due to unequal crossing-over (36). If spontaneous mutagenesis can result from errors in recombination, then this would explain the meiotic effect in that much more spontaneous recombination occurs during meiosis than during mitosis (e.g., 38). However, such a mechanism only explains a limited amount of spontaneous mutagenesis, since base-substitution reversions and other addition/deletion type reversions do not seem to be enhanced during meiosis (reviewed in reference 7). One way to resolve this question is to compare the genetic control of recombination with that for spontaneous mutagenesis. We have compared the available data on the genetic control of spontaneous recombination and of spontaneous mutagenesis in bacteria (21 genes) and fungi (22 genes) (reviewed in reference 1), and the results indicate that recombination errors do not play a major role in spontaneous mutagenesis. That is, there are many exceptions to the concept that an increase or decrease in the level of recombination should cause a similar change in the level of spontaneous mutagenesis.

REPAIR ERRORS

Bacteria   Mutations that sensitize cells to DNA-damaging agents have generally been shown to do so by reducing the cell's capacity for DNA repair. In this section we will evaluate mutations that affect DNA repair for their effects on spontaneous and experimentally-induced mutagenesis. Before doing this, however, it is helpful to understand the concepts of error-free and error-prone DNA repair. The uvrA, uvrB, and uvrC genes, which determine the UV "excinuclease" of E. coli (39), are required for the incision and excision steps in the excision repair of lesions that produce distortions in the structure of DNA, e.g., UV radiation-induced pyrimidine dimers. In general, DNA excision repair is considered to be largely error-free relative to the other major dark-repair process, postreplication repair (40). Thus, compared to wild-type strains, the uvrA, uvrB, and uvrC strains show enhanced mutability after UV irradiation (e.g., 40, 41).

The concept of error-prone repair resulted from the finding by Witkin (42) that a lexA (exrA) strain was not only deficient in the ability to survive UV irradiation, but was also deficient in UV radiation mutagenesis. The lexA gene product is a repressor for the recA gene, a gene required for UV radiation mutagenesis, and the classical lexA mutant is one in which the repressor protein is not removed under conditions that would normally cause derepression (reviewed in reference 43).

From a consideration of the mutations in bacteria and fungi that affect DNA repair (36 and 26 genes evaluated, respectively, as reviewed in reference 1), there is a good correlation in that those mutations that enhance a cell's sensitivity to experimentally-induced mutagenesis also enhance spontaneous mutagenesis, and those mutations that reduce a cell's sensitivity to experimentally-induced mutagenesis also reduce spontaneous mutagenesis. For example, the enhancement of spontaneous mutagenesis in mutants deficient in error-free repair was demonstrated in one study (44) using both uvrA and uvrB strains, and using several base-substitution and frameshift mutation assays. Depending upon the assay used, the spontaneous mutation rate per bacterium per cell division ranged from 1.9- to 6.2-fold greater for uvrA and uvrB strains than for isogenic wild-type strains. Such data suggest that excisable, cryptic lesions exist in the DNA, and, if not excised, they induce mutations with increased probability.

Mutations that inhibit error-prone repair in UV-irradiated cells also inhibit the enhanced spontaneous mutagenesis seen in uvrB strains. Specifically, uvrB strains carrying lexA, recA, umuC, or the uvrD and recB mutations in combination, have spontaneous mutation rates about 10-fold lower than the uvrB control strains (44). Mutations at recA and lexA reduce the spontaneous mutation rate by about 2-fold in uvr+ strains (reviewed in reference 44), suggesting that about half of the spontaneous base substitutions in a DNA repair-proficient strain are the result of error-prone repair. The notion that error-prone repair acts on DNA damage, and is not merely affecting replication or recombination, is supported by two pieces of data. (1) Replication-error processes have generally been categorized by their recA independence (reviewed in reference 5), yet, as noted above, about half of spontaneous mutagenesis is recA-dependent. (2) A recombination-error process seems to be ruled out for base-substitution data because the umuC antimutator is recombination proficient (44), and the recombination-deficient recB recF strain shows normal spontaneous mutagenesis (45).

Mutations that enhance error-prone repair, e.g., tif and dnaB, also enhance spontaneous mutagenesis (28, 29).

Similar conclusions concerning the important role that DNA repair plays in spontaneous mutagenesis can be made from the wealth of genetic data that are available for yeast (reviewed in reference 46).

Mammalian Cells Few spontaneous mutagenesis data are available for DNA-damage-sensitive lines of mammalian cells. Liu et al. (47, 48) described a line of Chinese hamster ovary cells that has a mutant form of DNA polymerase. These cells exhibit enhanced UV radiation sensitivity and mutagenesis and enhanced rates of spontaneous mutagenesis, with several forward mutation assays. These cells are not thought to be deficient in excision repair, but only preliminary results are available (49).

One prediction from the conclusion that uvrA and uvrB strains of E. coli are mutators was that cells from individuals with xeroderma pigmentosum (XP) should show a higher rate of spontaneous mutagenesis (44), because such cells are deficient in nucleotide excision repair (reviewed in reference 50). It was also predicted, because of the correlations between mutagenesis and carcinogenesis (e.g., 51), that individuals with XP would show a higher rate of spontaneous carcinogenesis. While the spontaneous mutation rate data for XP cells are not yet available, it is of interest to note that XP individuals have recently been shown to be prone to certain forms of cancer that would not be predicted from their sensitivity to light (52).

SPONTANEOUS DNA DAMAGE

What could be the source of the "spontaneous" mutagenic DNA damage postulated to explain the enhanced spontaneous mutagenesis in DNA repair-deficient strains of bacteria and yeast? One source includes factors present in any mutation assay procedure. The growth rate of the cells, the aeration rate of the culture, the pH and the temperature of the culture medium all have an effect on spontaneous mutagenesis (e.g., 53, 54). The near-UV radiation component of ambient light is known to be mutagenic, either directly (55) or indirectly through its effects on growth media (56). Oxygen apparently induces DNA damage (57) and is mutagenic (reviewed in reference 58), it causes chromosomal aberrations in Fanconi's anemia cells (59), and has been implicated in spontaneous carcinogenesis (60). Ames (61) has listed numerous mutagens that are present in a wide variety of foods, and these mutagens may also be present in culture media.

Convincing evidence has been presented that spontaneous base-substitution hotspots result from the spontaneous deamination of 5-methylcytosine residues to yield thymine residues, thus causing GC$\leftrightarrow$AT transitions (62). Spontaneous depurination (63) and targeted DNA N-glycosylase action (reviewed in reference 64) should induce mutations, because apurinic and apyrimidinic sites tend to result in the insertion of purines (especially adenine) in the nascent DNA (65). The bypass of such lesions requires protein synthesis, i.e., it is an inducible process, and it is associated with mutagenesis, i.e., the bypass process is error-prone (66).

The oxidation of cellular fatty acids could be an important source of "spontaneous" mutagens (reviewed in reference 61). Growth in the presence of phenylalanine, but not the other common amino acids, produces excisable DNA damage that produces mutations in E. coli via error-prone repair (67). Similarly, cysteine (as well as glutathione) is mutagenic in the Ames tester strains if mammalian subcellular preparations are included in the assay (68). As a more general example, a model system exists, using horseradish peroxidase and aromatic pyruvates, for an enzymatic reaction that requires oxygen to produce excited-state molecules (i.e., "UV-like") that can damage DNA (69).

There is also evidence with mammalian cells for the metabolic production of chemical species that damage DNA. Fibroblasts from patients with Bloom's syndrome produce a clastogenic factor that causes chromosomal aberrations in normal human blood lymphocytes, while fibroblasts from normal individuals have no such effect (70). Bloom's syndrome-cells also show enhanced frequencies of spontaneous chromosomal aberrations and sister chromatid exchanges (71), and enhanced spontaneous mutagenesis (72). Such metabolic damage to DNA has also been postulated to explain the characteristics of some other autosomal recessive diseases (73).

In addition, since it appears that DNA can be damaged by normal metabolic reactions such that the damage is recognized by error-prone repair systems (see above), it seems reasonable that damage could also be produced that causes coding errors during replication. For example, although recA strains are nonmutable by X or UV radiation, they are mutable by certain chemicals (e.g., ethyl methanesulfonate and N-methyl-N'-nitro-N-nitrosoguanidine) that produce damage that is presumed to cause miscoding errors during replication (3). Therefore, normal metabolic damage to DNA may also contribute to spontaneous mutagenesis by causing errors in DNA replication.

SUMMARY, CONCLUSIONS AND SPECULATIONS

Spontaneous Mutagenesis   There appears to be no dearth of mechanisms to explain spontaneous mutagenesis. For spontaneous base-substitution mutagenesis, data for E. coli and Saccharomyces cerevisiae suggest important roles in spontaneous mutagenesis for the error-prone repair of DNA damage (to produce mutations) and for the error-free repair of DNA damage (to avoid mutagenesis). Data from the very limited number of studies on the subject suggest that about 50% of the spontaneous base substitution mutagenesis in E. coli, and perhaps 90% in S. cerevisiae is due to error-prone DNA repair. On the other hand, spontaneous frameshift and deletion mutagenesis seem to result from mechanisms involving recombination and replication. Spontaneous insertion mutagenesis has been shown to be important in the strongly polar inactivation of certain loci, but it is less important at other loci.

While most studies have concentrated on mutator mutations, the most conclusive data for the actual source of spontaneous mutations has come from the study of antimutator mutations. Further study in this area, perhaps along with an understanding of the many chemical antimutators and antimutagens, should be invaluable in further clarifying the basis of spontaneous mutagenesis. Perhaps with continued study, the term "spontaneous mutagenesis" will be replaced by more specific terms such as 5-methylcytosine deamination mutagenesis, fatty acid oxidation mutagenesis, phenylalanine mutagenesis, and imprecise-recombination mutagenesis.

Spontaneous Carcinogenesis   The idea that metabolically-induced lesions in DNA are important determinants in spontaneous mutagenesis is also of importance in understanding the molecular basis of spontaneous carcinogenesis. Although there is currently much attention being focused upon oncogenes as the ultimate producers of the carcinogenic state, in general, they are "turned on" by a mutation (reviewed in reference 74). The idea that normal metabolism can provide the agents for producing spontaneous mutagenesis provides a mechanism for turning on oncogenes to produce spontaneous carcinogenesis. In support of this concept, the spontaneous activation of a human proto-oncogene has been reported (75).

The concepts in this review on the origins of spontaneous mutagenesis and spontaneous carcinogenesis are diagramed in Figure 1 and described below. Normal metabolic reactions produce products that can damage DNA. The genetic requirements for the repair of this damaged DNA in E. coli suggest that metabolically-produced DNA damage is "UV-like" and not "X-ray-like", and presumably arises through the action of excited-state molecules. This type of damage can presumably be prevented by detoxification, e.g., by the quenching of these metabolically-produced excited states by molecules other than DNA. DNA is also damaged by metabolic stress (e.g., depurination). Depending on the nature of the damage and the repair capacity of the cell, three things can happen: (1) the damage is repaired in an error-free manner and no mutations are produced, (2) the damage is repaired by an error-prone process that can produce a mutation, and (3) the damage changes the coding properties of a base such that normal replication past this altered base produces a mutation. Since these mutations arise without any treatment being applied to the cells, they are called spontaneous mutations. Spontaneous mutations can also arise via replication errors (i.e., the DNA template is undamaged). If a spontaneous mutation occurs in an appropriate gene, then cells can become transformed, and unless the immune system removes these transformed cells, spontaneous carcinogenesis can be the end product of this series of metabolic events.

Figure 1 also demonstrates that there are many mechanisms to explain a person's predisposition to spontaneous carcinogenesis. A person could be a genetic overproducer of products that damage DNA, or be an underproducer of the agents that can detoxify these products. They could be deficient in error-free repair, possess DNA replication enzymes that are error-prone, or be immunologically deficient.

If this model, which is well supported by the bacterial and yeast data for spontaneous mutagenesis, can be confirmed in mammalian cells, then one way of reducing the level of spontaneous carcinogenesis is to identify those enzymatic reactions that modify essential metabolites such that they produce damage to DNA, and then search for nontoxic molecules that can detoxify these reactions, and thus reduce the amount of damage produced in DNA.

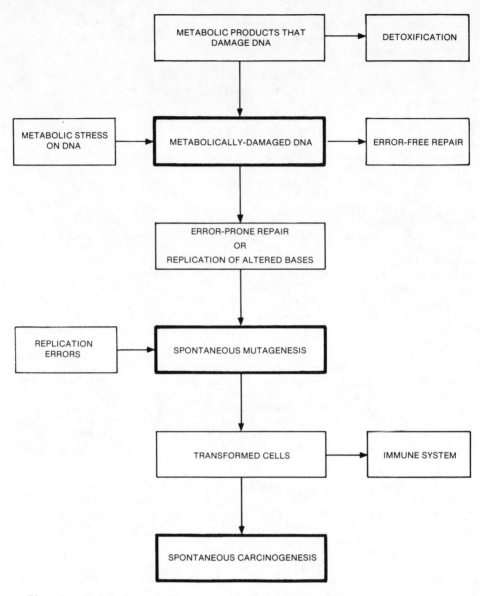

Fig. 1. Model for spontaneous carcinogenesis via spontaneous mutagenesis. See text for discussion.

The world has gone through the phase of identifying environmental
carcinogens, and is in the process of cleaning up the environment. The
next phase should be to identify the enzymatic reactions that can produce
carcinogens from essential metabolites, and begin to clean up or at least
detoxify our internal milieu.

REFERENCES

1. N. J. Sargentini and K. C. Smith, Spontaneous mutagenesis: The roles of DNA repair, replication, and recombination, _Mutation Res._ 154:1-27 (1985).

2. R. C. von Borstel, On the origin of spontaneous mutations, _Japan J. Genet. (Suppl. 1)_ 44:102-105 (1969).

3. S. Kondo, H. Ichikawa, K. Iwo, and T. Kato, Base-change mutagenesis and prophage induction in strains of _Escherichia coli_ with different DNA repair capacities, _Genetics_ 66:187-217 (1970).

4. S. Kondo, Evidence that mutations are induced by errors in repair and replication, _Genetics. Suppl._ 73:109-122 (1973).

5. E. C. Cox, Bacterial mutator genes and the control of spontaneous mutation, _Annu. Rev. Genet._ 10:135-156 (1976).

6. L. A. Loeb and T. A. Kunkel, Fidelity of DNA synthesis, _Annu. Rev. Biochem._ 51:429-457 (1982).

7. C. W. Lawrence, Mutagenesis in _Saccharomyces cerevisiae_, _Adv. Genet._ 21:173-254 (1982).

8. J. W. Drake, B. W. Glickman, and L. S. Ripley, Updating the theory of mutation, _Amer. Scientist_ 71:621-630 (1983).

9. P. E. Hartman, Z. Hartman, R. C. Stahl, and B. N. Ames, Classification and mapping of spontaneous and induced mutations in the histidine operon of _Salmonella_, _Adv. Genet._ 16:1-34 (1971).

10. J. D. Watson and F. H. C. Crick, The structure of DNA, _Cold Spring Harbor Symp. Quant. Biol._ 18:123-131 (1953).

11. M. D. Topal and J. R. Fresco, Complementary base pairing and the origin of substitution mutations, _Nature_ 263:285-289 (1976).

12. B. K. Duncan and J. H. Miller, Mutagenic deamination of cytosine residues in DNA, _Nature_ 287:560-561 (1980).

13. B. A. Kunz, Genetic effects of deoxyribonucleotide pool imbalances, _Environ. Mutagenesis_ 4:695-725 (1982).

14. G. G. Hillebrand and K. L. Beattie, Template-dependent variation in the relative fidelity of DNA polymerase I of _Escherichia coli_ in the presence of Mg^{2+} versus Mn^{2+}, _Nucleic Acids Res._ 12:3173-3183 (1984).

15. J. E. Patten, A. G. So, and K. M. Downey, Effect of base-pair stability of nearest-neighbor nucleotides on the fidelity of deoxyribonucleic acid synthesis, _Biochemistry_ 23:1613-1618 (1984).

16. G. Streisinger, Y. Okada, J. Emrich, J. Newton, A. Tsugita, E. Terzaghi, and M. Inouye, Frameshift mutations and the genetic code, _Cold Spring Harbor Symp. Quant. Biol._ 31:77-84 (1966).

17. L. S. Ripley, Model for the participation of quasi-palindromic DNA sequences in frameshift mutation, _Proc. Natl. Acad. Sci. USA_ 79:4128-4132 (1982).

18. L. S. Ripley and B. W. Glickman, Unique self-complementarity of palindromic sequences provides DNA structural intermediates for mutation, Cold Spring Harbor Symp. Quant. Biol. 47:851-861 (1982).

19. E. M. Witkin, Ultraviolet mutagenesis and inducible DNA repair in Escherichia coli, Bacteriol. Rev. 40:869-907 (1976).

20. J. Wildenberg and M. Meselson, Mismatch repair in heteroduplex DNA, Proc. Natl. Acad. Sci. USA 72:2202-2206 (1975).

21. G. Mohn and F. E. Wurgler, Mutator genes in different species, Humangenetik 16:49-58 (1972).

22. J. F. Speyer, J. D. Karam, and A. B. Lenny, On the role of DNA polymerase in base selection, Cold Spring Harbor Symp. Quant. Biol. 31:693-697 (1966).

23. Z. W. Hall and I. R. Lehman, An in vitro transversion by a mutationally altered T4-induced DNA polymerase, J. Mol. Biol. 36:321-333 (1968).

24. J. W. Drake and E. F. Allen, Antimutagenic DNA polymerases of bacteriophage T4, Cold Spring Harbor Symp. Quant. Biol. 33:339-344 (1968).

25. J. W. Drake, E. F. Allen, S. A. Forsberg, R. Preparata, and E. O. Greening, Spontaneous mutation. Genetic control of mutation rates in bacteriophage T4, Nature 221:1128-1132 (1969).

26. N. Muzyczka, R. L. Poland, and M. J. Bessman, Studies on the biochemical basis of spontaneous mutation. I. A comparison of the deoxyribonucleic acid polymerases of mutator, antimutator, and wild type strains of bacteriophage T4, J. Biol. Chem. 247:7116-7122 (1972).

27. G. C. Walker, Mutagenesis and inducible responses to deoxyribonucleic acid damage in Escherichia coli, Microbiol. Rev. 48:60-93 (1984).

28. D. W. Mount, A mutant of Escherichia coli showing constitutive expression of the lysogenic induction and error-prone DNA repair pathways. Proc. Natl. Acad. Sci. USA 74:300-304 (1977).

29. E. M. Witkin, Thermal enhancement of ultraviolet mutability in a dnaB uvrA derivative of Escherichia coli B/r: Evidence for inducible error-prone repair, in: "Molecular Mechanisms for Repair of DNA, Part A," P. C. Hanawalt and R. B. Setlow, eds., Plenum, New York (1975), pp. 369-378.

30. J. R. Geiger and J. F. Speyer, A conditional antimutator in E. coli, Mol. Gen. Genet. 153:87-97 (1977).

31. H. A. Erlich and E. C. Cox, Interaction of an Escherichia coli mutator gene with a deoxyribonucleotide effector, Mol. Gen. Genet. 178:703-708 (1980).

32. E. M. Witkin, Thermal enhancement of ultraviolet mutability in a tif-1 uvrA derivative of Escherichia coli B/r: Evidence that ultraviolet mutagenesis depends upon an inducible function, Proc. Natl. Acad. Sci. USA 71:1930-1934 (1974).

33. B. W. Glickman and M. Radman, Escherichia coli mutator mutants deficient in methylation-instructed DNA mismatch correction, Proc. Natl. Acad. Sci. USA 77:1063-1067 (1980).

34. M. Meuth, N. L'Heureux-Huard, and M. Trudel, Characterization of a mutator gene in Chinese hamster ovary cells, Proc. Natl. Acad. Sci. USA 76:6505-6509 (1979).

35. G. Weinberg, B. Ullman, and D. W. Martin, Jr., Mutator phenotypes in mammalian cell mutants with distinct biochemical defects and abnormal deoxyribonucleoside triphosphate pools, Proc. Natl. Acad. Sci. USA 78:2447-2451 (1981).

36. G. E. Magni, The origin of spontaneous mutations during meiosis, Proc. Natl. Acad. Sci. USA 50:975-980 (1963).

37. I. Machida and S. Nakai, Induction of spontaneous and UV-induced mutations during commitment to meiosis in Saccharomyces cerevisiae, Mutation Res. 73:59-68 (1980).

38. D. H. Maloney and S. Fogel, Mitotic recombination in yeast: Isolation and characterization of mutants with enhanced spontaneous mitotic gene conversion rates, Genetics 94:825:839 (1980).

39. A. Sancar and W. D. Rupp, A novel repair enzyme: UVRABC excision nuclease of Escherichia coli cuts a DNA strand on both sides of the damaged region, Cell 33:249-260 (1983).

40. E. M. Witkin, Radiation-induced mutations and their repair, Science 152:1345-1353 (1966).

41. M. H. L. Green, M. A. Rothwell, and B. A. Bridges, Mutation to prototrophy in Escherichia coli K-12: Effect of broth on UV-induced mutation in strain AB1157 and four excision-deficient mutants, Mutation Res. 16:225-234 (1972).

42. E. M. Witkin, Mutation-proof and mutation-prone modes of survival in derivatives of Escherichia coli B differing in sensitivity to ultraviolet light, Brookhaven Symp. Biol. 20:17-55 (1967).

43. E. M. Witkin, From Gainesville to Toulouse: The evolution of a model, Biochimie 64:549-555 (1982).

44. N. J. Sargentini and K. C. Smith, Much of spontaneous mutagenesis in Escherichia coli is due to error-prone DNA repair: Implications for spontaneous carcinogenesis, Carcinogenesis 9:863-872 (1981).

45. T. Kato, R. H. Rothman, and A. J. Clark, Analysis of the role of recombination and repair in mutagenesis of Escherichia coli by UV irradiation, Genetics 87:1-18 (1977).

46. R. H. Haynes and B. A. Kunz, DNA repair and mutagenesis in yeast, in: "Molecular Biology of the Yeast Saccharomyces: Life Cycle and Inheritance," Cold Spring Harbor Laboratory, Cold Spring Harbor, New York (1981), pp. 371-414.

47. P. K. Liu, C. Chang, and J. E. Trosko, Association of mutator activity with UV sensitivity in an aphidicolin-resistant mutant of Chinese hamster V79 cells, Mutation Res. 106:317-332 (1982).

48. P. K. Liu, C. Chang, J. E. Trosko, D. K. Dube, G. M. Martin, and L. A. Loeb, Mammalian mutator mutant with an aphidicolin-resistant DNA polymerase α, Proc. Natl. Acad. Sci. USA 80:797-801 (1983).

49. P. K. Liu, J. E. Trosko, and C. Chang, Hypermutability of a UV-sensitive aphidicolin-resistant mutant of Chinese hamster fibroblasts, Mutation Res. 106:333-345 (1982).

50. E. C. Friedberg, U. K. Ehmann, and J. J. Williams, Human diseases associated with defective DNA repair, Adv. Radiat. Biol. 8:85-174 (1979).

51. J. McCann, N. E. Spingarn, J. Kobori, and B. N. Ames, Detection of carcinogens as mutagens: Bacterial tester strains with R factor plasmids, Proc. Natl. Acad. Sci. USA 72:979-983 (1975).

52. K. H. Kraemer, M. M. Lee, and J. Scotto, DNA repair protects against cutaneous and internal neoplasia: Evidence from xeroderma pigmentosum, Carcinogenesis 5:511-514 (1984).

53. D. Savva, Spontaneous mutation rates in continuous cultures: The effect of some environmental factors, Microbios 33:81-92 (1982).

54. C. H. Clarke and D. M. Shankel, Antimutagenesis in microbial systems, Bacteriol. Rev. 39:33-53 (1975).

55. R. B. Webb, Lethal and mutagenic effects of near-ultraviolet radiation, Photochem. Photobiol. Rev. 2:169-261 (1977).

56. R. B. Webb and J. Lorenz, Toxicity of irradiated medium for repair-deficient strains of Escherichia coli, J. Bacteriol. 112:649-652 (1972).

57. M. Morimyo, Anaerobic incubation enhances the colony formation of a polA recB strain of Escherichia coli K-12, J. Bacteriol. 152:208-214 (1982).

58. M. Kelley and J. M. Baden, Oxygen mutagenicity, Mutation Res. 77:185-188 (1980).

59. H. Joenje, F. Arwert, A. W. Eriksson, H. de Koning, and A. B. Oostra, Oxygen-dependence of chromosomal aberrations in Fanconi's anaemia, Nature 290:142-143 (1981).

60. J. R. Totter, Spontaneous cancer and its possible relationship to oxygen metabolism, Proc. Natl. Acad. Sci. USA 77:1763-1767 (1980).

61. B. N. Ames, Dietary carcinogens and anticarcinogens. Oxygen radicals and degenerative diseases, Science 221:1256-1264 (1983).

62. R. Y.-H. Wang, K. C. Kuo, C. W. Gehrke, L.-H. Huang, and M. Ehrlich, Heat- and alkali-induced deamination of 5-methylcytosine and cytosine residues in DNA, Biochim. Biophys. Acta 697:371-377 (1982).

63. T. Lindahl and B. Nyberg, Rate of depurination of native deoxyribonucleic acid, Biochemistry 11:3610-3618 (1972).

64. T. Lindahl, DNA repair enzymes, Annu. Rev. Biochem. 51:61-87 (1982).

65. D. Sagher and B. Strauss, Insertion of nucleotides opposite apurinic/apyrimidinic sites in deoxyribonucleic acid during in vitro synthesis: Uniqueness of adenine nucleotides, Biochemistry 22:4518-4526 (1983).

66. R. M. Schaaper, T. A. Kunkel, and L. A. Loeb, Infidelity of DNA synthesis associated with bypass of apurinic sites, Proc. Natl. Acad. Sci. USA 80:487-491 (1983).

67. N. J. Sargentini and K. C. Smith, Mutagenesis by normal metabolites in Escherichia coli: Phenylalanine mutagenesis is dependent on error-prone DNA repair, Mutation Res. (1986) in press.

68. H. Glatt, M. Protic-Sabljic, and F. Oesch, Mutagenicity of glutathione and cysteine in the Ames test, Science 220:961-963 (1983).

69. G. Cilento, Photochemistry in the dark, Photochem. Photobiol. Rev. 5:199-228 (1980).

70. I. Emerit and P. Cerutti, Clastogenic activity from Bloom syndrome fibroblast cultures, Proc. Natl. Acad. Sci. USA 78:1868-1872 (1981).

71. R. S. K. Chaganti, S. Schonberg, and J. German, A manyfold increase in sister chromatid exchanges in Bloom's syndrome lymphocytes, Proc. Natl. Acad. Sci. USA 71:4508-4512 (1974).

72. S. T. Warren, R. A. Schultz, C. Chang, M. H. Wade, and J. E. Trosko, Elevated spontaneous mutation rate in Bloom syndrome fibroblasts, Proc. Natl. Acad. Sci. USA 78:3133-3137 (1981).

73. C. D. Lytle, R. E. Tarone, S. F. Barrett, J. D. Wirtschafter, J. Dupuy, and J. H. Robbins, Host cell reactivation by fibroblasts from patients with pigmentary degeneration of the retina, Photochem. Photobiol. 37:503-508 (1983).

74. R. A. Weinberg, A molecular basis of cancer, Scientific American 249:126-142 (1983).

75. E. Santos, E. P. Reddy, S. Pulciani, R. J. Feldmann, and M. Barbacid, Spontaneous activation of a human proto-oncogene, Proc. Natl. Acad. Sci. USA 80:4679-4683 (1983).

A METHOD FOR THE DETECTION OF NEO-ANTIGENS IN X-RAY INDUCED THYMOMAS OF

C57BL/6 MOUSE

A. Artus, B. Guillemain, E. Legrand, R. Mamoun,
T. Astier-Gin, and J. F. Duplan

INSERM, U. 117
Unite de Radiobiologie Experimentale et de Cancerologie
229, cours de l'Argonne
33076 Bordeaux Cedex, France

SUMMARY

Retroviruses are often encountered in radio-induced (X-rays) thymomas of the C57BL/6 mouse. Several viral strains, collectively referred to as "RadLVs", were shown, upon injection to normal mice to mimic the "radio-induced disease". However, the hypothesis of the role of radiations in activating endogenous non-pathogenic retroviruses leading (via recombination) to pathogenic RadLVs which in turn would be the etiological agents of the disease is not demonstrated. Indeed, RadLVs were detected in only a few instances.

Thus, instead of searching systematic association between tumor induction and virus expression, we tried to reveal radio-induced tumor antigens whatever their origin, viral or cellular. For this, we looked if radio-induced tumors harbored antigen(s) that could be recognized by gammaglobulins produced in the irradiated animal itself. Because of the need of large amounts of such specific immunoglobulins, we hybridized the own lymphocytes of the diseased animal with myeloma cells in order to obtain monoclonal antibodies (MoAb). As determined by ELISA, a large number of hybridoma cultures were found to secrete specific tumor antibodies.

When a number of such clonal antibodies were assayed for their ability to recognized different tumor cell extracts, it was found that only a few of them were specific of only one extract whereas the other cross-reacted with variable numbers of tumors. This was taken as an indication that radio-induced antigens were polymorphic in nature and differently expressed in distinct tumors.

INTRODUCTION

After the discovery by Gross (1951) of the first murine leukemic virus in cell extracts of AKR mice, leukemogenic retroviruses were harvested from radiation-induced (RX 4 x 1.75 Gy) thymic lymphosarcomas of C57BL mice (15). Then a number of investigators (4, 11) attempted to elucidate the role of these viruses in the leukemogenic process (15, 13, 10, 16). In the C57BL/6 mouse a number of viral agents, referred as "RadLV"(s) (Radiation leukemia virus) were isolated from radio-induced thymomas and upon injection to non-irradiated animals they were shown to mimic the radio-induced disease. It was then proposed (12) that irradiation acted in activating a cryptic RadLV which in turn was the etiological agent of the disease.

The origin of such a RadLV,-(VL3)-, was investigated by Decleve and coworkers (1978) who demonstrated that this virus arose via recombinational events between the two endogenous non-pathogenic retroviruses of the C57BL/6 strain, namely, the N ecotropic and the xenotropic (X) viruses, leading to an exogenous B-ecotropic virus (RadLV). However, latter studies (3, 6, 9, 2) showed that, in a number of instances, several B-ecotropic retroviruses could be harvested in tumor extracts but they could not be termed "RadLV" in view of their particular pathogenicity (latency period, polymorphism of the tumors induced).

Furthermore, radio-induced tumors were frequently shown not to produce any retrovirus; and among virus-positive tumors, RadLVs were not systematically detected. Therefore the hypothesis of the RadLV as the etiological agent of the radio-induced disease is not firmly established. Nevertheless, a number of reasons could explain the lack of detention of RadLVs in thymomas, among them it is conceivable that such agents are produced in an amount too low to be detectable or that they express only a part of their genetic information. Finally, it is also possible that the maintenance of the tumoral state do not depend on the expression of the virus which initiated cell transformation as described in another system by Grunwald (1982).

Thus, it seemed to us that a new approach of the problem could be of interest. We report here experiments aimed at the detection of new or superabundant antigenicities harbored (whatever their origin, viral or cellular) by T lymphocytes derived from radio-induced thymomas.

Because the searched antigens could differ from one to another tumor, we looked if tumoral cells harbored antigenicities that could be recognized by gammaglobulins produced in the irradiated animal itself. In view of the need of large amounts of such specific immunoglobulins, we hybridized the own lymphocytes of the diseased animal with myeloma cells with the aim to obtain monoclonal antibodies (MoAb). This allowed us to avoid immunizations of normal mice with tumor cells, a method which could have resulted in a loss of specific radio-induced antigens (see below).

RESULTS

In a first step, one month old mice (C57BL/6) were whole body irradiated (RX, 1.75 Gy four times at weekly intervals) as described by Latarjet and Duplan (13). After thymoma occurrence in one hand the lymphocytes of the spleen were hybridized and in the other hand, thymic tumor cells were used in part to be grafted into normal C57BL/6 mice and in part to establish continuous cell lines. The immortalized tumor cells could then be used to test the specificity of the MoAb by an ELISA technique.

The continuous cell lines were established according to the following procedure. Tumor cells were suspended in SFM-2 medium (a serum-free formulation chemically defined and without growth factors, developed in our laboratory) and seeded on a monolayer of established normal thymic

374

Table 1. Typing of cultured cells derived from radio-induced tumors.

Cell lines	Igs	θ	Ly-1.2	Ly-2.2
2945	0	93*	90	3
3302	0	77/95	0	0
3309	0	+	9	18
3316	0	80	27	22
3317	0	87	+**	56
3320	0	96	-	-
3324	0	97,8	+	4,5
3334	0	95	-	-
3438	0	95,6/100	0	85
3350	0	93	-	-
3541	0	90	-	-
4072	0	13	5	0
4638	0	+	17	22
4701	0	100	52	46
4708	0	98	+	54
4721	0	52	+	44
4745	0	92	+	87

* Percent of fluorescent cells using specific antisera.

** + or - means a positive or a negative result obtained
when the viability of the cells was too low to express
precise quantitative data.

epithelial cells (TAC7) which do not survive in the above medium. After 2
to 3 passages, the thymoma cells were only maintained in the serum-free
conditions. Among 35 established cell lines, 17 were more extensively
studied. Cells were typed by the use of specific antisera as described
previously (14). The results presented in Table 1 indicate that in every
case the thymic lymphoid origin of all cultured cells was demonstrated in
view of the systematic presence of antigens and of the complete lack of Ig
secretion. In addition, the analysis of the differentiation antigens
Ly-1.2, Ly-2.2) harbored by these cells revealed significant differences
according to the cell lines, thus suggesting that radio-induced tumor cells
differ in their phenotype with regard to their degree of maturation.

It was also shown that in vitro grown thymoma cells retained their
tumoral nature as indicated by their ability to induce tumors in grafted
animals (Table 2). In addition, grafted cells also retained their Ig and Ly
antigenic phenotypes.

The expression of retroviruses released by cultured thymoma cells in
the culture medium was investigated by the use of exogenous reverse
transcriptase assay (1). As indicated in Table 3, seven out of 19 cell

Table 2. Tumoral nature of in vitro estabished thymoma cells and maintenance of their phenotype after in vivo passage.

Cell lines	no tumorous animals/ no injected animals	Latence/ (days)	Phenotype of injected cells			Phenotype of resulting tumour cells		
			Ig	θ	Ly-1.2	Ig	θ	Ly-1.2
2945	3/3	23	0	93*	90	0	86	78
3302	3/3	23	0	77/95	0	0	81	9
3316	3/3	23	0	80	27	0	87	28
3317	3/3	23	0	87	+**	0	85	0
3334	3/3	23	0	95	-	0	97	24
3350	2/3	31	0	93	-	0	84	0
3438	3/3	23	0	96/100	0	0	97	28
4745	3/3	31	0	92	+	0	97	28

* Percent of fluorescent cells using specific antisera.

** + or - means a positive or a negative result obtained when the viability of the cells was too low to express precise quantitative data.

Table 3. Detection of type C retroviruses in the culture medium by the exogenous reverse transcriptase assay.

Cell lines		Incorporation[*]	N° assays
Controls	SFM-2	0.14	3
	TAC 98[**]	1.42	1
	TAC 7	0.15	2
Thymomas	2945	2.89	5
	3302	4.01	5
	3308	0.08	1
	3316	0.095	2
	3317	3.38	4
	3324	3.49	4
	3350	1.01	1
	3438	4.86	5
	3541	0.09	2
	4064	0.22	1
	4065	7.24	1
	4069	0.37	1
	4072	1.29	2
	4073	0.42	1
	4638	11.63	5
	4701	11.05	5
	4708	1.54	6
	4721	6.77	6
	4745	0.30	8

* ^{3}HTMP incorporated (pMole $\times$ hr^{-1} $\times$ ml^{-1}).

** TAC 98 thymic epithelial cells chronically infected with T98/B virus.

lines were found negative thus confirming that not all radio-induced thymomas derived cell lines produced "RadLV" like viruses.

The counterpart of these cell lines was the obtainment of MoAb able to specifically recognize radio-induced tumor associated antigens. For this microplate (96 wells) were seeded with Balb/c peritoneal macrophages (5 $\times$ 10^3 cells per well) in 100 μl SFM-2 containing 10% fetal calf serum (FCS) and incubated 24 hours (37°C, 5% CO_2). C57BL/6 mice with radio-induced thymomas were splenectomized and the splenocytes harvested; 10^7-10^8 splenocytes were fused with 10^7 myeloma cells SP2/0-Ag 14 (18) with polyethyen glycol 6000 according to Nowinsky (1979). An amount of 4/5 and of 1/5 of the resulting hybrids were seeded respectively in 5 microplates containing macrophages under 100 μl SFM-2 containing HAT. After 2 and 7 days incubation (37°C, 5% CO_2), 50 μl SFM-2 HT were added. On day 14, the presence of Igs in the culture medium of the hybrids was monitored by an ELISA technique using peroxidase conjugated sheep anti-mouse IgG (H + L).

As an average, 82% of the wells contained hybrid cultures of which 67% were Ig positive. The positive cultures were then tested for their content in antibodies directed against tumor cells. Tumor cells extracts (either from grafted tumors or from <u>in vitro</u> cultured tumor cells) were prepared by homogenization in 1 ml of N-octyl glucoside buffer (Tris-HCl pH 7.6; 50 mM; Mg acetate, 3 mM; sucrose, 0.25 M; N-octyl glucoside, 0.2%; phenyl-methyl-sulfonyl-fluoride, 0.1 mM) and centrifugated (600 g, 6 mn); the supernatant was stored, the pellet was resuspended in the same buffer but without N-octyl glucoside and recentrifugated (600 g, 6 mn), this supernatant was mixed with the former and dyalized against phosphate buffered saline. Such cell extracts were used to coat (1 μg per well) microplate wells (96), the hybride culture media to be tested for the presence of specific MoAb were then deposited (100 μl per well) and incubated for two hours. The wells corresponding to positive cultures were finally revealed as above. Finally, the tumor specific Ig releasing hybridoma cultures were cloned twice in SFM-2. After development of the clonal cultures, the MoAb were produced in SFM-2.

The results obtained showed that 46% of the Ig secreting hybridoma cultures contained specific antibodies directed against the tumor cells which arose in the same mouse (i.e., Autologous system). This confirmed the hypothesis according to which mice with radio-induced tumors develop a high antibody response to their own tumor associated antigens. To prove the specificity of these antibodies, the ELISA test was repeated but using a normal thymus as a source of antigen. Interestingly, 22% of the preceding hybridoma cultures secreted antibodies able to recognize such a normal

Table 4. Pattern of recognition of different tumor extracts by mono-clonal antibodies.

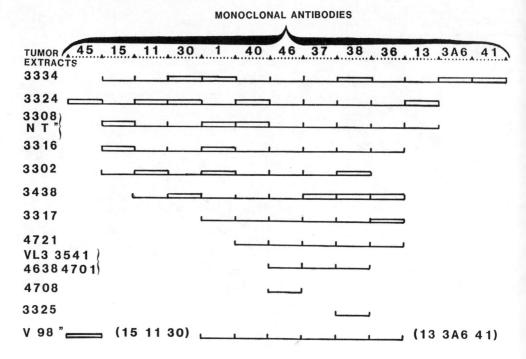

"N T : NORMAL THYMUS

"V 98 : B ECOTROPIC VIRUS OF THE C57BL/6 MOUSE : T98/B

⊏⊐ , ⌊___⌋ : + +, + E.L.I.S.A. ASSAYS

378

tissue. This allow to conclude that 78% antibodies were specific of the tumoral state. Among the antibodies directed against to the autologous tumor, a number could also recognize all or only a fraction of homologous thymomas. In these conditions, one must conclude that radio-induced thymomas are polymorphic in nature.

We also obtained antibodies directed against common antigenicities present in the normal thymus and in some homologous tumors (but not to the autologous tumor), a finding strongly suggesting that some tumor antigens, absent from leukemic cells, appeared during a preleukemic stage at an in usual high level. Finally, another class of antibodies, detected antigens only in homologous tumor cells (which are absent in autologous tumor cells), this would mean that such antigens were present in the autologous tumor at a preleukemic state but that their expression switched off thereafter. It is noticeable that these last two classes of antibodies would not have been detected by use of the classical hybridization technique which utilize the splenocytes of an experimentally preimmunized mouse.

In preliminary experiments and because the endogenous retroviruses and their recombinants are often expressed in radio-induced thymomas, we investigated the possibility that the tumor associated antibodies could recognize viral proteins. For this we used as a source of antigens a preparation of disrupted virus T98/B (9), a recombinant between the two endogenous retrovirus of the C57BL/6. It clearly appeared that only 20% of antibodies recognized viral antigenicities in autologous tumor cells. Thus, it may be concluded that irradiation leads mainly to the expression of tumor associated antigens which are specific of tumor cells and which are not related to the expression of retroviral genomes. A schematic representation of the different specificities of some MoAb is summarized in Table 4. Studies are now in progress to isolate and characterize such antigens.

ACKNOWLEDGEMENTS

We thank J. P. Porteil for the excellent technical assistance and Miss L. Couillaud for typing the manuscript.

This work was performed with the financial participation of the European Atomic Energy Commission (Contract No. BIO 371 F).

REFERENCES

1. T. Astier, B. Guillemain, and J. F. et Duplan, Proprietes biochimiques d'un virus des radioleucoses de la souris C57BL, C.R. Acad. Sci. (Paris), 282:1225 (1976).

2. T. Astier, B. Guillemain, F. Laigret, R. Mamoun, and J. F. et Duplan, Serological characterization of C-type retrovirus endogenous to the C57BL/6 mouse and isolated in tumors induced by radiation leukemia virus (RadLV-Rs), J. Gen. Virol. 61:55 (1982).

3. L. E. Benade, J. N. Ihle, and A. Decleve, Serological characterization of B-tropic viruses of C57BL mice: Possible origin by recombination of endogenous N-tropic and xenotropic viruses, Proc. Natl. Acad. Sci. (USA) 73:4675 (1978).

4. A. Decleve, M. Lieberman, J. N. Ihle, and H. S. Kaplan, Biological and serological characterization of radiation leukemic virus, Proc. Natl. Acad. Sci. (USA) 73:4675 (1976).

5. A. Decleve, M. Lieberman, J. N. Ihle, N. Rosenthal, M. L. Lung, and H. S. Kaplan, Physiochemical, biological and serological properties of leukemogenic virus isolated from cultured RadLV-induced lymphomas of C57BL/6 mice, Virology 90:23 (1978).

6. J. W. Gautsch, J. H. Elder, J. Schindler, F. C. Jensen, and R. A. Lerner, Structural markers on protein p30 of murine leukemia virus: Functional correlation with Fv-1 tropisme, Proc. Natl. Acad. Sci. (USA) 75:4553 (1978).

7. D. J. Grunwald, B. Dale, J. Dudley, W. Lamph, B. Sugden, B. Ozanne, and R. Risser, Loss of viral gene expression and retention of tumorigenicity by Abelson lymphoma cells, J. Virol. 43:92 (1982).

8. L. Gross, "Spontaneous" leukemia developing in C3H mice following inoculation, in infancy, with AK-leukemic extracts, or AK-embryos, Proc. Soc. Exp. Biol. 76:27 (1951).

9. B. Guillemain, T. Astier, R. Mamoun, and J. F. Duplan, Production and titration assays of B-tropic retroviruses isolated from C57BL Mouse tumors induced by radiation leukemic virus (RadLV-Rs): Effect of dexamethansone, Intervirology 13:65 (1980).

10. N. Haran-Ghera, Leukemogenic activity of centrifugates from irradiation mouse thymus and bone marrow, Int. J. Cancer 1:81 (1966).

11. N. Haran-Ghera, M. Ben-yaakou, and A. Peled, Immunological characteristics in relation to high and low leukemogenic activity of radiation-leukemia virus variants, Immunology 118:600 (1977).

12. H. S. Kaplan, Interaction between radiation and viruses in the induction of murine thymic lymphomas and lymphatic leukemias, in: "Radiation-induced leukemogenesis and related viruses, Vol. 1," J. F. Duplan, ed., Elsevier, North Holland - Amsterdam (1977), pp. 18.

13. R. Latarjet and J. F. Duplan, Experiment and discussion on leukemogenesis by cell free extracts of radiation-induced leukaemia in mice, Int. J. Rad. Biol. 5:339 (1962).

14. E. Legrand, B. Guillemain, R. Daculsi, and F. Laigret, Leukemogenic activity of B-ecotropic C-type retroviruses isolated from tumors induced by radiation leukemic virus (RadLV-Rs) in C57BL/6 mice, Int. J. Cancer 30:241 (1982).

15. M. Lieberman and H. S. Kaplan, Leukemogenic activity of filtrates from radio-induced lymphoid tumors of mice, Science 130:387 (1959).

16. P. B. Mistry and J. F. Duplan, Proprietes biologiques d'un virus isole d'une radioleucemie C57BL. Premiers passages du virus natif, Bull. Cancer 60:287 (1973).

17. R. C. Nowinsky, M. E. Lostrom, M. R. Tam, M. R. Stone, W. N. et Burnette, The isolation of hybrid cell lines producing monoclonal antibodies against p15(E). Protein of ecotropic murine leukemia viruses, Virology 93:111 (1979).

18. M. Schulman, C. D. Wilde, and G. et Kohler, A better cell line for making hybridomes secreting specific antibodies Nature 269:276 (1978).

VISIBLE LIGHT INDUCED KILLING AND MUTATION OF ACRIFLAVINE SENSITIZED

CHINESE HAMSTER CELLS

Tapan Ganguly and Sukhendu B. Bhattacharjee

Crystallography and Molecular Biology Division
Saha Institute of Nuclear Physics
AF/I, Salt Lake, Calcutta-700 0/64
India

INTRODUCTION

The acridine dyes are perhaps the most well studied photosensitizers both in vivo and in vitro. Exhaustive in vivo studies with these dyes have been made only with bacteria and bacteriophages but not with mammalian cells. The photodynamic effects in mammalian cells have been investigated mainly with the drugs hematoporphyrin, furocoumarins like 8-methoxypsoralen and chlorpromazine (6, 2, 1). Basic information regarding the target of visible light induced damage as well as the mechanism by which this damage occurs in acriflavine sensitized mammalian cells is important due to the application of these dyes in photochemotherapy.

The mode of photodynamic inactivation is not unique and varies from dye to dye. Even for a particular dye, there may not be a unique specificity for the site of its action (9). For example, damage to DNA is not the sole cause of photodynamic killing induced by DNA-binding acridines in E. coli (14, 15). Thus, the relative contributions of the dye sensitized photodamages at different cellular sites need to be ascertained.

The fundamental mechanism for the photooxidation of various cell components by a dye can involve either a free radical (Type I) or a singlet oxygen (Type II) intermediate. Singlet oxygen plays a very important role in most of the photodynamic effects at conditions favorable for the diffusion of molecular oxygen. Azide ions quench singlet oxygen and deuterated water (D_2O) lengthens their lifetimes. Experiments to estimate the role of singlet oxygen in the photodynamic action are usually done in the presence of these substances (10, 12). The involvement of singlet oxygen in the photodynamic effects has been shown in mammalian cells by using D_2O as the test chemical (11, 7).

In this report, we have studied the visible light induced killing and mutation of acriflavine sensitized V-79, Chinese hamster cells. Attempts have also been made to get an idea of the relative contributions of the photodynamic damage at DNA and non-DNA sites in cell lethality and the role of singlet oxygen in the process.

381

MATERIALS AND METHODS

Chemicals   Acriflavine, 8-Azaguanine and Neomycin sulphate were
purchased from Sigma (USA). Penicillin and Streptomycin sulphate were
supplied by local pharmaceutical companies. Stock solution of acriflavine
was prepared immediately before use by dissolving in Eagle's MEM (4)
without phenol red (PR). The aza stock solution (3 mg/ml) was prepared by
dissolving in DMSO.

Cells and Culture Conditions   Details of the culture conditions,
media, etc. for the V-79 Chinese hamster cells have already been published
(5). Cells were grown in MEM complete with all non-essential amino acids,
vitamins, penicillin (100 units/ml), streptomycin sulphate (100 g/ml),
neomycin sulphate (50 g/ml) and supplemented with 10% dialyzed goat serum.

Dye-sensitization and Exposure to Visible Light   Survival experiment:
The details of the techniques used have been given in the earlier report
(5). In brief, exponential cells after trypsinization were plated on
plastic petri dishes at required numbers. After cell attachment, the
growth medium was replaced with fresh growth medium (without PR) and the
dye solution was added to the cells in the dark. Exposure of the dye
sensitized cells to visible light was done under two conditions, unwashed
and washed. In the unwashed condition, the dye sensitization was done in
the dark for 20 min. and the dye containing medium was removed after
different periods of visible light exposure in presence of the dye. In the
washed condition, the dye containing medium was removed with washing after
the dye treatment (50 min.) but before the visible light exposure.
Following exposures in both cases, medium was replaced with fresh growth
medium (with PR). The dishes were then incubated in the dark at $37^{\circ}C$ in
CO_2 atmosphere for colony formation and the subsequent determination of
viability.

To investigate the role of singlet oxygen in the photodynamic killing,
acriflavine and sodium azide were simultaneously added to the cells and
both were removed after visible light exposure in the unwashed condition.
The pH dependence of the inactivation was studied by adding growth medium
(without PR) of pH 8.5 to the cells during exposure in the washed
condition. Exposures from two daylight 10W fluorescent tubes were made in
5% humidified CO_2 atmosphere in a specially made visible light chamber; the
exposure intensity was 2 W/m^2 on the top of the dish and 1.45 W/m^2 at the
surface of the medium as measured with a luxmeter (5).

Mutation experiment: Mutation to 8-azaguanine resistance was detected
following the procedures described earlier (3). About 10^6 exponential
cells were treated with dye plus light in the unwashed condition. 24 hr.
after the photodynamic treatment, the cells were trypsinized, seeded in
appropriate numbers and allowed to grow for 7-9 days in growth medium for
mutation expression with 3-4 subcultures during this period. After
expression, cells were replated at 5×10^5 cells/dish, in 5 Corning dishes
(100 mm) in selection medium containing 3 µg/ml 8-aza in complete growth
medium. Resistant clones were counted after 14 days. 250 cells were also
plated in triplicate in normal growth medium for viable cell count and the
colonies were counted after 7 days.

RESULTS AND DISCUSSION

The survival of acriflavine sensitized cells on visible light
exposures in washed and unwashed conditions have been shown in Figure 1.
In the former case, the dye bound washed cells kept in the dark under
identical conditions except for visible exposures served as control.

382

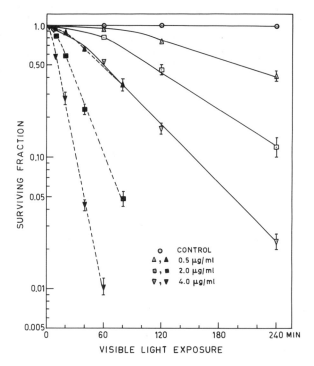

Fig. 1. Survival of acriflavine sensitized washed (continuous curves) and unwashed (dotted curves) V-79
cells on visible light exposures.

Visible light exposure up to 240 min. had no effect on the viability of
normal untreated cells. But the cells treated with both acriflavine and
visible light underwent inactivation in concentration and dose dependent
manner (continuous curves). The dotted curves represent the photodynamic
inactivation in unwashed condition. Here also the control cells had all
treatments identical but for visible light exposure. It is quite evident
from the figure that when cells were exposed in the presence of the dye in
the medium, they had much higher photodynamic sensitivity compared to the
cells exposed in the absence of the dye.

Though acriflavine is primarily a DNA intercalating dye, it also
binds, when added to a cell, to non-DNA sites; binding to DNA being the
strongest. During exposure of cells after dye removal, the dye molecules
may gradually be released from the non-DNA components, but those bound to
DNA remain almost equally bound. This is based on the assumption that dye
binding with DNA is not dependent upon the continuous presence of the dye
in the medium within the limited period of 240 min. On this assumption,
the higher sensitivity of the cells in the unwashed condition must be due
to damage at the non-DNA components of the cells and for exposure in the
washed condition, the site of damage could be mainly DNA.

Table 1. Proposed contribution of DNA damage in cellular inactivation.

AF concentration μg/ml.	Slope of the survival curve		Difference (a - b) ($\times 10^{-3}$)	Contribution from DNA* b/a (%)
	In unwashed condition (a) ($\times 10^{-3}$)	In washed conditioned (b) ($\times 10^{-3}$)		
0.5	15.3	5.3	10.0	34.6
2.0	44.8	10.8	34.0	24.1
4.0	83.0	17.0	66.0	20.5

* Including contributions due to disturbances in chromosomal protiens if any.

Estimates on the relative contributions of damages at DNA and non-DNA sites in cell killing can be made from the differences in the slopes of the survival curves under the two conditions (Table 1). Column 5 of this table shows that with increasing dye concentration DNA damage was playing a minor role or in other words, non-DNA damage was the principal factor in the photodynamic inactivation in the unwashed condition.

The influence of sodium azide on the photodynamic killing of dye sensitized unwashed cells has been shown in Figure 2. At concentrations above 4 mM, sodium azide itself is somewhat toxic to V-79 cells (data not shown) and to take into account this toxicity, azide, and dye treated unwashed cells in the dark were held as control. Figure 2 indicates that sodium azide inhibited the killing in a concentration dependent manner, thus providing evidence of the involvement of singlet oxygen in the process.

The role of singlet oxygen can also be ascertained indirectly by studying the pH dependence of the photodynamic killing (8). Table 2 represents the influence of pH during the visible light exposure on the survival of dye sensitized washed cells. Here also the washed cells kept at a pH 8.5 in the dark had a loss in viability compared to the washed cells kept at the physiological pH 7.5 in the dark. So the cells of the former condition was taken as control for the washed cells exposured at a pH 8.5. It is clearly seen that for a particular exposure time at the higher pH, the survival was much less compared to that of the cells exposed at the pH 7.5 and such difference was more pronounced at higher concentrations of acriflavine. The enhanced photodynamic sensitivity of the cells at the higher pH could be due to the increase in the yield of singlet oxygen with pH (13). The pH dependence of the yield of singlet oxygen and similar dependence of the photodynamic inactivation also implicate the role of singlet oxygen.

The mutagenicity of the dye plus light treatment for V-79 cells was studied by using the CH/HGPRT cell mutation system and 8-azaguanine as the selecting drug. The involvement of singlet oxygen was also studied by photodynamic treatment of the cells in the presence of sodium azide. Table 3 gives the mutagenicity of acriflavine and sodium azide in the dark.

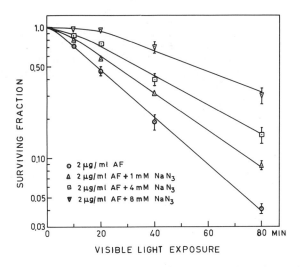

Fig. 2.   Influence of sodium azide on the photodynamic inactivation of acriflavine sensitized unwashed cells.

Table 2. Survival of acriflavine (AF) sensitized washed
cells for exposure at pH 8.5.

AF concentration µg/ml	Visible light exposure min.	Survival for exposure at	
		pH 8.5	pH 7.5 (from Fig.1)
0.5	60	0.67	0.95
	120	0.14	0.74
	240	0.025	0.42
2.0	60	0.29	0.82
	120	0.055	0.46
	240	0.004	0.12
4.0	60	0.083	0.52
	120	0.016	0.18
	240	0.0007	0.023

Acriflavine up to a concentration of 2 µg/ml and a treatment time of 140 min. was not mutagenic to V-79 cells but on addition of azide the mutant frequency increased moderately. The effect of visible light on the yield of mutants have been illustrated in Table 4. Like acriflavine, visible light itself was also not mutagenic to normal untreated cells. But the

Table 3. Mutagenicity of acriflavine and sodium azide in the dark for V-79 cells.

Treatment.	Treatment time min.	Surviving fraction.	Mutant frequency per 10^5 viable cells with standard error.
Control	–	1.00	0.11 ± 0.10
AF, 0.5 µg/ml	140	0.90 ± 0.01	0.15 ± 0.13
AF, 2.0 µg/ml	140	0.74 ± 0.02	0.41 ± 0.12
AF, 2.0 µg/ml, and sodium azide, 4 mM in conjunction.	60	0.85 ± 0.03	0.50 ± 0.18
	100	0.75 ± 0.03	1.29 ± 0.24
	140	0.70 ± 0.02	1.46 ± 0.22

Table 4. Mutagenicity of acriflavine and sodium azide in the presence of visible light for V-79 cells.

Treatment.	Visible light exposure min.	Surviving fraction.	Mutant frequency per 10^5 viable cells with standard error.
Control	40	1.0	0.17 ± 0.10
	80	1.0	0.22 ± 0.13
	120	1.0	0.30 ± 0.14
AF, 0.5 µg/ml	40	0.66 ± 0.01	1.87 ± 0.35
	80	0.34 ± 0.03	2.42 ± 0.56
	120	0.16 ± 0.02	3.75 ± 0.50
AF, 2.0 µg/ml	40	0.28 ± 0.05	3.29 ± 0.82
	80	0.05 ± 0.02	4.66 ± 0.73
	120	0.009 ± 0.0003	6.51 ± 0.71
AF, 2.0 µg/ml, and sodium azide, 4 mM in conjunction.	40	0.52 ± 0.03	0.58 ± 0.21
	30	0.28 ± 0.02	1.38 ± 0.33
	120	0.17 ± 0.05	1.71 ± 0.53

combined dye plus light treatment in the unwashed condition resulted in significant induction of mutants depending on the dye concentration and the period of exposure. The induced mutation was suppressed by sodium azide just as in the case of survival studies. The inhibitory effect of sodium azide demonstrated the photodynamic origin of mutation as well as the participation of singlet oxygen. The result seems to indicate that the apparent small role of DNA in cell killing could be critical so far as the genetic effect was concerned.

REFERENCES

1. M. J. Ashwood-Smith, A. T. Natarajan, and E. A. Poulton, J. Natl. Cancer Inst. 69:189-197 (1982).

2. E. Ben-Hur, A. Prager, M. Green, and I. Rosenthal, Chem. Biol. Interact. 29:223-233 (1980).

3. S. B. Bhattacharjee and B. Pal, Mutat. Res. 101:329-338 (1982).

4. H. Eagle, Science 130:432-437 (1959).

5. T. Ganguly and S. B. Bhattacharjee, Photochem. Photobiol. 38:65-69 (1983).

6. J. Gomer and D. M. Smith, Photochem. Photobiol. 32:341-348 (1980).

7. N. Greuner and M. P. Lockwood, Biochem. Biophys. Res. Commun. 90:460-465 (1979).

8. T. Ito, Photochem. Photobiol. 25:47-53 (1977).

9. T. Ito and K. Kobayashi, Photochem. Photobiol. 26:581-587 (1977).

10. K. Kobayashi and T. Ito, Photochem. Photobiol. 23:21-28 (1976).

11. J. Moan, E. O. Pattersen, and T. Christensen, Br. J. Cancer 39:398-407 (1979).

12. J. Piette, C. M. Calberg-Bacq, and A. Van de Vorst, Photochem. Photobiol. 26:377-382 (1977).

13. R. Pottier, R. Bonneau, and J. Houssot-Dubien, Photochem. Photobiol. 22:59-61 (1975).

14. S. Wagner, W. D. Taylor, A. Keith, and W. Snipes, Photochem. Photobiol. 32:771-779 (1980).

15. S. Wagner, A. Feldman, and W. Snipes, Photochem. Photobiol. 35:73-81 (1982).

ONCOGENES ACTIVATED IN RADIATION-INDUCED RAT SKIN TUMORS

S. J. Garte, M. J. Sawey, and F. J. Burns

Institute of Environmental Medicine
New York University Medical Center
550 First Avenue
New York, N.Y. 10016

ABSTRACT

Male, Sprague-Dawley rats were exposed at four weeks of age to 0.8 MeV electron radiation in single or fractionated doses ranging from 800 to 1600 rads. A sample of 6 tumors was excised at 50 or 74 weeks of age. The DNA from three carcinomas produced transformed foci by transfection in NIH3T3 cells. In 4 transfectants a rat tumor derived K-ras Eco R1 fragment was seen by Southern blot analysis. The DNA of four cancers showed myc gene amplification in each case compared to normal rat liver DNA. Hybridization with an H-ras probe showed no significant amplification of this gene in any of the tumors. Northern blot analysis of poly A$^+$ RNA demonstrated a major increase of myc gene expression in a tumor which was active in the transfection assay. Analogous experiment using the same mRNA samples showed no differences in H-ras gene expression between normal skin and any tumor. These data demonstrate simultaneous activation of oncogenes from myc and ras complementation groups in a single tumor.

INTRODUCTION

Ionizing radiation is a potent and well characterized carcinogen for the rat skin (1). Several types of carcinomas develop in rat skin following localized exposure to single or fractionated doses of ionizing radiation (2). These skin tumors are classified on the basis of their differentiation patterns into three principle categories: keratinized, sebaceous, and nondifferentiated tumors (2). The histologic type of the tumor presumably reflects the cell type of origin.

The molecular mechanism(s) by which ionizing radiation lead to tumorigenesis are not known. Breaks in the deoxyribophosphate strand are one important way that ionizing radiation damages DNA (1). The consequence of double-strand DNA breaks could include repair or misrepair in a way that leads to gene amplification, chromosomal rearrangements, and translocations (3). Translocation and gene amplification have been proposed as mechanisms to activate cellular oncogenes (4-8).

Cellular oncogenes of two distinct complementation groups represented by myc and the ras family are capable together of transforming primary

389

fibroblasts in vitro (9). Whereas ras genes, which have NIH3T3 cell transforming activity, are mutationally activated (10–18), most examples of active myc genes involve chromosomal translocations and/or gene amplification (4-6, 19). Guerrero et al. (18) have demonstrated the activation of a c-k-ras oncogene by somatic mutation in mouse lymphomas induced by gamma radiation. Mouse skin carcinomas chemically induced by the 2-stage initiation-promotion protocol (20) or by the direct acting alkylating agent β-propiolactone (Hochwalt and Garte, unpublished observations) contain activated H-ras oncogenes. We now report evidence for activation of both c-K-ras and c-myc oncogenes in individual rat skin tumors induced by ionizing radiation.

MATERIALS AND METHODS

Radiation Induction of Rat Skin Tumors

Male, Sprague Dawley rats were exposed at four weeks of age to 0.8 MeV electron radiation (maximum skin penetration - 1.0 mm) in single or fractionated doses ranging from 800-1600 rads. The skin tumors arising 46 or 70 weeks later were excised and frozen in liquid nitrogen immediately after sacrifice of the animal. A section of each tumor was examined for histologic diagnosis.

DNA Isolation

All tumors and tissues used for DNA isolation were pulverized to a powder in liquid nitrogen and high molecular weight DNA was extracted by a phenol-chloroform extraction method and precipitated with ethanol. The concentration and purity of the DNA was determined by spectrophotometric analysis at 260 and 280 nm.

DNA Transfection Assays

Aliquots of tumor DNA (30-40 µg) were co-precipitated with calcium phosphate and transfected into subconfluent NIH3T3 cells according to the method of Wigler et al. (21). Two days after transfection, plates were subcultured at 1:3. Cultures were maintained in DMEM Supplemented with 10% fetal calf serum for three weeks, after which time foci were picked with cloning cyclinders and/or coded plates were stained with Giemsa and scored double blind. Negative (NIH3T3) and positive (T24 human bladder carcinoma) control DNAs were run in each assay.

Southern Blot Hybridization

DNA (15 µg) from RAD tumors and NIH3T3 transfectants were digested to completion with EcoR1, electrophoresed on a 0.8% agarose gel, and transferred to a nitrocellulose filter (22). The K-ras probe (P.ras.2 from ONCOR) DNA (0.2 µg) was nick translated to 4×10^6 CPM/µg with dCTP^{32} and hybridized to the transfectant DNA filter in 2X Denharts solution, 6X SSC, at 64°C for 18 hours. The filter was washed to a final stringency of 0.5X SSC and 0.1% SDS at 60°C and exposed to X-ray film. The filters containing the RAD tumor DNAs were hybridized with H-ras (pHBI) and myc (MC413) as described above except that probes had a final specific activity of 10^7 CPM/µg, and filters were washed to a final stringency of 1X SSC at 60°C.

RNA Isolation

Normal rat skin was obtained from 28 day old male Sprague-Dawley CD rats. The epidermis was separated from the whole rat skin using the heat shock method of Marrs and Voorhees (23). The normal rat epidermal tissue

Table 1. Oncogene Activation in Radiation Induced Tumors

Tumor Number	Tumor Type	No. Foci/ No. Plate	No. Foci/ g DNA	K-ras in Foci	myc Amplification
		Transfection of Tumor DNA in NIH3T3 Cells			
NIH3T3	____	0/24	0.003	N.A.	N.A.
T24	Human Bladder Carcinoma	22/24	0.102	N.A.	N.A.
RAD 1	Poorly Differentiated Clear Cell Carcinoma	22/18	0.100*	N.D.	+
RAD 2	Well Differentiated Cornified Squamous Cell Carcinoma	0/18	0.005	N.A.	N.D.
RAD 3	Basal Cell Carcinoma	0/18	0.005	N.A.	N.D.
RAD 4	Sebaceous Carcinoma (necrotic)	4/18	0.019*	+	+
RAD 5	Poorly Differentiated Clear Cell Carcinoma	10/18	0.051*	+	+
RAD 6	Fibroma	1/18	0.005	N.A.	+

* Transfection positive (by chi square analysis)
N.A. - Not applicable.
N.D. - Not determined.

and RAD tumors were pulverized to a powder in liquid nitrogen and total cellular RNA isolated by the guanidinium/hot phenol method (24). Poly A$^+$ mRNA was selected by chromatography on oligo (dT) cellulose (25, 26).

Northern Blot Hybridization

Poly A$^+$ RNA (20 µg) was denatured in glyoxal, ran on a 1% agarose gel, transferred to nitrocellulose (27, 28), and hybridized to c-myc and H-ras probes as described above.

RESULTS

Transfection of Rat Tumor DNA

Purified DNA from radiation induced tumors of various histologic types were tested in the NIH3T3 focus assay. Histologic diagnosis of each tumor (shown in Table 1) was confirmed independently by three investigators. Each tumor DNA was run in at least two experiments and coded plates were scored for foci double blind.

Table 1 shows the results of these experiments. Of the 6 tumor DNAs tested, 3 were positive in the transfection assay, and foci from 2 of these tumor DNAs were picked and grown to mass culture. The transformed phenotype of one such focus was confirmed by subcutaneous injection of 5 x

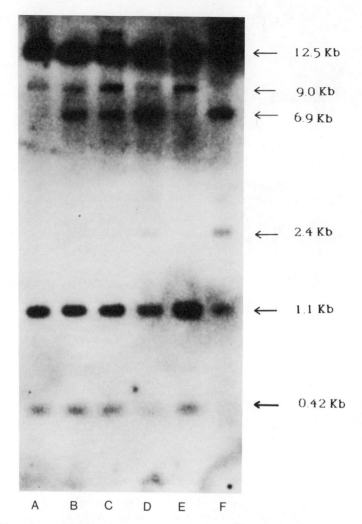

					← 12.5 Kb
					← 9.0 Kb
					← 6.9 Kb
					← 2.4 Kb
					← 1.1 Kb
					← 0.42 Kb

A   B   C   D   E   F

Fig. 1.   Southern blot analysis of NIH3T3 transfectant
           DNA, hybridized to a K-ras probe. Lane A -
           NIH3T3; Lane B - transfectant 407-5 from
           -tumor RAD 4; Lane C - transfectant 407-46
           from tumor RAD 4; Lane D - transfectant 407-
           47 from tumor RAD 5; Lane E - transfectant
           407-52 from tumor RAD 5; and Lane F - rat
           liver.

10^6 transfectant cells into five nude mice, each of which developed
sarcomas at the injection site within two weeks.

The frequency of positive transfection in this system is similar to
that found in other experimental animal models (14, 18, 20). It appears
from Table 1 that the poorly differentiated tumors were more likely to
contain active NIH3T3 transforming genes although the number of tumors
tested so far is insufficient to provide convincing evidence for tissue
specificity.

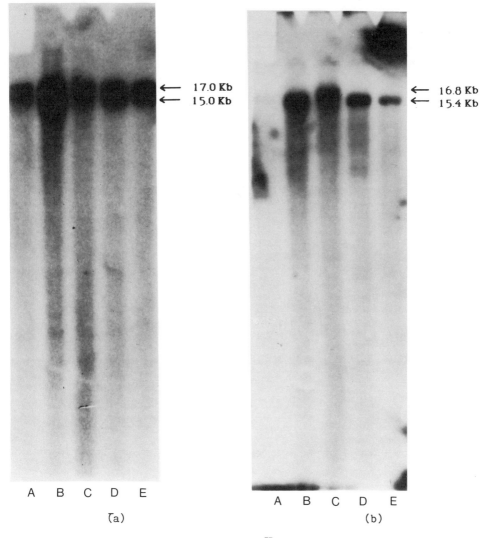

Figure 2. Southern blot analysis of RAD tumor DNA. Hybridization
probes were: (a) H-ras (pHBI) or (b) c-myc (pMC413). DNAs
for (a) and (b) were from: Lane A - rat liver; Lane B - RAD
1; Lane C - RAD 4; Lane D - RAD 5; and Lane E - RAD 6.

Identification of Active Transforming Oncogene

Southern blot analysis of the DNA from 4 NIH3T3 transfectants using a
K-ras probe showed that each contained at least one rat-derived Eco R1 DNA
fragment at 6.9 kb; transfectant #407-47, which was derived from RAD 5
tumor DNA also contained a rat band at 2.4 kb (Figure 1). Similar
experiments, using N- and H-ras probes revealed only the endogenous mouse
fragments in transfectant DNA (data not shown). These transfectants were
originally derived from tumor 4 (407-5 and 407-46) and tumor 5 (407-47 and
407-52), indicating that both of the positive tumors tested contained the
same activated member of the ras gene family. Transfectants from tumor 1
DNA were not picked.

Evidence for myc Amplification and Enhanced Expression

The original tumor DNA's were also examined by Southern analysis using oncogene probes. As shown in Figure 2, each tumor shows approximately the same Eco R1 banding pattern for H-ras as is seen in rat liver, whereas when a myc probe (Figure 2b) was used with the same DNA samples, each of the 4 radiation tumors tested showed clear indication of 5- to 10-fold gene amplification (based on densitometric analysis of the data in Figure 2b). RAD 4 tumor DNA also exhibited a restriction polymorphism of the major band from 15.4 kb to 16.8 kb. Amplification of myc was seen in tumors that were both positive and negative in transfection, and of different histologic types (see Table 1).

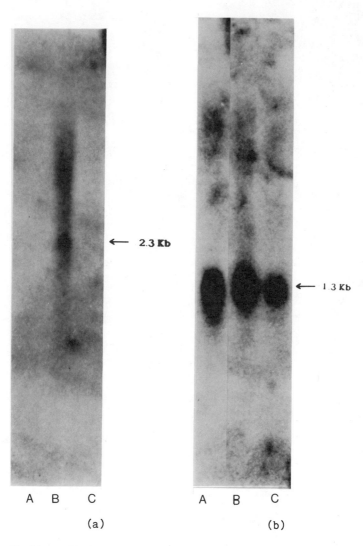

Fig. 3. Northern blot analysis of RAD tumor Poly A$^+$ RNA. Hybridization probes were: a) c-myc (pMC413) or b) H-ras (pHBI). RNA samples for (a) and (b) were isolated from: Lane A - rat epidermis; Lane B - RAD 5; and Lane C - RAD 6.

A portion of three tumors (RAD 4, 5, and 6) had been set aside for preparation of poly A$^+$ RNA. Northern blot analysis of RAD 5 and RAD 6 RNAs, and of a sample of normal rat epidermal RNA, is shown in Figure 3. The necrotic RAD 4 tumor did not yield usable poly A$^+$ RNA, as determined by the absence of any signal with Northern hybridization to several probes (data not shown). Under the conditions used, virtually no myc gene expression was detected in rat epidermis. In contrast, tumor RAD 5 showed clear expression of a 2.3 kb band. A faint signal was also detected for RAD 6 (Lane C). When the same RNA samples were hybridized with an H-ras probe (Figure 3b), no increase in poly A$^+$ RNA over normal skin levels was seen for either tumor. Thus, two of the radiation induced rat skin tumors examined contained an amplified myc oncogene as well as a activated K-ras oncogene (Table 1), and at least one of these (RAD 5) also exhibited enhanced myc expression. No correlation was seen between oncogene activation parameters and the size or growth rate of tumors, or with radiation dose or age of animal at sacrifice.

DISCUSSION

The reported genotoxic effects of ionizing radiation include primarily chromosomal aberrations, and DNA strand breaks (1) as opposed to the point mutations often found with certain chemical carcinogens, such as NMU (29). Chromosomal translocations of the type that could occur as a result of the genotoxic effects of radiation on target cells have been shown to result in activation of the myc oncogene by promoter insertion in Burkitts lymphoma (6). The findings of gene amplification, restriction polymorphism, and enhanced expression of the radiation tumor myc gene is therefore consistent with the known effects of ionizing radiation on target DNA and the known mechanisms of myc activation. A more precise understanding of the role of myc gene activation in radiation carcinogenesis will depend on further research, including analysis of the rat skin myc gene at various times after irradiation.

It may be significant that the same transforming oncogene (K-ras) was activated in these rat skin carcinomas, as was found in mouse thymic lymphomas, the only other report of transforming oncogene activation n radiation induced tumors (18, 30). In contrast, chemically induced mouse skin carcinomas (20, 31) as well as the other tumors of epithelial origin (11, 14) contain activated H-ras. These results imply selectivity toward activation of particular ras genes by specific carcinogenic agents, such as ionizing radiation. Evidence for carcinogen specificity in transforming oncogene activation in experimental tumors has been observed in other systems (18, 32, 33).

Of the 6 malignant skin tumors tested in the NIH3T3 transfection assay, the 3 whose DNA were positive were of a similar poorly differentiated, non-keratinizing histologic type. The possibility that this model system can be used to examine the question of tissue specificity of oncogene activation within a single carcinogenic protocol in a single organ is being addressed by testing a larger panel of radiation induced rat skin tumors of different histologic types.

There is a great deal of evidence that carcinogenesis is a multistep process (34, 35). The finding that at least two active oncogenes are required to transform primary fibroblasts (9) has led to the hypothesis that particular stages of tumorigenesis are associated with activation of different oncogene classes. Balmain and his colleagues, for example, have found that the H-ras oncogene is mutationally activated in the pre-malignant papilloma stage of mouse skin chemical carcinogenesis (31).

Using the same tumor system we have found that the Moloney Murine Leukemia Virus LTR gene is expressed only in late stage malignant carcinomas (36).

Rat skin radiation carcinogenesis is clearly an excellent model for the study of activation of multiple oncogenes in individual etiologically defined tumors. Extension of the experiments reported here to a larger number of these tumors may provide useful information regarding the dynamics of activation of different oncogene classes during tumorigenesis.

The authors thank Dr. Peter D'Eustachio for his invaluable support and Drs. Arthur Upton and Arthur Penn for critical review of the manuscript. This work was supported by grant CA36342 from the National Cancer Institute and Contract #DE-AS02-76-EV03380 from DOE, and by Center Programs CA13343, from the National Cancer Institute and ES00260, from the National Institute of Environmental Health Sciences.

REFERENCES

1. F. J. Burns and R. E. Albert, in: "Radiation Carcinogenesis," A. Upton, F. Burns, and R. Shore, eds., Elsevier Science Publishing Co., New York, New York (1985), in press.

2. R. E. Albert, M. E. Phillps, P. Bennett, F. Burns, and R. Heimbach, Cancer Res. 29:658-668 (1969).

3. H. P. Lennhouts and K. H. Chadwick, Theor. Appl. Genet. 44:167-172 (1974).

4. W. S. Hayward, B. G. Neel, ad S. M. Astrin, Nature 290:475-480 (1981).

5. K. B. Marcu, et al., Proc. Natl. Acad. Sci. (USA) 80:519-523 (1983).

6. R. Dalla-Favera, S. Martinotti, and R. C. Gallo, Science 219:963-967 (1983).

7. G. Klein, Cell 32:311-315 (1983).

8. J. Cairns, Nature 289:353-357 (1981).

9. H. Land, L. F. Parada, ad R. A. Weinburg, Nature 304:596-602 (1983).

10. C. J. Tabin, et al., Nature 300:143-152 (1982).

11. J. Fujita, O. Yoshida, Y. Yuasa, J. S. Rhim, M. Hatanaka, and S. A. Aaronson, Nature 309:464-466 (1984).

12. A. Hall, C. J. Marshall, N. K. Spurr, ad R. A. Welss, Nature 303:396-400 (1983).

13. A. Eva and S. A. Aaronson, Science 220:955-956 (1983).

14. S. Sukumar, V. Notario, D. Martin-Zanca, and M. Barbacid, Nature 306:658-661 (1983).

15. E. P. Reddy, R. K. Reynolds, E. Santos, ad M. Barbacid, Nature 300:149-152 (1982).

16. E. Taparowsky, Y. Suard, O. Fasano, K. Shimizu, M. Goldfarb, and M. Wigler, Nature 300:762-765 (1982).

17. K. Shimizu, et al., Proc. Natl. Acad. Sci. (USA) 80:2112-2116 (1983).

18. I. Guerrero, P. Calzava, A. Mayer, and A. Pellicer, Proc. Natl. Acad. Sci. (USA) 81:202-205 (1984).

19. G. S. Payne, J. M. Bishop, and H. E. Varmus, Nature 295:209-214 (1982).

20. A. Balmain and I. B. Pragnell, Nature 303:72-74 (1983).

21. M. Wigler, A. Pellicer, S. Silverstein, R. Axel, G. Urlaub, and L. Chosin, Proc. Natl. Acad. Sci. (USA) 76:1373-1376 (1979).

22. E. M. Southern, J. Mol. Biol. 98:503-517 (1975).

23. J. M. Marrs and J. J. Voorhees, Invest. Dermatol. 56:174-181 (1971).

24. J. R. Feramisco, D. M. Helfman, J. E. Smart, K. Burridge, G. P. Thomas, J. Biol. Chem. 257:11024-11031 (1982).

25. M. Edmonds, M. H. Vaughn, and H. Nakazato, Proc. Natl. Acad. Sci. (USA) 68:1336-1340 (1971).

26. H. Aviv and P. Ceder, Proc. Natl. Acad. Sci. (USA) 69:1408-1412 (1972).

27. G. K. McMaster and G. G. Carmichael, Proc. Natl. Acad. Sci. (USA) 74:4835-4838 (1977).

28. P. S. Thomas, Proc. Natl. Acad. Sci. (USA) 77:5201-5205 (1980).

29. G. P. Margison and P. J. O'Connor, in: "Chemical Carcinogenesis and DNA, Vol. 1," P. L. Grover, CRC Press, Boca Raton, Florida (1979), pp. 111-159.

30. I. Guerrero, A. Villasante, V. Corces, and A. Pellicer, Science 225:1159-1162 (1984).

31. A. Balmain, M. Ramsden, G. T. Bowden, and S. Smith, Nature 307:658-660 (1984).

32. S. J. Garte, A. T. Hood, A. E. Hochwalt, C. A. Snyder, and A. Segal, Proc. Amer. Assoc. Cancer Res. (1985), in press.

33. H. Zarbl, S. Sukumar, A. V. Arthur, D. Martin-Zanca, and M. Barbacid, Nature 315:382-385 (1985).

34. I. Berenblum, and P. Shubik, Br.J. Cancer 1:388 (1947).

35. R. K. Boutwell, Crit. Rev. Toxicol. 2:419-443 (1974).

36. G. Hausey, P. Kirschmeier, S. J. Garte, F. J. Burns, W. Troll, and I. B. Weinstein, Biochem. Biophys. Res. Commun. 127:391-398 (1985).

MUTAGENESIS IN MAMMALIAN GERMS CELLS BY RADIATION OR NITROGEN

MUSTARD--A COMPARATIVE STUDY*

Lawrence S. Goldstein

Department of Radiation Oncology
University of California
San Francisco, CA 94143

ABSTRACT

The dominant lethal mutant rate was determined in mouse embryos
fertilized by spermatozoa that were derived from spermatogonia treated with
nitrogen mustard, gamma radiation or accelerated neon ions. The doses
chosen (2.0 mg/kg nitrogen mustard, 1.8 Gy ^{137}Cs and 0.65 Gy neon) gave an
isoeffect when the dominant lethal mutant rate was evaluated in embryos
fertilized by spermatozoa that were treated in the sensitive spermatid
stage.

An in vitro methodology was employed. Male mice were mated 35 or more
days after treatment. The 2-cell stage embryos were removed from the
female and cultured for a total of 7 days during which time they develop to
an early postimplantation stage. The frequency of successful development to
the trophectoderm outgrowth stage was used as the index of mutation
induction.

Although each treatment gave essentially the same mutant rate in
treated spermatids, the mutant rate in treated spermatogonia seemed to be
different. These rates were 1.5% for cesium, -2.7% for neon, and 8.3% for
nitrogen mustard. Although none of these rates were significantly
different than controls, other data suggest that neon and nitrogen mustard
do induce dominant lethal mutations in spermatogonia. When a higher dose of
neon was tested, the dominant lethal rate increased to 19%. When a more
sensitive endpoint (the frequency of inner cell mass differentiation) was
used to evaluate nitrogen mustard induced mutations, a rate of 11% was
found. Both these rates are significant.

These results indicate that the in vitro method can detect mutagenesis
by drugs or radiation at clinically relevant doses.

*This work supported by Grant CA 30995 from the National Cancer Institute,
Department of Human and Health Services.

INTRODUCTION

Patients who have been cured of their primary neoplasm by aggressive radiotherapy or chemotherapy are at a substantially higher risk for secondary neoplasms than are patients treated with less aggressive approaches. The risk of a second neoplasm is especially high in patients treated with more than one modality, either for the management of primary disease or for adjuvant therapy to prevent a future recurrence (1). While an aggressive approach increases curability, this treatment-related carcinogenic risk must be addressed when considering the quality of life in the cured patient.

Treatment-related neoplasms have been well documented in Hodgkin's patients who have been cured of their disease (2). Often the neoplasm is a leukemia that histologically is characterized by numerous structural and numerical chromosome aberrations. Similar clastogenic changes can be induced by chemotherapeutic drugs or radiation in spermatogonial stem cells and can be detected as dominant lethal mutations in offspring fertilized by spermatozoa derived from damaged progenitor cells (3-5). Analysis of dominant lethal mutations might therefore be a useful way by which potential carcinogen risk can be accurately predicted.

Dominant lethal mutations are expressed as developmental arrest of the embryo before or soon after implantation. In vivo it is difficult to separate mutational events from non-fertilization since both are manifest as a reduction in the average number of implantations. A system has been developed to overcome this problem: embryos sired by treated or control males are removed surgically from the female soon after fertilization. The embryos are then grown in vitro using media that permit normal growth and differentiation through an early implantation stage. The frequency of successful development in vitro is used as the measure of dominant lethality. This assay has been applied to studies of mutation induction by radiation (3) or drugs (4, 5).

In this study I compare the dominant lethal mutant rate in spermatogonia treated with gamma radiation, densely ionizing charged particle radiation, or the chemotherapeutic drug mechlorethamine (nitrogen mustard) to one another. I have attempted to tailor the doses to levels that cause the same amount of initial mutagenic damage in the testis. The data indicate that the mutagenic risk to the spermatogonial stem cell is different for these different mutagens.

MATERIALS AND METHODS

Male ICR mice were divided into three treatment groups. The first group was irradiated in a self-contained 2000 Ci ^{137}Cs source. The dose rate, determined with LiF thermoluminescent dosimeters in paraffin phantoms was 2.17 Gy/min. Groups of 40 were irradiated with 0.90, 1.80, 2.70, 3.60, or 4.50 Gy; 40 unirradiated mice served as controls. The second group was irradiated with accelerated neon ions generated by the Bevalac accelerator of the Lawrence Berkeley Laboratory of the University of California. A 557 MeV/amu beam of ions was scattered by a 3/64-inch thick lead filter to a spot size of 5 cm. The Bragg peak was spread to 10 cm by a rotating spiral brass ridge filter. Mice were localized in the distal peak region and irradiated with a pelvic field. Doses of 0.65, 1.25, 1.90, 2.50, and 3.15 Gy were administered at a dose rate of approximately 1.2 Gy/min. The dose and dose rate were measured by ion chambers set in the beam path. 200 experimental and 40 control mice were used. The third group of mice was injected with nitrogen mustard to final doses of 0.3, 1.2, 2.1, 3.0, and

3.9 mg/kg body weight. Injections were by the tail vein. The size of the groups was in the irradiation experiments.

Eight days after treatment and for the next two weeks (to assay damage to the spermatid stage), the males were mated to females that has been induced to superovulate by injection with 5.0 IU Pregnant Mares' Serum followed 48 hours later by 5.0 IU of human Chorionic Gonadotrophin. On the morning following mating, the females were checked for the presence of a vaginal plug. Plugged females were housed for an additional day. They were then killed and their oviducts removed and placed in drops of modified L-15 medium (6). Embryos at the 2-cell stage were removed by gently irrigating the oviducts with modified L-15. The embryos were counted and transferred in groups of about 150 to organ culture dishes containing 0.5 ml Standard Egg Culture Medium (after Biggers, ref. 7). They were incubated for 3 days during which time they normally develop to the blastocyst stage. Blastocysts were counted and transferred in groups of 20 to each well of an 8-chambered tissue culture slide containing 0.25 ml Modified Eagles' Medium (8). After an additional 4 days of incubation, the number of blastocysts that developed to the trophectoderm outgrowth (TBOG) stage was determined. All incubations were at $37^{\circ}C$ in 5% CO_2.

Matings and embryo culture were performed 8, 11, 15, 18, and 21 days after treatment. The data for each treatment group for these days were pooled and the dominant lethal mutant rate determined by:

$$1 - \frac{(\text{TBOG/2-cell stage, exp})}{(\text{TBOG/2-cell stage, cont})}$$

The doses necessary to give a dominant lethal mutant rate of 20% were determined and mice in these irradiation groups were retained for further study. Nitrogen-mustard-treated mice could not be retained and a new group of mice (40 experimental and 40 control) were enrolled. Matings were reinitiated 35, 38, 42, 45, 49, 52, 56, 59, 63, 66, and 70 days after treatment using the above protocol. The dominant lethal mutant rate was determined for pooled data from these matings.

RESULTS AND DISCUSSION

Dominant lethality was detected in offspring of males treated 8 to 21 days earlier with ^{137}Cs, accelerated neon ions and mechlorethamine. The dominant lethal mutant rate increased linearly with increasing dose (Figure 1). The shape of the induction curve is consistent with the single-event nature of the presumed damage. Primary damage of this kind includes deletions, inversions, and acentric fragments. Another interpretation is that the repair of mutagenic lesions is defective in post-meiotic stages and that the induction curve approaches linearity with increasing dose. Spermatids treated with alkylating agents have been reported to be defective in unscheduled DNA synthesis, a measure of repair (9).

Often primary damage (i.e., damage to a single chromosome) is lethal in replicating cells. If the treatments caused cell killing in spermatids, it was not of sufficient magnitude to impair fertilization since the fertilization rate (the ratio of 2-cell stage embryos to total ova) was unaffected, even at the highest doses. In the absence of cell killing, and because even grossly genomically imbalanced spermatozoa have a normal fertilization rate (10), the dominant lethal mutant rate in embryos fertilized by spermatozoa derived from treated spermatids can serve as an index of the clastogenicity of the test treatment. Taking this argument one step further, an isoeffect level of mutation induction in this stage may be an indicator of equal levels of initial chromosomal damage by these agents.

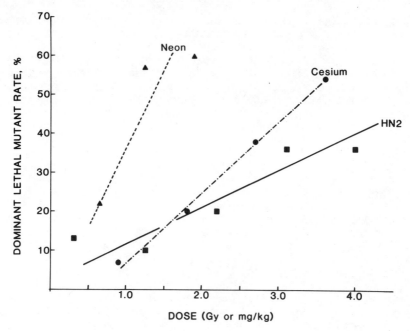

Fig. 1. The dominant lethal mutant rate for spermatozoa derived from spermatids treated with ^{137}Cs (0.9-4.5 Gy)●, accelerated neon ions (0.65-1.90 Gy)▲, or mechlorethamine (HN$_2$, 0.3-3.9 mg/kg)■.

When mouse embryos are irradiated directly, the time of developmental arrest is correlated with dose. As the dose increases, the embryos arrest at progressively earlier stages (11). This suggests that forms of damage that prevent cell division require more than one hit or involve damage to more than one chromosome. Because I find that the dominant lethal mutations are expressed at all developmental stages and not preferentially in an early developmental stage over the range of radiation and chemical doses tested, I conclude that the fertilizing spermatozoa carry primary chromosomal damage and damage to more than one chromosome or multiple damage within a single chromosome do not contribute significantly to the dominant lethal mutant rate in spermatids.

The dominant lethal mutant rates for spermatozoa derived from spermatogonia treated with 1.80 Gy of ^{137}Cs, 0.65 Gy of accelerated neon ions and 2.0 mg/kg mechlorethamine (the doses that gave a dominant lethal mutant rate of 20% in spermatids (Figure 1) were determined. The rate of dominant lethal mutants for spermatogonia treated at these doses was much less than that found for treated spermatids (Table 1). This observation has been reported for radiation (3) and drugs (12) and reflects the culling of primary chromosomal damage in mitosis and meiosis. Although oligospermia was almost certainly induced, the fertilization rate was not affected. The mutant rates were not significant by parametric (t-test) or non-parametric (Man-Whitney u-test) evaluations.

Other data (not shown) suggest that a 1.25 Gy dose of accelerated neon ions results in a significant 19% dominant lethal mutant rate. Higher doses gave higher rates. The kinetics of induction can be described adequately by a linear function of dose, and it seems likely that if a study were undertaken to specifically demonstrate mutagenesis by a 0.65 Gy dose, significant mutation induction would be detected.

Table 1. Dominant lethal mutant rate in spermatogonia

TREATMENT (DOSE)	DLM RATE
CESIUM (1.8 Gy)	-2.1%[1] $1.4 \pm 4.6\%$[2]
NEON IONS (0.65 Gy)	3.4%[1] $-2.7 \pm 6.2\%$[2]
NITROGEN MUSTARD (2.25 mg/kg)	7.9%[1] $8.3 \pm 4.2\%$[2]

[1] determined by considering data from 35-70 days post-treatment as a single sample i.e.

$$dlm = 1 - \left[\frac{(\Sigma TBOG/\Sigma 2\text{-cell})\ exp.\ day\ 35\text{-}70)}{(\Sigma TBOG/\Sigma 2\text{-cell})\ cont.\ day\ 35\text{-}70)} \right]$$

[2] determined from the dlm rates from data for days 35-70 post-treatment i.e.

$$dlm = \frac{(dlm\ day\ 35 + dlm\ day\ 39 + ... + dlm\ day\ 70)}{n}$$

where n is the number of samplings; uncertainties are standard errors.

Improvements in the culture system allowed me to use the criteria of inner cell mass formation in the TBOG as a measure of dominant lethality in mice treated with mechlorethamine. This endpoint is more sensitive than TBOG formation, and a highly significant ($p = .002$, u-test) 13% mutant rate was detected in spermatogonia treated with 2.0 mg/kg mechlorethamine.

Dominant lethal mutants were not detected in offspring of Cesium-irradiated mice even at doses as high as 4.50 Gy.

Because dominant lethality in spermatogonia is thought to reflect secondary damage (i.e., reciprocal translocations and other two-event aberrations), I conclude that mechlorethamine and accelerated neon ions either induce these kinds of clastogenic damage more readily than does ^{137}Cs, or that fewer cells with secondary chromosomal damage are culled during spermatogenesis when mechlorethamine or accelerated neon ions is the damaging agent. The higher mutant rate may, therefore, be due to quantitative or qualitative differences in the nature of induced chromosomal damage.

These studies indicate that clinically relevant levels of accelerated neon radiation or mechlorethamine can result in detectable levels of stable chromosomal damage to the stem cell spermatogonia. It seems reasonable to conclude that mutagenic damage would also be induced in somatic cells and that this damage could result in neoplastic transformation.

REFERENCES

1. C. N. Coleman, Adverse effects of cancer therapy: The risk of secondary neoplasms, Am. J. Pediatr. Hematol. Oncol. 4:103-111 (1982).

2. C. N. Coleman, Secondary neoplasms in patients treated for cancer: Etiology and perspective, Radiat. Res. 92:188-200 (1984).

3. L. S. Goldstein, A. I. Spindle, and R. A. Pedersen, Detection of X-ray-induced dominant lethal mutations in mice: An in vitro approach, Mutat. Res. 41:289-296 (1976).

4. L. S. Goldstein, Methyl methanesulfonate-induced dominant lethal mutations in male mice detected in vitro. Mutat. Res. 42:135-138 (1977).

5. L. S. Goldstein, Dominant lethal mutations induced in mouse spermatogonia by antineoplastic drugs, Mutat. Res. 140:193-197 (1984).

6. A. Leibovitz, The growth and maintenance of tissue cell cultures in free gas exchange with the atmosphere, Amer. J. Hyg. 78:173-180 (1963).

7. L. S. Goldstein, A. I. Spindle, and R. A. Pedersen, X-ray sensitivity of the preimplantation mouse embryo in vitro, Radiat. Res. 62:276-287 (1975).

8. A. I. Spindle and R. A. Pedersen, Hatching, attachment and outgrowth of mouse blastocysts in vitro: Fixed nitrogen requirements, J. Exptl. Zool. 186:305-318 (1973).

9. G. A. Sega, Unscheduled DNA synthesis in the germ cells of male mice exposed in vivo to the chemical mutagen ethyl methane sulfonate, Proc. Natl. Acad. Sci. (USA) 71:4955-4959 (1974).

10. C. E. Ford, Gross genome imbalance in mouse spermatozoa: Does it influence the capacity to fertilize?, in: "Proc. Int. Symp. The Genetics of the Spermatozoon," R. A. Beatty and S. Gluesksonh-Waelsch, eds., Churchill, London (1972), pp. 359-369.

11. L. B. Russell, Death and chromosome damage from irradiation of preimplantation stages, in: "Preimplanatation Stages of Pregnancy," G. E. W. Wolstenholme and M. O'Conner, eds., Churchill, London (1965), pp. 217-241.

12. U. H. Ehling, Differential spermatogenic response of male mice to the induction of mutations by antineoplastic drugs, Mutat. Res., 26:285-295 (1974).

GENE AMPLIFICATION IN MAMMALIAN CELLS AFTER EXPOSURE TO IONIZING RADIATION AND UV

Christine Lucke-Huhle and Peter Herrlich

Kernforschungszentrum Karlsruhe
Institut fur Genetik und Toxikologie
P.O. Box 3640
D-7500 Karlsruhe 1
Federal Republic of Germany

Since the initial observations (1, 2), gene amplifications have been detected in several organisms and cell cultures (review: 3). One system has been studied extensively: The development of resistance to methotrexate (MTX). This resistance is associated with the amplification of the gene for the methotrexate target enzyme, dihydrofolate reductase (4). In this system, the spontaneous rate of gene amplification has been determined to 10^{-3} events per cell division (5). Amplification is enhanced not only by MTX treatment but also by other agents which affect nucleotide metabolism (3), or by treatment of cells with tumor promoters or mutagens (6, 7). The amplification goes along with the appearance of unstable chromosomal structures called double minute chromosomes (8), or of stably integrated homogeneously staining regions (9).

Our interest is concentrated on early genetic responses to carcino-genic treatment that occur at higher frequency than mutation (10). Gene amplifications are much more frequent than point mutations. They have also been detected in the end products of carcinogenic pathways: in human tumors (11).

Our study is directed towards characterizing the mechanism of gene amplification induced by irradiation. We report here that: (1) various types of ionizing radiation and ultraviolet light induce the amplification of integrated SV40 sequences in Chinese hamster cells (in the absence of virus production), (2) human skin fibroblasts of a patient with Ataxia telangiectasia amplify the DHFR gene in response to 4 MeV alpha irradiation while amplification of the gene in fibroblasts of a normal individual was below detection level, and (3) the amplification of genes seems to be mediated by a TRANS acting mechanism.

AMPLIFICATION OF INTEGRATED SV40 DNA IN CHINESE HAMSTER EMBRYO CELLS

In order to compare and quantitate the effect of different types of radiation on gene amplification, a cell line is used that has been shown to reach high degrees of amplification after treatment with chemical

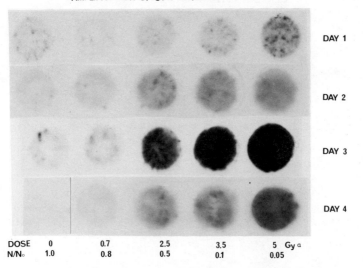

AMPLIFICATION OF SV40 SEQUENCES AFTER α

DAY 1

DAY 2

DAY 3

DAY 4

DOSE	0	0.7	2.5	3.5	5 Gy α
N/Nₒ	1.0	0.8	0.5	0.1	0.05

Fig. 1.   Autoradiogram showing the increase in SV40 DNA in
Chinese hamster embryo cells (Co631) after
exposure to 3.4 MeV alpha particles. At various
times after irradiation cells were trypsinized and
samples of 5×10^5 cells were trapped on
nitrocellulose filters. Cells were lysed and
their DNA was denatured and hybridized against
^{32}P-SV40 DNA as described by Lavi et Etkin (12).
The cpm of the filters were determined by liquid
scintillation spectrometry.

carcinogens (12): SV40 transformed Chinese hamster embryo cells (Co 631;
courtesy S. Lavi). Co 631 cells contain 5 SV40 copies per haploid cell
genome. These SV40 sequences are taken as an example for an endogenous
gene. The amplification is measured by the dispersed-cell-assay (12). As
will be shown (Figures 1-3), all types of radiation used: alpha particles,
gamma rays, and UV induce amplification of integrated SV40 sequences in a
dose-dependent manner. Amplification is not accompanied by virus
production.

241-AMERICIUM ALPHA PARTICLES

Monolayers of Co 631 cells are exposed to alpha particles through the
bottom of the culture dish (13). The energy of the particles at the bottom
surface is 3.4 MeV corresponding to 120 keV/μm, the dose rate being 0.35
Gy/min. The cells react with a rapid increase in the amount of SV40
sequences per cell (Figure 1). The increase is dose-dependent and already
detectable at day 1 after irradiation. Maximum amplification is reached at
day 3 (15 fold after 5 Gy).

COBALT-GAMMA-RAYS

Co 631 cells amplify the SV40 sequences also after exposure to 60-
Cobalt gamma rays (1.1 Gy/min). The amplification is dose dependent but
starts more slowly as compared to alpha irradiation (Figure 2). Maximum
amplification is reached at day 6 (20 fold after 12 Gy). The number of SV40
copies decreases thereafter (not shown).

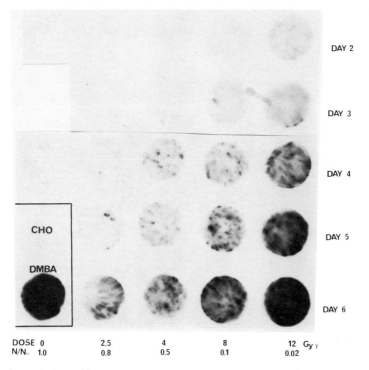

Fig. 2.   Autoradiogram showing the increase in SV40 DNA in Chinese hamster embryo cells (Co631) after exposure to ^{60}Cobalt-γ-rays. Cells were assayed as described in Figure 1. Two additional controls (see insert) are included: (1) background control with 5×10^5 untransformed Chinese hamster ovary cells (CHO) and (2) positive control after treatment with the chemical carcinogen DMBA (Dimethylbenz(a)anthrazene).

UV LIGHT

Increasing doses of UV light lead to amplification already detectable at day (1) (Figure 3). With $5 \ J/m^2$ a dose optimum is reached, larger doses are less effective. Maximum copy number is found at day 3 (28 fold after 5 J/m^2).

A comparison (at equal survival level) between all three types of radiation used, show UV light to amplify most efficiently the integrated SV40 sequences. Altogether, however, the results with Co 631 cells demonstrate that various types of DNA damage, caused by either ionizing radiation or UV, can trigger amplification. We have not been able to detect amplification of the DHFR or ACTIN gene in this cell lines.

IMPORTANCE OF INTACT VIRAL ORIGIN OF REPLICATION AND LARGE T ANTIGEN

For the amplification process, a functional origin of replication of the viral replicon is required. Chinese hamster cells transformed with SV40 mutants, of which either the viral origin of replication is deleted or

407

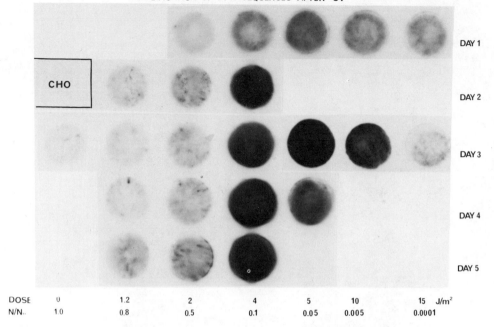

AMPLIFICATION OF SV40 SEQUENCES AFTER UV

DOSE	0	1.2	2	4	5	10	15 J/m²
N/N₀	1.0	0.8	0.5	0.1	0.05	0.005	0.0001

Fig. 3. Autoradiogram showing the increase in SV40 DNA in Chinese hamster embryo cells (Co631) after exposure to UV light (2537 Å). Cells were assayed as described in Figure 1. Background control (insert): untransformed CHO cells.

the viral A gene carries a mutation rendering its gene product thermosensitive in its ability to initiate viral replication, are incapable of amplifying SV40 DNA. In case of the temperature sensitivity, only at the permissive temperature of 33°C SV40 DNA is amplified and not at 39°C. We conclude from that, that it is the viral origin of replication which is initiated again and again by DNA damage.

GENE AMPLIFICATION - A CIS OR TRANS EFFECT?

The characteristic energy distribution of the alpha particles permits to derive from calculations a rough estimate of whether the amplification is caused by damage within or near the SV40 sequences, or whether DNA damage distant from the amplified site leads to the observed amplification.

If the nucleus is considered to extend 8 μm in diameter and the DNA packing density to be 4.6%, a dose of 2.5 Gy corresponds to about 250 hits within the mammalian DNA (1 hit is defined as the traverse of an alpha particle through one DNA fiber). Assuming a statistical distribution of the hits, it is rather improbable that SV40 sequences are hit directly in a significant number of cells. This is easily seen in considering the following comparison:

$$\text{SV40 genome:} \qquad \sim 5 \times 10^3 \text{bp}$$

$$\text{total target if 5 SV40 copies:} \qquad \sim 2.5 \times 10^4 \text{bp}$$

$$\text{mammalian cell DNA:} \qquad \sim 5 \times 10^9 \text{bp}$$

$$\text{hit Probability for SV40 sequences:} \qquad \underline{1 : 1000\ 000}$$

408

A DOT HYBRIDIZATION:

GM637

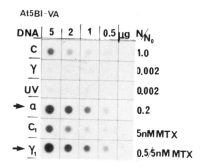

DNA	5	2	1	0.5 µg	N/N_0
C					1.0
γ					0.04
UV					0.002
a					0.2
a					0.002
C_1					5nM MTX
C_2					50nM MTX
Y_1					0.5/5nM MTX

At5BI-VA

DNA	5	2	1	0.5 µg	N/N_0
C					1.0
γ					0.002
UV					0.002
→ a					0.2
C_1					5nM MTX
→ Y_1					0.5/5nM MTX

B SOUTHERN B

GM637

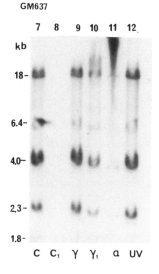

At5BI-VA

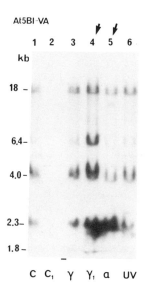

Fig. 4. A) Autoradiogram showing dot hybridization of total DNA from SV40-transformed human skin fibroblasts (GM637) and SV40 transformed Ataxia cells (At5BI-VA), isolated 3 days after exposure to various types of radiation (α = 3.4 MeV alpha particles, γ = [60]Cobalt- -rays, UV = UV light, C = unirradiated control). Various amounts of cellular DNA (0.5-5 µg) were trapped on nitrocellulose, denatured by alkali and hybridized to ^{32}P-labelled DHFR (dihydrofolate reductase) c-DNA. MTX = methotrexate.

B) Autoradiogram of Southern blots: The same DNA's as in Figure 4A were digested with restriction endonuclease EcoRI. Total DNA fragments (10 µg) were loaded onto a 0.8% agarose gel, separated by electrophoresis, transferred to nitrocellulose and hybridized to ^{32}P-labelled DHFR c-DNA. The scale in kilobases was derived from the location of restriction fragments of known length detected in a separate track of the same gel.

We conclude, that the amplification of genes is mediated by a TRANS acting mechanism. DNA damage at any site in the mammalian genome induces amplification of the integrated SV40 sequences.

GENE AMPLIFICATION IN ATAXIA CELLS

Since gene amplification might be a step in carcinogenesis, we examined cells from a patient with the high-cancer-risk syndrome Ataxia telangiectasia for their ability to amplify genes in response to radiation. SV40 transformed Ataxia cells (AT5BI-VA, courtesy A. Lehman) and SV40-transformed skin fibroblasts from a healthy donor (GM637) were irradiated with either alpha particles, gamma rays or UV light. The DNA was examined 3 days after irradiation by dot blot and Southern transfer hybridization (Figure 4). By using a DHFR (dihydrofolate reductase) gene probe for hybridization, no amplification is detectable in the normal fibroblasts (GM637). In Ataxia cells, however, the DHFR gene is amplified about 4 fold after alpha irradiation or following gamma irradiation with subsequent selection by 5 nM methotrexate. We have not been able to detect amplification of SV40 sequences, possibly due to a defective origin of replication. Digestion of the various DNA's with restriction enzyme Eco RI yields 5 bands of 18, 6.4, 4.0, 2.3, and 1.8 kb. While methotrexate selection enforces the amplification of all fragment (Figure 4, track 4), alpha irradiation alone leads to an increase of the 2.3 kb band mainly (track 5). Possibly this fragment is closest to an origin of replication, amplification does not necessarily include the complete replicon.

DISCUSSION

The recognition of ionizing radiation as a carcinogen evolved soon after the discovery by Roentgen in 1895. Oncogenic transformation is a complex process (14): It involves at least two steps: An initiation step - presumably an irreversible DNA alteration - and a second promotion step leading to the characteristic morphological changes of a tumor cell. According to current ideas, one could imagine that amplification of oncogenes themselves, or rearrangement of sequences subsequent to amplification (15) and the change in the expression of critical genes in the neighborhood, leads to the formation of a cancer cell.

ACKNOWLEDGEMENTS

We wish to thank Professor H. Dertinger for helping with the hit calculations and Miss Monika Pech for her excellent technical assistance.

REFERENCES

1. F. M. Ritossa, Natl. Acad. Sci. (USA) 60:509-516 (1968).

2. D. D. Brown and I. B. Dawid, Science 160:272-280 (1968).

3. R. T. Schimke, Cell 37:705-713 (1984).

4. R. T. Schimke, F. W. Alt, R. E. Kellems, R. Kaufman, and J. R. Bertino, Cold Spring Harbor Symp. Quant. Biol. 62:649-657 (1978).

5. R. N. Johnston, S. M. Beverley, and R. T. Schmike, Proc. Natl. Acad. Sci. (USA) 80:3711-3715 (1983).

6. A. Varshavsky, _Cell_ 25:561-572 (1981).

7. S. Lavi, _Proc._ _Natl._ _Acad._ _Sci._ _(USA)_ 78:6144-5148 (1981).

8. J. L. Biedler and B. A. Spengler, _Science_ 191:185-187 (1976).

9. G. Balaban-Malenbaum and F. Gilbert, _Science_ 198:739-742 (1977).

10. P. Herrlich, P. Angel, C. Lucke-Huhle, N. Harth, A. Eades, and H. J. Rahmsdorf, _Adv._ _in_ _Enzyme_ _Regulation_ 25: (1986) in press.

11. J. Whang-Peng, C. S. Kao-Shan, E. C. Lee, P. A. Bunn, D. N. Carney, A. F. Gazdar, C. Portlock, and J. D. Minna, _in:_ "Gene Amplification," Cold Spring Harbor Laboratory (1982), pp. 107-113.

12. S. Lavi and S. Etkin, _Carcinogenesis_ 2:417-423 (1981).

13. C. Lucke-Huhle, W. Comper, L. Hieber, and M. Pech, _Radiat._ _Environm._ _Biophys._ 20:171-185 (1982).

14. J. Cairns, "UCLA Symposium on Molecular and Cellular Biology New Series, Vol. 2," Alan R. Liss, Inc., New York (1982), pp. 559-562.

15. C. J. Bostock and C. Tyler-Smith, _in:_ "Gene Amplification," Cold Spring Harbor Laboratory (1982), pp. 15-21.

REGULATION OF GENE EXPRESSION AT THE TRANSLATIONAL LEVEL IN PLANT EMBRYO

A. S. N. Reddy, S. Gunnery, and A. Datta

Molecular Biology Unit
School of Life Sciences
Jawaharlal Nehru University
New Delhi - 110 067
India

ABSTRACT

In barley embryos certain mRNAs are synthesized during embryogenesis and stored to be utilized during germination. This kind of temporal separation of transcription and translation involves a fine regulation at the level of translation. In our attempt to understand the regulation of translation of stored messages, we have isolated translation inhibitors (protein and RNA) from barley embryos. The presence of these translational inhibitors could be the reason for inefficiency of the barley embryo cell-free translation system, in spite of the presence of stable translatable mRNA, large store of eukaryotic initiation factor-2 (a rate limiting initiation factor of protein synthesis), ribosomes and other components of translational machinery. Protein inhibitor is a cAMP-independent protein kinase which resembles mammalian casein kinase II. A protein of molecular weight of 52,000, isolated from barley extract by using purified protein kinase-immobilized column, serves as much better substrate than exogenous substrates. Antibodies against protein kinase have been raised to study the molecular mechanism of inhibition. RNA inhibitor is a small weight species (smaller than tRNA) that inhibits initiation of translation. It is a single stranded RNA with no long poly(A) sequence. In the light of the above findings, regulation of gene expression at the translational level in plant embryo is discussed.

INTRODUCTION

The existence of stored mRNA in higher plant seeds has been well established (see review 1). This stored mRNA is synthesized during embryogenesis and utilized for protein synthesis during germination. However, the manner by which mRNA is stored is not known. Moreover, the phenomenon of temporal separation of transcription and translation which is found to be associated with many developing organisms (2, 3), serves as a good model system to study the regulation of gene expression at the translational level.

413

In this paper we show that barley embryo has processed and translatable stored mRNA. We have also demonstrated the presence of two translational inhibitors in barley embryo - a cAMP - independent protein kinase and a small molecular weight RNA.

EXPERIMENTAL PROCEDURES

Embryos were excised manually from barley seeds for germination experiments, whereas for preparative purposes, embryos were isolated as described by Marcus (4). Incorporation of (^{3}H)-Leucine (1.3 Ci/mmole) and (^{3}H)-uridine (7.5 Ci/mmole) into proteins and RNA during germination was measured as described earlier (5). Poly(A)-RNA was isolated by the method of Brawerman (6). S_{30} extract of wheat germ (Nilback, Rochester, N.Y.) was prepared (7) and translation of Poly(A) mRNA was carried out as described (5). Eukaryotic initiation factor-2 (eIF-2) was assayed by monitoring ternary complex formation (eIF-2. GTP. Met-tRNA) as described (8). Protein kinase assay was done using casein as substrate based on the method of Datta et al. (9). Rabbit reticulocyte lysate was prepared according to the procedure of Gilbert and Anderson (10). Translation assays were done as described earlier (11). Reticulocyte lysate was only used to investigate the effect of protein kinase and small molecular weight RNA. ^{32}P labelled ATP was synthesized according to Glynn and Chappel (12) with slight modifications. Sepharose 6B was activated with cyanogen bromide (13) and casein was coupled to activated Sepharose 6B as described by Thornberg and Lindell (14).

Purification of Protein Kinase 15 gm of embryos were ground in PK buffer (20 mM Tris-HCl, pH 7.6, 3 mM Mg(OAC)$_2$ and 1 mM DTT) and the homogenate was centrifuged at 35,000 xg for 30 min. The supernatant containing 1580 mg of protein was filtered through muslin cloth and applied onto a casein-Sepharose column (1.5 x 10 cm) which was previously equilibrated with PK buffer. The column was extensively washed with PK buffer and bound material was eluted with PK buffer containing 0.5 M KCl. Peak fractions of activity were pooled and dialyzed. Precipitate that was formed during dialysis was removed by centrifugation at 5000 xg for 5 min. The dialyzed preparation was then applied onto a DE52 column (1.5 x 8 cm) which was previously equilibrated with PK buffer. The column was washed with buffer and eluted with 100 ml of 0-500 mM linear KCl gradient in PK buffer. 2.5 ml fractions were collected and assayed for activity. Bound protein eluted as single peak at 0.2-0.3 M KCl concentration with which enzyme activity was correlated. The endogenous substrate for this kinase was isolated as described (15).

Isolation of Inhibitor RNA Embryos were homogenized in a buffer containing 20 mM Tris-Cl, pH 7.6, 10 mM KCl and 200 µg/ml heparin and centrifuged at 27,000 x g for 15 min. Supernatant was collected and centrifuged at 150,000 x g for 4.5 h. The resultant supernatant was again centrifuged at 255,000 x g for 4 h. and RNA was extracted from 255,000 x g supernatant by the method of Palmiter (16) with some modifications. The ratio of A260 to A280 of the RNA is about 2 indicating the absence of protein as a contaminant. The RNA was electrophoresced on 12% polyacrylamide gel containing 6 M urea and ethidium bromide stained bands were cut and RNA was eluted by shaking overnight in 100 mM Tris-Cl pH 7.5, 500 mM NaCl and 0.01% SDS at 37°C. Eluted RNA was precipitated with ethanol at -20°C overnight. The precipitate was dried and dissolved in sterile water.

For sucrose density gradient analysis, 100 µl translation assay mixture was incubated at 30°C for 10 min. The reaction was stopped, layered on a linear 15-30% sucrose density gradient and centrifuged as

414

described by Darnbrough et al (17). Fractions were collected and
absorbance at 260 nm of 50 µl of each fraction in 1 ml water was taken. 50
l of each fraction was also precipitated in 1 ml cold 5% TCA and kept in a
boiling water bath for 20 min. The precipitate was then collected on
Whatman GF/C filter, dried, and counted.

<u>Antisera Preparation</u> Purified protein kinase (240 µg) was emulsified
with little over one volume of Freund's complete adjuvant and injected
subcutaneously at multiple sites on the back of New Zealand white rabbit.
A second injection of 160 µg protein kinase in incomplete Freund's adjuvant
was injected in the same way after a gap of 3 weeks. Rabbit was bled from
the ear and serum was separated. Ouchterlony immunodiffusion tests were
done as described (18).

RESULTS AND DISCUSSION

Incorporation studies with (^{3}H-leucine and (^{3}H)-uridine into proteins
and RNA, respectively in presence and absence of inhibitors demonstrated
that (i) in barley embryos, protein synthesis starts within 15 min of
commencement of germination. Actinomycin D (20 µg/ml), a known inhibitor
of RNA synthesis and cordycepin (20 µg/ml), an inhibitor of polyadenylation
of mRNA, have no effect on protein synthesis whereas cyclohexamide inhibits
the same (Figure 1A). (ii) The synthesis of RNA starts after a lag period
of 2 h. However, mRNA synthesis (α-amanitin sensitive RNA) is detectable
only after 8 h of germination. RNA synthesis during the period of 2-8 h of
germination is insensitive to α-amanitin indicating the synthesis of
ribosomal RNA (Figure 1B). We have also observed that early protein

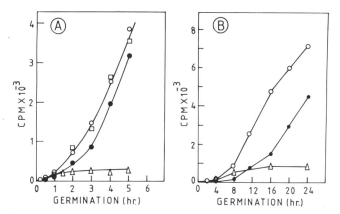

Fig. 1. A: Effect of protein and RNA Synthesis inhibitors on
incorporation of (^{3}H)-leucine into proteins by barley embryos
during germination. Control (O—O), with cycloheximide
(△—△), with actinomycin D (□—□) and with cordycepin (●—●).

B: Effect of α-amanitin and cylcloheximide on incorporation of
(^{3}H)-uridine into RNA during germination of barley embryos. The
α-amanitin sensitive fraction was calculated by subtacting the
resistant values from the total counts. With cycloheximide
(△—△), α-amanitin resistant (O—O) α-amanitin sensitive
(●—●).

synthesis is essential for RNA synthesis. These observations clearly
suggest that barley embryos contain stored mRNA which is polyadenylated and
protein synthesis during early phase of germination (0-8h) is due to the
presence of this stored mRNA.

It is not known as to how the messages are selectively recruited and
stored and also how the translation of stored mRNA is prevented until
germination. In order to understand the regulation of translation of
stored mRNA, we have investigated (i) whether the stored mRNA is processed
and translatable; (ii) the levels of eukaryotic initiation factor (eIF-2),
an important protein factor involved in initiation of protein synthesis,
during embryogenesis and germination and (iii) the presence of
translational inhibitors.

We could isolate poly(A)-mRNA from dry embryos using poly(U) Sepharose
column which is active in wheat germ cell-free translation system (Table
1). This result gives further evidence for the fact that stored mRNA in
barley embryos is processed and translatable. However, in case of cotton

Table 1. *In vitro* protein synthesis by poly (A)-RNA from dry embryo.

RNA added (μg)	Counts/min
0	620
1.5	3,866
3	8,308
6	15,820

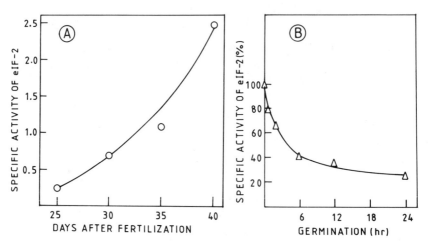

Fig. 2. eIF-2 activity in barley embryos during (A) embryogenesis
and (B) germination. 100% corresponds to a specific
activity (number of pmoles of (^{3}H)Met-tRNA$_i$ retained on
nitrocelulose filter per milligram protein) of 2.06 at 0h
germination.

416

cotyledons it has been reported that stored mRNA is not processed until germination (19).

As shown in Figure 2A, the amount of eIF-2 activity during early stages of embryogenesis is very low but increases rapidly after 30 days of fertilization resulting in high amount of eIF-2 in dry embryos. However, this high level of eIF-2 in dry embryos falls to 40% by 6 h and to 25% by 24 h of germination when the rate of protein synthesis is maximum (Figure 2B). Hence, there is no correlation between eIF-2 level and protein synthesis. Macrae et al. (20) also reported that rate of protein synthesis has no correlation with eIF-2 levels in _Artemia salina_. Our results suggest that dry embryos store excess of eIF-2 so that the embryo during germination does not have to replenish the stock during early hours of germination, the period when more crucial germination specific proteins are being synthesized.

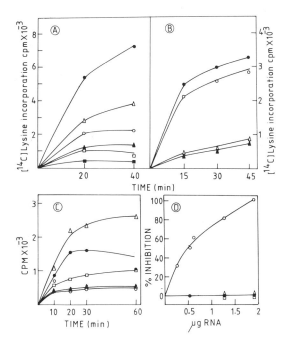

Fig. 3. Inhibition of translation by protein kinase (A and B) and iRNA (C and D). A: without hemin (▲——▲), with 30 μM hemin (●——●), hemin plus 0.7 μg PK (△——△), hemin plus 1.4 μg PK (○——○), hemin plus 3.6 μg PK (□——□), hemin plus 7.3 μg PK (■——■). B: without hemin (▲——▲) with 30 μM hemin (●——●), hemin plus 2.2 μ g PK (△——△), hemin plus 2.2 μM heat treated PK (○——○). C: without hemin (▲——▲), with 20 μM hemin (△——△), hemin plus 0.64 μ g RNA (●——●), hemin plus 1.28 μg RNA (□——□), hemin plus 1.92 μ g RNA (○——○). D: without hemin (●——●), with 20 μg hemin (○——○), hemin plus alkali digested RNA (△——△), hemin plus pancreatic RNase treated RNA (□——□).

Investigations from various laboratories have clearly established that cAMP-independent protein kinases and small molecular weight RNAs are involved in the regulation of translation (21, 22). In our attempts to find such translational inhibitors in barley embryos, we have isolated a cAMP-independent protein kinase and a small molecular weight RNA that inhibits _in vitro_ protein synthesis.

Cyclic AMP-independent protein kinase is purified by using affinity and ion exchange column chromatography. The purified enzyme has an estimated native mol. wt. = 95,000 with two non-identical subunits of 58,000 and 39,000 daltons. This enzyme shows similar properties as casein kinase type II of animals. It prefers acidic proteins over basic proteins. Purified enzyme strongly inhibits protein synthesis in rabbit reticulocyte lysates (Figure 3A). Heat treatment of the enzyme abolishes both its catalytic activity as well as inhibitory activity (Figure 3B), suggesting the cause of inhibition is due to phosphorylation. In order to understand the role of this kinase in depth, we have isolated an endogenous substrate by using purified protein kinase immobilized column. The mol. wt. of this substrate is 52,000 as determined by SDS-PAGE. This endogenous substrate acts as a very efficient phosphate acceptor as compared to exogenous substrates. It is possible that the substrate might have some pivotal role in translation as the enzyme inhibits translation. Antibodies against purified kinase have been raised in rabbits (Figure 4) to study the molecular mechanisms of action of protein kinase and the levels of the enzyme during different stages of embryogenesis and germination.

All these results clearly demonstrate that the inefficiency of translation in barely embryos extract is not due to lack of processed mRNA or initiation factor 2 (eIF-2). Hence, we searched for a probable translational inhibitor.

We have isolated, for the first time from a plant system, a small molecular weight RNA (hereafter referred as iRNA) that inhibits translation in hemin containing lysates but not in hemin-deficient lysates indicating that iRNA is acting at the level of initiation of protein synthesis and has no effect on elongation (Figure 3C). Sucrose density gradient analysis of hemin-deficient and containing lysates in presence and absence of iRNA has confirmed our observation that it acts at initiation step (Figure 5). iRNA

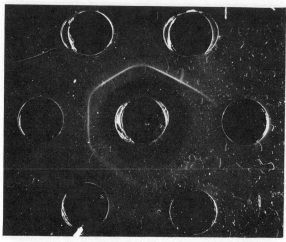

Fig. 4. Reactivity of protein kinase with rabbit antiserum as assayed by Ouchterlony immunodiffusion. The center well contains antiserum and the surrounding wells contain different concentrations (0.4-9µg) of purified protein kinase.

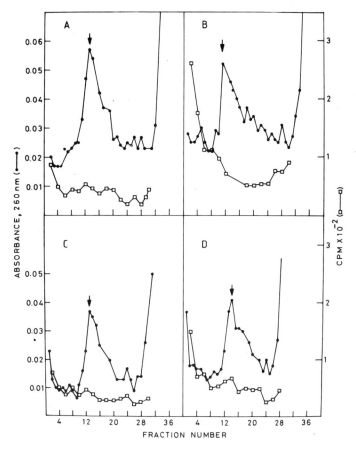

Fig. 5. Analysis of translationally active polysomes by sucrose
density gradient centrifugation. A: hemin-deficient lysate.
B: hemin-containing lysate. C: hemin-deficient lysate plus
1.28 µg RNA. D: hemin-containing lysate plus 1.28 µg RNA.
Experimental details are discussed in Materials and Methods.

has no long poly(A) sequence as judged by its inability to bind oligo d(T)
cellulose column. Abolition of translation inhibitory activity of iRNA by
alkali (0.3 N KOH) and pancreatic RNase treatment (Figure 3D) shows that
inhibition is not due to any DNA or protein contaminants and the RNA is
single stranded. Presence of these translational inhibitors could be the
reason for yielding a poor in vitro translation system from barley extract
- an observation made by us and others (23). Finally, the role of these
inhibitors in mRNA conservation cannot be ruled out. The involvement of
small mol. wt. RNA in the suppression of translation of stored mRNA in
early stage of muscle development has already been reported by Heywood (2,
24). Work in our laboratory is in progress to determine the possibility of
such a role of iRNA in this plant developmental system and also the mode of
action of these translational inhibitors.

ACKNOWLEDGEMENTS

This work is supported by DST, New Delhi and Hindustan Lever Ltd.,
Bombay. Travel assistance is provided by DST and CSIR, New Delhi to Dr. A.

S. N. Reddy to attend the NATO Advanced Study Institute and for presenting this work.

REFERENCES

1. P. I. Payne, Biol. Rev. 51:329-363 (1976).

2. D. S. Kennedy, E. Siegel, and S. M. Heywood, FEBS Lett. 90:209-214 (1978).

3. J. M. Sierra, D. Meier, and S. Ochoa, Proc. Natl. Acad. Sci. (USA). 71:2693-2697 (1974).

4. A. Marcus, D. Effron, and D. P. Weeks, Methods Enzymol. 30:749-754 (1974).

5. S. K. Sopory, M. Puri Avinashi, N. Deka, and A. Datta, Plant Cell Physiol. 21:649-657 (1980).

6. G. Brawerman, Methods Enzymol. 30:605-612 (1974).

7. B. E. Roberts and B. M. Paterson, Proc. Natl. Acad. Sci. (USA) 70:2330-2334 (1973).

8. S. Gunnery, A. S. N. Reddy, and A. Datta, Plant Cell Physiol. 24:565-568 (1983).

9. A. Datta, C. DeHaro, J. M. Sierra, ad S. Ochoa, Proc. Natl. Acad. Sci. (USA) 74:1463-1467 (1977).

10. M. J. Gilbert and W. H. Anderson, J. Biol. Chem. 245:2342-2349 (1970).

11. A. S. N. Reddy, S. Gunnery, and A. Datta, Biochem. Int. 7:9-13 (1983).

12. I. M. Glynn and J. B. Chappel, Biochem. J. 90:147-149 (1964).

13. J. Porath, Methods Enzymol. 34:13-30 (1974).

14. W. Thornberg and T. J. Lindell, J. Biol. Chem. 252:6660-6665 (1977).

15. A. S. N. Reddy and A. Datta, Biochem. Int. 9:77-82 (1984).

16. R. D. Palmiter, Biochem. 13:3606-3615 (1974).

17. C. Darnbrough, T. Hunt, and R. J. Jackson, Biochem. Biophys. Res. Comm. 48:1556-1564 (1972).

18. J. S. Garvery, N. E. Cremer, and D. H. Sussdorf, in: "Methods Immunology, 3rd Edition," (1977), pp. 313-327.

19. L. S. Dure III, Ann. Rev. Plant Physiol. 26:259-278 (1975).

20. T. H. Macrae, M. R. Chowdhury, K. J. Houston, C. L.Woodley, and A. J. Wahba, Eur. J. Biochem. 100:67-76 (1970).

21. S. Ochoa, Arch. Biochem. Biophys. 223:325-349 (1983).

22. M. M. Winkler, C. Lashbrook, J. W. B. Hershey, A. K. Mukherjee, and S. Sarkar, J. Biol. Chem. 258:15141-15145 (1983).

23. A. R. Carlier and W. J. Peumans, Biochim. Biophys. Acta 447:436-444 (1976).

24. T. L. McCarthy, E. Siegel, B. Mroczkowski, and S. M. Heywood, Biochemistry 22:935-941 (1983).

PROOXIDANT STATES AND PROMOTION*

Peter A. Cerutti

Swiss Institute for Experimental Cancer Research
Chemin des Boveresses 155 - CH - 1066 EPALINGES

SUMMARY

There is considerable evidence that increased concentrations of active
oxygen, organic-peroxides and organic-radicals (prooxidant states),
can promote initiated cells to neoplastic growth. Prooxidant states can be
caused by different classes of agents, including, hyperbaric oxygen,
ionizing radiation, xenobiotic metabolites, Fenton-type reagents, modulators of
cytochrome P450 electron transport, peroxisome proliferators,
inhibitors of the antioxidant defense, and membrane-active agents. Many of
these agents cause chromosomal damage by indirect action, but the role of
this damage in carcinogenesis remains unclear. Prooxidant states can be
prevented or suppressed by the enzymes of the cellular antioxidant defense
and low molecular weight scavenger molecules. Many antioxidants are
antipromoters and anticarcinogens. Prooxidant states may modulate the
expression of a family of "prooxidant genes" which are related to cell
growth and differentiation by inducing alterations in DNA structure or by
epigenetic mechanisms, e.g., by poly ADP-ribosylation of chromosomal
proteins (1).

ACKNOWLEDGEMENTS

During the writing of this article, I have profited from discussions
with Drs. D. Borg, I. Emerit, P. Hornsby, W. Kozumbo, C. Richter, and J.
Seegmiller. Original work reported here was supported by the Swiss National
Science Foundation and the Swiss Association of Cigarette Manufactures.

REFERENCE

1. Cerutti, P.A. Prooxidant states and promotion. Science 227:375-381
   (1985).

---

*Only the summary of this paper appears here; the full length version was
published as an article in Science.

MOLECULAR ASPECTS OF DNA DAMAGE AND ITS MODIFICATION*

P. O'Neill and E. M. Fielden

Division of Molecular Processes
MRC Radiobiology Unit
Harwell, Didcot
Oxon Ox11 ORD
United Kingdom

INTRODUCTION

The time scale of radiation induced events in a biological system is illustrated in Figure 1. The initial energy deposition events occur on a time scale related to the passage of a particle moving at the velocity of light crossing an atomic diameter, i.e., of the order of 10^{-16} seconds. Starting from that moment there is a period in which the deposited energy is redistributed among the energy levels of several molecules, bonds are broken and secondary electrons thermalized. From about 10^{-12} seconds after the initial energy deposition, recognizable and observable chemical events take place. Because the free radicals produced initially often have strongly oxidizing or reducing properties, these initial radical reactions may be very rapid and complete within microseconds. The products of these reactions themselves are usually radicals, but of a less reactive nature, and thus a chain of chemical reactions is initiated which ultimately, within the space of $\sim$ 1 second, leads to a relatively stable chemical modification of biological molecules. Cells and organisms have various ways in which they deal with such insults, which may be either wholly repaired or may lead to modified biological function; be it cell death or permanent modification of genetic material. Thus, the biological changes induced by radiation, which may be only expressed or observed hours or even years after exposure to radiation, are a consequence of radiation induced chemical events taking place on a much shorter time scale.

These events may be strongly influenced by the presence of chemical modifiers such as radiosensitizers and radioprotectors. Indeed, a knowledge of the effects of chemical modifiers of altering radiation-induced damage to DNA should assist in the identification of the types of lesions which may be responsible for cellular inactivation and may lead to a better understanding of the mutagenic effects of ionizing radiation.

It has recently been demonstrated using cellular systems that endogenous non-protein thiol levels results in significant modification of

---

*Dedicated to Professor Schulte-Frohlinde on the occasion of his 60th birthday.

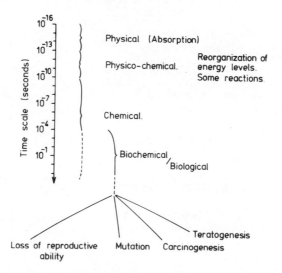

Fig. 1. The time scale of radiation action.

the response of cells to ionizing radiation in the presence and absence of
oxidants (1, 2, 3). The basis for the 'free radical repair' of the
cellular damage was suggested to be mediated through H-atom donation by the
thiol resulting in reconstitution of the target molecule (3-7).
Furthermore, glutathione has also been suggested (1) to play a role in the
detoxification of oxygen damage by acting as a substrate for important
enzyme systems. In the 'free radical repair' model (7), it is envisaged
that radiation-induced radicals produced on critical biomolecules, e.g.,
DNA, undergo competitive reactions either with O_2 (or oxidants) leading to
fixation of damage or with reductants, e.g., thiols, leading to potential
repair.

$$R^{\cdot} + O_2 \longrightarrow R - O_2^{\cdot} \text{ fixation} \tag{1}$$

$$R^{\cdot} + -SH \longrightarrow RH + -S^{\cdot} \text{ repair} \tag{2}$$

Much of the quantitative information concerning the feasibility of such
reactions has been obtained using the pulse radiolysis technique. Indeed,
such information is essential to the mechanistic understanding of
radiobiological effects.

In this presentation, we will be concerned mainly with the role of
reductants in the modification of radiation-induced damage of DNA using the
information obtained from interaction of water radiolysis radicals with
model systems. The 'free-radical repair' model will be discussed in the
light of the relative reactivities of the specific DNA radicals with O_2 and
reductants.

PRODUCTION AND REACTIONS OF WATER-RADIOLYSIS RADICALS

Production of Radicals

The indirect effect of ionizing radiation in radiobiology refers to
the action of the primary species produced on the radiolysis of water
(e.g., mammalian cells contain $\sim$ 70% water). The water radicals may produce
damage by virtue of their diffusion to and interaction with critical
targets. On the radiolysis of water, three main primary species are

426

produced; the hydrated electron (e⁻aq), the hydrogen atom (H·) and the hydroxyl radical (·OH) together with the molecular products, H_2O_2 and H_2.

$$H_2O \longrightarrow\!\!\bigwedge\!\!\bigwedge\!\!\bigwedge\!\!\longrightarrow \cdot OH,\ H\cdot,\ e^-aq$$

The yields of ·OH radicals and of e⁻aq are about the same whereas the yield of H-atoms is about 20% that of ·OH.

Furthermore, the number of free radicals produced in a given system produced by radiation is directly related to the dose of radiation given. If a stable product is sought, which is derived from the reactions of the primary radicals, e.g., OH, H, and e⁻, then increasing the dose may increase the yield of the derived product, but it will also increase the number and yield of undesired products. Thus, as the radiation dose is increased the yield of product does not increase proportionately and it is unrealistic to expect the linearity between dose and product yield to extend much beyond 30% conversion of starting materials.

The primary radical products of water radiolysis mentioned above are highly reactive and in general will react with most impurities just as easily as with a desired solute. In the case of the hydroxyl radical, for example, any organic material present will act as a scavenger of these radicals with biomolecular rate constants in the range of 10^7–10^{10} dm^3 $mol^{-1}\ s^{-1}$. Thus, in designing experiments in which it is desired to detect the products of an OH-solute reaction, it is important that any other material added to the system, such as buffers, must be known not to react with OH and the scavenging power of the solute (scavenging power is proportional to the product of solute concentration and rate constant of its reaction with OH radicals) should greatly exceed that of any adventitious material. This latter point can be particularly difficult to achieve when one is working with very small volumes of liquid in order to keep the concentration of solute high, e.g., samples of specific DNA. The techniques used to prepare such solutions may involve elution from columns of organic material or dialysis in bags of organic material with a large surface area to volume ratio. It may then be very difficult to limit the amount of adventitious organic material and hence to quantify the amount of products seen in relation to the amount of OH produced by the radiation.

In order to study the interactions of the primary radicals of water radiolysis, systems have been developed whereby these primary radicals may be selectively removed or scavenged. Readers are referred to reference 8 for a review of these systems.

b. Reactions of Water-Radiolysis Radicals with DNA

(1) Hydrated Electrons: The reaction of e⁻aq with DNA proceeds predominately (9) by interaction with the bases since the sugar-phosphate backbone would be expected to be relatively inert to attack by e⁻aq. In aerated systems, the resulting electron-adducts of the DNA bases may interact with O_2 via an electron transfer process as shown in reactions 3 and 4 where B represents one of the bases.

$$B + e^-aq \longrightarrow B\cdot^- \tag{3}$$

$$B\cdot^- + O_2 \longrightarrow B + O_2^- \tag{4}$$

Reaction 4 may also compete with alternative modes of decay of B·⁻, such as rearrangement, whereby interaction with O_2 becomes less favoured. Reaction 4 represents protection against the effects of e⁻aq, and will not be discussed in further detail. Indeed, e⁻aq-adducts of the DNA bases would not be expected to interact with reductants unless the adduct radicals

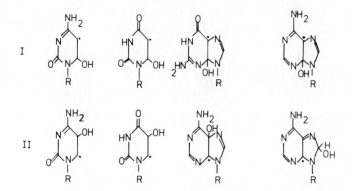

Fig. 2. The proposed structures of the hydroxyl-radical-adducts of purines (13, 16) and pyrimidines (14, 15) with oxidizing (I) and reducing (II) properties.

rearrange to yield oxidizing radicals as has been demonstrated (10) with uracils.

(2) <u>Hydroxyl</u> <u>Radicals</u> <u>and</u> <u>H·-atoms</u>: The interaction of the sugar-phosphate of DNA with ·OH-radicals and H-atoms proceeds via an H-atom abstraction pathway as shown in reaction 5. It is generally considered (11) that ∿20%

$$R-H + \cdot OH \ (H\cdot) \longrightarrow R\cdot + H_2O(H_2) \tag{5}$$

of the ·OH-radicals interact with the sugar-phosphate backbone. In the case of H-atoms, there is evidence that attack occurs preferentially at the bases of DNA (12).

In the interaction of the ·OH-radical with the base moieties of DNA, it has been demonstrated (13, 14, 15) using model systems that the resulting ·OH-radical adducts of the bases possess different redox properties depending upon the position of addition of the ·OH radical to the purine and pyrimidine ring systems. For instance, addition of an ·OH-radical to C_4 of the purines and to C_6 of the pyrimidines results in radicals with oxidizing properties whereas addition to C_5 and C_8 of the purines and C_5 of the pyrimidine bases results in radicals with reducing properties (13, 14, 15). The different types of OH-adduct of the DNA bases are presented in Figure 2. The relative yields of these oxidizing and reducing radicals of the DNA bases are presented in Table 1. It should be noted that the OH radical adduct derived from adenine with oxidizing properties is only produced through the spontaneous conversion of the C_4-adduct, which has reducing properties, into an oxidizing radical (16).

H-atom addition to the DNA bases has also been shown (10) to result in H-atom adducts with different redox properties. At present, the relative yields of the various H-atom adducts of the DNA bases have not been characterized to the same extent as those for the OH-radical adducts of the DNA bases.

428

Table 1. Yield of reducing and oxidizing radicals produced on intereaction of ·OH radicals with DNA bases

Base	Reducing radicals[a]	Oxidising radicals[a]
dGMP	56[b]	51[b]
dAMP	78[b]	32[b]
Thymine	65[c]	31[c]
Cytosine	87[d]	10[d]

a) expressed as a percentage of G(OH)   b) ref. 13
c) ref. 14   d) ref. 15

Repair of Sugar-Phosphate Radicals

Sugar-phosphate radicals produced by H-atom abstraction may interact with thiols involving H-atom transfer. Such a process would result in the reconstitution of the sugar-phosphate (reaction 2). This type of reaction has been demonstrated (4, 5, 6, 17, 18) to occur with a variety of model substances using the technique of pulse radiolysis to monitor the interactions. A series of rate constants for repair of radicals produced by H-atom abstraction are presented in Table 2. The rate constants for the 'repair' of the radicals derived from 2-methyl-propan-2-ol and 2-deoxyribose have been determined using the method of Wolfenden and Willson (17). The rate constants for repair of the sugar moiety of a series of nucleotides by cysteine have also been determined (19) to be 10^8 dm^3 mol^{-1} s^{-1}. The verification that reaction 2 proceeds via an H-atom transfer was obtained from the pH dependence of the reactivity (4). Since H-atom abstraction from the deoxyribose portion of the DNA has been implicated (20, 21) as the precursor leading to strand-breakage, then interaction of thiols via H-atom donation with the sugar radicals should reduce the probability of strand-breakage in model aqueous systems.

The repair of alkanol radicals by H-atom donation by a series of reductants, e.g., ascorbate, vitamin E, NADH was demonstrated (22, 23) to be inefficient or may not occur. It is, therefore, considered that these reductants do not directly modify DNA damage by H-atom donation.

The importance of radicals derived from the sugar-phosphate backbone of DNA is the fact that O_2 may also interact efficiently with these radicals (k 10^7-10^9 dm^3 mol^{-1} s^{-1}) so that a competition will exist (reactions 2 and 3) between repair by thiols and fixation of damage by O_2. Based upon rate data information for interaction of O_2 (24, 25) and thiols (24) with DNA, the concentration of thiols would have to exceed that of O_2 by at least a factor of 200. In fact, many cell survival studies using various additives to reduce intracellular thiol levels have indicated (1, 2, 3) that, under aerobic conditions, radiosensitivity is only slightly effected whereas under hypoxic conditions, radiosensitivity increases on reducing the levels of endogenous thiol levels. Furthermore, naturally occurring amino-thiols in glutathione-deficient cells appear (2) to be inefficient as glutathione-substitutes. Based upon the similar efficiencies of H-atom donation by the thiols, the above findings could indicate additional roles of glutathione in radioprotection such as the ability to act as a substrate for specific enzymatic repair systems.

Table 2. Rate constants for interaction of thiols with a series of radicals derived from alcohols on interaction with OH radicals at pH = 7

Substrate	$10^{-8} \times k/dm^3 \ mol^{-1} \ s^{-1}$	
2-propanol[a]	4.2	(3.3[a])
ethanol[a]	1.4	(1.7[c])
glucose[a]	0.32	
t-butanol[a]	0.18	
2-deoxyribose[b]	0.20	
t-butanol[b]	0.52	

a) ref. 4 with cytseamine   b) this work - with cysteine
c) ref. 17 cysteine

Modification of DNA Base Radicals

As mentioned earlier, the hydroxyl-radical adducts of the DNA bases have different redox properties (13, 14, 15, 16) depending on the position of addition of ·OH to the ring system. In the case of guanine, thymine, and cytosine, the oxidizing and reducing radical adducts are probably formed directly (see Figure 2) whereas in the case of adenine it has been proposed (16) that the radical with oxidizing properties is formed on dehydration of the C_4-radical. The following discussion will be subdivided according to the redox properties of the OH-radical adducts.

(1) Oxidizing ·OH-adducts of DNA Bases: It has previously been demonstrated (13, 14, 15) using N,N,N',N'-tetramethyl-p-phenylenediamine (k 10^9 dm^3 mol^{-1} s^{-1}) as the reductant that a certain percentage of the OH-radical adducts of the DNA bases have oxidizing properties (see Table 1). In Tables 3 and 4, representative rate constants are presented for the interaction of a series of reductants with OH-adducts of dGMP and dAMP with oxidizing properties. These rate constants were determined (16, 26, 27) from the first order rate of change of optical absorption at a wavelength where the one-electron oxidized reductant absorbs.

From the observed variation in these rate constants based upon the ease of oxidation of the reductants (26, 27), it is apparent that the interaction of the OH-adducts with oxidizing properties with reductants proceeds via an electron transfer process. This mechanism is consistent with the reported (22, 23, 26) inefficient H-atom donation by these reductants and the formation of one-electron oxidized species of the reductant. From preliminary investigations with poly G, it is inferred that the corresponding interactions of the reductants, TMPD and resorcinol, with the OH-radical adducts of poly G do occur, however, the rate constants are at least 50% less than those shown in Table 3 for interaction with dGMP. From these initial qualitative observations with poly G, it is inferred that similar interactions to those observed with the nucleotides may occur with polynucleotide macromolecules.

The rate constants for interaction of thiols with the OH-adduct of dGMP possessing oxidizing properties have previously been determined (13) to be 0.36 - 1.8 x 10^8 dm^3 mol^{-1} s^{-1} at pH ~9.5-10.5. In fact, it was shown that the reactivity of the thiols increase at pH > 7.5 from which it

Table 3. Rate constants for interaction of reductants with OH-radical adducts of dGMP with oxidizing properties together with the redox potentials of the reductants

Substrate	$k \times 10^{-8}/dm^3\ mol^{-1}\ s^{-1}$	E^2_{-7}/mV [d]
N,N,N',N'-tetramethyl-p-phenylene diamine	15 [a]	270
Ascorbate	4.8 [a]	300
p-phenylenediamine	17.3 [b]	310
p-aminophenol	12.9 [b]	410
Hydroquinone	9.0 [c]	460
p-methoxyphenol	8.6 [b]	600
Catechol	4.9 [c]	530
Resorcinol	3.4 [c]	810

a) ref. 13   b) ref. 26   c) ref. 27   d) ref. 28

Table 4. Rate constants for interaction of reductants with the OH-radical adducts of dA(dAMP) with oxidising properties (from ref. 16)

Reductant	$k \times 10^{-8}/dm^3\ mol^{-1}\ s^{-1}$	
	dA	dAMP
TMPD	~20	10
ABTS	40	9.0
Ascorbate		1.6
Trolox C	3.5	
Chlorpromazine	1.4	
Resorcinol		0.6

was suggested (13) that this interaction involves predominantly the thiolate ion in an electron transfer process. The pH dependence determined for the nucleotide base radicals is essentially the reverse of that determined (4) for reactions involving H-atom donation by thiols. With dA, the oxidizing radical of which absorbs strongly at $\lambda \leq 320$ nm no increase in this absorption is observed if cysteine is present at pH 7. From this observation, it is inferred that the thiol may interact with the dA-adduct with oxidizing properties. The rate constant for this interaction is estimated to be $\sim 10^7$ dm^3 mol^{-1} s^{-1} at pH 7 (O'Neill, unpublished data). Previous estimates of the rate constant for interaction of thiols with ·OH-adducts of thymidine and of uracil were determined (4) to be $< 10^7$ dm^3 mol^{-1} s^{-1}.

There is now increasing information that the ·OH–adducts of DNA bases with oxidizing properties may interact, via electron transfer, with reductants and with the thiolate ion. In fact, preliminary indications show that these types of interactions also pertain to poly-nucleotides.

The question arises as to how may reductants modify radiation–induced DNA base damage? The following scheme illustrates a possible repair process of those DNA base radicals with oxidizing properties when produced in the presence of reductants. This concept of repair has been extended to include the H-atom adducts of the bases which could have oxidizing properties based on the rationale developed for the OH-radical adducts (13, 14, 15).

$$(\text{base-OH})^{\cdot}_{ox} \qquad (\text{Red}) \tag{6}$$

$$(\text{base-OH})^{-} \qquad (\text{Red})^{\cdot +}$$

$$-OH^{-} \diagup \qquad \diagdown +H^{+}$$

$$\text{base} \qquad\quad \text{hydrated base}$$

On interaction of ·OH radicals and ·H-atoms with the DNA bases, those adducts with oxidizing properties may interact with a reductant via electron transfer whereby the subsequent species could then eliminate OH⁻ resulting in restoration of the base. A protonation step followed by dehydration of the resulting hydrated base is an alternative pathway leading to base repair.

$$(7)$$

This mode of interaction represents potential repair of a DNA base radical via electron transfer in contrast to the repair of sugar damage by thiol involving H-atom transfer (4, 5, 6, 7).

Of further interest is the apparent inefficient interaction of O_2 (k $< 1 \times 10^7$ dm^3 mol^{-1} s^{-1}) with at least some of those OH-radical adducts with oxidizing properties. In the case of thymine (14) and guanosine (13), the yield and rate of formation of the one-electron oxidized species of the reductants on interaction with the oxidizing OH-adducts of these bases are independent of the presence of O_2. In the case of adenine (16), O_2 has been shown to interact with the precursor radical yielding the oxidizing radical via a H_2O elimination reaction. Therefore, based upon a 'competitive repair' mechanism of the OH-adducts with oxidizing properties, O_2 should not compete efficiently with reductants, with the exception of adenosine, in contrast to the known efficient competition for sugar radicals based on rate constant data. These efficiencies do not take into account possible electrostatic effects when considering highly charged macromolecules. In the case of adenosine, O_2 could, however, effectively prevent formation of the oxidizing radical and, therefore, the restitution of the intact base by intercepting the precursor radical with reducing properties.

(2) <u>Reducing OH-adducts of DNA bases</u>: It has previously been demonstrated using tetranitromethane (13, 14, 15) that with the exception of guanine, the majority of the radicals of DNA bases produced on interaction with ·OH radicals, have reducing properties as witnessed from the formation of the nitroform anion. In the studies with reductants (13, 14, 16, 28, 29), it is apparent that the ·OH-radical adducts of DNA bases with reducing properties do not interact efficiently with reductants (k < 5 x 10^6 dm^3 mol^{-1} s^{-1}). On the other hand, O_2 has been shown (14, 15, 29, 30) to interact with these types of OH-radical adducts to produce peroxyl intermediates with the possible exception of the purines. It is generally inferred that the interaction with O_2 results in the production of a peroxyl radical via O_2 addition and that the resulting radical has oxidizing properties (14, 15) in the case of the pyrimidines. From our preliminary investigations with guanosine (Handman and O'Neill), it is inferred that on interaction of O_2 with the reducing OH-adduct of guanosine, superoxide or a peroxyl radical is produced which does not have oxidizing properties.

In previous studies, it has been shown that OH-adducts of pyrimidines with reducing properties reduce/or form adducts with ferricyanide (31), benzoquinone (32), and a series of nitroaromatics (33, 34, 35). Therefore, in the presence of O_2 or oxidants, it is proposed that enhancement of damage of DNA bases with reducing properties may occur as shown.

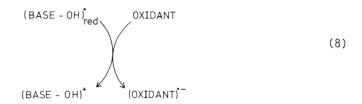

$$(8)$$

If electron transfer occurs between (Base-OH)·$_{red}$ and the oxidant, the resulting carbocation may interact with $H_2O(OH^-)$ to yield glycolic products which cannot dehydrate to restore the base. In the case of peroxyl radical formation in the presence of O_2, organic peroxides are the probable product especially if interaction of the oxidizing peroxyl radical with a reductant occurs. As stated earlier, 'competitive interactions' of these reducing OH-adducts between oxidants and reductants should favour interactions with the oxidants.

In a cellular system, the interactions described may lead to enhancement of base damage, the repair of which would have to rely upon the biochemical repair systems of the cell. Such systems may misrepair such damage resulting in enhancement of permanent chemical damage of the DNA. Such damage may be important in the development of radiation-induced mutagenesis. A further important concept, which has been recently developed (36) using poly U, is the fact that base radicals may ultimately by an, as yet, unknown mechanism result in a strand break. The OH-radical adduct of the base which is responsible for the strand breakage has not been identified so that the possible enhancement of such a process by oxidants cannot be assessed. From these latter findings, it is implied that the production of 'direct' strand breakage is not unique to sugar radicals and that the involvement of DNA base damage should be considered for both the mutagenic effects of radiation and also cell lethality.

Synergistic Effects of Reductants in Repair Processes

Even though thiols may repair radicals via H-atom donation as discussed for the repair of sugar-phosphate radicals, it is apparent that reductants (see Table 3) may also indirectly repair carbon centered radicals via the intermediate involvement of thiols. This 'indirect' repair is based upon the fact that thiyl radicals may interact with ascorbate and other reductants (22, 26, 26, 37, 38) via an electron transfer process. Therefore, as shown in the scheme a radical produced on

$$R^{\cdot} \quad -SH \quad (reductant)^{\cdot +}$$
$$H^{+}$$
$$RH \quad -S^{\cdot} \quad (reductant)$$

(9)

H-atom abstraction ($R^{\cdot}$) may be repaired, as discussed above, by an H-atom donation from a thiol. The resulting thiyl radical then interacts with a reductant via an electron transfer process to regenerate the thiol at the expense of the reductant. The efficiency of this process will be related to the ease of oxidation of the reductant. Such synergistic effects may be of importance whereby reductants may maintain the level of endogenous thiols within the vicinity of specific target sites. The level of thiols may be critical when considering the competition with O_2 and oxidants for radiation-induced bioradicals produced by H-atom abstraction. Synergistic effects and modification of DNA damage by thiols and reductants may also be important in restitution of DNA following direct energy deposition within nuclear DNA. As a result of an ionization event, electron capture by O_2 or an oxidant is envisaged (39) whereby a positive centre remains upon the DNA. This centre would be expected to have electrophilic properties and, therefore, be susceptible to attack by reductants. Such an interaction would result in repair of DNA damage as shown. Of course, relaxation of the positive centre within DNA could yield a neutral radical which may still have electrophilic character. At present, sufficient information is not available to assess the repairability of 'direct' damage of DNA by thiols and reductants.

$$\underset{RS^{-}}{\overset{\cdot +}{\downarrow}} \qquad \underset{O_2}{\overset{e^{-}}{\downarrow}}$$

repair O_2^{-}
(electron transfer)

(10)

CONCLUSIONS

In conclusion, it has been the authors intention to draw attention to the potential modifications to radiation-induced DNA damage brought about by interactions of reductants and oxidants with specific DNA radicals. Some of the interactions discussed may lead to reconstitution of the DNA whereas interactions with oxidants may lead to enhanced DNA damage. The involvement of reductants other than thiols in a fast free radical repair of radiobiological damage (including synergistic effects) has been highlighted. It is also becoming apparent that not all radiation-induced DNA radicals interact efficiently with O_2 as has previously been thought to be the case. It is hoped that some of the concepts developed will assist in the interpretation of fundamental models of radiation-induced carcinogenesis in which the redox state of the cell is altered by the manipulation of thiol levels, etc..

ACKNOWLEDGEMENTS

This work was funded partly by the EEC (Grant BIO,C.363-81-UK(H)). We also thank NATO for financial support.

REFERENCES

1. J. E. Biaglow, M.E. Varnes, E. P. Clark, and E. R. Epp, Symposium: thiols. The role of thiols in cellular response to radiation drugs, Radiat. Res. 95:437-455 (1983).

2. L. Revesz and M. Edgren, Mechanism of radiosensitization and protection studied with glutathione-deficient human cell lines, in: "Prog. in Radio-Oncol II," K. H. Karcher, et al., ed., Raven Press, New York (1982), pp. 235-242.

3. C. J. Koch, Competition between radiation protectors and radiation sensitizers in mammalian cells, in: "Radioprot. Anticarcinog.," F. Nygaard and M. G. Simic, eds., Academic Press, New York (1983), pp. 275-295.

4. G. E. Adams, G. S. McNaughton, and B. D. Michael, Pulse radiolysis of sulphur compounds, Part 2 - Free radical "repair" by hydrogen transfer from sulphydryl compounds, J.C.S. Faraday Trans. 64:902-910 (1968).

5. L. Revesz and E. P. Malaise, Significance of cellular glutathione in radioprotection and repair of radiation damage, in: "Functions of Glutathione: Biochemical, Physiological, Toxicological and Clinical Agents," A. Larsson, et al., eds., Raven Press, New York (1983), pp. 163-173.

6. P. Alexander and A. Charlesby, Physico-chemical methods of protection against ionizing radiations, in: "Radiobiology Symposium 1954," Z. M. Bacq and P. Alexander, eds., Butterworths, London (1955), pp. 49-59.

7. G. E. Adams, R. C. Armstrong, A. Charlesby, B. D. Michael, and R. L. Willson, Pulse radiolysis of sulphur compounds, Part 3 - Repair by hydrogen transfer of a macromolecule irradiated in aqueous solution, J. C. S. Faraday Trans. 65:732-742 (1969).

8. G. E. Adams and P. Wardman, Free radicals in biology: The pulse radiolysis approach, in: "Free Radicals in Biology, Vol. III," Academic Press, New York (1977), pp. 53-95.

9. G. Scholes, Primary events in the radiolysis of aqueous solutions of nucleic acids and related substrates, in: Effects of Ionizing Radiation on DNA,: J. Huttermann, W. Kohnlein, R. Teoule, and A. J. Bertinchamps, eds., Springer, Berlin (1978), pp. 153-203.

10. S. Das, D. J. Deeble, M-N Schuchmann, and C. von Sonntag, Pulse radiolytic studies on uracil and uracil derivatives. Protonation of their electron adducts at oxygen and carbon, Int. J. Radiat. Biol. 46:7-9 (1984).

11. C. von Sonntag and D. Schulte-Frohlinde, Radiation-induced degradation of the sugar in model compounds and in DNA, in: "Effects of Ionizing Radiation on DNA," J. Huttermann, W. Kohnlein, R. Teoule, and A. J. Bertinchamps, eds., Springer Verlag, Berlin (1978), pp. 204-225.

12. G. Scholes and M. Simic, Radiolysis of aqueous solutions of DNA and related substances: reactions of hydrogen atoms, Biochim. Biophys. Acta 166:255 (1968).

13. P. O'Neill, Pulse radiolytic study of the interaction of thiols and ascorbate with OH-adducts of dGMP and dG: Implications for DNA repair processes, Radiat. Res. 96:198-210 (1983).

14. S. Fujita and S. Steenken, Pattern of ·OH radical addition to uracil and methyl- and carboxyl-substituted uracils. Electron transfer of OH adducts with N,N,N',N'-tetramethyl-p-phenylenediamine and tetranitromethane, J. Am. Chem. Soc. 103:2540-2545 (1981).

15. D. K. Hazra and S. Steenken, Pattern of OH radical addition to cytosine and 1-, 3-, 5-, and 6-substituted cytosines. Electron transfer and dehydration reactions of the OH adducts, J. Amer. Chem. Soc. 105:4380-4386 (1983).

16. P. O'Neill, P. W. Chapman, and D. G. Papworth, Repair of hydroxyl radical damage of dA by antioxidants, Chemistry Life Reports, 3:62-69 (1985).

17. B. S. Wolfenden and R. L. Willson, Radical cations as reference chromogens in kinetic studies of one-electron transfer reactions: pulse radiolytic studies of 2,2'-azinobis-(-3 ethylbenzthiazoline-6-sulphonate), J. C. S. Perkin Trans. 2:805-812 (1982).

18. M. Tambe and M. Quintiliani, Kinetic studies of reactions involved in hydrogen transfer from glutathione to carbohydrate radicals, Radiat. Phys. Chem. 23:259-263 (1984).

19. C. L. Greenstock and I. Dunlop, Reactions of nucleic acid radicals with radiation modifiers, in: "Fast Processes in Radiation Chemistry and Biology," G. E. Adams, E. M. Fielden, and B. D. Michael, eds., J. Wiley and Sons, Bristol (1975), pp. 247-258.

20. J. F. Ward, Deoxynucleotides - models for studying mechanisms of strand breakage in DNA. I. Protection by sulphydryl compounds, Int. J. Radiat. Phys. Chem. 3:239-249 (1971).

21. D. Schulte-Frohlinde, Kinetics and mechanism of polynucleotide and DNA strand break formation, in: "Radioprot. Anticarcinogens," F. Nygaard and M. G. Simic, eds., Academic, New York (1983), pp. 53-71.

22. R. L. Willson, Free radical repair mechanisms and the interaction of glutathione and vitamins C and E, in: "Radioprotectors and Anticarcinogens," F. Nygaard and M. G. Simic, eds., Academic Press, New York (1983), pp. 1-22.

23. J. L. Redpath and R. L. Willson, Reducing compounds in radioprotection and radiosensitization: model experiments using ascorbic acid, Int. J. Radiat. Biol. 23:51-65 (1973).

24. B. D. Michael, K. D. Held, and H. A Harrop, Biological aspects of DNA radioprotection, in: "Radioprot. Anticarcinogens," F. Nygaard and M. G. Simic, eds., Academic Press, New York (1983), pp. 325-338.

25. P. O'Neill, T. C. Jenkins, and E. M. Fielden, Interaction of oxygen and nitroxyls with radiation-induced radicals of DNA and related bases in aqueous solution, Radiat. Res. 82:55-64 (1980).

26. P. O'Neill and P. W. Chapman, Potential repair of free radical adducts of dGMP and dG by a series of reductants. A pulse radiolytic study, Int. J. Radiat. Biol., 47:71-80 (1985).

27. P. O'Neill, Hydroxyl radical damage: potential repair by sulphydryls, ascorbate, and other anti-oxidants, Life Chemistry Reports, pp. 337-341 (1984).

28. S. Steenken and P. Neta, One-electron redox potentials of phenols. Hydroxy- and aminophenols and related compounds of biological interest, J. Phys. Chem. 86:3661 (1982).

29. R. L. Willson, The reaction of oxygen with radiation-induced free radicals of DNA and related compounds, Int. J. Radiat. Biol. 17:349-358 (1970).

30. M. Isilder, M. N. Schuchmann, D. Schulte-Frohlinde, and C. von Sonntag, Oxygen uptake in the radiolysis of aqueous solutions of nucleic acids and their constituents, Int. J. Radiat. Biol. 41:525-533 (1982).

31. K-D Asmus, D. J. Deeble, A. Garner, I. Ali, and G. Scholes, Chemical aspects of radiosensitization. Reactions of sensitizers with radicals produced in the radiolysis of aqueous solutions of nucleic acid components, Br. J. Cancer 37(Suppl. 3):46-49 (1978).

32. M. Simic and E. Hayon, Comparison between the electron transfer reactions from free radicals and their corresponding peroxyl radicals to quinones, Biochem. Biophys. Res. Commun. 50:364-369 (1973).

33. A. J. Varghese, Sensitization of thymine and uracil to ionizing radiation by p-nitroacetophenone, Int. J. Radiat. Biol. 28:477-484 (1975).

34. S. Nishimoto, H. Ide, T. Wada, and T. Kagiya, Radiation-induced hydroxylation of thymine promoted by electron-affinic compounds, Int. J. Radiat. Biol. 44:585-600 (1983).

35. C. L. Greenstock and I. Dunlop, Pulse radiolysis studies of nitrofurans: chemical radiosensitization, Radiat. Res. 56:428-440 (1973).

36. D. G. E. Lemaire, E. Bothe, and D. Schulte-Frohlinde, Yields of radiation-induced main chain scission of poly U in aqueous solution: strand break formation via base radicals, Int. J. Radiat. Biol. 45:351-358 (1984).

37. P. O'Neill, Interaction of the ·OH-radical adduct of dGMP with a series of anti-oxidants: implication for DNA repair processes, in: Proc. 7th ICRR, Amsterdam (1983), Abstract A3-33.

38. L. G. Forni, J. Monig, V. O. Mora-Arellano, and R. L. Willson, Thiyl free radicals: direct observations of electron transfer reactions with phenothiazines and ascorbate, J. C. S. Perkin Trans. 2:961-965 (1983).

39. G. E. Adams and M. D. Cooke, Electron-affinic sensitization I. A structural basis for chemical radiosensitizers in bacteria, Int. J. Radiat. Biol. 15:457-471 (1969).

5-HYDROXYMETHYL URACIL: A PRODUCT OF IONIZING RADIATION AND TRITIUM TRANSMUTATION FORMED IN DNA

K. Frenkel*, A. Cummings and G. W. Teebor

Department of Pathology
New York University Medical Center
550 First Avenue
New York, N.Y. 10016

ABBREVIATIONS

HMUra, 5-hydroxymethyl uracil; HMdU, 5-hydroxymethyl-2'-deoxyuridine; TG, thymine glycol, 5,6-dihydroxy-5,6-dihydrothymine; dTG, thymidine glycol, 5,6-dihydroxy-5,6-dihydrothymidine; HMH, 5-hydroxy-5-methyl hydantoin; AP, apurinic/apyrymidinic; HPLC, high pressure liquid chromatography; ODS, octadecylsilane; ss, single-stranded, ds, double-stranded; 1 krad, 10 Gy.

The mutagenic and carcinogenic properties of ionizing radiation are thought to be a consequence of DNA damage it causes (1). Such DNA damage includes single- and double-strand breaks, DNA-protein crosslinks, base loss with formation of AP sites and chemical modification of bases (2-6). Among the bases, the thymine moiety appears to be the most susceptible to the modifying effects of ionizing radiation (7, 8). One of the most studied derivatives formed through the action of ionizing radiation, thymine glycol (TG), is formed by the oxidation of the 5,6-double bond of thymine (Figure 1) (2, 9-13). TG is susceptible to further oxidation by radiogenically-derived hydroxyl radicals. It leads to the opening of the ring and formation of an unstable N'-formyl-N-pyruvyl urea (FPU) which either fragments or cyclizes and becomes 5-hydroxy-5-methyl hydantoin (HMH) (9, 10, 14). The other thymine derivative, 5-hydroxymethyl uracil (HMUra), is formed by oxidation of the methyl group of thymine (Figure 1) (15-17). In contrast to TG, HMUra is chemically stable (18). Therefore, it is possible that HMUra will serve as a marker of exposure to ionizing radiation in the same way as cyclobutane pyrimidine dimers became markers of exposure to UV radiation.

HMUra is a natural constituent of some B. subtilis phages such as SP01, SP08 and SP12 (19-21). However, when administered as the 2-deoxyribonucleoside HMdU, it is mutagenic and cytostatic to mammalian and bacterial cells (22, 23). Both HMUra and HMdU can be incorporated into DNA (22, 24), and both are potent inducers of λ prophage from E. coli WP2$_s$( )

---

*Presently Departments of Pathology and Environmental Medicine.

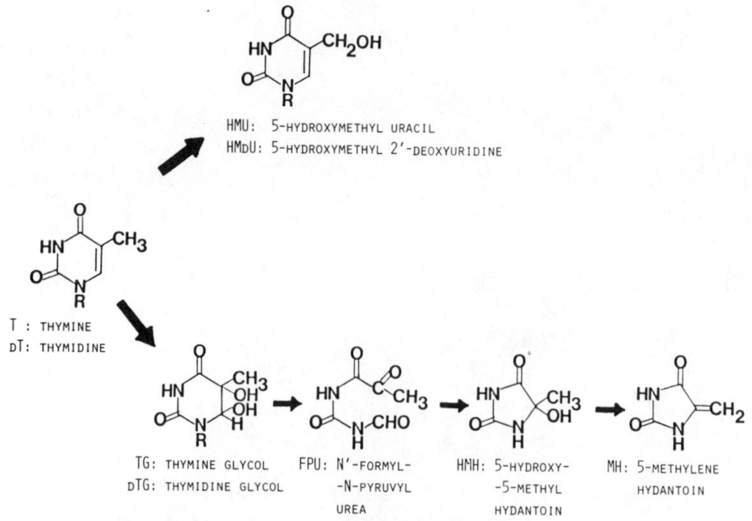

Fig. 1. Structures of thymine derivatives formed through the
         action of ionizing radiation.

uvrA⁻ strain (Rossman and Frenkel, unpublished data). When injected into
mice, HMdU causes diarrhea and leukopenia which are characteristic of acute
radiation sickness (23). Since many properties of HMdU mimic those of
ionizing radiation, it is possible that formation of this particular
thymidine derivative is responsible for at least some of those properties.
Our laboratory has found that HMdU is indeed formed in cellular DNA when
HeLa cells are γ-irradiated (25).

     HeLa cells grown in the presence of (6-³H)thymidine were either γ-
irradiated from a ¹³⁷Cs source or used as an unirradiated control (25).
DNA was extracted, enzymatically digested to 2'-deoxyribonucleosides and
analyzed by HPLC on the ODS column (12, 25). The hydrolysate of DNA
obtained from the control cells contained only negligible amounts of ³H
eluting together with marker HMdU. In contrast, the hydrolysate obtained
from cells irradiated with 14 krads contained small but reproducible
amounts of ³H-containing material which co-eluted with marker HMdU (Figure
2). The identity of this peak as HMdU was confirmed by acetylation and
subsequent HPLC analysis of the derivative (25, 26). The (³H)HMdU peak
constituted 6×10^{-4}% of the total ³H applied to the ODS column. After 28
krads of radiation, the HMdU content increased to 13×10^{-4}% of the total
³H. This increased amount of HMdU was the first indication that HMdU could
possible serve as a marker of exposure to ionizing radiation.

     To determine the suitability of HMdU as a marker, solutions of DNA
isolated from E. coli grown in the presence of (6-³H)thymidine were
irradiated in water with increasing doses (14, 28, 42 and 56 krads) of γ-
radiation (26). (³H)DNA was enzymatically hydrolyzed and the resultant
2'deoxyribonucleosides analyzed by HPLC. Fractions co-eluting with marker
HMdU were combined, acetylated and the derivatives analyzed again by HPLC.
The experiments were designed to answer three questions. The first was
whether HMdU is formed in a dose-dependent manner. The second question was
whether the conformation of DNA influences the amount of HMdU formed; for
this reason solutions of both ss and ds DNA were irradiated at each dose.
The third question was whether HMdU was primarily formed through the
indirect action of ionizing radiation. To answer the last question, DNA
solutions of two concentrations (25 and 250 g DNA/ml) were γ-irradiated.

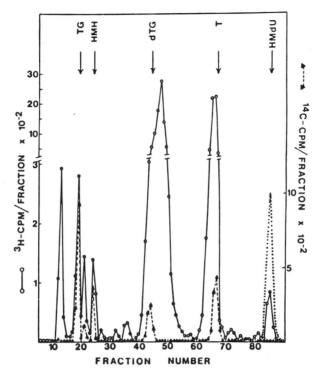

Fig. 2. HPLC analysis of an enzymatic hydrolysate (2'-deoxyribonucleosides) of (6-^{3}H)thymidine-labeled DNA (O) isolated from γ-irradiated (14 krad) HeLa cells in the presence of marker compounds (^{14}C)TG, (^{14}C)HMH, (^{14}C)dTG, and (^{14}C)thymine (▲) and unlabeled HMdU (●●●).

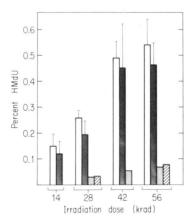

Fig. 3. Percent HMdU formed in gamma-irradiated (^{3}H)DNA. At 25 μg DNA/ml: ☐ -ss DNA and ▨ -ds DNA. At 250 μg DNA/ml: ▨ -ss DNA ▨ and -ds DNA. Vertical lines represent standard error of the means.

441

As can be seen in Figure 3, at both concentrations of DNA, HMdU content increased in a linear manner but leveled off between 42 and 56 krads. Such leveling off probably can be explained by the increasing release of bases by the increased doses of radiation (3, 6) leading to a progressive fragmentation of DNA and a loss of some HMUra moieties from the DNA backbone, resulting in fewer HMdU molecules. There was no significant difference between the extent of HMdU formation in ss and ds DNA at either concentration. However, there was a 10-fold difference in % HMdU formed at each radiation dose depending upon whether 25 or 250 g DNA/ml samples were irradiated. This 10-fold difference in the % HMdU formed means that the same <u>absolute</u> <u>number</u> of HMdU molecules were formed at both DNA concentrations. These results prove that it is indeed the indirect action (27) of ionizing radiation which is responsible for HMdU formation at this particular concentration range of DNA.

It appears that in the experiments using 25 and 250 µg DNA/ml, HMdU was formed only by the indirect effects of radiation because the calculated G value of 0.002 (which in this case reflects the number of HMdU molecules formed per 100 eV of radiation) was the same for both concentrations. However, the G value for HMdU formation in the DNA of irradiated HeLa cells was 0.03 which is higher than anticipated from the indirect effects alone. It is possible that at the high concentration of DNA within the nucleus (60 mg DNA/ml assuming 8 µ diameter), the direct effects of ionizing radiation and/or endogenous radiosensitizers are responsible for this high G value.

HMdU can be formed through the interaction of radiogenically-derived hydroxyl radicals with thymidine. It can also be formed by transmutation as the result of the β decay of ^{3}H located in the methyl group of thymidine (25). In compounds which have ^{3}H bound to carbon, the emission of an electron (β particle) from a neutron located in the nucleus of ^{3}H leads to the formation of the nucleus of ^{3}He. The bond linking ^{3}He to C is very unstable with a half life of 10^{-4} to 10^{-5} sec. The neutral ^{3}He is released by asbtracting an electron from C which leaves a very reactive carbocation (28). When such a carbocation is formed in the methyl group of thymidine, it reacts with a hydroxide ion of water generating (^{3}H)HMdU as the stable product (25). This mechanism of HMdU formation is illustrated in Figure 4.

When cells were labeled with thymidine containing three ^{3}H atoms in the methyl group, formation of (^{3}H)HMdU was detected in the cellular DNA (12, 25). Figure 5 shows an HPLC profile of DNA isolated from the non-

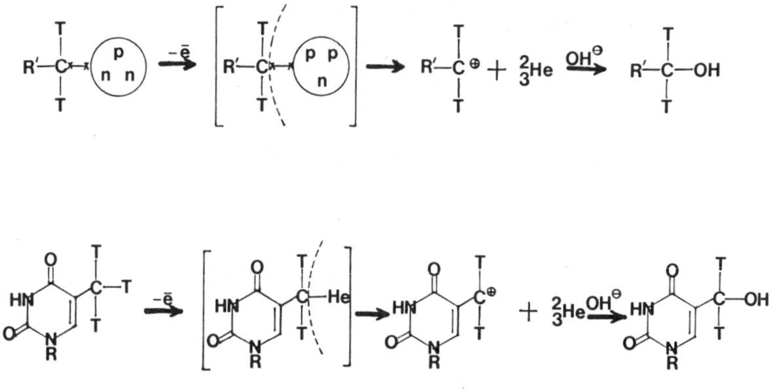

Fig. 4. Proposed mechanism of formation of HMdU from (<u>methyl-</u> ^{3}H) thymidine as a result of the transmutation of ^{3}H to ^{3}He. p, Proton; n, neutron; e$^-$, electron; T, tritium; R = H or 2'-doxyribose, R' = alkyl or aryl moiety.

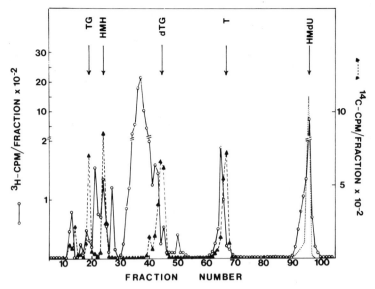

Fig. 5.   HPLC aalysis of an enzymatic hydrolysate (2'-
deoxyribonucleosides) of (methyl-3H)thymidine-
labeled DNA (O) isolated from non-irradiated HeLa
cells in the presence of marker compounds (14C)TG,
(14C)dTG, and 14C) thymine (▲) and unlabeled HMdU
(●●●).

irradiated control HeLa cells prelabeled with (methyl-3H)thymidine. As can
be seen at fractions 90-100, this DNA hydrolysate contained relatively
large amounts of (3H)HMdU. In contrast, there was practically no 3H-
containing material co-eluting with HMdU marker in the hydrolysate of DNA
isolated from (6-3H)thymidine-prelabeled cells (not shown). The high
(3H)HMdU amounts in DNA of non-irradiated cells prelabeled with (methyl-
3H)thymidine accumulated during the time needed to label cells, extract,
digest and analyze DNA. The formation of (3H)HMdU through transmutation
occurs at the rate of which is decay 0.017% per day (3H half life is
12.25 years). This mechanism of its formation was further proven when E.
coli DNA labeled with (methyl-3H)thymidine and stored for 17 months at
4°was assayed for the presence of (3H)HMdU. It contained 8% of its 3H as
HMdU, the exact amount expected from the rate of β decay. Since HMdU
cannot be formed by transmutation when thymidine is labeled with 3H in the
position 6, we have used (6-3H)thymidine-prelabeled cells for the
determinations of HMdU formation through the action of ionizing radiation.

It already has been shown that labeling of E. coli or Chinese hamster
ovary cells with 3H-containing thymidine caused mutations (29, 30). The
mutagenic properties of (3H)thymidine were in part related to the position
of 3H within the thymine moiety. Therefore, 3H transmutation products,
HMdU among them, may contribute to the known mutagenic and carcinogenic (31,
32) effects of (3)thymidine and may constitute a cumulative biological
hazard when incorporated into the DNA or long-lived cells.

ACKNOWLEDGEMENT

This investigation was supported by PHS Grant Number CA 16669, awarded
by the National Cancer Institute, DHHS.

443

REFERENCES

1. A. Upton, in: "Cancer," F. F. Becker, ed., Plenum Press, New York and London (1975), pp. 387-403.

2. P. A. Cerutti, in: "Photochemistry and Photobiology of Nucleic Acids, Vol. 2, " S. Y. Wang, ed., Academic Press, New York (1976), pp. 375-401.

3. J. F. Ward and I. Kuo, Radiat. Res. 66:485-498 (1976).

4. B. Dunlap and P. Cerutti, FEBS Lett. 51:188-190 (1975).

5. G. Scholes, J. F. Ward, and J. Weiss, J. Mol. Biol. 2:379-391 (1960).

6. H.-J. Rhaese and E. Freese, Biochim. Biophys. Acta 155:476-490 (1968).

7. G. Scholes, in: "Photochemistry and Photobiology of Nucleic Acids, Vol. 1," S. Y. Wang, ed., Academic Press, New York (1976), pp. 521-577.

8. J. Cadet and R. Teoule, Photochem. Photobiol. 28:661-667 (1978).

9. R. Teoule, A. Bonicel, C. Bert, J. Cadet, and M. Polverelli, Radiat. Res. 57:46-58 (1974).

10. R. Teoule, C. Bert, and A. Bonicel, Radiat. Res. 72:190-200 (1977).

11. K. Frenkel, M. S. Goldstein, N. Duker, and G. W. Teebor, Biochemistry 20:750-754 (1981).

12. K. Frenkel, M. S. Goldstein, and G. W. Teebor, Biochemistry 20:7566-7571 (1981).

13. G. W. Teebor, K. Frenkel, and M. S. Goldstein, Prog. Mutat. Res. 4:301-311 (1982).

14. J. Cadet, M. Berger, and R. Teoule, Sov. J. Quantum Electron. 11:1576-1582 (1981).

15. B. Ekert, Nature 194:278-279 (1962).

16. L. S. Myers, Jr., J. F. Ward, W. T. Tsukamoto, D. E. Holmes, and J. R. Julca, Science 148:1234-1235 (1965).

17. J. Cadet and R. Teoule, Bull. Soc. Chim. Fr. 3-4:891-895 (1975).

18. R. E. Cline, R. M. Fink, and K. Fink, J. Am. Chem. Soc. 81:2521-2527 (1959).

19. R. G. Kallen, M. Simon, and J. Marmur, J. Mol. Biol. 5:248-250 (1962).

20. D. H. Roscoe and R. G. Tucker, Biochem. Biophys. Res. Commun. 16:106-110 (1964).

21. S. Okubo, B. Strauss, and M. Stodolsky, Virology 24:552-562 (1964).

22. J. B. Meldrum, V. S. Gupta, and J. R. Saunders, Antimicrob. Ag. Chemother. 6:393-396 (1974).

3. S. Waschke, J. Reefschlager, D. Barwolff, and P. Langen, Nature (London) 255:629-630 (1975).

24. E. Matthes, D. Barwolff, B. Preussel, and P. Langen, in: "Antimetabolites in Biochemistry, Biology and Medicine," J. Skoda and P. Langen, eds., Pergamon Press, Oxford (1978), pp. 115-126.

25. G. W. Teebor, K. Frenkel, and M. S. Goldstein, Proc. Natl. Acad. Sci. (USA) 81:318-321 (1984).

26. K. Frenkel, A. Cummings, J. Solomon, J. Cadet, J. J. Steinberg, and G. W. Teebor, Biochemistry, 24:4527-4533 (1985).

27. Z. M. Bacq and P. Alexander, in: "Fundamentals of Radiobiology," Pergamon Press, Oxford, London, New York, Paris (1961), pp. 45-55.

28. L. E. Feinendegen and V. P. Bond, in: "Tritium," A. A. Moghissi and M. W. Carter, eds., Messenger Graphix, Phoenix, AZ (1973), pp. 221-231.

29. S. Person, W. Snipes, and F. Krasin, Mutat. Res. 34:327-332 (1976).

30. J. E. Cleaver, Genetics 87:129-138 (1977).

31. H. Licso, R. Baserga, and W. E. Kisieleski, Nature 192:571-572 (1961).

32. D. J. Mewissen and J. H. Rust, in: "Tritium," A. A. Moghissi and M. W. Carter, eds., Messenger Graphix, Phoenix, AZ (1973), pp. 252-267.

CHARACTERIZATION OF TWO CHO VARIANTS IN RESPECT TO MNNG-INDUCED CELL

KILLING, MUTATIONS, AND REPAIR OF METHYLATED DNA BASES*

R. Goth-Goldstein and M. Hughes

Biomedical Division
Lawrence Berkeley Laboratory
University of California
Berkeley, CA 94720

ABSTRACT

Two Chinese hamster ovary (CHO) cell variants differ substantially in their sensitivity to N-methyl-N'-nitro-N-nitrosoguanidine (MNNG). The resistant clone (Cl 3) was isolated from the sensitive parent line (Cl 9) after treating Cl 9 cells with a highly cytotoxic dose of MNNG. In contrast to their different sensitivity to the toxic effect of MNNG, the two variants are equally sensitive to its mutagenic effect. MNNG methylates DNA of Cl 9 and Cl 3 to the same extent. Loss of the two methylated purines N3-methyladenine and N7-methylguanine from DNA occurs at the same rate. O^6-methylguanine is not repaired in either clone. We conclude that the increased resistance of Cl 3 is neither due to a reduced uptake or binding of MNNG, nor due to an increased repair of the major methylated bases in DNA.

INTRODUCTION

N-nitroso compounds are a class of potent carcinogens which have been well characterized in respect to their reaction products with cellular DNA. So far, 12 sites in DNA have been identified as targets with which these agents can react (1). Less is known about the biological relevance of these alterations. There is much evidence that alkylation of DNA bases at exocyclic oxygens yields potentially mutagenic lesions (2). What constitutes a potentially lethal lesion is much less understood. Using mutants which affect the repair of specific DNA lesions, 3-methyladenine and 3-methylguanine have been identified as lethal lesions in Escherichia coli (3, 4). In mammalian cells no particular methylated DNA base correlates with cell killing (5). The inability of alkylating agent-sensitive human tumor strains of the Mer⁻ phenotype to repair O^6-methylguanine suggests that O^6-methylguanine which in bacteria is solely a mutagenic lesion, might be a lethal lesion in mammalian cells (6).

We are studying the mechanism of cell killing by alkylating agents by using variants of mammalian cells with altered sensitivity to these agents.

*This work was supported by NIH Grants ES01916 and ES03603.

MATERIALS AND METHODS

Cell Culture   The CHO subclone Cl 9 has been described previously (7). Cl 3 was isolated from a Cl 9 population which survived an MNNG-treatment of 3 g/ml.   Cl 9 and Cl 3 have the same growth rate and the same modal chromosome number of 21.   Cells are grown in McCoy's 5A medium supplemented with 7.5% fetal calf serum, 100 IU/ml penicillin, 100 g/ml streptomycin, and 1 mM Hepes buffer in open plastic tissue culture flasks in a CO_2 incubator at $37^{\circ}C$.

MNNG-treatment   MNNG (Aldrich Chemical Co., Milwaukee, WI) was dissolved in 100 mM acetate buffer, pH 5 at 1 mg/ml and frozen down in aliquots until needed.   MNNG-treatment was performed in 75 cm^2 flasks with about 4×10^6 exponentially growing cells.   Appropriate amounts of MNNG solution were added to 10 ml serum free medium in the culture flasks and cells were incubated with the drug at 37° for 1 hr.

Cell Survival Assay   After the MNNG-treatment cells were trypsinized and aliquots plated into 90 mm tissue culture dishes to determine the plating efficiency.   After 10 days of growth colonies were stained with 1% methylene blue.   The effect of MNNG on cell survival was expressed as percent cloning efficiency relative to untreated controls.   The plating efficiency for untreated cultures was between 75% and 85%.

Selection for 6-thioguanine Resistant (6TG^r) Mutants   Clones resistant to 6TG were determined after continuous exponential growth of cells for 8 days after MNNG-treatment.   At that time, 10^5 cells were plated per dish in medium containing 5 g/ml 6TG.   The plating efficiency of cells in drug-free medium at this time was also measured and mutation frequencies were corrected for cell survival at the time of drug challenge.

Determination of Methylated Purine Bases   Cells were seeded into half gallon roller bottles and prelabeled overnight with 0.0025 Ci (^{3}H)-thymidine per ml (8.27 Ci/mmol; New England Nuclear, Boston, Mass.).   The next morning cells were treated for 30 min. with 1.2 g per ml (methyl-^{14}C) MNNG (13.9 Ci/mol, 10 Ci in 0.1 ml methylenechloride, New England Nuclear).   Then cells were rinsed with saline and received fresh medium. After 0, 4, 22 hr. cells from 2 bottles were harvested.   DNA isolation, DNA hydrolysis and chromatographic separation of the purine bases on a Sephadex G-10 column were performed as described previously (8, 9).   The absorption at 260 nm and the radioactivity of each fraction were determined.   The amount of methylated base was expressed as c.p.m. eluted in the respective peak relative to the concentration of the parent base.   The 22 hr. values were corrected for dilution by cell proliferation by calculating from the loss of ^{3}H specific activity of DNA in the 22 hr. interval a dilution factor (0.9 for Cl 9 and 0.62 for Cl 3) by which the calculated concentrations of parent bases were multiplied.

RESULTS

Survival as a function of the MNNG dose is qualitatively and quantitatively different in the two CHO variants Cl 9 and Cl 3 (Figure 1). Cl 3 cells are much more resistant to the toxic effects of MNNG than Cl 9 cells.   In Cl 3 cells survival is a simple exponential function of the MNNG dose, whereas Cl 9 cells have a biphasic response consisting of an initial steep drop followed by a flatter component with a slope similar to that of Cl 3.   This second component does not seem to be due to a resistant subpopulation, because any subclone derived from a single cell of Cl 9 shows again a biphasic survival curve (Goth-Goldstein, in preparation).

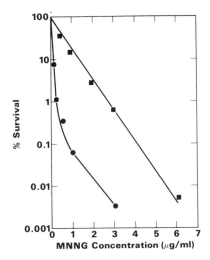

Fig. 1.   Cell survival after MNNG in parent line Cl 9 (●)
          and Cl 3 (■).

The increased resistance of Cl 3 to the toxic effect of MNNG was stable for
seven months in continuous culture.

To further characterize Cl 3 its mutability by MNNG was compared to
that of Cl 9 measuring induction of resistance to 6TG. MNNG induces 6TG^r
mutants linearly with dose and to the same extent in Cl 9 and Cl 3 (Figure
2). Other genetic markers, resistance to ouabain and diphtheria toxin,
seem to be induced by MNNG also at the same frequency in the two variants,
even though there is more scatter in the data, because these mutations are
induced at a much lower frequency.

The increased resistance of Cl 3 to MNNG is not due to a decreased
uptake of MNNG by Cl 3. If cells are treated with (methyl-^{14}C)MNNG, acid
precipitable material of Cl 9 and Cl 3 contains the same amount of ^{14}C
activity (data not shown). ^{14}C-MNNG also methylates the DNA of both cell

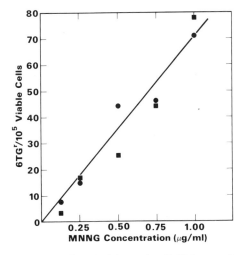

Fig. 2.   MNNG-induced mutations to 6-thioguanine resistance
          in Cl 9 (●) and Cl 3 (■).

Table 1. Relative amounts of methylated purine bases in the DNA of CHO cells treated for 30 min. with ^{14}C-MNNG

Clone	N3-methyladenine (cpm/µM A)	N7-methylguanine (cpm/ µM G)	0^6-methylguanine (cpm/ µM G)
9	57	1388	203
3	65	1225	185

Table 2. Loss of methylated purine bases from DNA expressed as fraction of 0-hr. value remaining in DNA.

Clone	Posttreatment Incubation [hr]	N3-methyladenine	N7-methylguanine	0^6-methylguanine
9	4	0.31	0.94	0.81
	22	<0.15	0.41*	0.98*
3	4	0.36	0.81	0.94
	22	<0.13	0.55*	1.0*

* Values corrected for dilution by cell proliferation

lines to the same extent with the same amounts of 3-methyladenine, 7-methylguanine and 0^6-methylguanine being formed (Table 1). The loss of these methylated purine bases from DNA during a 4 hr. or 22 hr. posttreatment incubation was also measured, and is given as fraction of the 0 hr. value remaining in DNA in Table 2. The values for Cl 9 and Cl 3 are very similar and compare well with data previously reported for Cl 9 after MNU treatment (9). The fractions of 3-methyladenine and 7-methylguanine remaining in DNA after 22 hr. are lower than what would be expected if they were lost by spontaneous depurination alone, indicating that these bases are also removed by cellular repair processes. In contrast, the amount of 0^6-methylguanine which is a stable product in DNA is unchanged after 22 hr. in both cell lines. Therefore, the different MNNG sensitivity of the two variants is not due to a different repair of these three major DNA methylation products.

DISCUSSION

Two CHO variants were compared in respect to their sensitivity to the cytotoxic effects of MNNG in which they differ considerably, and in respect to their mutability by MNNG, in which they are undistinguishable. A similar set of variants has been described for HeLa S3 cells where the resistant clone was obtained after treatment of the sensitive line with ethyl methanesulfonate (10). These findings demonstrate that cell killing and mutation induction by alkylating agents are separable events.

450

There are only few examples in the literature of mutants that are specifically hypersensitive to alkylating agents, where the hypersensitivity could be correlated to a biochemical alteration: the E. Coli tag and alkA mutants and Mer⁻ human tumor cells. The E. coli mutants lack a specific N-glycosylase, a repair enzyme which removes either specificially N3-methyladenine (tag) or has a broad substrate specificity for bases methylated at a ring nitrogen (alkA). Several human tumor cell strains are deficient in supporting the growth of adenovirus treated with MNNG and they are hypersensitive to killing by MNNG and other alkylating agents. All cell strains of this phenotype, termed Mer⁻, are also unable to repair O^6-methylguanine. The different MNNG sensitivity of the two CHO variants described here does not seem to be due to a different repair of the methylated purine bases. N3-methyladenine is removed readily in both lines and is no longer detectable after 22 hr. O^6-methylguanine is not repaired in either line.

As the biochemical difference of the CHO variants does not lie in the repair of the major methylated bases of DNA, there must be other factors which mediate cytotoxicity of MNNG which are altered in Cl 3 and lead to its increased survival after MNNG.

REFERENCES

1. B. Singer, N-nitroso alkylating agents: formation and persistence of alkyl derivatives in mammalian nucleic acids as contributing factors in carcinogenesis, J. Natl. Cancer Inst. 62:1329-1339 (1979).

2. A. E. Pegg, Formation and metabolism of alkylated nucleosides: Possible role in carcinogenesis by nitroso compounds and alkylating agents, Adv. Cancer Res. 25:195-269 (1977).

3. P. Karran, T. Lindahl, T. Ofsteng, G. B. Evensen, and E. Seeberg, Escherichia coli mutants deficient in 3-methyladenine-DNA glycosylase, J. Mol. Biol. 140: 101-127 (1980).

4. P. Karran, T. Hjelmgren, and T. Lindahl, Induction of a DNA glycosylase for N-methylated purines is part of the adaptive response to alkylating agents, Nature 296:770-773 (1982).

5. D. T. Beranek, R. H. Heflich, R. L. Kodell, S. M. Morris, and D. A. Casciano, Correlation between specific DNA methylation products and mutation induction at the HGPRT locus in Chinese hamster ovary cells, Mutation Res. 110:171-180 (1983).

6. R. S. Day, III, C. H. J. Ziolkowski, D. A. Scudiero, S. A. Meyer, A. S. Lubiniecki, A. J. Giradi, S. M. Galloway, and G. D. Bynum, Defective repair of alkylated DNA by human tumor and SV40-transformed human cell strain, Nature 288:724-727 (1980).

7. R. D. Wood and H. J. Burki, Repair capability and the cellular age response for killing and mutation induction after UV, Mutation Res. 95:505-514 (1982).

8. R. Goth-Goldstein, Repair of DNA damaged by alkylating carcinogens is defective in xeroderma pigmentosum derived fibroblasts, Nature 267:81-82 (1977).

9. R. Goth-Goldstein, Inability of Chinese hamster ovary cells to excise O^6-alkylguanine, Cancer Res. 40:2623-2624 (1980).

10. R. M. Baker, W. C. Van Voorhis, and L. A. Spencer, HeLa cell variants that differ in sensitivity to monofunctional alkylating agents with independence of cytotoxic and mutagenic response, Proc. Natl. Acad. Sci. (USA) 76:5249-5253 (1979).

INVESTIGATION OF THE SENSITIVITY OF ORIENTED φX-174 DNA TO IONIZING RADIATION

P. D. McCormack[1] and C. Swenberg[2]

[1]Division of Cancer Diagnosis and Biology
National Cancer Institute
National Institutes of Health
Bethesda, Maryland 20205

[2]Chief, Division of Physical Radiobiology
Armed Forces Radiobiology Research Institute
Bethesda, Maryland 20814

ABSTRACT

Application of an external electric field to an aqueous solution of φX-174 DNA is shown to result

a. in specific reduced dichroism changes which saturate at a field strength of 15,000 V/cm.

b. in increased sensitivity to damage by gamma-radiation estimated by agarose gel electrophoresis as single strand breaks.

Due to the mobility of the DNA, the maximum voltage used was 400 (2400 V/cm) and the percentage increase in yield (of SSBs per molecule) was 38%. At this field strength, theory predicts that only about 10% of the molecules are oriented by the field. The increase in damage must therefore be largely attributed to the conformational changes (unfolding) in the molecules induced by the applied electric field.

INTRODUCTION

Much effort has been made to increase the effectiveness of radiation in the treatment of tumors, by the use of the oxygen effect (1), hyperthermia and radiation sensitizing drugs. The latter are electron affinic compounds which can sensitize cells to radiation damage by fixation of the free radicals in DNA by oxidation. Neurotoxicity is dose limiting, and at this time there is no clinically effective method of radiation sensitization in regular use in radiation therapy. The object of the work to be described here is to establish whether or not orientation of DNA in electric fields could result in significant increase its sensitivity to damage by ionizing radiation.

The particular DNA chosen for study was ϕX-174. A considerable amount of research has been done on the effects of radiation on this DNA, and a further advantage is the well separated and simple band pattern which it produces in agarose gel electrophoresis for the damaged and undamaged forms.

Before any therapeutic value can be ascribed to the use of electric fields, a positive effect would have to be demonstrated for intracellular DNA and for tumor cells in animals, with a differential in the effect in favor of tumor versus normal cells. Aside from these clinical aspects, the results will have their own intrinsic value in relation to the general sphere of interest involving DNA/radiation interaction and the environmental aspect of exposure to strong electric fields.

ELECTRIC FIELD FORCES IN MOLECULES

A necessary condition for major electric field induced changes in molecules is the presence of permanent and/or induced dipoles, or ions or ionized groups. The primary effects of electric fields on molecules are:

a. Orientation of dipolar species.

b. Deformation of polarizable systems.

c. Movement of ionic species (electrophoresis).

Among the most successful use of electric fields for probing ionic structures and electrical and optical anisotropies, has been the case of linear polyelectrolytes. These are macromolecules with many ionizable groups. In solution they dissociate into polyvalent macro-ions (polyions) and a large number of small ions of opposite charge (counter-ions). Linear polyelectrolytes, and particularly polynucleotides and DNA, are electrically anisotropic. They are also optically anisotropic and give rise to the phenomena of electric birefringence and dichroism.

Electric Dichroism Of Macromolecules In Solution

By analogy with the definition of birefringence, the electric dichroism parallel, A_{11}, and perpendicular, A_1, to the field (E) of an assumbly of macro-ions in aqueous are defined as,

$$A_{11} = A_{11}(E) - A(0) \tag{1}$$

$$A_1 = A_1(E) - A(0) \tag{2}$$

where $A_{11}(E)$ and $A_1(E)$ are the optical absorbances of the solution for light polarized parallel and perpendicular to the field, with light propagation being perpendicular to the field. $A(0)$ denotes the isotropic absorbance measured at zero field. A more useful concentration independent quantity is the reduced parallel dichroism, defined as

$$A_{11}/A(0) = (A_{11}(E) - A(0))/A(0) \tag{3}$$

which is used here in reporting experimental results. For an ensemble of macro-ions in aqueous solution, the reduced parallel dichroism can be written as the product of an optical term $G(\theta)$ and an orientational function (2).

$$A_{11}/A(0) = G(\theta)\phi \tag{4}$$

The optical spectrum for the dilute solution of ϕX-174 DNA used in the experiments reported here, is shown in Figure 1. The characteristic DNA peak at a wavelength of 260 nm is clearly seen, and is due to the optical transitions of the nucleic acid bases. The variation of reduced parallel dichroism with field strength (for the same solution) is shown in Figure 2. The wavelength used for the measurements was 260 nm. The results indicate that,

   a. the reduced dichroism is not linearly related to either the field strength or to its square, at least to the lowest field strengths used (about 1200 V/cm).

   b. satuation sets in at about 15,000 V/cm.

A specific theory of optical activity for circular molecules is currently lacking. A least squares fit of the function arc tan is shown in Figure 2, but several other functions fit equally well.

By use of relaxation measurements to determine the rotational diffusion coefficient, Chen et al (3) determined that the length of the polynucleotide, dGm^{5}dC increased significantly during the change from the B- to the Z-form. Similarly, extension of the polyelectrolyte's dimensions generally accompanies the application of an external electric field (4). With such electric field effects on the conformation and orientation of polyelectrolytes such as DNA, it would not be surprising to find a concomitant effect on the interaction of oriented DNA and ionizing radiation.

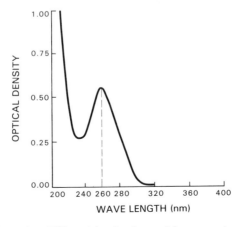

Fig. 1. DNA optical absorption spectrum.

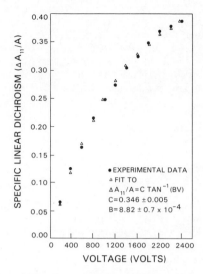

Fig. 2.   DNA electric dichroism field effect.

Effects Of Ionizing Radiation On DNA In Solution

It is now well established that the cell's DNA is the major target for radiation damage leading to cell death. Types of damage include single strand breaks, double strand breaks and cross-linking (Figure 3).

Ionizing radiation interacts with DNA in two ways:

a.   Direct - via a number of primary processes such as excitation, ionization, etc., which involve sites on the DNA molecule itself.

b.   Indirect - due to the action of small diffusible radicals (OH$\cdot$, H$\cdot$, and $_{aq}e^-$) released by the action of the radiation on the solvent (water).

In dilute aqueous solution of DNA, the indirect effect predominates (5) and the OH$\cdot$ radical produces most of the damage (6, 7, 8). Double strand breaks will result in biological inactivation and the biological yield, G_b, is defined as

$$G_b = (100/rD_{37})N_o \qquad (4)$$

where N_o = DNA concentration in number of molecules per ml.

   r   = number of eV deposited per gram per rad = 6.25×10^{13}

   D_{37} = 37% survival dose. At DNA concentrations below 0.7 mgm/ml the biological yield is $G_b = 0.9$.

Braams and Ebert (9, 10) have shown that the reaction rates between the free radical $_{aq}e^-$ and proteins such as ribonuclease increase with unfolding of the macromolecule. They analyzed this in terms of the collision frequency of $_{aq}e^-$ radicals with molecules modelled as extended rigid rods and spheres. Theory predicts that for molecular weights over 10^4 the collision frequencies for spherical molecules are much less than those for rod-like molecules. ϕX-174 DNA is a circular molecule and under

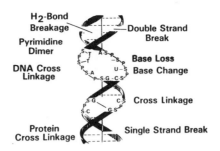

Fig. 3. Types of DNA radiation damage.

normal conditions of pH and ion concentration exists in a supercoiled form. Application of an external electric field would result in some uncoiling to occur, with increased exposure of reactive sites to the radiation produced free radicals. An increase in G value would therefore be expected, more on the basis of electric field conformation changes than of orientation.

Yield of Single Strand Breaks for ϕX-174 DNA

Consider the electrophoretic gel band pattern for ϕX-174 DNA illustrated in Figure 4. The undamaged supercoiled form, called the Replicative Form I has the greatest mobility in the gel and is the lowest band designated as RF-I, Band No. 1. One single strand break releases the tension in the molecule and produces the 'nicked' circular form, with the lowest mobility and is the top band designated as Band No. 3. A double strand break causes the circle to open up and produces the Linear form, designated as Band No. 2. In these experiments the yields were computed in terms of single strand breaks and the intensities of bands 1, 2, and 3 were monitored. To allow monitoring by scintillation counting, the DNA was tritiated, Then if,

RFI_O = counts/min, in the RFI band at zero dose = N_O

RFI_D = counts/min. in the RFI band at dose D(rad) = N, then using target theory

$$RFI_D/RFI_O = \exp(-n_{SSB/mol.})$$ (5)

or

$$n_{SSB/mol.} = \ln(RFI_O/RFI_D)$$ (6)

where $n_{SSB/mol.}$ is the number of single strand breaks per molecule. After irradiation of DNA in dilute solutions, the number of single strand breaks per nucleotide is proportional to the dose,

$$B_{SSB/nT} = kD$$ (7)

where k is the probability of a break per nucleotide per rad. At a DNA concentration of 0.2 mgm/ml, the value found for k was 415×10^{-t} rad^{-1} (11). Now, for ϕX-174 DNA, the molecular weight is 3.4×10^6 daltons, and with 3.5×10^2 daltons per nucleotide this gives about 10^4 nT/RFI molecule, where nT stands for nucleotide. Hence, the number of single strand breaks in ϕX-174 DNA for a dose of D rad is,

$$B_{\phi X} = 4.15 \times 10^{-3} \text{ D per molecule}$$ (8)

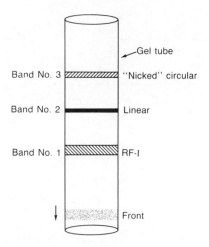

Fig. 4. Sketch of gel band patterns in φX-174 DNA.

Radiation Experiments

The experimental plan, in outline, was as follows:

1. Determination of the variation of the specific reduced dichroism of φX-174 DNA in aqueous solution, buffered with TRIS agent, with applied field voltage. This has been described and discussed Section 2.

2. Exposure of buffered tritiated φX-174 DNA in a Kerr cell (Figure 5) to a range of electrical voltages, in order to establish the loss of DNA through deposition on the steel electrodes. This determined the feasible range of voltages to be used in the radiation experiments.

3. Exposure of buffered tritiated φX-174 DNA in a Kerr cell to an intense source of ^{60}Co gamma radiation, while subjected to a range of electric field strengths.

4. Estimation of the variation of DNA damage with increasing field strength. Agarose gel electrophoresis was used to separate out the various damaged and undamaged fractions of the DNA. Quantitative estimation of the damage--in the form of single strand breaks and corresponding yield, or G values--was obtained by dissecting out the bands from the gels, determining the relative amounts present by scintillation counting, and using the formulas developed in Section 2.

φX-174 DNA

A pure (cloned) replicative form of φX-174 DNA was used in these experiments. As mentioned previously, it was tritiated. The concentration of DNA in the source solution was 0.75 mgm/ml. Electrophoresis showed the presence of a small amount of the nicked circular form. In the experiments, optical densities between .15 and .20 were required and so the procedure was to make up batches of 20 mls of solution (it took 1.3 mls to fill the Kerr cell) formed of,

a. 200 µl of DNA source solution diluted to 18 mls with pure water.

b. 2 mls TRIS buffer (millimolar).

c. 100 µl EDTA buffer (millimolar).

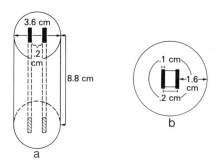

Fig. 5. Kerr cell. A: Cylinder - side view. B: Cylinder - top view

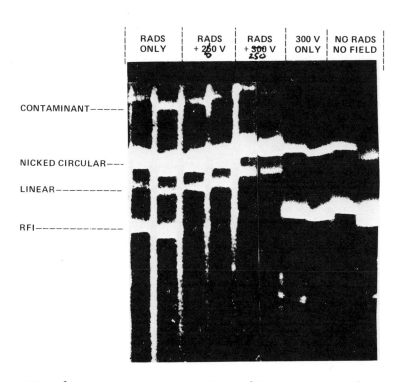

Fig. 6. Experimental gel pattern (Experiment No. 1).

The TRIS and EDTA were made up into a standard buffer solution, which then could be used as the 'background' solution in the spectrophotometer measurements. Optical densities varied over the experiments as follows:

WAVELENGTH	260 nm	280 nm
OPTICAL DENSITY	.18-.19	.091-.096

Gel band patterns for the solutions used (zero volts/zero radiation - 'background' cases) are shown in Figures 6 and 7.

KERR CELL AND RADIATION EXPOSURE

The DNA solution was placed in the Kerr cell. This cell had been designed by Elliott Charney at the National Institutes of Health in Bethesda, for use in his electric dichroism work. It is a high quality lucite cylinder, 8.8 cms long and 3.6 cms diameter (Figure 5). A rectangular cavity was cut out of the cylinder along an equatorial plane and this was lined with two stainless steel plates spaced about 1.5 mms apart. The ends of the cavity were sealed with two lucite plates screwed down to impinge on teflon seals. Two steel pins connected the electrodes via external leads to the power supply.

To compute the dose to the solution in the cell when exposed ^{60}CO source, the tissue-to-air ratio (TAR) was determined experimentally and theoretically (using the Bragg-Gray Principle governing small cavity ionization). With the steel plates pointed towards the source and the Kerr cell vertical, the TAR value computed for the cell was 0.94 and this was confirmed by experiment. For an air dose rate of 7005 rad/min., this gives a solution dose rate of 6585 rad/min. There was an added dose of 487 rad which allowed for the time taken to raise and lower the source. In the series of radiation exposures (experiments number 1 and 2) the total exposure time was 2 minutes, giving a total dose to the DNA solution of 13,627 rad.

Electric Field Apparatus

The electric field voltage was supplied from a stabilized power supply which could supply up to 2,000 volts at currents up to 100 m.a. The mobility of DNA in solution is quite high - of the order of 5×10^{-4} cm./sec. volt at 10 mM sodium ion concentration (Ref.12). At 1000 volts, for example, a terminal velocity of about 3 cm./sec. would be expected. With an electrode spacing of .15cm., removal of all the DNA to the positive electrode would occur in about 50 millisecs. At 400 volts this would increase to about 125 millisecs. To reduce this electrophoretic loss of DNA, field reversal was used. The vacuum relay which accomplished the reversal had a switching time of about 150 millisecs and so a practical upper limit of 400 volts for the applied field was indicated and this was substantiated by experimental results.

AGAROSE GELS

The only points of note here were that,

a. TRIS-acetate buffer was used to make the gels.

b. Tube gels were made.

c. Ethidium Bromide dye was added after the electrophoresis was complete.

d. 25 μl DNA solution plus bromophenol blue was poured on top of each tube.

The gel patterns were examined under UV light and photographed. The bands were then dissected out of the gels, placed in containers with 20 mls of scintillator 'cocktail' and the relative DNA contents measured in an automatic scintillation counting unit.

INVESTIGATION OF DNA LOSS BY ELECTRIC FIELD EFFECT ALONE

This experiment involved subjecting the buffered φX-174 DNA solution in the Kerr cell to field voltages from 200 to 400 (field strengths from 1200 to 2400 V/cm), without irradiation, for periods of two minutes. Percentage loss of DNA was subsequently determined by taking 2 μl samples of the exposed DNA and adding them to 10 mls of scintillator 'cocktail' for counting. Figure 8 (top graph) shows that at 400 volts there was a very large loss of DNA (almost 100%). It was found that by switching the field ON and OFF every ten seconds, the loss of DNA was reduced (to about 80% at 400 volts). The loss was further reduced by using an interval of five seconds (30% loss at 400 volts). In the first radiation experiment a continuous voltage was applied to the electrodes, but the maximum voltage used was 250 volts. Corrections were made for 'field' losses in computing yields. In the second radiation experiment voltages up to 400 were used, but the field was switched ON and OFF at five second intervals. As the field was only on for one minute, less field effect would be expected. Again, corrections to computed yield values for 'field' losses of DNA were made.

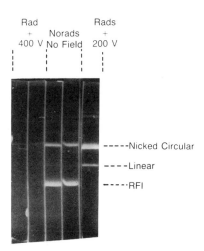

Fig. 7.   Experimental gel pattern (Experiment No. 2)

FIRST RADIATION EXPERIMENT

In this experiment there were three radiation exposures of the DNA solution in the Kerr cell. The exposures were of two minutes exposure with a total absorbed dose of 13,627 rad each. The conditions for the exposure were:

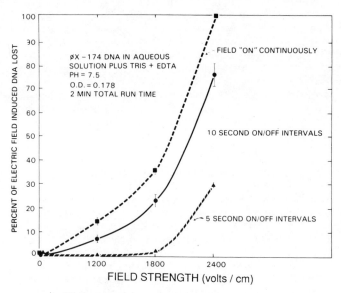

Fig. 8. Electric field induced DNA losses.

Number 1   Radiation +250 volt field.

Number 2   Radiation +200 volt field.

Number 3   Radiation only.

A further three control measurements were made as follows:

Number 4   250 volt field only.

Number 5   200 volt field only.

Number 6   Background —zero radiation/zero field.

A photograph of the gel electrophoresis patterns is shown in Figure 6. A summary of the results obtained in counts/min., for each of the bands obtained in each run, is shown in Table 1. A small amount of contaminant was present and this produces the top (fourth) band. Band No. 3 is the nicked circular; 2 is the linear; 1 is the RFI.

Using Equation 6 for the number of single strand breaks per ϕX molecule, the yield G was computed from Table 1 for the three radiation runs. These are given in Column 1 of Table 2 and are designated as uncorrected. The corrected values, based on the 'field' losses as given by Runs 4 and 5 are give in Column 2. The field induced increases in single strand breaks are given in Column 4 and are 40% at 250 volts (1500 V/cm) and 27% at 200 volts (1200 V/cm).

SECOND RADIATION EXPERIMENT

The procedures described in Experiment No. 1 were largely repeated in this series. Voltages of 200, 250, 300, 350, and 400 were used. As mentioned earlier, to minimize the 'field' loss of DNA the field was switched ON for five seconds and then OFF for five seconds over the two minute exposure interval. Some reduction in yield would be expected and the results of Experiments No. 1 and 2 are not exactly comparable.

Table 1. Scintillation counts/min. - Experiment No. 1

Run No.	Band No. 4	3	2	1
1. RAD+250V	810	7,100	806	1,612
2. RAD+200V	680	12,700	218	2,238
3. RAD	640	25,400	4,500	5,455
4. 250V	791	1,100	484	18,621
5. 200V	740	950	640	20,500
6. Background	868	7,140	545	31,221

Table 2. Single strand break yields in Experiment No. 1

Run No.	G Value Uncorrected	Corrected	% Increase
1. RAD+250V	2.96	2.44	40
2. RAD+200V	2.63	2.21	27
3. RAD	1.74	-	-

Table 3. Radiation results - Experiment No. 2

Run No.	Band No. 3	2	1	G Value Uncorr.	Corr.	%Increase in G Uncorr.	Corr.
1. Background	1500	560	8,300	-	-	-	-
2. Radiation	6350	1250	1,500	1.71	-	-	-
3. 400V	1250	940	3,800	-	-	-	-
4. RAD+400V	4620	850	358	3.14	2.36	83	38

Figure 7 shows the gel patterns obtained for the 400V , 300V, and background cases. Table 3 presents the background, 400V and 400V plus radiation results. The uncorrected and corrected G values and the % increases in single strand breaks due to the electric field effect are shown.

Figure 9 shows the percent increase in single strand breaks per molecule plotted versus field voltage (multiply by 6 to get approximate field strength). The increases in the 250/300 volt region are less than those recorded in Experiment No. 1, reflecting the reduced electric field exposure time in Experiment No. 2. The dichroism field effect results have been also entered in Figure 9 and the increase in yield of SSB's (single strand breaks) appear to follow the increase in specific reduced dichroism.

In Equation 8 the predicted number of SSB per ϕX molecule, at a concentration of .2 mgm/ml, was given as

$$G = 4.15 \times 10^{-3} D$$

where D is the dose in rad, and taking 10^4 as the approximate number of nucleotides in the ϕX molecule. For a total dose of 13,627 rad, this would predict a yield of about 56 single strand breaks per molecule. The concentration of DNA used in these experiments was only 0.008 mgm/ml--about 1/25th the above value. Scaling linearly for concentration reduction, a G value here of about 2 would be expected. Values obtained in the 'radiation only' runs in Experiments No. 1 and 2 above, were in the region of 1.7. Within experimental error, the correspondence is close enough to confirm the reliability of the results obtained here.

The effect of Joule heating of the DNA solution during each run has not so far been addressed. To minimize, the Kerr cell was chilled before each experiment and during the exposures rested on solid CO_2 which acted as a heat sink. Temperature rises, measured by a thermistor immersed in the DNA solution, in dummy runs using the electric field alone, were limited to less than 8°C.

CONCLUSIONS

The results demonstrate a significant increase in gamma radiation damage to ϕX-174 DNA in dilute aqueous solution in the presence of quite

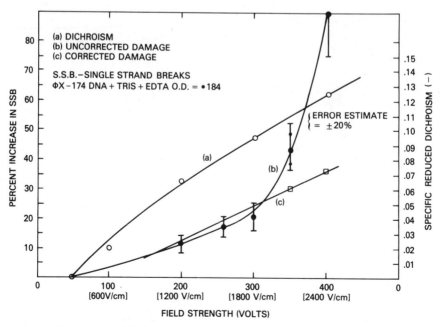

Fig. 9.   DNA damage versus electric field strength.

moderate field strengths. At a field strength of 2400 V/cm (400V) the increase is about 38%. Dichroism results indicate that only about 10% of the DNA molecules are aligned with the external field at this field strength. Thus, field induced conformational changes must be the source of this large effect.

Linear extrapolation of the damage versus field strength curve to the saturation value of 15,000 V/cm would predict an increase of the order of 250%. This would need to be verified by extending the range of field strengths used to much higher values, which would necessitate the use of electronic field switching. The results are promising enough to warrant a similar investigation using intracellular DNA and it is planned to do this shortly. The phenomena of electric birefringence and dichroism have already been established for chromatin subunits (13, 14) and so it is not unreasonable to expect that an external electric field could sensitize the intracellular DNA to damage by ionizing radiation.

ACKNOWLEDGEMENTS

Dr. Percival D. McCormack gratefully acknowledges the award of a Senior Staff Fellowship at the National Cancer Institute, National Institutes of Health, which made this work possible and the encouragement given by Drs. DeLisi and Jernigan of the National Cancer Institute. The authors acknowledge the valuable assistance given by Major M. Hagan, Ph.D., U. S. Army and the Armed Forces Radiobiology Research Institute, as is the willing and efficient assistance of Mr. Golightly and Lt. Dooley of the AFRRI Staff in the Division of Radiological Physics. The assistance and advice of Drs. Charney, Chen and Rau of the Department of Chemical Physics, National Institutes of Health is also very much appreciated.

REFERENCES

1. L. W. Brady, T. L. Phillips, and T. H. Wasserman, in: "Progress in Radio-Oncology, II," K. H. Karcher, ed., Raven Press, New York, (1982), pp. 834-842.

2. E. Charney and K. Yamaoka, Biochemistry 21:834-842 (1982).

3. H. H. Chen, E. Charney, and D. Rau, Nucleic Acids Research 10:3561-3571 (1982).

4. R. Jernigan and S. Miyazawa, in: "Molecular Electro-Optics," S. Krause, ed., Plenum Press (1981), pp. 163-179.

5. W. Gunther and H. Jung, Z. Naturforsch 22b:313 (1967).

6. J. Blok and H. Loman, Current Topics in Rad. Res. Quart. 9:165 (1973).

7. G. Scholes, Prog. Biophys. Mol. Biol. 13:597 (1963).

8. J. Ward, Int. J. Rad. Phys. Chem. 3:239 (1971).

9. R. Braams and M. Ebert, Adv. Chem. Ser. 81:464-471 (1968).

10. R. Braams and M. Ebert, Int. J. Rad. Biol. 13:195 (1967).

11. U. Hagen, Biochim. Phys. Acta 134:45 (1967).

12. P. H. Johnson and L. J. Grossman, Biochemistry 16:4217 (1977).

13. J. McGhee, D. Rau, E. Charney, and G. Felsenfeld, _Cell_ 22(Pt. 1):87 (1980).

14. H. Wu, N. Dattagupta, M. Hogan, and D. Crothers, _Biochemistry_ 18:3960 (1979).

RADIOSENSITIZERS AND THYMINE BASE DAMAGE

Joyce F. Remsen

Laboratory for Energy-Related Health Research
University of California
Davis, California

ABSTRACT

The use of radiosensitizers in the therapy of cancer in conjunction with radiation has been of considerable interest. The mechanism by which they act, however, is not clear. Because these compounds have an electron affinity similar to oxygen and/or are free radicals, it was postulated that their presence might have an effect on the formation of DNA base damage induced by radiation. The effect of three sensitizers, misonidazole, p-nitroacetophenone and 4-hydroxy-2,2,6,6-tetramethylpiperidino-1-oxy (TMPN), on formation of thymine damage of the 5,6-dihydroxydihydrothymine type by irradiation with gamma rays was characterized in HeLa cells. The three sensitizers have different electron affinities, or, in the case of TMPN, are a stable free radical. The formation of thymine base damage was measured in the presence of increasing concentrations of each of the three sensitizers with and without 500 Gy of cobalt-60 gamma rays, at ice temperature. Each sensitizer gave a different result. Increasing concentrations of misonidazole suppressed the formation of base damage in air but had no apparent effect under hypoxia. In the presence of p-nitroacetophenone, similar amounts of base damage were formed under both aerobic and hypoxic conditions. TMPN, on the other hand, resulted in a complex pattern, with suppression at higher concentrations (60 mM). The overall conclusion is that the sensitizers do not result in increased base damage but, if anything, suppress its formation. Therefore, the mechanism by which they sensitize under hypoxic conditions, such as found in solid tumors, is not by an increase in thymine base damage.

INTRODUCTION

Radiosensitizers are compounds which increase the sensitivity of cells to radiation under hypoxic conditions, such as found in the center of solid tumors where vascularization is poor. A major class of sensitizers contain an imidazole ring as exemplified by misonidazole (Ro-07-0582, 1-(2-nitroimidazole-1-yl)-3-methoxypropan-2-ol), a nitroimidazole. The effectiveness of the nitroimidazoles is influenced by the side chains and their positions on the imidazole ring and is correlated with electron affinity. In general, the higher the electron affinity, the greater the sensitization. Two other compounds which have been shown to enhance sensitivity of specific cell systems under hypoxic conditions are p-nitroacetophenone, also an electron-affinic compound, and 4-hydroxy-2,2,6,6-tetramethylpiperidino-1-oxy (TMPN), a stable free radical. Much of the information on the biological effectiveness of these sensitizers has come from studies on survival of cells in culture. Although some information is available about their metabolism and reaction with the product of radiolysis of water, little is understood about the mechanism by which they sensitize. Although there is some evidence for covalent bonding with DNA, indirect effects are also possible.

Past research has indicated that DNA damage from ionizing radiation is largely due to indirect action of the products of the radiolysis of water and that damage is greater under aerobic conditions than under hypoxia. Since sensitizers react with the products of radiolysis, have electron affinity similar to oxygen, and are free radicals, it was postulated that one mechanism by which they could exert their biological effect was by altering the amount of damage. One type of damage which can readily be measured is thymine base damage of the 5,6-dihydroxydihydrothymine type. This damage is formed primarily by the hydroxyl radical produced by the radiolysis of water in cells (2). In addition, metabolism of sensitizers (specifically misonidazole) differs under aerobic and hypoxic conditions. Also, thymine base damage is less when cells are irradiated under hypoxic conditions (3). The effect of the three sensitizers on the formation of thymine base damage when present during irradiation with gamma rays from a cobalt-60 source was studied under aerobic and hypoxic conditions.

METHODS

HeLa cells were prelabeled with ^{3}H-thymine for 20 hours. Cells were irradiated with 500 Gy of gamma rays in the presence of increasing concentrations of each of the three sensitizers. Controls consisted of unirradiated cells, cells receiving radiation alone, and cells exposed to sensitizers but no irradiation. All manipulations were at ice temperature. Cells were irradiated under aerobic or hypoxic conditions. For aerobic conditions, the dose was fractionated with mixing of the cell suspensions to reaerate. For hypoxia, cell suspensions were gassed for 30 minutes with nitrogen in stoppered tubes and, while the dose was fractionated so that the cells could be resuspended, the sealed tubes were not opened. Four fractionations were used. At the end of the irradiation period, aliquots of cells were added to an equal volume of 10% TCA and the precipitate assayed for thymine base damage of the 5,6-dihydroxydihydrothymine type (1). Viability as determined by trypan blue dye exclusion was the same at the termination of the experiment as at the beginning.

RESULTS

The effects of the three sensitizers on formation of thymine base damage when present during irradiation with cobalt-60 gamma rays were different. This is not surprising because of the difference in structure, electron affinity and metabolism. Misonidazole depressed formation of base damage at higher concentration (15 mM) under aerobic conditions with no apparent effect under hypoxia; no net base damage was detected. Misonidazole alone with no irradiation resulted in the formation of some product which was detected by the alkaline-acid degradation assay used for thymine damage (Remsen, Radiat. Res., in press). The structure of this compound is not known but could represent a covalent adduct formed via free radical interactions.

Para-nitroacetophenone yielded similar amounts of damage due to radiation under both conditions and that amount increased significantly in a dose dependent manner. The amount of assayable product without irradiation was minor compared with radiation-induced damage. With the nitroxy free radical, TMPN, the pattern of formation of product was complex in that at low concentrations, assayable product was decreased but it increased at higher concentrations. The net effect of TMPN at 60 mM was to decrease the radiation-induced damage under both aerobic and hypoxic conditions.

CONCLUSIONS

The three sensitizers effect formation of thymine base damage in different ways. Since either the formation of 5,6-dihydroxydihydrothymine type lesions is the same under both conditions of irradiation or is suppressed, it is concluded that thymine base damage plays a minor role, if any, in the sensitization of hypoxic cells to sensitizers and, therefore, is not a major mechanism by which sensitizers exert their action.

ACKNOWLEDGEMENT

This research was supported by Grant PHS CA34861-02 of the National Cancer Institute.

REFERENCES

1. P. V. Hariharan and P. A Cerutti, Proc. Natl. Acad. Sci. (USA) 71:3532 (1974).

2. J. F. Remsen and J. L. RotiRoti, Int. J. Radiat. Biol. 32:191 (1977).

3. J. L. RotiRoti and P. Cerutti, Int. J. Radiat. Biol. 25:413 (1974).

HUMAN CANCER-PRONE DISORDERS, ABNORMAL CARCINOGEN RESPONSE, AND DEFECTIVE DNA METABOLISM[1]

M. C. Paterson, M. V. Middlestadt, M. Weinfeld,
R. Mirzayans and N. E. Gentner*

Molecular Genetics and Carcinogenesis Laboratory
Department of Medicine, Cross Cancer Institute, Edmonton
Alberta, Canada T6G 1Z2
*Health Sciences Division
 Chalk River Nuclear Laboratories
 Atomic Energy of Canada Limited
 Chalk River, Ontario, Canada K0J 1J0

INTRODUCTION

Insight into cancer, one of the principal scourges of modern man, has increased slowly but steadily over the years. Epidemiologists concur that most human malignancies are caused, at least in part, by environmental determinants over which an individual can exercise some control; in principle then, the disease is preventable to some extent (10). In practice, however, the goal of cancer prevention by large-scale efforts to minimize exposure to the causal agents would seem to be unattainable, as judged by societal experience with two major 'life-style' factors, habitual tobacco usage and sunbathing. Although an ultimate aim is to develop other more socially acceptable prevention strategies, there exists in the interim a requirement for improved diagnostic techniques and more rational treatment protocols. Each of these approaches to cancer control will almost certainly necessitate clearer understanding of the fundamental mechanisms underlying the etiology and pathogenesis of the disease.

One burgeoning line of exploration into the carcinogenic process is the investigation of human genetics as it pertains to mankind's susceptibility to cancer. Although as many as 90% of all human malignant neoplasms are said to have environmental causes (21), by far the most potent risk factor is the genetic component. There exists a repertoire of loci in the human genome, any one of which, in its mutated form, can confer

---

[1]This article is substantially similar to one published in the proceedings of the NATO/ENEA Advanced Science Institutes Course on "Epidemiology and Quantitation of Environmental Risk in Humans from Radiation and Other Agents," (A. Castellani, ed.), San Miniato, Italy, 1984 September 02-11, Plenum Press, New York (1985), pg. 235.

a marked increase in cancer risk (37). In fact, ecogenetics, involving the study of individual variation in response to an environmental factor (37), is rapidly emerging as a profitable experimental approach for unravelling the origins of cancer.

A particularly enlightening ecogenetic inquiry concerns the application of laboratory models (derived primarily from microbial systems) to the in vitro investigation of cells from patients in whom astute clinicians have noted an untoward response to a recognized carcinogen (35). These patients, for the most part, are afflicted with Mendelian monogenic traits characterized by a propensity to develop malignancy. Cultured cells from subjects with many of these rare hereditary disorders display enhanced sensitivity to inactivation by the pertinent etiological agent; in several syndromes, this carcinogen hypersensitivity is, in turn, associated with anomalies in the enzymatic processes that repair, replicate past, or otherwise tolerate lesions introduced into DNA by the same carcinogenic agent (14, 26, 44). Such correlations provide telling evidence that fully functional DNA metabolic systems form an integral part of the host machinery which Homo sapiens routinely marshals in defense against the development of cancer.

EXPERIMENTAL STRATEGIES AND PRIMARY AIMS

This chapter describes our own particular laboratory studies into the various molecular mechanisms that underlie the predisposition to cancer seen in certain hereditary and familial conditions. In each of these undertakings, primary emphasis has been placed on evaluating the role of carcinogen-induced injury to cellular DNA and the faulty enzymatic repair of this damage as a contributing factor in the multistep process whereby a normal somatic cell may undergo malignant conversion.

In general, our experimental approach has entailed subjecting dermal fibroblast strains, derived from selected donors, to a battery of assays which are designed to detect specific biological and/or biochemical abnormalities following exposure to an etiologically relevant carcinogen. Normally a given fibroblast strain was monitored first for reproductive survival, as judged by retention of colony-forming ability (CFA), in response to a panel of appropriate carcinogens; if a strain responded abnormally to any of these agents, a search was then undertaken for anomalies in either the initial induction or the subsequent metabolic processing of specific lesions induced in DNA by the pertinent agent(s). Two disorders--xeroderma pigmentosum (XP), a skin disease characterized by striking sensitivity to solar ultraviolet (UV) light, and ataxia telangiectasia (AT), its ionizing radiation-sensitive, neurovascular counterpart, served as archetypes for our investigations. Both of the foregoing are rare, autosomal recessively inherited syndromes in which cancer proneness and carcinogen hypercytotoxicity have been closely linked with defects in lesion processing (for review, see 26, 44). In charting this experimental course, our intent has been four-fold: (1) to extend current knowledge of known DNA repair deficiency disorders; (2) to identify other cancer-prone ecogenetic traits, and then to define their molecular basis; (3) to utilize these mutant strains to assist in delineating the normal sequence of reactions in different DNA repair processes and in other cellular processes germane to carcinogenesis; and (4) to assess the contribution of heterozygous carriers of genes for malignancy-associated autosomal recessive syndromes in general and AT in particular to the overall cancer burden in the general population.

STATUS REPORT ON OUR OWN ECOGENETIC STUDIES

Our progess thus far in seven specific ecogenetic investigations is now summarized (for background information, see refs. 41, 42, 44). Space restrictions necessarily preclude all but cursory reference to parallel studies in other laboratories.

New Insight into the Molecular Defect in XP

A major breakthrough in our understanding of environmental-hereditary interactions in cancer causation occurred when Cleaver (5) provided evidence that dermal fibroblasts from XP patients are defective in handling cyclobutyl pyrimidine dimers. These DNA lesions, which are formed by the covalent joining of adjacent intrastrand pyrimidine bases upon absorption of UV radiation, are believed to be largely responsible for the lethal, mutagenic, and carcinogenic effects of sunlight (32, 50). Since Cleaver's seminal disclosure some 17 years ago, many advances have been made in defining the DNA repair deficiencies displayed by cultured XP cells after exposure to UV rays and certain chemical carcinogens (for details regarding the overall laboratory picture in XP, including the impairments in post-UV colony survival and DNA metabolism typical of cells from affected donors, see refs. 6, 14, 26, 44). In this characterization, fibroblast strains from 119 unrelated XP patients have been allocated to nine genetically distinct groups on the basis of a biochemical complementation test, using a conventional somatic cell fusion technique. As can be seen in Table 1, 98 of the strains have been assigned to eight mutually complementing groups, designated A-H. The primary biochemical anomaly in each of these strains is apparently a deficiency in the ability to execute the nucleotide mode of excision repair. The remaining 21 XP strains have been pooled together to form the ninth complementation group, the so-called variant. The most striking anomaly in these latter strains appears to be a marked deficiency in performing post-replication or daughter-strand repair, an ill-defined process that is presently thought to be instrumental in permitting the de novo DNA synthesis machinery to replicate past pyrimidine dimers and other non-coding alterations in template DNA.

Table 1. DNA repair properties of xeroderma pigmentosum complementation groups[a]

| | | Excision Repair (% of normal) as judged by | | |
Group	No. of Cases	UV Endonuclease Site Removal	UV-induced Repair Synthesis	Postreplication Repair
A	49	~0	<5[b]	partly deficient
B	1	<10	3-7	partly deficient
C	32	15-35	10-25	partly deficient
D	9	~0	20-55	partly deficient
E	1	60	40-60	proficient
F	3	70	10-20	?[c]
G	2	~0	<5	partly deficient
H	1	?	30	partly deficient
Variant	21	100	60-100	markedly deficient
Total	119			

[a] Adapted from Paterson et al. (1984b)

[b] One strain (XP8LO) displays 30% of normal repair synthesis

[c] Unknown

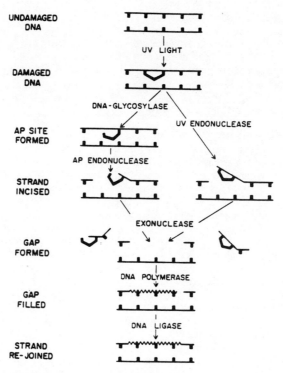

Fig. 1. Proposed model for the two distinct mechanisms by which the nucleotide mode of excision repair is known to occur in different microbial systems. In this mode a carcinogen-induced defect (illustrated here as a cyclobutyl pyrimidine dimer) in either chain of the double helix is excised within an oligonucleotide, as detailed in the text. The designation nucleotide excision distinguishes it from another general excision repair mode termed base excision. (In the latter, a carcinogen-damaged or nonconventional base is released by a highly specific DNA glycosylase, after which the resultant AP site is restored by co-ordinated strand incision/AP site excision/repair synthesis/strand ligation reactions (for details, consult refs. 13 and 30)).

The current model for the nucleotide excision repair process has been derived principally from the more extensive and sophisticated studies possible in simple prokaryotes (see refs. 13, 20, 43, 51). As shown schematically in Figure 1, two distinct pathways for this intricate multienzymatic process have been identified to date. The first pathway, originally described in Escherichia coli almost two decades ago, is composed of the following sequential reactions: (1) the damage-containing strand is incised upstream from (i.e., on the 5'-side of) the lesion by a damage-recognizing endonuclease (e.g., a so-called UV endonuclease in the case of the pyrimidine dimer); (2) a second nick is made downstream from (i.e., on the 3'-side of) the lesion by an exonuclease, facilitating the release of the lesion within a short oligonucleotide (in E. coli, at least, the first two steps are, in fact, performed in concert by an 'excinuclease complex' and may be followed by 5'→3' exonucleolytic removal of 5'-deoxyribonucleoside monophosphates); (3) the resultant gap is filled in with nucleotides complementary to those in the opposite, intact strand by a

474

DNA polymerase, in a procedure termed repair synthesis; and finally (4) the pre-existing and newly synthesized strand termini are covalently joined by a DNA ligase.

The second pathway by which nucleotide excision repair may proceed is found in, for example, Micrococcus luteus and bacteriophage T4. Their 'UV endonucleases' accomplish incision at a dimer-containing site by the sequential action of a pyrimidine dimer-DNA glycosylase activity and an apyrimidinic/apurinic (AP) endonuclease activity. The former cleaves the N-glycosyl bond between the 5'-pyrimidine member of a dimer and its corresponding deoxyribose, and the latter then hydrolyzes a phosphodiester bond 3' to the newly formed AP site. In all probability, the incised site is subsequently mended as in the first nucleotide excision pathway--that is, site removal, repair synthesis and strand ligation.

By virtue of their abnormality in excision repair, XP strains belonging to groups A-H are also inept, where tested, in handling a variety of other bulky lesions, such as those induced by reactive metabolites of the following potent chemical carcinogens: benzo(a)pyrene, N-acetoxy-2-acetylaminofluorene and 4-nitroquinoline 1-oxide (4NQO) (26, 44). What is more, these eight genetic forms of the disease all seem to be blocked, inexplicably, at the same stage (incision step) in the excision repair process.

In general, strains belonging to a given excision repair-defective complementation group display a similar degree of repair deficiency. This holds irrespective of the particular DNA repair assay used, including those presumed to monitor early or late reactions in the excision-repair process. As a case in point, group A strains appear to be severely defective in executing dimer repair, as exemplified by the following two deficits: (1) negligible ability to perform the initial incision event in the removal of dimer-containing sites (detected as UV-induced sites susceptible to subsequent strand incision in vitro by the action of a UV endonuclease contained in a crude protein extract of M. luteus, and hereafter referred to as UV endonuclease-sensitive sites); and (2) pronounced impairment in the capacity to carry out UV-induced repair synthesis (measured as unscheduled DNA synthesis (UDS) or DNA repair replication) (see Table 1). In several other excision repair-defective groups (e.g., C), although a reduced ability to perform dimer repair is apparent, a significant residual level clearly remains; this is true for both assays in Table 1.

XP group D, however, constitutes a glaring exception to the inter-assay uniformity in quantitating the residual repair capacity of representative strains from patients with the disorder (see Table 1). Strains assigned to this group are markedly, if not totally, impaired in effecting the elimination of UV endonuclease-sensitive sites, but nonetheless manage to carry out a substantial amount of UV-induced repair synthesis, ranging from 20-55% of normal, depending upon which laboratory's results are cited. (A second exception is evident in another group, namely, F; in contradistinction to group D, strains in this group appear to act on many more UV endonuclease-sensitive sites than expected from their repair synthesis deficiency.)

One possible explanation for the peculiar excision repair properties of group D fibroblasts is that, following UV exposure, these mutant cells may act in an aberrant manner on a fraction of the dimer-containing sites, inserting repair patches while failing to excise the photoproducts themselves. To test whether some of the dimers are modified but not removed in group D strains, we measured the photoreactivability (a well-documented diagnostic probe of dimer authenticity (19)) of UV endonuclease-sensitive sites in extracted DNA from normal and group D strains as a

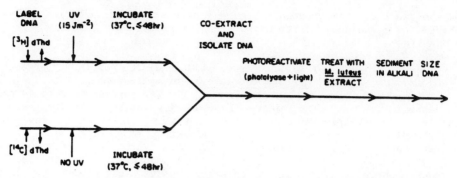

Fig. 2.   Experimental scheme designed to detect aberrant repair of UV-
           induced pyrimidine dimers in XP group D fibroblasts. The
           treatment protocol was virtually identical to that followed in
           a conventional enzymatic assay for dimer quantification (48),
           except for the introduction of an enzymatic PR step (thus
           converting remaining dimers back to normal monomers in situ)
           prior to treatment of the naked DNA with an M. luteus protein
           extract containing dimer-recognizing UV endonuclease. The
           ^{14}C-labelled DNA from non-UV-irradiated cultures served as an
           internal control which permitted correction for non-specific
           strand breakage stemming from the various physical
           manipulations and enzymatic treatments prescribed in the
           assay.

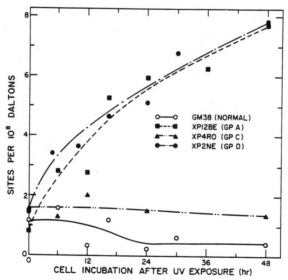

Fig. 3.   Incidence of novel sites accumulating in the DNA
           of normal and XP strains as a function of post-UV
           incubation time. The experimental protocol is
           outlined in Figure 2. Each datum point is the
           mean of multiple determinations (SE <15%).

function of cell incubation time after exposure to 15 J m^{-2} of far UV
(chiefly 254 nm) light. Our assay protocol is depicted in Figure 2.
Following post-UV incubation, each cell culture was lyzed; the extracted

DNA was subjected to exhaustive enzymatic photoreactivation (PR) treatment (using highly purified Streptomyces griseus photolyase which, in the presence of fluorescent light, simply ruptures the cyclobutane ring of a pyrimidine dimer, thereby regenerating two normal monomeric pyrimidines in situ without any additional modification to the site, and was then probed by incubation with an M. luteus extract containing UV endonuclease activity. In short, this series of treatments was expected to detect any dimer-containing sites which had been altered so as to render them refractory to photoenzymatic monomerization but still susceptible to incision by UV endonuclease. Lastly, the number of extract-induced single-strand breaks, and thus the incidence of apparently unrepaired sites remaining in the DNA, was determined by velocity sedimentation in alkaline sucrose gradients.

Our results, presented in Figure 3, demonstrated the appearance of altered sites in the DNA of XP group D (XP2NE) cells specifically with incubation after UV exposure (also see ref. 40). These sites did not arise in similarly treated control (GM38) cells, suggesting that their occurrence in the XP strain arose from unsuccessful attempts to repair UV-induced pyrimidine dimers. These novel sites in the DNA of XP2NE fibroblasts reached an incidence approaching 8 per 10^8 daltons by 48 hrs; this number was equivalent to ~15% of the dimers initially introduced, and was similar in magnitude to the residual level of UV-stimulated repair synthesis (15-20% of normal) arising in the XP strain. Accumulation of novel sites after UV irradiation was not confined to XP group D. As illustrated in Figure 3, sites also appeared in the UV-damaged DNA of incubated group A (XP12BE) cells, with kinetics very similar to those in group D cells. On the other hand, a representative group C strain, XP4RO, behaved very much like the normal GM38 strain.

In both XP groups A and D strains, there was no decrease (compared to the number originally induced) in total UV endonuclease-sensitive sites or in the number of dimers actually remaining in DNA (16), but there was an apparent decrease in the number of UV endonuclease-sensitive sites subject to restoration by enzymatic PR (Figure 3). One interpretation of these findings is that the photoenzymatic treatment gives rise to strand breaks at these seemingly metabolically modified dimer-containing sites (that is, the same sites that are normally recognized by UV endonuclease). If so, then these sites should be detectable as frank single-strand breaks if extracted DNA was subjected to enzymatic PR alone (that is, without ensuing M. luteus extract treatment). We have now demonstrated that this is indeed the case. This intriguing observation is consistent with the notion that during post-UV incubation of group A and D fibroblasts, a phosphodiester bond between the two dimer-forming pyrimidines may be cleaved, and that at these modified sites individual DNA chains are then held together solely by the cyclobutane ring (i.e., -p-T̄-p-T̄-p- ⟶ -p-T̄ p-T̄-p- or -p-T̄-p T-p-). It seems that the excision repair process tends to abort at this stage in group A cells since they carry out little repair synthesis, whereas in group D cells the intradimer backbone cleavage is apparently accompanied by aberrant insertion of a repair patch, presumably proximal to the unexcised photoproduct. To test this hypothesis, we performed photochemical reversal on the dimer-containing excision fragments isolated from post-UV incubated normal cells, and were able to observe the release of both free thymidine and thymidine monophosphate molecules. Their combined yield proved to be essentially stoichiometric with the number of dimers photoreversed, signifying that most of the excised oligonucleotide fragments did indeed contain a dimer at one end, with an internal phosphodiester break (e.g., T̄ p-T̄-p-N- and p-T̄ p-T̄-p-N- ⟶T, pT and p-T-p-N-) (17).

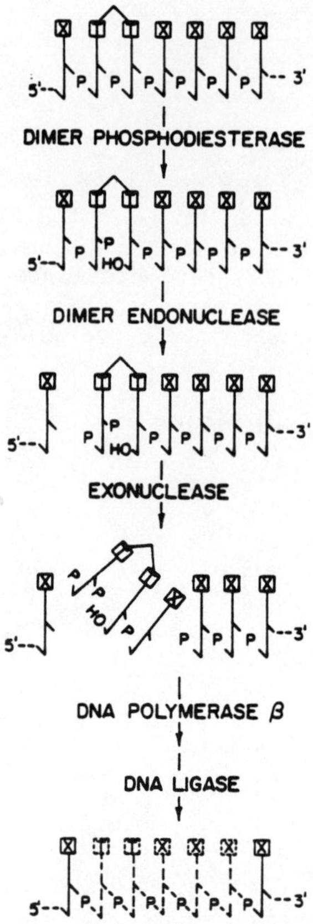

Fig. 4.　New model for the nucleotide mode of excision repair
operating on UV-induced cyclobutyl pyrimidine dimers in
cultured human skin fibroblasts. Note that only the
dimer-containing strand of the DNA duplex is shown
here. The essential difference between this model and
that for prokaryotes in Figure 1 is that here the
initial reaction is catalyzed by a putative pyrimidine
dimer-DNA phosphodiesterase rather than by either a dimer-
DNA glycosylase, as in M. luteus and phage T4, or an
'excinuclease' complex, as in E. coli. In the scheme
show here, the dimer is depicted at the 5'-end of the
excision fragment and the cleavage of the intradimer
phosphodiester linkage is assumed to yield 3'-P and 5'-
OH termini. Other possibilities clearly exist and the
exact location and nature of the breaks associated with
dimer removal await determination.

　　　Our inability to detect the release of free thymine upon direct
photoreversal of dimer-containing excision products corroborates the
earlier report by LaBelle and Linn (27) that human cells do not initiate
dimer excision by hydrolysis of the N-glycosyl bond of one member of the
dimerized pyrimidines, as do M. luteus and bacteriophage T4. Rather,
cleavage of the intradimer phosphodiester linkage would seem to be the
first step in the human nucleotide excision repair process, followed by
classical strand incision/lesion excision/repair synthesis/strand ligation
steps. In this new mode, depicted in Figure 4, the proposed function of
the putative pyrimidine dimer-DNA phosphodiesterase is to induce a

localized structural change at the dimer-containing site such that the site is then recognizable by a generalized 'bulky lesion-repair complex', perhaps analogous to the UVRABC excinuclease complex which is active in E. coli on a host of chemically disparate lesions (51). Breakage of the phosphodiester bond between dimerized pyrimidines in human cells may additionally serve to relieve regional conformational stress imparted by the intradimer cyclobutane bridge, thus restoring hydrogen bonding to adjoining base pairs in the double-stranded helix and, in so doing, presumably enhancing the fidelity of de novo DNA synthesis on a UV-damaged template. Investigation into these and other ramifications of the new model are in progress.

Defective Repair of 4NQO Lesions in AT Cells

A considerable portion of our research effort over the past decade has been devoted to elucidating the primary biochemical defect(s) in ataxia telangiectasia (reviewed in refs. 41, 42, 44). Persons inheriting this complex neurovascular and immunological disorder are prone to lympho-proliferative neoplasia and react adversely (sometimes fatally) to conventional radiotherapy. Cultured cells from these patients also exhibit enhanced radiosensitivity, as judged by impaired CFA and elevated levels of chromosomal aberrations after X irradiation. In our studies fibroblasts from most AT donors were found to be defective in the ability to repair certain (as of yet chemically undefined) types of alkali-stable DNA radioproducts, as indicated by (1) a deficiency in executing γ ray-stimulated DNA repair synthesis and (2) a reduced capacity to remove radiogenic DNA lesions (assayed as sites sensitive to damage-recognizing endonucleases and DNA glycosylases in a crude M. luteus extract). These data led us to propose that such AT strains may harbor an anomaly in an excision repair pathway operating on particular classes of alkali-stable radioproducts (e.g., altered base or sugar residues); these strains have consequently been designated exr⁻. However, other AT strains, although themselves as radiosensitive as the exr⁻ strains and established from donors presenting typical hallmarks of the disease, exhibited no demonstrable deficiency in repairing radiogenic damage to their DNA; they have accordingly been denoted exr⁺.

Two independent lines of evidence from other investigators have substantiated our division of AT strains into two major classes (exr⁻ and exr⁺) on the basis of DNA repair capability. Firstly, Scudiero (52) has convincingly demonstrated that the capacity of AT strains to undertake DNA repair synthesis after treatment with the alkylating agent N-methyl-N'-nitro-N-nitrosoguanidine (MNNG) mimics that observed after γ ray exposure-- that is, exr⁻ strains are deficient and exr⁺ strains are proficient. Secondly, Jaspers and Bootsma (24) have made the intriguing observation that, whereas in normal cells pretreatment with X radiation has no effect on the amount of DNA repair synthesis induced by subsequent exposure to UV light, the same preirradiation of AT cells serves to modify the level of UV-induced repair synthesis, acting as an inhibitor in exr⁻ strains and as a stimulus in exr⁺ strains.

An earlier study in our laboratory provided one of the first pieces of evidence that the putative DNA repair deficiency may not be confined to damage introduced by ionizing radiation (59). A class of guanyl adducts induced by 4NQO was shown to be removed more slowly in two AT strains-- namely, AT2BE and AT4BI--than in a normal control, a finding consistent with the hypersensitivity of these two particular AT strains to the cytotoxic effect of this chemical carcinogen.

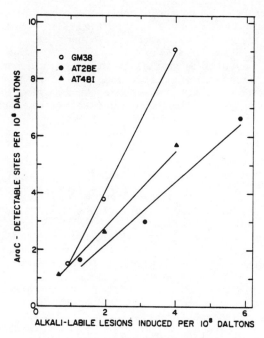

Fig. 5.   4NQO dose-dependent incidence of strand breaks
          accumulating in the DNA of normal and AT strains due to
          araC-induced abortive repair during post-treatment
          incubation. The experimental protocol was patterned
          after that of Mirzayans and Waters (36).   4NQO
          treatments (< 10 μM) were administered for 30 min at
          37°C in serum-free growth medium. Note that the doses
          received by each strain have been expressed in terms of
          alkali-labile lesions formed in DNA from cultures which
          were allowed no time for repair, thereby normalizing
          for any interstrain differences in lesion formation.

     In a current follow-up study, we have used 1-β-D-arabinofurano-
sylcytosine (araC), a metabolic inhibitor of DNA synthesis, to
intentionally block completion of the excision repair process operating on
4NQO-purine adducts in DNA.   In this approach, which has been popularized
by Collins and Johnson (7), the extent of strand break accumulation during
post-4NQO incubation with araC becomes a measure of the efficiency of the
excision repair process. As depicted in Figure 5, the level of araC-
detectable sites that were repaired during 2 hr after treatment with
different 4NQO concentrations proved to be significantly higher in GM38
(normal) cells than in AT2BE and AT4BI cells. This observation provides
additional proof that at least two AT strains are indeed faulty in
processing 4NQO-purine adducts in DNA.

     Since the four major reaction products formed in DNA by 4NQO can be
readily detected by various chromatographical methods (23), we are
presently assaying the normal and AT strains for their ability to excise
these chemically distinct adducts. This strategy should permit us to
confirm, and extend in a more direct and detailed manner, this specific DNA
repair anomaly associated with certain AT genotypes. In view of the
disturbing interlaboratory discrepancies in the DNA repair properties of
cultured AT fibroblasts (for review, see ref. 28), such confirmation would
be a welcome addition to the literature.

Faulty Repair of O^6-Methylguanine Lesions in Nontransformed Cells from Cancer Patients

Of the reaction products formed in DNA by MNNG and N-methyl-N-nitrosourea (MNU), O^6-methylguanine (O^6-MeGua) residues in particular have been strongly implicated in the mutagenic, carcinogenic and possibly lethal potency of these two methyl-N-nitroso compounds (30, 55). These guanyl adducts are repaired in cultured human fibroblasts in the same manner as initially proposed in E. coli (39), i.e., by the direct transfer of the offending methyl group from the O^6-position of the purine base to a cysteine residue in the protein, termed O^6-methylguanine-DNA transmethylase (49). The reaction is highly unusual among recognized DNA repair processes, being stoichiometric and suicidal, rather than catalytic and regenerating. That is, each transmethylase molecule is consumed in the reaction as its activity is exhausted upon S-alkylation of its acceptor cysteine residue.

Approximately 20% of all established human tumor cell lines are said to display the Mer⁻ phenotype, as defined by the following criteria: (1) reduced capacity to support the growth of MNNG-treated adenovirus; (2) enhanced susceptibility to MNNG-induced cell inactivation; (3) increased sensitivity to MNNG-induced production of sister chromatid exchanges; and (4) depressed constitutive levels of O^6-methylguanine-DNA transmethylase (9, 56, 69). The remaining tumor lines are similar to all nontransformed human fibroblast strains reported to date, and are thus designated Mer⁺ (53).

In collaboration with Dr. D. M. Parry and her colleagues in the Clinical and Environmental Epidemiology Branches of the U.S. National Cancer Institute in Bethesda, MD, we have recently identified a number of nontransformed fibroblast strains that display impaired CFA in response to MNU treatment (see Table 2). Included are strains from the following subjects, all of whom are either afflicted with or predisposed to neoplasia: (1) three affected members of a family with Gardner syndrome (GS), an autosomal dominant trait characterized by premalignant colonic polyps, soft tissue tumors, and cystic lesions of the skin (33); (2) a patient suffering from acquired immune deficiency syndrome (AIDS), which manifests itself as life-threatening opportunistic infections and/or malignancies, especially Kaposi sarcoma (4); and (3) a patient with Hodgkin's disease (HD) who developed multiple primary neoplasms subsequent to receiving conventional chemotherapy (D. M. Parry, personal communication). We present here a brief description of the in vitro properties of these strains.

Gardner Syndrome Family   In our search for environmental-hereditary interactions predisposing to gastrointestinal cancer, we previously reported MNNG hypercytotoxicity in vitro in one of four GS families studied (47). Surprisingly, this defect in post-MNNG CFA was observed, without exception, in strains from affected females whereas strains from affected males were indistinguishable from clinically normal donors. To confirm this apparent sex-dependent variability in cellular expression of enhanced susceptibility to an N-methyl-N-nitroso chemical, we have measured loss of colony-forming ability as a function of MNU treatment (1 hr at 37°C in serum-free, HEPES-buffered Ham's F12 medium) in strains from five affected core members of the MNNG-hypersensitive GS family and from two healthy volunteers. The CFA assay practiced by us was essentially that described by Paterson and coworkers (46). Our findings, summarized in Table 2, indicated that strain GM3314, derived from the proband in the family, was markedly sensitive to MNU, as reflected by a dose reduction factor (DRF) of 6 (using D_{10}, i.e., dose that reduces colony survival to 10%, as the quantitative measure of a given strain's response to the cytotoxic agent). Strains GM3944 (proband's affected sister) and GM3946 (proband's affected

Table 2. Relation between post-MNU survival and O^6-methylguanine-DNA transmethylase activity in strains from normal or cancer-predisposed subjects

| Strain | Donor | | | | MNU $D_{10} \pm SE$[b] (mM·hr) | O^6-MeGua-DNA Transmethylase Activity[c] (x10^{-5}) |
	Clinical Status[a]	Age	Sex	Relation		
GM38	normal	9	female	proband	1.31 ± 0.05	1.3 ± 0.13
GM969	normal	2	female	proband	1.57 ± 0.04	1.3 ± 0.14
GM3314	GS	48	female	proband	0.23 ± 0.08 (S)[d]	0.069 ± 0.018
GM3944	GS	38	female	sib	0.68 ± 0.06 (S)	0.63 ± 0.027
GM3946	GS	22	female	child	0.63 ± 0.07 (S)	0.57 ± 0.027
GM3948	GS	30	female	child	1.15 ± 0.07	1.2 ± 0.037
GM3954	GS	24	male	child	1.33 ± 0.04	1.2 ± 0.045
3638T	HD, tonsilar & colonic carcinomas	65	male	proband	0.90 ± 0.41 (S)	0.52 ± 0.026
3652T	AIDS	32	male	proband	0.69 ± 0.14 (S)	0.32 ± 0.063

[a] GS, Gardner syndrome; HD, Hodgkin's disease; AIDS, acquired immune deficiency syndrome

[b] Dose reducing survival to 10% ± standard error of the mean

[c] Methyl acceptor sites per cell

[d] Sensitive, using the two-tail t test of Tarone et al. (1983) to compare the D_{10} of the indicated strain to the mean (1.44 ± 0.08) of the two normal strains and taking p = 0.05 as the level of significance

daughter) also displayed impaired post-MNU CFA; however, their impairment (DRF ∿2) was considerably less than in GM3314. On the other hand, the two remaining strains (GM3948 and GM3954), one of which was obtained from an afflicted female, formed colonies at normal rates after MNU treatment (Table 2).

To investigate a probable biochemical basis for the observed cellular chemosensitivity segregating in family members presenting the affliction, we measured constitutive levels of O^6-methylguanine-DNA transmethylase in sonicates of cultured fibroblasts from these individuals. The assay adopted by us was an adaptation of that described by Olsson and Lindahl (39). The data, given in Table 2, indicated that the level of transmethylase protein in GM3314 was only ∿5% (6.9 x 10^3 molecules per cell) of that present in the two normal controls. The other two MNU-hypersensitive strains (GM3944 and GM3946) each possessed ∿50% of the normal complement, implying a possible gene dosage effect. In these three GS strains, then, the deficiency in the methyl-acceptor protein correlated closely with the impairment in post-MNU colony survival. Parallel experiments also demonstrated that the five GS strains examined here all had normal amounts of DNA glycosylase activities for 7-methylguanine and 3-methyladenine, two other major reaction products formed by N-methyl-N-nitroso compounds. We thus propose that a malfunction in the repair of O^6-MeGua residues may be largely, if not completely, responsible for the MNU hypersensitivity exhibited by strains from certain affected members of this GS family.

Other Cancer-Prone Patients   Cell sonicates of strains 3638T and 3652T, derived from the HD and the AIDS patient, respectively, contained reduced quantities of O^6 methylguanine-DNA transmethylase (Table 2). As seen previously in the GS family, the residual methyl-acceptor protein in these strains was consistent with their moderate susceptibility to MNU-induced killing; again, a transmethylase deficiency offers a likely explanation for the observed hypercytotoxicity to MNU.

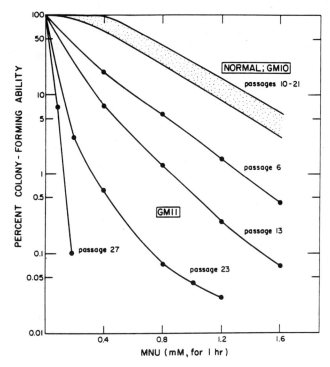

Fig. 6. MNU dose-response curves for two age-matched fetal
fibroblast strains as a function of culture age. The
stippled area is bounded by the steepest and shallowest
curves obtained for normal (GM10) cultures ranging from
passages 10-21.

Follow-up studies are currently underway to determine (1) if other
factors, in addition to reduced constitutive levels of transmethylase
activity, contribute to the chemosensitivity seen in these two strains (as
well as in the three MNU-hypersensitive GS strains discussed above), and (2)
if there is complementation among the various mutant strains with respect
to transmethylase expression.

Fetal Strain Displaying Age-Dependent Increase in MNU Toxicity

Our laboratory has discovered yet another nontransformed fibroblast
strain which displays defective colony-forming ability upon exposure to
MNU (34). The strain, GM11, was originally derived from an eight-week-old
fetus; it was described as apparently normal in the supplier's current
catalog (38). Our discovery was made fortuitously when the strain was
selected as one of the normal controls in our investigation into the post-
MNU CFA of the GS strains summarized previously. GM11 cells proved to be
exquisitely sensitive to MNU compared to control (GM10) cells, age-matched
in vivo and in vitro (see Figure 6). Moreover, the magnitude of the
enhancement in chemosensitivity was dependent upon the age of the cells in
culture, increasing from a DRF of approximately 2 at passage 6 to greater
than 10 at passage 23. Of additional significance was the fact that the
dose-response curve generated for GM11 at passage 23, for example, was
clearly nonlinear, as typified by a steep initial slope (at low
concentrations of MNU) which tailed off to a more gradual decline at higher
concentrations; the final slope closely paralleled the survival response of

normal cells. We interpret such biphasic curves as reflecting the presence of two cell populations, one hypersensitive to MNU and the other normal. The former population appears to increase from ∿25% of the total culture at passage 6 to >99% by passage 23.

This age-dependent increase in MNU-induced cytotoxicity contrasted sharply with the 1.6-fold hypersensitivity, irrespective of culture age, to killing by methyl methanesulfonate (MMS). Since MNU produces considerable quantities of O^6-MeGua adducts in DNA, whereas MMS forms relatively little (31), we assayed cell sonicates of GM11 for O^6-methylguanine-DNA transmethylase content. Reduced amounts of O^6-methyl-acceptor protein, but normal levels of DNA glycosylases active on 3-methyladenine and 7-methylguanine, were found. In fact, at passage 10 or greater, sonicates of all GM11 cultures possessed a negligible capacity to accept methyl groups from a test DNA substrate containing donor O^6-MeGua residues. At earlier culture ages, however, appreciable amounts of transmethylase protein were present; for example, sonicates from passage 4 cultures, the youngest assayed to date, contained approximately 25-30% of the level found in age-matched controls.

We are currently extending these studies to the youngest cultures available (passage 2) in order to quantitate accurately the in vitro age-dependent increase in O^6-methylguanine-DNA transmethylase activity vis-a-vis changes in colony-forming ability and mutation induction after MNU treatment. This may possibly enable us to correlate a deficiency in the removal of O^6-MeGua adducts with specific lethal and mutagenic events. Furthermore, aside from providing new insight into the genetic control of transmethylase expression, this intriguing fetal strain may ultimately assist in clarifying the role of the Mer⁻ phenotype in the transformation process.

Other Conditions Linking Cancer Proneness with Carcinogen Hypersensitivity

Using the clinical pictures in XP and AT as paradigms, we have uncovered a number of additional Mendelian single-gene disorders in which cancer predisposition evident in the clinic is similarly associated with carcinogen hypercytotoxicity observable in the laboratory. Examples of these newly described ecogenetic traits (with the pertinent carcinogen(s) given in brackets) include: Rothmund Thomson syndrome (γ rays; 60); combined hereditary cutaneous malignant melanoma/dysplastic nevus syndrome (4NQO and UV rays; 57, 58); and tuberous sclerosis (γ rays; 46). Thus far, only in the first syndrome has the observed carcinogen susceptibility been linked with a biochemical anomaly, namely, a particular malfunction in an excision-repair pathway acting on base/sugar radioproducts.

The preceding disorders are characterized by a well-defined genetic etiology. Our search for new human models of nature-nurture interactions in the genesis of neoplastic transformation has not been restricted to such source material, however. In the course of our six-year collaboration with U.S. NCI, we have assessed the post-carcinogen CFA and DNA repair properties of fibroblast strains from an assortment of cancer-prone subjects; these include special patient groups, unusual individual patients, and, in particular, members of 'cancer families' (summarized in refs. 41, 42). These latter families have been so designated because of an excessive occurrence of neoplasia, generally of specific histologic types, in kindred related by blood or environment. In many of these kinships, cancer has developed following documented exposure to a known biospheric, occupational or therapeutic carcinogen, raising the possibility that the individual may be genetically predisposed to the neoplastic effects of the agent. Two notable associations disclosed thus far between predisposition to familial malignancy and cellular hypersensitivity to an etiologically relevant carcinogen are the following:

a. A 42-year-old woman, who lost four of her six offspring (two daughters and two sons) and several blood relatives to acute myelogenous leukemia, presented rectal carcinoma 14 years following radiotherapy for uterine cervical cancer. Dermal cells from the woman and her two leukemic daughters exhibited impaired colony survival in response to γ rays, whereas those from her husband, the two remaining unaffected sons, and a sister with breast cancer displayed normal γ ray tolerance (2). Consequently, in this family there is a good correlation between cancer occurrence in vivo and elevated radiosensitivity in vitro. The latter trait may therefore be a direct cellular expression of a 'leukemogenic factor' segregating through the maternal side of the family.

b. A 30-year-old male with bilateral gynecomastia (and a well-documented family history of diverse malignancies) presented adenocarcinoma of the breast three decades following irradiation for an enlarged thymus. Cultured fibroblasts from the patient displayed diminished colony survival after exposure to either γ rays or bleomycin, a free radical-generating (and hence radiomimetic) chemical (18). Elevated radiosensitivity in cells from the patient's normal mother and hypersensitivity to bleomycin in cells from his unaffected sister add support to the suspicion that genetic susceptibility contributed to an increased risk of radiogenic neoplasia in the patient.

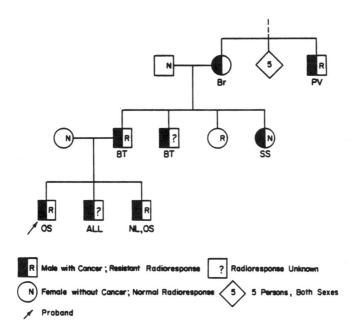

Fig. 7. Abridged pedigree of a cancer family with diverse malignancies (including two of possible radiogenic origin). The clinical status and cellular radioresponse are compared for each member. Abbreviations used: OS, osteosarcoma; ALL, acute lymphoblastic leukemia; NL, neurilemoma; SS, soft-tissue sarcoma; BT, brain tumor; Br, breast cancer; and PV, polycythemia vera.

485

While the foregoing clinical-laboratory investigations have demonstrated that enhanced sensitivity to carcinogen-induced cell killing may often be correlated with propensity to develop specific malignancies, we have also observed just the converse--that is, enhanced resistance to carcinogen toxicity in fibroblasts from persons at high risk of familial malignancy. We now outline our findings to date on two cancer families in which this unprecedented correlation has been made.

In Vitro Radioresistance in a Family Prone to Diverse Cancers. The first family is characterized by an unusual clustering of divergent types of malignancies, such as bone and soft-tissue sarcomas, breast and brain cancers, and leukemia (see Figure 7 for an abridged pedigree; (3)). The distribution of neoplasms observed is not unlike that seen in the Li-Fraumeni familial syndrome of breast cancer and soft-tissue sarcoma (29). The cancers in this first family have appeared over six generations in a pattern explicable by transmission of a partially penetrant, autosomal dominant gene with pleiotropic effects. The family was of particular significance because two members presented clinical abnormalities attributable to previous radiation exposure: (1) an adolescent brother of the proband developed a vertebral osteosarcoma in the field of radiotherapy administered 12 years earlier for bilateral malignant neurilemomas; and (2) his paternal great-uncle contracted polycythemia vera five years after occupational exposure to radioactive heavy water.

Pertinent clinical and laboratory characteristics are indicated in Figure 7 for various members in this cancer family (for details, see ref. 1). Of eight family members assayed by us for post-γ ray CFA, significantly increased radioresistance (RR) was seen in four members with neoplasia (including two having a history of radiation exposure) and a fifth without, but not in a member with leiomyosarcoma or in two normal spouses. In brief, the RR phenotype was detected in five of the six members in the cancer-prone lineage, but not in two spouse controls, implying that increased tolerance to the lethal effects of radiation may be a cellular manifestation of a genetically determined susceptibility factor common to diverse forms of cancer.

Biochemical delineation of this novel RR trait may possibly uncover a new mechanism of carcinogenesis underlying a number of common malignancies. On this premise, conventional DNA repair assays have been performed on the following RR strains: 2675T (proband with osteosarcoma), 2673T (his father with astrocytoma), 2674T (his brother with malignant neurilemoma and radiogenic osteosarcoma) and 2800T (his paternal great-uncle with radiogenic polycythemia vera). To determine intrinsic cellular capacity to repair radiogenic DNA damage in general, we measured the amount of DNA repair synthesis performed by these four RR strains in the 2-hr period following exposure to 500 Gy of γ radiation (41). The amount of repair synthesis induced in these strains did not differ significantly from that occurring in normal controls. Likewise, both the initial yield and the subsequent rate of disappearance of single-strand breaks and of M. luteus extract-sensitive sites proved to be similar in an RR (2674T) compared to a control (GM38) strain. Together, these data imply strongly that RR strains both sustain and repair radiogenic DNA damage at normal rates.

To characterize further the DNA metabolic properties of representative RR strains, DNA replicative synthesis was monitored in 2675T and 2800T fibroblasts after γ ray exposure. As demonstrated in Figure 8, both the extent of initial inhibition of de novo synthesis induced by the radiation treatment and the time interval before its subsequent recovery were much greater in 2800T cells than in normal (GM38) cells. Furthermore, the

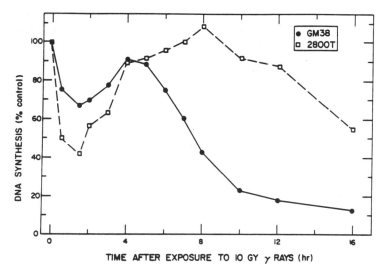

Fig. 8. γ ray-induced inhibition and recovery of DNA replicative
synthesis in normal (●) and RR (□) fibroblasts.
Exponentially growing cultures were prelabelled with ^{14}C-
thymidine (dThd) and divided into two groups; one
received 10 Gy of γ rays while the other received none.
At each indicated time during subsequent incubation, a
culture from each group was labelled with ^{3}H-dThd for 10
min and then lyzed, after which the DNA was collected
and its radioactivity counted. The ratio of ^{3}H/^{14}C
values for corresponding irradiated and non-irradiated
cultures served as a measure of the extent of radiogenic
inhibition of de novo DNA synthesis in each strain.

degree of recovery was more extensive and was maintained for longer times
in the RR strain than in the normal control. A similar pattern of post-
radiation DNA replication has also been observed in 2675T (data not shown).
The increased and protracted depression in replicative synthesis after
γ ray treatment in RR strains may promote cellular recovery by 'buying
additional time' during which repair processes can act on potentially
lethal radioproducts and, by so doing, may leave an exceptionally low
number of noncoding lesions for the replication machinery to navigate past.

It is noteworthy perhaps that the abnormality in radiation-induced
depression of DNA semi-conservative synthesis observed in the RR strains is
the exact opposite of that universally displayed by radiosensitive AT
strains. In the latter, the extent to which ionizing radiation inhibits de
novo DNA synthesis is appreciably diminished compared to that arising in
similarly treated normal cells (see, e.g., ref. 22).

We have previously proposed that the RR phenotype may result from an
increased activity of an error-prone DNA metabolic process which
facilitates elevated survival but at the expense of an increased mutation
load (1). To test this working hypothesis, our laboratory is in the
process of measuring the frequency of γ ray-induced 6-thioguanine-
resistance in RR compared to normal strains.

Table 3. Post-carcinogen colony-forming ability of skin fibroblasts from normal subjects and members of a multiple polyposis-sarcoma family

| Strain | Clinical Status | Donor | | | MNU $D_{10} \pm SE^a$ (mM·hr) | MMC $D_{10} \pm SE^a$ (µg/ml·hr) |
		Age	Sex	Relation		
"Normal"[b]	normal	2-83	male/female		1.37 ± 0.03	0.420 ± 0.038
3437T	glioblastoma, ANL[c]	26	female	proband	1.34 ± 0.03	2.36 ± 0.23 (R)[d]
3701T	endometrial carcinoma	75	female	paternal aunt	1.40 ± 0.35	1.06 ± 0.12 (R)
3702T	normal	66	male	paternal uncle	1.36 ± 0.06	0.526 ± 0.42
3703T	normal	60	female	mother	1.27 ± 0.13	0.414 ± 0.043
3704T	normal	52	female	paternal aunt	1.26 ± 0.27	0.823 ± 0.149 (R)

[a] Dose reducing survival to 10% ± standard error of the mean

[b] Average survival response of 15 control strains from unrelated normal donors

[c] Acute nonlymphocytic leukemia

[d] Reistant, using the two-tail t test of Tarone et al. (1983) to compare the D_{10} of the indicated strain to that of the "Normal" and taking p = 0.05 as the level of significance

In Vitro Resistance to MMC in a Multiple Polyposis-Sarcoma. The cardinal features of the second family are colonic polyps prone to malignant transformation in coexistence with malignant extra-alimentary sarcomas (12). The pattern of malignant involvement in the kinship is compatible with autosomal dominant inheritance of a single mutant, pleiotropic gene of high penetrance. Our initial interest in the family was stimulated in part by the appearance of a suspected cytotoxic drug-induced cancer in a 28-year-old female member who had undergone combined therapy for a glioblastoma three years earlier. Following treatment, which included 1,3-bis(2-chloroethyl)-1-nitrosourea, the patient developed a fatal nonlymphocytic leukemia, a recognized sequela of alkylating agent therapy. Consequently, strain 3437T from this patient along with strains from four other family members were assayed for colony-forming ability upon exposure to the model alkylating agent MNU and other DNA-damaging agents.

As shown in Table 3, all five strains responded normally to the lethal action of MNU. Somewhat surprisingly, however, three of the strains--namely 3701T, 3704T and 3437T--exhibited enhanced resistance to the inactivating effects of another antineoplastic chemical, mitomycin C (MMC). 3437T cells proved to be especially drug resistant, yielding a D_{10} value for post-MMC CFA which was ~ 5.5 times greater than that found for normal controls. It is noteworthy that all three MMC-resistant strains were derived from family members either with or at high risk of cancer (i.e., in the cancer-prone lineage). Of the remaining two strains, which displayed normal levels of post-MMC colony survival, one of the donors served as a spouse control while the other was asymptomatic. Thus, in this kinship, there was complete concordance between cancer predisposition in vivo and cellular hyperresistance to MMC in vitro.

MMC is a potent inducer of cross-links between the complementary strands of the double helix (see, e.g., ref. 15). These cross-links, and not the numerically greater monoadducts, appear to be the prime contributors to the cytotoxic, and perhaps the carcinogenic, potential of this agent. On a priori grounds, such interstrand cross-links are expected to constitute an effective block to de novo replicative synthesis and (unless successfully circumvented by repair processes) should therefore be tantamount to reproductive death. To determine whether an enhanced ability

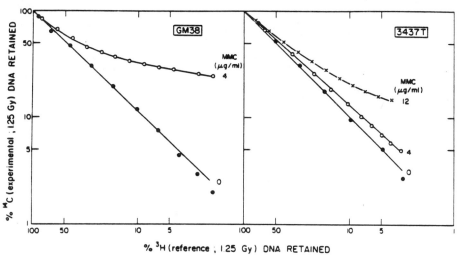

Fig. 9. Assay by alkaline elution of the interstrand cross-links
induced by MMC in the DNA of normal cells (left panel) and
MMC-hyperresistant cells (right panel). Experimental
cultures, labelled with ^{14}C-dThd, were treated (1 hr, 37°C)
with serum-free growth medium containing the indicated
concentrations of MMC. Following MMC treatment, the cells
were collected and exposed to 1.25 Gy of [60]Co γ rays, and
each cell sample was mixed with an equal number of reference
[3]H-labelled cells that had received the same γ ray exposure.
Cell mixtures were then lyzed on filters and their DNAs were
assayed by alkaline elution for rate of unwinding, as
detailed in van der Schans et al. (66). For each elution
point, the percentage of total ^{14}C-experimental DNA retained
on the filter was plotted versus the percentage of [3]H-
reference DNA retained. As expected, in the absence of
interstrand cross-links in the experimental DNA, a slope of -
1 was found. Cross-links induced in the ^{14}C-experimental DNA
by the MMC treatment resulted in a diminished rate of ^{14}C-DNA
compared to ^{3}H-DNA elution. A 'cross-link factor' may be
calculated (not shown) which suggests that ∿20 µg/ml MMC
treatment would be required with 3437T to achieve the same
level of cross-linking as results from 4 µg/ml MMC
administered to GM38.

to repair specifically this class of lesions was responsible for the MMC-
resistant phenotype, colony survival of 3437T versus normal cells was
compared after treatment with two other well-known DNA cross-linking
agents, cis-diamminedichloroplatinum II (cis-DDP) and 8-methoxypsoralen
(activated by UV-A light). For both agents, the post-treatment CFA for
3437T cells was similar to that exhibited by control cells, indicating that
3437T did not owe its MMC hyperresistance to any 'super-proficient' ability
to repair DNA cross-links. This strain has also been shown to be ∿5 times
more resistant than normal controls to the lethal effects of 4NQO, another
agent which, like MMC, requires metabolic reduction for activation (63,
65). Hence, these survival experiments raised the possibility that 3437T
cells were resistant to MMC- and 4NQO-induced cytotoxicity because they
lacked the normal complement of reductases responsible for the conversion
of these compounds to activated intermediates capable of damaging DNA. (An
alternative explanation, namely, reduced capacity to take up drugs, seemed

remote in view of the normal response of 3437T cells to inactivation by MNU, cis-DDP and photoactivated psoralen.) That diminished bioreduction might indeed account for most, if not all, of the cross-resistance to MMC and 4NQO has been surmised from the following three observations:

a. Using the alkaline elution method, we have demonstrated that 3437T cells must be exposed to ∿5 times as much MMC as GM38 cells in order to sustain comparable levels of interstrand cross-linking (see Figure 9).

b. Following identical 4NQO treatments, the incidence of both alkali-labile and alkali-stable adducts (a measure of drug dosimetry) was at least three times lower in 3437T cells than in normal cells.

c. Extracts of 3437T cultures have been shown to contain only about 25% of the 4NQO reductase activity that is present in normal cell extracts.

It is known that enzyme-mediated bioreduction reactions may be directed towards the destruction or the activation of potential genotoxins, depending upon the particular chemical (68). It is quite conceivable then, that under certain conditions individuals with a specific bioreductive enzyme deficiency may carry an amplified 'carcinogen load' compared to the general population. Furthermore, changing cellular biochemistry has been implicated in the stepwise development of cancer. In particular, Farber (11) has championed a resistant hepatocyte model for liver carcinogenesis in which an initiated cell, due to altered enzymology, acquires resistance to the genotoxic effects of various carcinogens. We are presently examining the similarities, if any, between their findings and ours, to determine if carcinogen resistance may have played a role in cancer development in the polyposis-sarcoma family.

AT Heterozygotes: A Cancer-Prone Subgroup Exhibiting Cellular
Hypersensitivity to Chronic γ Radiation In Vitro

Genetic variability dictates that people may differ, perhaps considerably, in their susceptibility to environmental carcinogens (37). A disproportionately large contribution to the human cancer burden may be made by heterozygous carriers of genes coding for certain rare recessive syndromes with neoplastic tendencies. As a case in point, the harmful impact of the AT gene on public health is thought to derive almost totally from its cancer-predisposing potential when present in single dosage. More specifically, a comprehensive retrospective analysis of cancer incidence in 27 AT families led Swift and his coworkers (62) to predict that as many as 5% of all fatal malignancies before age 45 may occur in carriers of the disease. This provocative prediction, determined from the product of the estimated frequency of heterozygotes (1% of the general population, in accordance with the Hardy-Weinberg equilibrium principle) and their relative mortality rate (five times normal), is in all likelihood conservative. Classical cell hybridization studies have identified at least four and perhaps as many as nine complementation groups in 17 unrelated patients with the affliction, suggesting that the AT phenotype can result from a recessive mutation at any one of many gene loci (25). If correct, it then follows that the incidence of AT heterozygotes among cancer fatalities in early adulthood could be 10% or more. Moreover, the ill health impact of heterozygosity for AT may not be limited to cancer development. As an extension of their earlier work, Swift and his associates (61, 67) have reported that AT gene carriers may also be predisposed to assorted congenital malfunctions and developmental anomalies, as well as ischemic heart disease.

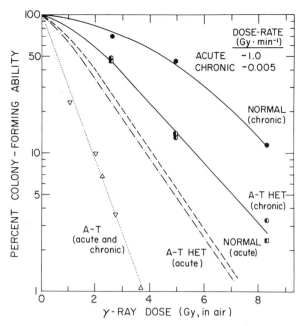

Fig. 10. Radiation response, expressed as percentage of survival of colony-forming ability, of confluent (density-proliferation inhibited) dermal fibroblasts from a normal volunteer (closed circles, GM38); two AT homozygous patients (triangles, AT3BI; inverted triangles, AT5BI), and two asymptomatic AT heterozygous carriers (half-open circles; ATH80CTO; half-open squares, ATH96CTO) as a function of chronic treatment with ^{60}Co γ radiation administered under oxia. For comparative purposes, survival curves of the same strains after acute γ ray exposure are also indicated (broken lines). Note that 1 Gray (Gy) = 100 rads. (From Paterson et al. (42) with permission of Raven Press)

The non-availability of a definitive marker -- for example, a telltale clinical abnormality or a simple laboratory assay -- for unequivocal detection of AT heterozygotes in the general population has hitherto prevented substantiation of the proposed disease-predisposing property of the AT heterozygous state. Given the consistent striking radiosensitivity of cultured cells harboring an AT gene in double dosage (e.g., ref. 41), we were prompted to explore the possibility of impaired post-γ ray CFA as an in vitro hallmark of an AT gene in single dosage. Some 25 dermal fibroblast strains from healthy volunteers and from afflicted AT homozygous children and their asymptomatic parents (i.e., presumed obligatory heterozygotes) in seven randomly selected families have been included thus far in this on-going feasibility study.

While conventional ^{60}Co γ ray treatment (i.e., delivered acutely under oxic conditions) killed cells derived from the parents at normal rates in all strains tested, radiation administered under hypoxia affected the CFA of these obligatory AT heterozygotes to an extent intermediate between that of the normal controls and the AT homozygotes in five of the seven families (45).

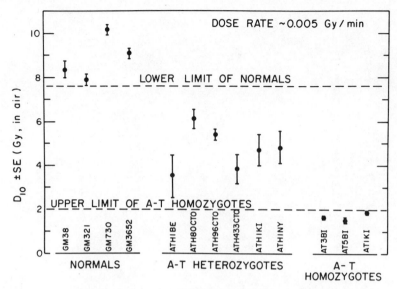

Fig. 11. Reproductive survival after chronic exposure to oxic γ radiation, expressed as D_{10} (in Gy) with an associated standard error (SE; vertical bars), of dermal fibroblast strains cultured from four clinically normal subjects, six presumed AT heterozygous carriers and three AT homozygous patients. (From Paterson et al. (45) with permission of Alan R. Liss, Inc.)

To define further the influence of one or two copies of a defective AT gene on the response of human fibroblasts to ionizing radiation, we assayed the effect of dose rate on γ ray-induced cytotoxicity in AT homozygous and heterozygous strains relative to normal controls. As is readily apparent in Figure 10, reduction of the dose rate of oxic radiation from 1.0 Gy/min to ∿0.005 Gy/min resulted in a twofold elevation in reproductive survival in the normal strain, that is, the D_{10} (dose reducing overall CFA to 10%) increased from 4.1 to 8.5 Gy. In sharp contradistinction, protraction of the dose rate had no measurable effect on the post-radiation reproductive capacity of the two AT homozygous strains. This finding, first reported by Cox (8), strongly implies that harboring an AT gene in double dosage severely inhibits the ability of a human cell to recover from (and, by inference, to repair) sublethal damage introduced by γ radiation.

That the normal radiation response of heterozygous strains in two of the seven AT families discussed earlier merely reflects the limited resolving power of acute γ ray treatment (as opposed to, for example, false paternity) is also evident in Figure 10. The 200-fold reduction in dose rate resulted in these two "worst case" heterozygous strains becoming intermediate between that of representative normal and AT homozygotes. For these and other presumed heterozygotes, D_{10} data depicted in Figure 11 illustrate the sensitivity of chronic exposure in resolving interstrain differences in cytotoxic response to γ rays.

Although the post-chronic γ ray CFA assay is far too labor intensive and time consuming for widespread screening purposes, our results may well point the way to the development of a practical diagnostic test for identification of asymptomatic carriers of AT. Our findings to date are certainly consistent with the postulate that an appreciable portion of society-at-large may be prone to malignant transformation and to other disease states owing to an inherited hypersensitivity to ionizing radiation and/or radiomimetic chemicals in the environment (see also ref. 54).

CONCLUSION

The take-home message is clear. By studying the biochemical basis for abnormal carcinogen responsiveness in rare individuals who are at increased risk of cancer because of some peculiarity in their personal or familial medical history, we are attempting to gain new insight into the origins of human neoplasia and, more importantly, into fundamental mechanisms of carcinogenesis such as may apply to common malignancies in society-at-large. Continued studies along the lines of those outlined here promise to assist in predicting and treating, and eventually in preventing, neoplastic transformation in man.

ACKNOWLEDGMENTS

Our research was financed by Atomic Energy of Canada Limited and the U.S. National Cancer Institute through Contracts N01-CP-21029 (Basic) and N01-CP-9100 with the Clinical and Environmental Epidemiology Branches, National Cancer Institute, Bethesda, MD. M.C.P. is a Heritage Medical Scientist and R. M. and M. W. are Postdoctoral Fellows of the Alberta Heritage Foundation for Medical Research. We are most grateful to L. D. Johnson, S. J. MacFarlane, R. S. McWilliams, G. M. Norton, and B. P. Smith for excellent technical assistance; and to A. Stewart for her patience and persistence in the preparation of the manuscript. The senior author wishes to express his sincere thanks to Drs. W. A. Blattner, J. F. Fraumeni, Jr., M. H. Greene, F. P. Li, R. W. Miller, J. J. Mulvihill, D. J. Tollerud, and especially D. M. Parry of the Clinical and Environmental Epidemiology Branches of the U.S. National Cancer Institute for their wise counsel and unfailing encouragement during the course of the studies described here.

REFERENCES

1. N. T. Bech-Hansen, W. A. Blattner, B. M. Sell, E. A. McKeen, B. C. Lampkin, J. F. Fraumeni, Jr., and M. C. Paterson, Transmission of in-vitro radioresistance in a cancer-prone family, Lancet 1:1335 (1981).

2. N. T. Bech-Hansen, B. M. Sell, J. J. Mulvihill, and M. C. Paterson, Association of in vitro radiosensitivity and cancer in a family with acute myelogenous leukemia, Cancer Res. 41:2046 (1981).

3. W. A. Blattner, D. B. McGuire, J. J. Mulvihill, B. C. Lampkin, J. Hananian, and J. F. Fraumeni, Jr., Genealogy of cancer in a family, JAMA 241:259 (1979).

4. Center for Disease Control, Opportunistic infections and Kaposi's sarcoma among Haitians in the United States, Morbid. Mortal. Weekly Rep. 31:353 (1982).

5. J. E. Cleaver, Defective repair replication of DNA in xeroderma pigmentosum, Nature 218:652 (1968).

6. J. E. Cleaver, DNA damage, repair systems and human hypersensitive diseases, J. Environ. Pathol. Toxicol. 3:53 (1980).

7. A. R. S. Collins and R. T. Johnson, Use of metabolic inhibitors in repair studies, in: "DNA Repair: A Laboratory Manual of Research Procedures, Vol. 1, Part B," E. C. Friedberg and P. C. Hanawalt, eds., Marcel Dekker, Inc., New York (1981), pg. 341.

8. R. Cox, A celluar description of the repair defect in ataxia-telangiectasia, in: "Ataxia-Telangiectasia -- A Cellular and Molecular Link between Cancer, Neuropathology, and Immune Deficiency", B.A. Bridges and D.G. Harnden, eds., John Wiley & Sons, Chichester (1982), pg. 141.

9. R. S. Day, III, C. H. J. Ziolkowski, D. A. Scudiero, S. A. Meyer, A. S. Lubiniecki, A. J. Girardi, S. M. Galloway, and G. D. Bynum. Defective repair of alkylated DNA by human tumor and SV40-transformed human cell strains, Nature 288:724 (1980).

10. R. Doll and R. Peto, The causes of cancer, J. Natl. Cancer Inst. 66:1191 (1981).

11. E. Farber, Cellular biochemistry of the stepwise development of cancer with chemicals: G. H. A. Clowes Memorial Lecture, Cancer Res. 44:5463 (1984).

12. J. F. Fraumeni, Jr., C. L. Vogel, and J. M. Easton, Sarcomas and multiple polyposis in a kindred: A genetic variety of hereditary polyposis?, Arch. Intern. Med. 121:57 (1968).

13. E. C. Friedberg, T. Bonura, J. D. Love, S. McMillan, E. H. Radany, and R. A. Schultz, The repair of DNA damage: Recent developments and new insights, J. Supramolec. Struct. Cell. Biochem. 16:91 (1981).

14. E. C. Friedberg, U. K. Ehmann, and J. I. Williams, Human diseases associated with defective DNA repair, Adv. Radiat. Biol. 8:85 (1979).

15. Y. Fujiwara, Defective repair of mitomycin C crosslinks in Fanconi's anemia and loss in confluent normal human and xeroderma pigmentosum cells, Biochim. Biophys. Acta, 699:217 (1982).

16. N. E. Gentner, B. Rözga, B. P. Smith, M. C. Paterson, and J. Cadet, Proc. 9th Annual Meeting Am. Soc. Photobiol., (1981), pg. 164 (abstr.).

17. N. E. Gentner, M. Weinfeld, L. D. Johnson, and M. C. Paterson, Incision of the phosphodiester bond internal to the pyrimidine dimer-forming bases may occur during excision repair of UV-induced damage in human fibroblasts, Env. Mutag. 6:429 (1984) (abstr.).

18. M. H. Greene, J. J. Goedert, N. T. Bech-Hansen, D. McGuire, M. C. Paterson, and J. F. Fraumeni, Jr., Radiogenic male breast cancer with in vitro sensitivity to ionizing radiation and bleomycin, Cancer Invest. 1:379 (1983).

19. H. Harm, Repair of UV-irradiated biological systems: Photoreactivation, in: "Photochemistry ad Photobiology of Nucleic Acids, Vol. 2," S. Y. Wang, ed., Academic Press, New York (1976), pg. 219.

20. W. A. Haseltine, Ultraviolet light repair and mutagenesis revisited, Cell 33:13 (1983).

21. J. Higginson and C. S. Muir, Environmental carcinogenesis: Misconceptions and limitations to cancer control, J. Natl. Cancer Inst. 61:1291 (1979).

22. J. Houldsworth and M. F. Lavin, Effect of ionizing radiation on DNA synthesis in ataxia telangiectasia cells, Nucleic Acids Res., 8:3709 (1980).

23. M. Ikenaga, M. Tada, and Y. Kawazoe, Measurement of base damage caused by 4-nitroquinoline 1-oxide, in: "DNA Repair: A Laboratory Manual of Research Procedures, Vol. 1, Part A," E. C. Friedberg and P. C. Hanawalt, eds., Marcel Dekker, Inc., New York (1981), pg. 187.

24. N. G. J. Jaspers and D. Bootsma, Abnormal levels of UV-induced unscheduled DNA synthesis in ataxia telangiectasia cells after exposure to ionizing radiation, Mutat. Res. 92:439 (1982).

25. N. G. J. Jaspers, R. B. Painter, M.C. Paterson, C. Kidson, and T. Inoue, Complementation analysis of ataxia-telangiectasia, in: "Ataxia-Telangiectasia: Genetics, Neuropathology, and Immunology of a Degenerative Disease of Childhood," R. A. Gatti and M. Swift, eds., Alan R. Liss, Inc., New York (1985), pg. 147.

26. K. H. Kraemer, Heritable diseases with increased sensitivity to cellular injury, in: "Update: Dermatology in General Medicine," T. B. Fitzpatrick, A. Z. Eisen, K. Wolff, I. M. Freedberg, and K. F. Austen, eds., McGraw-Hill Book Co., New York (1983), pg. 113.

27. M. LaBelle and S. Linn, In vivo excision of pyrimidine dimers is mediated by a DNA N-glycosylase in Micrococcus luteus but not in human fibroblasts, Photochem. Photobiol. 36:319 (1982).

28. A. R. Lehmann, M. R. James, and S. Stevens, Miscellaneous observations on DNA repair in ataxia-telangiectasia, in: "Ataxia-telangiectasia--A Cellular and Molecular Link between Cancer, Neuropatholgy and Immune Deficiency," B. A. Bridges and D. G. Harnden, eds., John Wiley & Sons, Chichester (1982), pg. 347.

29. F. P. Li and J. F. Fraumeni, Jr., Soft-tissue sarcomas, breast cancer, and other neoplasms: A familial syndrome?, Ann. Intern. Med. 71:747 (1969).

30. T. Lindahl, DNA repair enzymes, Ann. Rev. Biochem. 51:61 (1982).

31. G. P. Margison and P. J. O'Connor, Nucleic acid modification by N-nitroso compounds, in: "Chemical Carcinogens and DNA, Vol. 1," P. L. Glover, ed., CRC Press, Florida (1979), pg. 111.

32. J. J. McCormick, K. C. Silinskas, S. A. Kateley, J. E. Tower, and V. M. Maher. The induction of anchorage independent growth and tumor formation of diploid human fibroblasts by carcinogens, Proc. Am. Assoc. Cancer Res. 22:122 (1981) (abstr.).

33. V. A. McKusick, "Mendelian Inheritance in Man: Catalogs of Autosomal Dominant, Autosomal Recessive, and X-linked Phenotypes (Fifth Ed.)," The Johns Hopkins University Press, Baltimore (1978).

34. M. V. Middlestadt, G. Norton, and M. C. Paterson, Absence of O^6methylguanine-DNA methyltransferase activity in a nontransformed human fetal fibroblast line, Env. Mutag. 6:430 (1984) (abstr.).

35. R. W. Miller, Clinical clues to interactions in carcinogenesis, in: "Genetic and Environmental Factors in Experimental and Human Cancer," H. V. Gelboin et al., eds., Japanese Scientific Societies Press, Tokyo (1980), pg. 351.

36. R. Mirzayans and R. Waters, DNA damage and its repair in human normal or xeroderma pigmentosum fibroblasts treated with 4-nitroquinoline 1-oxide or its 3-methyl derivative, Carcinogenesis 2:1359 (1981).

37. J. J. Mulvihill, Clinical observations of ecogenetics in human cancer, Ann. Intern. Med. 92:809 (1980).

38. NIGMS Human Genetic Mutant Cell Repository (Eleventh Ed.), U.S. Department of Health and Human Services, Bethesda (1984).

39. M. Olsson and T. Lindahl, Repair of alkylated DNA in Escherichia coli: Methyl group transfer from O^6-methylguanine to a protein cysteine residue, J. Biol. Chem. 255:10569 (1980).

40. M. C. Paterson, Accumulation of non-photoreactivable sites in DNA during incubation of UV-damaged xeroderma pigmentosum group A and group D cells, Prog. Mutat. Res. 4:183 (1982).

41. M. C. Paterson, N. T. Bech-Hansen, W. A. Blattner, and J. F. Fraumeni, Jr., Survey of human hereditary and familial disorders for γ ray response in vitro: Occurrence of both cellular radiosensitivity and radioresistance in cancer-prone families, in: "Radioprotectors and Anticarcinogens," O. F. Nygaard and M. G. Simic, eds., Academic Press, New York (1983), pg. 615.

42. M. C. Paterson, N. T. Bech-Hansen, P. J. Smith, and J. J. Mulvihill, Radiogenic neoplasia, cellular radiosensitivity and faulty DNA repair, in: "Radiation Carcinogenesis: Epidemiology and Biological Significance," J. D. Boice, Jr. and J. F. Fraumeni, Jr., eds., Raven Press, New York (1984), pg. 319.

43. M. C. Paterson and N. E. Gentner, Introduction: Environmentally induced DNA lesions and their biological consequences, in: "Repairable Lesions in Microorganisms," A. Hurst and A. Nasim, eds., Academic Press, New York (1984), pg. 1.

44. M. C. Paterson, N. E. Gentner, M. V. Middlestadt, and M. Weinfeld, Cancer predisposition, carcinogen hypersensitivity and aberrant DNA metabolism, J. Cell. Physiol. Suppl. 3:45 (1984).

45. M. C. Paterson, S. J. MacFarlane, N. E. Gentner, and B. P. Smith, Cellular hypersensitivity to chronic γ-radiation in cultured fibroblasts from ataxia-telangiectasia heterozygotes, in: "Ataxia-Telangiectasia: Genetics, Neuropathology, and Immunology of a Degenerative Disease of Childhood," R. A. Gatti and M. Swift, eds., Alan R. Liss, Inc., New York (1985), pg. 73.

46. M. C. Paterson, B. M. Sell, B. P. Smith, and N. T. Bech-Hansen, Impaired colony-forming ability following γ irradiation of skin fibroblasts from tuberous sclerosis patients, Radiat. Res. 90:260 (1982).

47. M. C. Paterson, B. P. Smith, A. J. Krush, and E. A. McKeen, In vitro hypersensitivity to N-methyl-N'-nitro-N-nitrosoguanidine in a Gardner syndrome family, Radiat. Res. 87:483 (1981) (abstr.).

48. M. C. Paterson, B. P. Smith, and P. J. Smith, Measurement of enzyme-sensitive sites in UV- or γ-irradiated human cells using Micrococcus luteus extracts, in: "DNA Repair: A Laboratory Manual of Research Procedures, Vol. 1, Part A," E. C. Friedberg and P. C. Hanawalt, eds., Marcel Dekker, Inc., New York (1981), pg. 99.

49. A. E. Pegg, M. Roberfroid, C. von Bahr, R. S. Foote, S. Mitra, H. Bresil, A. Likhachev, and R. Montesano, Removal of O^6-methylguanine from DNA by human liver fractions, Proc. Natl. Acad. Sci. USA 79:5162 (1982).

50. J. H. Robbins, Hypersensitivity to DNA-damaging agents in primary degenerations of excitable tissue, in: "Cellular Responses to DNA Damage," E. C. Friedberg and B. A. Bridges, eds., Alan R. Liss, Inc., New York (1983), pg. 673.

51. A. Sancar and W. D. Rupp, A novel repair enzyme: UVRABC excision nuclease of Escherichia coli cuts a DNA strand on both sides of the damaged region, Cell 33:249 (1983).

52. D. A. Scudiero, Decreased DNA repair synthesis and defective colony-forming ability of ataxia telangiectasia fibroblast cell strains treated with N-methyl-N'-nitro-N-nitrosoguanidine, Cancer Res. 40:984 (1980).

53. D. A. Scudiero, S. A. Meyer, B. E. Clatterbuck, M. R. Mattern, C. H. J. Ziolkowski, and R. S. Day, III, Relationship of DNA repair phenotypes of human fibroblast and tumor strains to killing by N-methyl-N'-nitro-N-nitrosoguanidine, Cancer Res. 44:961 (1984).

54. Y. Shiloh, E. Taber and Y. Becker, The response of ataxia-telangiectasia homozygous and heterozygous skin fibroblasts to neocarzinostatin, Carcinogenesis 3:815 (1982).

55. B. Singer, N-nitrosoalkylating agents: Formation and persistence of alkyl derivatives in mammalian nucleic acid as contributing factors in carcinogenesis, J. Natl. Cancer Inst. 62:1329 (1979).

56. R. Sklar and B. Strauss, Removal of O^6-methylguanine from DNA of normal and xeroderma pigmentosum-derived lymphoblastoid lines, Nature 289:417 (1981).

57. P. J. Smith, M. H. Greene, D. Adams, and M. C. Paterson, Abnormal responses to the carcinogen 4-nitroquinoline 1-oxide of cultured fibroblasts from patients with dysplastic nevus syndrome and hereditary cutaneous malignant melanoma, Carcinogenesis 4:911 (1983).

58. P. J. Smith, M. H. Greene, D. A. Devlin, E. A. McKeen, and M. C. Paterson, Abnormal sensitivity to UV-radiation in cultured skin fibroblasts from patients with hereditary cutaneous malignant melanoma and dysplastic nevus syndrome, Int. J. Cancer 30:39 (1982).

59. P. J. Smith and M. C. Paterson, Defective DNA repair and increased lethality in ataxia telangiectasia cells exposed to 4-nitroquinoline 1-oxide, Nature 287:747 (1980).

60. P. J. Smith and M. C. Paterson, Enhanced radiosensitivity and defective DNA repair in cultured fibroblasts derived from Rothmund Thomson syndrome patients, Mutat. Res. 94:213 (1982).

61. M. Swift and C. Chase, Cancer and cardiac deaths in obligatory ataxia-telangiectasia heterozygotes, Lancet 1:1049 (1983).

62. M. Swift, L. Sholman, M. Perry and C. Chase, Malignant neoplasms in the families of patients with ataxia-telangiectasia, Cancer Res., 36:209 (1976).

63. M. Tada and M. Tada, Seryl-tRNA synthetase and activation of the carcinogen 4-nitroquinoline 1-oxide, Nature 255:510 (1975).

64. R. E. Tarone, D. A. Scudiero, and J. H. Robbins, Statistical methods for in vitro cell survival assays, Mutat. Res. 111:79 (1983).

65. M. Tomasz and R. Lipman, Reductive metabolism and alkylating activity of mitomycin C induced by rat liver microsomes, Biochemistry 20:5056 (1981).

66. G. P. van der Schans, M. C. Paterson, and W. G. Cross, DNA strand break and rejoining in cultured human fibroblasts exposed to fast neutrons or gamma rays, Int. J. Radiat. Biol. 44:75 (1983).

67. K. Welshimer and M. Swift, Congenital malformations and developmental disabilities in ataxia-telangiectasia, Fanconi anemia, and xeroderma pigmentosum families, Am. J. Hum. Genet. 34:781 (1982).

68. A. S. Wright, The role of metabolism in chemical mutagenesis and chemical carcinogenesis, Mutat. Res. 75:215 (1980).

69. D. B. Yarosh, R. S. Foote, S. Mitra, and R. S. Day, III, Repair of O^6-methylguanine in DNA by demethylation is lacking in Mer⁻ human tumor cell strains, Carcinogenesis 4:199 (1983).

NEW DNA REPAIR SYSTEMS AND NEW INSIGHTS ON OLD SYSTEMS IN Escherichia coli

K. C. Smith, N. J. Sargentini, R. C. Sharma and T. V. Wang

Department of Radiology
Stanford University School of Medicine
Stanford, CA 94305

INTRODUCTION

One can deduce the extreme importance of maintaining the integrity of cellular DNA, simply by noting the numerous and diverse types of systems that a cell has at its disposal for the repair of damaged DNA (for reviews, see references 1-3). There is a repair system that requires visible light (i.e., photoreactivation), and several systems that can work in the absence of light. There are repair systems that can function in the absence of DNA replication (e.g., excision repair), and systems that can only function after damaged DNA has been replicated (i.e., postreplication repair). There are systems for the repair of DNA base damage, and systems for the repair of single-strand and double-strand breaks in DNA. Certain alterations in DNA can be repaired by more than one type of repair system, suggesting that cells have "backup" systems for DNA repair. Some of these repair systems are constitutive and some are inducible. Finally, some of these repair systems are error-free and some are error-prone (i.e., the repair is not accurate and, therefore, produces mutations). Within the space limitations for this review, we will describe some new DNA repair systems and discuss new insights on some old repair systems in Escherichia coli.

Excision Repair

Nucleotide Excision Repair   Although there has been general agreement since the late 1960's concerning the overall model for nucleotide excision repair in E. coli, a controversy has remained as to whether the DNA strand is cut on both sides of the lesion simultaneously ("cut and patch" model), or whether the DNA is cut on one side of the lesion followed by DNA synthesis and strand displacement, and then a cut is made on the other side of the lesion to complete the excision process ("patch and cut" model) (reviewed in reference 4). The most recent evidence, however, supports the "cut and patch" model. Sancar and Rupp (5) have shown that in vitro the uvrABC enzyme complex makes two cuts in UV-irradiated DNA. One cut is at the 8th phosphodiester bond on the 5' side of pyrimidine dimers, and the second cut is at the 4th or 5th phosphodiester bond on the 3' side. A revised model for the major pathway of excision repair is shown in Figure 1.

Base Excision Repair   A new excision repair process, base excision repair, was discovered in the late 1970's (reviewed in reference 2). In

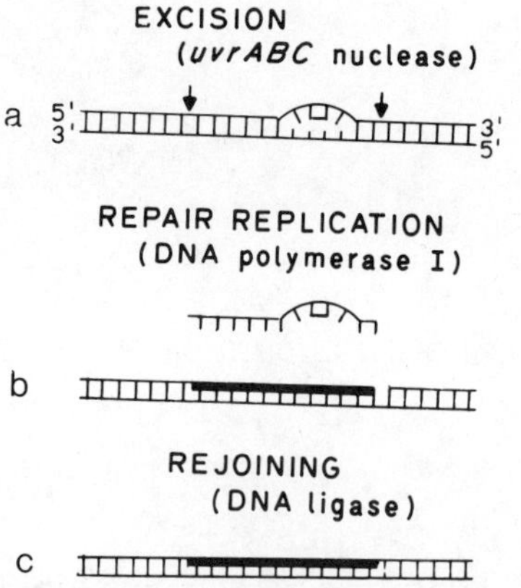

EXCISION
(*uvrABC* nuclease)

a $\begin{smallmatrix}5'\\3'\end{smallmatrix}$ [[[[[[[[[[[[[[[[[[[[[[[[[[[[[[[[[[$\begin{smallmatrix}3'\\5'\end{smallmatrix}$

REPAIR REPLICATION
(DNA polymerase I)

b [[[[[[[[[[[[[[[[[[[━━━━━━━━[[[[[[

REJOINING
(DNA ligase)

c [[[[[[[[[[[[[[━━━━━━━━━━━[[[[[

Fig. 1. A revised model for nucleotide excision repair in
E. coli. The uvrABC nuclease recognizes the lesion,
shown here as a cylobutyl pyrimidine dimer, and cuts on
both sides of the lesion. Repair replication (heavy
line) fills this gap using the opposite strand of DNA
as the template. Finally, the break in the repaired
DNA strand is sealed by DNA ligase (modified from
reference 5).

this process, a DNA glycosylase recognizes an altered purine or pyrimidine
base, and cleaves the glycosylic bond. This results in the removal of the
inappropriate base without the breakage of the sugar-phosphate backbone of
the DNA. So far, six DNA glycosylases that are specific for the removal of
altered bases have been described in E. coli, i.e., those for the removal
of uracil, hypoxanthine, 3-methyladenine, formamidopyrimidine, urea, and
thymine glycol.

Another type of enzyme, AP endonuclease, recognizes the apurinic or
apyrimidinic (AP) sites generated in DNA by the DNA glycosylases, and cuts
the DNA strand. There are two classes of AP endonucleases: Class I
enzymes cleave DNA on the 3' side of an AP site, and Class II enzymes
cleave on the 5' side. The subsequent steps of this repair process are
presumed to be similar to those depicted for nucleotide excision repair
(Figure 1).

Growth Medium-Dependent Excision Repair. In addition to the excision
repair process shown in Figure 1, a process that can proceed in cells held
in buffer (e.g., 6), there is another type of excision repair in E. coli
that can only proceed when the cells are incubated in complete growth
medium (7). At least a portion of this medium-dependent repair is the
"long patch" excision repair process (8). The growth medium-dependent
repair of incision gaps is dependent upon the recA, recB, lexA (7) and recF
genes (9). Because of the similarities in the genetic control of postreplication repair (see below) and of recA-dependent excision repair, it
has been proposed that recA-independent excision repair takes place
principally in the unreplicated portion of a chromosome, while recA-
dependent excision repair, which depends upon the same genes that control
genetic recombination, takes place only in the replicated portion of the
chromosome where sister duplexes are present, and, therefore,
recombinational repair can occur (9).

Postreplication Repair

A New Mechanism of Postreplication Repair. Rupp and Howard-Flanders
(10) observed that the DNA synthesized in UV-irradiated E. coli is
discontinuous. With subsequent incubation, however, these short pieces of
DNA are joined together to form DNA with a molecular weight equal to that
from unirradiated cells. A model for this postreplication repair process
is shown in Figure 2. According to this model, the DNA daughter-strand
gaps produced opposite the lesions are the substrates for postreplication
repair. The repair of these daughter-strand gaps is under the control of
the recA gene (11), and of the recF gene (12-14). The question was then
raised that if a uvrB recB strain is almost as sensitive to UV radiation as
a uvrB recF strain (Figure 3a), but shows almost no deficiency in the e
repair of DNA daughter-strand gaps (Figure 3b), then what type of postreplication repair is the recB gene product involved in?

If a daughter-strand gap is not repaired, the single-stranded DNA
opposite the gap might be cleaved by an endonuclease, resulting in a DNA
double-strand break. The transformation of a DNA daughter-strand gap into
a double-strand break would create a new type of lesion that needs to be
repaired. Wang and Smith (14) have observed the formation of DNA double-
strand breaks after UV irradiation in uvrB cells that are also deficient in
the repair of DNA daughter-strand gaps (i.e., carrying additional mutations
at recA, recF, or recF recB). These double-strand breaks are repaired in
uvrB recF cells, but not in uvrB recF recB cells. A model for this recB-
dependent pathway of postreplication repair, which is called sister duplex
recombination, suggests that the ends of the double-strand break can
initiate recombination in the adjacent sister duplex, with the subsequent
repair of the double-strand break or segregation of the lesions out of the
chromosome. Since uvrB recF cells and uvrB recB cells have nearly equal UV
radiation sensitivities, this suggests that the repair of DNA daughter-
strand gaps and of DNA double-strand breaks are of about equal importance
to cellular survival in UV-irradiated uvrB cells.

The interrelationship of the two major pathways of postreplication
repair is depicted in Figure 4. There is evidence for a third pathway
of postreplication repair (15, 16). Although this third process is also
for the repair of DNA daughter-strand gaps, it is independent of the recB
and recF genes (16).

Mammalian cells also exhibit a response resembling the repair of DNA
daughter-strand gaps (e.g., 17). However, in contrast with the case for E.
coli where parental strands containing lesions are joined to daughter-
strand DNA about 50% of the time (18), this is a rare event for mammalian
cells (17). Similar to the case for E. coli (14), the postreplicational
formation and repair of DNA double-strand breaks also occur in UV-
irradiated human cells (19).

Inhibition of Postreplication Repair by Rich Growth Medium. E. coli
cells deficient in excision repair show higher survival after UV irradiation
if they are plated on minimal medium instead of rich medium (e.g., yeast
extract plus nutrient broth). This phenomenon has been called Minimal
Medium Recovery (MMR) (20). This rich medium effect on viability can also
be duplicated with minimal medium to which a mixture of amino acids has
been added (Figure 5). At the molecular level, one consequence of the
extra amino acids is to interfere with the ability of cells to repair DNA
daughter-strand gaps. Rich medium inhibits all of the recB recF-
independent pathway of daughter-strand gap repair (16), but only a portion
of the recF-dependent (21) and recB-dependent pathways (22).

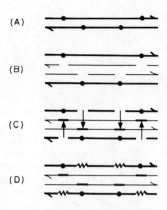

Fig. 2.   A model for the <u>recF</u> gene-dependent pathway of
postreplication repair (i.e., the repair of DNA
daughter-strand gaps) in <u>E. coli</u>. A. The dots
indicate lesions in the two parental strands of DNA
(heavy lines). B. DNA synthesis proceeds past these
lesions leaving gaps in the daughter strands (thin
lines). C. These daughter-strand gaps are filled with
material from the parental strands by a recombination
process. About half of the time, however, parental
strands that contain lesions are joined to the daughter
strands (18). This process is not shown in this
diagram. D. Repair of the gaps in the parental strands
by repair replication (wavy lines).

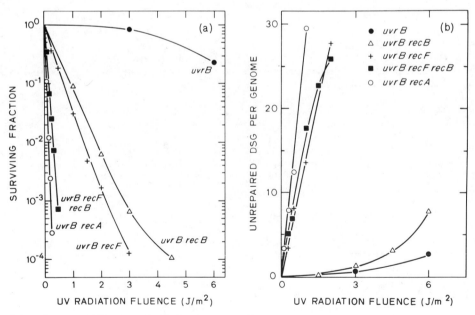

Fig. 3.   Effects of <u>recB</u>, <u>recF</u>, and <u>recA</u> mutations on cell survival
(a) and on the repair of DNA daughter-strand gaps (b) in
UV-irradiated <u>uvrB</u> strains of <u>E. coli</u>. Symbols for
strains: ● , <u>uvrB</u>; △ , <u>uvrB</u> <u>recB</u>; +, <u>uvrB</u> <u>recF</u>; □ , <u>uvrB</u>
<u>recF</u> <u>recB</u>; and o, <u>uvrB</u> <u>recA</u> (from reference 14).

When uvrB cells are UV irradiated and incubated in minimal medium, there is an abrupt cessation of bulk DNA synthesis, however, if the cells are incubated in rich medium there is only a temporary slowing of DNA synthesis (23). Apparently, the failure of UV-irradiated cells to cease bulk DNA synthesis in rich medium decreases their ability to perform post-replication repair. Since some signal must normally tell cells to stop their bulk DNA synthesis after irradiation, rich medium apparently interferes with this signal.

Certain cells deficient in DNA repair also appear to have lost this ability to know that they have been irradiated, and they do not shut off bulk DNA synthesis after irradiation even in minimal medium (24, 25). It has been reported that cells from patients with ataxia telangiectasia seem to be missing a signal that tells them when they have been X-irradiated (26). We have isolated a mutation, mmrA1 (27), that allows UV-irradiated E. coli cells to slow down their DNA synthesis even in the presence of rich medium. We hope that further work in this area will provide a better understanding of this presumed cellular radiation-damage-detection mechanism.

Inducible Repair

Medium Dependent Resistance (MDR)   Our laboratory is isolating new mutants of E. coli that are selectively sensitive to ionizing radiation in the hope of discovering new repair systems and/or learning more about known repair systems (28-30). While characterizing one of these new mutants, we discovered an inducible recovery phenomenon in wild-type cells that is selective for the repair of ionizing radiation damage to DNA (31). We have called this phenomenon Medium Dependent Resistance (MDR). The basic observation is that cells grown to logarithmic phase in rich growth medium and plated on rich medium are much more resistant to X and UV radiation than are cells grown to logarithmic phase in minimal medium and plated on minimal medium (Figure 6).

In contrast to MMR, where survival is only affected by the type of medium the cells are put into after irradiation, in MDR, survival is dependent, as well, on the type of medium that the cells are grown in before irradiation. Although, compared to UV irradiation, there is very

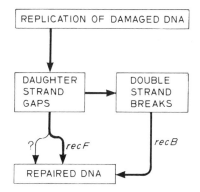

Fig. 4.   Schematic diagram of the interaction of the recF and the recB pathways of postreplication repair in E. coli. The pathway for the repair of DNA daughter-strand gaps marked with "?", is a minor pathway that functions in the absence of the recF and recB genes (15, 16).

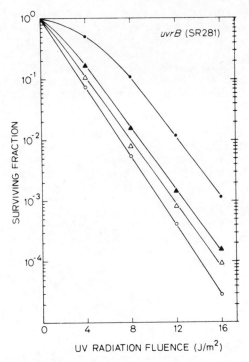

Fig. 5.   Minimal medium recovery in UV-irradiated E. coli uvrB.
Cells were grown to logarithmic phase in minimal
medium, UV irradiated in phosphate buffer, and then
plated on minimal medium (MM) (●), MM supplemented
with Casamino Acids (2 mg/ml) (△), MM supplemented
with 13 amino acids at the concentrations reported for
Casamino Acids (▲), and on yeast extract-nutrient
broth plates (○) (modified from reference 21).

little MMR after ionizing irradiation, the MDR phenomenon is about twice as
large after ionizing irradiation as after UV irradiation (Figure 6).

MDR is an inducible DNA repair process that is dependent upon
functional recA and lexA genes. It has a larger effect on cells X-
irradiated in air (3.7-fold) than in nitrogen (2.6-fold). MDR is
associated with a greatly increased ability to repair DNA single-strand
breaks and DNA double-strand breaks, and with reduced DNA degradation and
protein-synthesis retardation after X-irradiation (31-33).

While many laboratories are studying the transcriptional regulation of
inducible repair systems, (reviewed in reference 3), it is important to
remember that unless a cell has the capacity to synthesize proteins rapidly
after irradiation, the induction of new messenger RNA may have little effect
on cell survival. The enhanced survival observed in the MDR phenomenon
appears to be due to the fact that cells grown to logarithmic phase in rich
medium have more protein synthesizing capacity than do cells grown in
minimal medium (31), and thus are able to maximally express the induced
repair systems.

Town et al. (34) differentiated the repair of X-ray-induced DNA
single-strand breaks into Type I (ultrafast) repair (which has since been
shown to result from nonenzymatic "chemical restoration" processes (35-37),

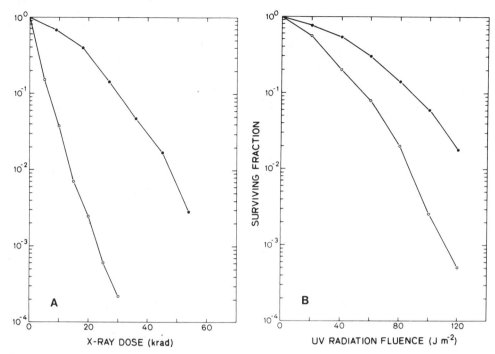

Fig. 6. Medium Dependent Resistance (MDR) in wild-type E. coli cells
after (A) X irradiation in air and (B) UV irradiation. Cells
were grown to logarithmic phase in rich medium ( ) or in
minimal medium (o) before treatment, and were plated on
homologous medium. The growth medium-dependent dose-
modification factor at 2% survival for MDR is 3.7 after X
irradiation, and 1.5 after UV irradiation (modified from
reference 31).

Type II (fast) repair (which is largely polA gene-dependent, and can occur
in cells held in buffer), and Type III (slow) repair (which is recA gene-
dependent, and does not occur in cells held in buffer).

As mentioned above, MDR enhances dramatically the capacity of cells to
repair X-ray-induced DNA single-strand breaks. It is Type III repair that
is enhanced, and not Type II repair. In addition, MDR enhances the
ability of cells to repair DNA double-strand breaks, and it was shown that
the Type III repair of DNA single-strand breaks is actually the repair of
DNA double-strand breaks (32, 33).

Based upon recent results with E. coli, it has been suggested that the
slow component for the repair of X-ray-induced DNA single-strand breaks in
mammalian cells (e.g., see reference 38) probably represents the repair of
DNA double-strand breaks, and the fast component is probably the repair of
true single-strand breaks (32).

Adaptive Response   Another recently-discovered DNA repair system (39)
is the adaptive response (reviewed in references 2, 3). The major mutagenic lesion in cells exposed to methylating agents is O^6-methylguanine.
Although E. coli cells normally have a limited capacity for removing this
lesion from their DNA, a repair system for this lesion can be induced in
cells that are pretreated with low concentrations of alkylating agents.
This error-free adaptive response can be induced in recA cells, and, there-

505

fore, cannot be one of the SOS responses (see below). The biochemical reaction of the adaptive response is the transfer of the methyl group of O^6-methylguanine to a cysteine group of a methyltransferase, which is rendered inactive upon accepting the methyl group from DNA. The existence of this unique repair system certainly was not predicted. Therefore, in view of all these recent discoveries of new DNA repair processes, one cannot help but wonder how many more DNA repair processes are still to be discovered.

The Genetic Control of Radiation Mutagenesis

Radiation-induced mutations are the result of inducible, error-prone DNA repair in E. coli. This process has been called "SOS" repair (for a recent review, see reference 3). Mutations that block this SOS process also block most radiation-induced mutations. Thus, E. coli recA cells can be killed by UV radiation, but they are not mutated by it. However, the SOS (recA lexA) system not only controls mutagenesis, but also a diverse set of physiological phenomena (reviewed in reference 3). Therefore, there may be genes that are under the control of the SOS process whose products actually perform the error-prone DNA repair that produces the mutations. A major candidate for such a gene is umuC, which was identified by Kato and Shinoura (40) as being required for UV radiation mutagenesis. Although it was also reported that the umuC gene is essential for ionizing radiation mutagenesis, this conclusion is inconsistent with other work in the literature (discussed in reference 41).

This question of the nonmutability of umuC strains was reinvestigated using an insertion mutation (umuC122::Tn5). Insertion mutations generally have a null phenotype, and offer a way to test if a particular point mutation in the same gene is leaky or not. In such a test, the original umuC36 mutation was indeed found to be somewhat leaky, but UV radiation mutagenesis still seemed to depend almost exclusively on the umuC gene. In contrast, there appear to be umuC-dependent and umuC-independent modes of ionizing radiation mutagenesis. Depending upon the mutation assay (e.g., ochre and frameshift reversion, and induction of drug resistance) and the radiation dose used, the deficiency of the umuC122::Tn5 strain in ionizing radiation mutagenesis varied from no deficiency to a 50-fold deficiency, compared to a wild-type strain (41). These results suggest that ionizing radiation produces a class of DNA damage that is site specific, and is "UV-like" in its requirements for repair.

SUMMARY

While it is understandable that everyone wants to know how DNA damage is repaired in mammalian cells, it should not be forgotten that the insights that currently guide the research on DNA repair in mammalian cells came from studies on DNA repair and mutagenesis in bacteria. The relatively rapid expansion in knowledge concerning DNA repair in bacteria (remember that thymine dimers were only discovered in 1960 (42)) has been due to the relative ease of working at the molecular level with the smaller chromosome of bacteria, the availability of extensive genetic information on E. coli (43), the availability of several techniques for moving genes from one cell to another, and the relative ease of isolating new mutations that confer radiation sensitivity.

Some people seem to feel that the DNA repair systems have all been discovered, and they are all fully understood in bacteria. If this were so, then there would be no need to do further research on bacteria, however, this perception is clearly incorrect. In fact, none of the DNA repair systems are fully understood even in bacteria. Furthermore, new repair systems are still being discovered in E. coli, and probably many more remain to be discovered. Bacteria continue to be "proper subjects for cancer research" (44).

REFERENCES

1. P. C. Hanawalt, P. K. Cooper, A. K. Ganesan, and C. A. Smith, DNA repair in bacteria and mammalian cells, Annu. Rev. Biochem. 48:783-836 (1979).

2. T. Lindahl, DNA repair enzymes, Annu. Rev. Biochem. 51:61-87 (1982).

3. G. C. Walker, Mutagenesis and inducible responses to deoxyribonucleic acid damage in Escherichia coli, Microbiol. Rev. 48:60-93 (1984).

4. K. C. Smith, The roles of genetic recombination and DNA polymerase in the repair of damaged DNA, Photophysiology 6:209-278 (1971).

5. A. Sancar and W. D. Rupp, A novel repair enzyme: uvrABC excision nuclease of Escherichia coli cuts a DNA strand on both sides of the damaged region, Cell 33:249-260 (1983).

6. M. Tang and K. C. Smith, The expression of liquid holding recovery in ultraviolet-irradiated Escherichia coli requires a deficiency in growth medium-dependent DNA repair, Photochem. Photobiol. 32:763-769 (1980).

7. D. A. Youngs, E. Van der Schueren, and K. C. Smith, Separate branches of the uvr gene-dependent excision repair process in ultraviolet-irradiated Escherichia coli K-12 cells; their dependence upon growth medium and the polA, recA, recB and exrA genes, J. Bacteriol. 117:717-725 (1974).

8. P. K. Cooper and P. C. Hanawalt, Role of DNA polymerase I and the rec system in excision-repair in Escherichia coli, Proc. Natl. Acad. Sci. (USA) 69:1156-1160 (1972).

9. K. C. Smith and R. C. Sharma, A model for recA-dependent excision repair in UV-irradiated Escherichia coli, Mutat. Res., submitted 1986).

10. W. D. Rupp and P. Howard-Flanders, Discontinuities in the DNA synthesized in an excision-defective strain of Escherichia coli following ultraviolet irradiation, J. Mol. Biol. 31:291-304 (1968).

11. K. C. Smith and D. H. C. Meun, Repair of radiation-induced damage in Escherichia coli. I. Effect of rec mutations on post-replication repair of damage due to ultraviolet radiation, J. Mol. Biol. 51:459-472 (1970).

12. A. K. Ganesan and P. C. Seawell, The effect of lexA and recF mutations on post-replication repair and DNA synthesis in Escherichia coli K-12, Molec. gen. Genet. 141:189-205 (1975).

13. R. H. Rothman and A. J. Clark, The dependence of postreplication repair on uvrB in a recF mutant of Escherichia coli K-12, Molec. gen. Genet. 155:279-286 (1977).

14. T. V. Wang and K. C. Smith, Mechanisms for recF-dependent and recB-dependent pathways of postreplication repair in UV-irradiated *Escherichia coli* uvrB, *J. Bacteriol.* 156:1093-1098 (1983).

15. T. V. Wang and K. C. Smith, recF-dependent and recF recB-independent DNA gap-filling repair processes transfer dimer-containing parental strands to daughter strands in *Escherichia coli* K-12 uvrB, *J. Bacteriol.* 158:727-729 (1984).

16. R. C. Sharma and K. C. Smith, A minor pathway of postreplication repair in *Escherichia coli* is independent of the recB, recC and recF genes, *Mutat. Res.* 146:169-176 (1985).

17. A. J. Fornace, Jr., Recombination of parent and daughter-strand DNA after UV-irradiation in mammalian cells, *Nature* 304:552-554 (1983).

18. A. K. Ganesan, Persistence of pyrimidine dimers during post-replication repair in ultraviolet light-irradiated *Escherichia coli* K-12, *J. Mol. Biol.* 87:103-119 (1974).

19. T. V. Wang and K. C. Smith, Postreplication repair in ultraviolet-irradiated human fibroblasts: formation and repair of DNA double-strand breaks, *Carcinogenesis* 7:389-392 (1986).

20. A. K. Ganesan and K. C. Smith, Recovery of recombination deficient mutants of *Escherichia coli* K-12 from ultraviolet irradiation, *Cold Spring Harbor Symp. Quant. Biol.* 33:235-242 (1968).

21. R. C. Sharma, T. R. Barfknecht, and K. C. Smith, Postreplication repair in uvrA and uvrB strains is inhibited by rich growth medium, *Photochem. Photobiol.* 36:307-311 (1982).

22. R. C. Sharma and K. C. Smith, Repair of DNA double-strand breaks in UV-irradiated *Escherichia coli* uvrB recF cells is inhibited by rich growth medium, *Mutat. Res.*, in press (1986).

23. R. C. Sharma and K. C. Smith, A mechanism for rich-medium inhibition of the repair of daughter-strand gaps in the deoxyribonucleic acid of UV-irradiated *Escherichia coli* K12 uvrA, *Mutat. Res.* 146:177-183 (1985).

24. K. C. Smith, DNA synthesis in sensitive and resistant mutants of *Escherichia coli* B after ultraviolet irradiation, *Mutat. Res.* 8:481-495 (1969).

25. Z. Trgovcevic, D. Petranovic, E. Salaj-Smic, M. Petranovic, N. Trinajstic, and Z. Jericevic, DNA replication past pyrimidine dimers in the absence of repair, *Mutat. Res.* 112:17-22 (1983).

26. R. B. Painter, Are lesions induced by ionizing radiation direct blocks to DNA chain elongation? *Radiat. Res.* 95:421-426 (1983).

27. R. C. Sharma, N. J. Sargentini, and K. C. Smith, New mutation(mmrA1) in *Escherichia coli* K-12 that affects minimal medium recovery and postreplication repair after UV irradiation, *J. Bacteriol.* 154:743-747 (1983).

28. W. P. Diver, N. J. Sargentini, and K. C. Smith, A mutation (radA100) in *Escherichia coli* that selectively sensitizes cells grown in rich medium to X- or U.V.-radiation, or methyl methanesulphonate, *Int. J. Radiat. Biol.* 42:339-346 (1982).

29. N. J. Sargentini and K. C. Smith, Characterization of an Escherichia coli mutant (radB101) sensitive to γ and UV radiation, and methyl methanesulfonate, Radiat. Res. 93:461-478 (1983).

30. I. Felzenszwalb, N. J. Sargentini, and K. C. Smith, Characterization of a new radiation-sensitive mutant, Escherichia coli K-12 radC102, Radiat. Res. 97:615-625 (1984).

31. N. J. Sargentini, W. P. Diver, and K. C. Smith, The effect of growth conditions on inducible, recA-dependent resistance to X rays in Escherichia coli, Radiat. Res. 93:364-380 (1983).

32. N. J. Sargentini and K. C. Smith, Growth-medium-dependent repair of DNA single-strand and double-strand breaks in X-irradiated Escherichia coli, Mutat. Res. 104:109-115 (1985).

33. N. J. Sargentini and K. C. Smith, Characterization and quantitation of DNA strand breaks requiring recA-dependent repair in X-irradiated Escherichia coli, Radiat. Res. 105:180-186 (1986).

34. C. D. Town, K. C. Smith, and H. S. Kaplan, The repair of DNA single-strand breaks in E. coli K-12 X-irradiated in the presence or absence of oxygen; the influence of repair on cell survival, Radiat. Res. 55:334-345 (1973).

35. I. Johansen, The radiobiology of DNA strand breakage, in: "Molecular Mechanisms for Repair of DNA," P. C. Hanawalt and R. B. Setlow, eds., Plenum Press, New York (1975), pp. 459-469.

36. O. Sapora, E. M. Fielden, and P. S. Loverock, The application of rapid lysis techniques in radiobiology. I. The effect of oxygen and radiosensitizers on DNA strand break production and repair in E. coli B/r, Radiat. Res. 64:431-442 (1975).

37. R. Roots and K. C. Smith, On the nature of the oxygen effect on X-ray-induced DNA single-strand breaks in mammalian cells, Int. J. Radiat. Biol. 26:467-480 (1974).

38. R. Roots and K. C. Smith, Rejoining of DNA single-strand breaks in mammalian cells incubated in buffer or in medium after aerobic or anaerobic X-irradiation, Int. J. Radiat. Biol. 27:595-602 (1975).

39. L. Samson and J. Cairns, A new pathway for DNA repair in Escherichia coli, Nature 267:281-282 (1977).

40. T. Kato and Y. Shinoura, Isolation and characterization of mutants of Escherichia coli defective in induction of mutations by ultraviolet light, Molec. gen. Genet. 156:121-131 (1977).

41. N. J. Sargentini and K. C. Smith, umuC-dependent and umuC-independent γ- and UV-radiation mutagenesis in Escherichia coli, Mutat. Res. 128:1-9 (1984).

42. R. Beukers and W. Berends, Isolation and identification of the irradiation product of thymine, Biochim. Biophys. Acta. 41:550-551 (1960).

43. B. J. Bachmann, Linkage map of Escherichia coli K-12, Edition 7, Microbiol. Rev. 47:180-230 (1983).

44. J. Cairns, Bacteria as proper subjects for cancer research, Proc. R. Soc. Lond. B208:121-133 (1980).

THE RELATIONSHIP OF DEFECTIVE RECOGNITION OF DNA DAMAGE TO CANCER IN

ATAXIA-TELANGIECTASIA

R. B. Painter

Laboratory of Radiobiology and Environmental Health
University of California
San Francisco, CA 94143

Ataxia-telangiectasia (A-T) is a human genetic disease that includes cancer proneness among its pathologies. Between 10 and 20% of A-T patients develop neoplastic disease, generally of the lymphoreticular system. Both the patients with A-T and their cells display hypersensitivity to ionizing radiation. This is accompanied by increased frequencies of radiation-induced chromosomal aberrations, which are almost certainly the cause of the increased cell killing (4). There is also an abnormally high frequency of spontaneous chromosomal aberrations, with a preferential involvement of chromosomes 7 and 14 in some patients (3).

Cells from A-T patients display another unique response to ionizing radiation: Their semiconservative DNA synthesis is not inhibited by exposure to ionizing radiation as it is in normal cells (Figure 1). This radioresistant DNA synthesis is primarily the result of the failure of some kind of damage-recognition factor to block the growing DNA replication forks when they approach radiation-induced DNA lesions (Figure 2). The initiation of whole clusters of replicons is blocked by radiation in normal cells, but only the initiation of the damaged replicon is blocked in A-T cells (6). It is probable that this difference is also caused by the defective damage-recognition factor. Furthermore, A-T fibroblasts exhibit a radiation-resistant mitotic delay; i.e., after X-irradiation A-T cells are delayed less in moving from G_2 into mitosis than are normal cells (9, 12). Again, a putative damage-recognition factor appears to fail in A-T cells. It is highly likely that the failure of each of these responses to X-radiation in A-T cells is the consequence of a single defective factor, because all of the processes fail only when the cell is homozygous recessive for the A-T phenotype.

I have suggested that this defective factor may cause the increased aberration frequency in A-T cells, either by allowing replication of DNA lesions (as a result of failure to inhibit DNA synthesis) or by permitting cells to enter mitosis before all pre-aberrational damage has been repaired, or both. However, there are data that indicate these ideas are

This work was supported by the Office of Health and Environmental Research, U.S. Department of Energy Contract No. DE-AC03-76-SF01012.

511

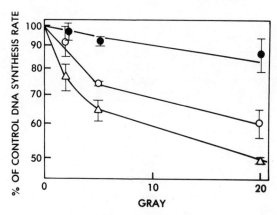

Fig. 1. Effects of ionizing radiation dose on rate of
DNA synthesis in human cells. ● , A-T
fibroblasts; ○ , normal human fibroblasts;
△ , fibroblasts from a patient with an
undiagnosed neurological disorder.

incorrect. Smith and Paterson (10) showed that incubation of A-T cells
with aphidicolin, which almost completely blocks semiconservative DNA
synthesis, does not enhance the survival of X-irradiated A-T cells. Under
the conditions of this experiment, the inhibition of DNA synthesis should
have allowed the cells to repair their DNA before the lesions were fixed by
replication. Cornforth and Bedford (1) showed that the restitution of X-
ray-induced chromosome fragments, observed by the premature chromosome
condensation (PCC) technique, is defective in A-T cells. Although the
number of induced fragments and their initial rate of repair were the same
in A-T cells as in normal cells, a much higher fraction remained unrepaired
in the A-T cells. This experiment was performed under conditions in which
the cells never left the G_1 phase. Therefore, it seems that the increased
frequency of chromosome aberrations, at least, can occur in A-T cells
without the intervention of the S phase or the transition from G_2 into
mitosis.

Despite the fact that these experiments cast doubt on my previous
proposal for mechanisms of enhanced aberration frequencies in A-T cells, it
is still probable that a defective damage-recognition factor is responsible
for them. DNA replication and progression from G_2 to mitosis are both so
intimately involved in control of the integrity of the genetic apparatus
that the changes observed in A-T must be a clue to an important process.
For instance, the failure of this factor may cause abortive chromosomal
restitution because a normally late step in repair begins before the
substrate for this step is available.

A particularly intriguing and unique feature of the differences
between chromosomal aberrations in normal and A-T cells is that relatively
high frequencies of chromatid aberrations are observed in A-T cells after
they have been irradiated in G_0 or G_1, whereas they are almost never
observed when normal cells are irradiated in G_0 or early G_1 (11). This
implies either that some kind of DNA damage persists in A-T cells, but not
in normal cells, until after entry into the S phase, or that DNA damage
persists in both A-T and normal cells through G_1 but is processed
successfully only in normal cells after reaching S phase. There is no
evidence for the first possibility, but there is evidence for the
difference in processing of damage in the two cell types. When normal
human cells are irradiated in plateau phase (with almost all cells in G_1)

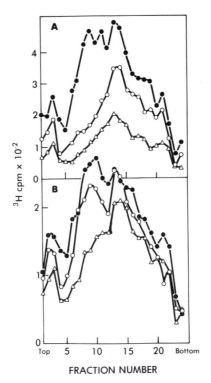

Fig. 2. Alkaline sucrose gradient profiles of DNA from
(A) normal diploid HS-27 cells and (B) AT5BI
cells irradiated with 0 (●), 5 (○), or 20
(△) Gy and pulse-labeled with (^{3}H)thymidine
30 min. later. Sedimentation is from left to
right. A dose-dependent inhibition of
initiation of replicons is deduced from
reduced radioactivity in low molecular weight
DNA (fractions 4-11). A dose-dependent
inhibition of chain elongation is deduced from
reduced radioactivity in high molecular weight
DNA (fractions 12-20). Note that A-T cells
show less inhibition of replicon initiation
and almost no inhibition of chain elongation.
(Reproduced from ref. 5 with permission of
Elsevier-North Holland Biomedical Press.)

and then released to progress through the cell cycle, there is a dose-
dependent increase in the time required for the cells to reach S phase and
a corresponding decrease in the number of cells that enter S phase. In
contrast, when A-T cells are so treated, all irradiated cells arrive at S
at the same time as unirradiated cells, and all enter S phase (4). Again,
a damage-recognition factor seems to fail in A-T cells. Saha and Tolmach
(8) showed that when HeLa cells are irradiated in early G_1, they enter S on
schedule (8 hr. later), but their rate of DNA synthesis is depressed;
recovery occurs 1-2 hr. after entry into S. Thus, throughout the G_1 phase
some kind of damage persists that requires semiconservative DNA synthesis
for its repair.

The results of these two experiments suggest the possibility that A-T
cells containing radiation-induced damage inflicted in G_0 or G_1 enter S
phase without pausing, as normal cells do, to allow proper processing of

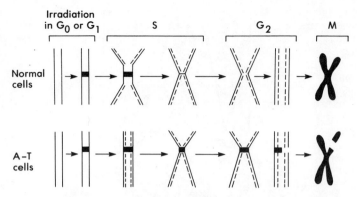

Fig. 3. Scheme for production of chromatid aberrations in A-T cells after irradiation in G_0 or G_1. The same lesion (crosslink?) is formed in normal and A-T cells in G_0 or G_1 phase. When cells reach S, DNA replication begins in both cell types. In normal cells the damage-recognition factor blocks replication in the region of the lesion until a putative processing converts the lesion to another form that can be completely repaired when the cells reach G_2. In A-T cells, however, the defective damage-recognition factor fails, DNA synthesis is not inhibited, and the DNA damage is fixed. This lesion cannot be successfully repaired when the cells are in G_2, and a chromatid aberration results upon entry into mitosis.

this damage, which is consequently converted into chromatid aberrations. In a possible scheme for this phenomenon (Figure 3), the precocious DNA replication in irradiated A-T cells may occur so rapidly upon entry into S that an early repair step that requires inhibition of DNA synthesis is bypassed, thus fixing the damage. A second repair step in G_2, which has been revealed by studies with chemicals (2) and with radiation (7), thus cannot occur in A-T cells, and a chromatid aberration is formed when the cells enter mitosis. Although this scheme is bound to be incorrect in some details, an S-dependent process that is defective in A-T cells may very well be the cause of the chromatid aberrations observed after A-T cells are irradiated in G_1.

Irrespective of the exact mechanisms by which the damage-recognition factor acts, there is little doubt that its failure in A-T cells is involved in the increased frequency of cancer observed in A-T patients. Therefore, it is highly likely that isolation and characterization of the genes and gene products responsible for the increased frequency of radiation-induced chromosome aberrations in A-T cells will also reveal a great deal about how ionizing radiation causes cancer in humans.

REFERENCES

1. M. N. Cornforth and J. S. Bedford, Science 227:1589-1591 (1985).

2. K. Hansson, B. A. Kihlman, C. Tanzarella, and F. Palitti, Mutat. Res. 126:251-258 (1984).

3. F. Hecht and B. Kaiser-McCaw, in: "Ataxia-Telangiectasia. A Cellular and Molecular Link Between Cancer, Neuropathology, and Immune Deficiency," B. A. Bridges and D. G. Harnden, eds., John Wiley and Sons, Chichester (1982), pp. 235-241.

4. H. Nagasawa and J. B. Little, Mutat. Res. 109:297-308 (1983).

5. R. B. Painter, Mutat. Res. 84:183-190 (1981).

6. R. B. Painter, in: "Ataxia-Telangiectasia: Genetics, Neuropathology and Immunology of a Degenerative Disease of Childhood," R. A. Gatti and M. Swift, eds., Alan R. Liss, New York (1985), pp. 89-100.

7. R. J. Preston, Mutat. Res. 69:71-79 (1980).

8. B. K. Saha and L. J. Tolmach, Radiat. Res. 66:76-89 (1976).

9. D. Scott and F. Zampetti-Bosseler, Int. J. Radiat. Biol. 42:679-683 (1982).

10. P. J. Smith and M. C. Paterson, Biochim. Biophys. Acta 739:17-26 (1983).

11. S. Wolff, Int. Rev. Cytol. 25:279-296 (1969).

12. F. Zampetti-Bosseler and D. Scott, Int. J. Radiat. Biol. 39:547-558 (1981).

MULTIFUNCTIONAL REPAIR ENZYMES EXCISE THYMINE AND ADENINE RESIDUES DAMAGED

BY IONIZING RADIATION FROM DNA

L. H. Breimer

Imperial Cancer Research Fund
Mill Hill Laboratories
London NW7 1AD
England

ABSTRACT

Aerobic metabolism is associated with the chance occurrence of reactive forms of oxygen, which may damage DNA (1-3). Analogous lesions are formed by ionizing radiation (4-6). It has been suggested that many dietary mutagens and carcinogens act through the production of oxygen radicals (7), and the deleterious free radical reactions involving oxygen have also been implicated in the genesis of spontaneous cancer in man (8) as well as in the aging process (9). It has been reported recently (10) that rats, which have a higher basal metabolic rate and shorter life span than humans, excrete in their urine 15 times more thymine glycol (an oxidation product of thymine) per unit body mass compared to humans, though what proportion of this that is derived from tRNA is not clear. Radiation-induced base damage in DNA is known to make an important contribution to the lethal and mutagenic effects observed in vivo (11, 12). Consequently, repair enzymes which act on DNA damaged by ionizing radiation and oxidizing agents are important in the preservation of the genome and prevention of mutagenesis and carcinogenesis.

As a model for the action of ionizing radiation on the nitrogenous bases in DNA, one can use oxidation by potassium permanganate (13). This is because it has an action similar to that of X-rays but less damaging to the sugar-phosphate backbone (14, 15). The chemistry of reactions of potassium permanganate with thymine has been extensively studied (14-19). At alkaline pH, there is saturation of the 5,6-double bond to give "thymine glycol" (5,6-dihydroxy-6-hydrothymine) but at neutral or acid pH saturation of the 5,6-double bond gives 5-hydroxy-5-methyl-barbiturate, but this compound is thought to be unstable when attached to deoxyribose, and the ring opens between N1 and C6 to give methyltartronylurea. Thymine glycol and methyltartronylurea may break down further, probably through pyruvylurea, which may either cyclise to give 5-hydroxy-5-methylhydantoin or decompose into urea. Methyltartronylurea may also decompose directly into urea (20). If alkaline osmium tetroxide is used instead of potassium permanganate only thymine glycol is formed (21, 22).

Adenine, on the other hand, is almost totally resistant to the action of these oxidizing agents (14, 15). Taking advantage of this, we used terminal transferase to synthesize a poly (dA.(2-^{14}C)dT) copolymer containing 2-4% thymine residues (13). The polymer was incubated with potassium permanganate to convert the thymine residues into urea and N-substituted urea derivatives. It was then annealed with an equimolar amount of poly (dT) to generate a double stranded polydeoxyribonucleotide containing scattered, fragmented, selectively labelled base residues. On incubation with crude cell extracts of E. coli, I found that free urea was released by DNA glycosylase action (13). (DNA glycosylases are enzymes which cleave the base-sugar bond of modified bases to initiate an excision repair process (23).)

The E. coli enzyme has now been purified 9,5000-fold to apparent homogeneity by phosphocellulose and DNA-cellulose chromatography, AcA54 gel filtration, heparin-sepharose and Affigel-blue chromatography (24). It is a monomeric globular protein of M_r = 25,000 and there are about 400 molecules in an E. coli cell. It acts on double stranded DNA, requires no cofactors and is not inhibited by urea. The enzyme excises not only urea but also methyltartronyurea, 5-hydroxy-5-methylhydantoin and thymine glycol from DNA, and cleaves the phosphodiester bond at the 3'-side of base-free sites. That is, it acts as an apyrimidinic endonuclease. The AP endonuclease activity and the DNA glycosylase activities for the oxidation products of thymine copurified at constant ratios throughout the purification procedure and are functions of the one protein seen on SDS-polyacrylamide gel electrophoresis in the final fraction. The enzyme is identical to E. coli DNA endonuclease III, an enzyme first described by Radman (25) as an activity which incises heavily UV-irradiated double stranded DNA. Its substrate specificity and reaction mechanism have been further studied by Linn's group (26, 27). They showed that it cuts DNA at thymine glycol and AP sites but not at pyrimidine dimers. Demple and Linn (28) showed that a partially purified fraction of endonuclease III could release thymine glycol by a DNA glycosylase mechanism. Our work (24) demonstrates that the DNA glycosylase activities for several oxidation products of thymine are functions of endonuclease III. This explains how urea, methyltartronylurea, 5-hydroxy-5-methylhydantoin and thymine glycol are released from damaged DNA. The enzyme presumably recognizes a structural feature common to all oxidized pyrimidine derivatives, such as the consequences of the absence of the 5,6 double bond. Katcher and Wallace (29) have proposed a similar model.

A similar enzyme exists in calf thymus and human fibroblasts (30) and rodent cells (31). I have partly purified and characterized the mammalian enzyme (30). It is similar to the bacterial enzyme but the activity on thymine glycol relative to urea is much less. A survey of human fibroblasts obtained from patients suffering from inherited disorders characterized by increased sensitivity to ionizing radiation and risk of malignancy did not reveal any enzyme deficient strain (30). The syndromes studied were: Fanconi's anaemia, ataxia telangiectasia, inherited retinoblastoma and basal cell nevus syndrome.

The homogeneous bacterial enzyme is now being used as a reagent enzyme to analyze the relative proportions of various thymine derivatives formed after different radiation insults to DNA.

Most studies on the effect of ionizing radiation on the bases in DNA have been concerned with the fate of thymine residues. Purine residues are also sensitive to ionizing radiation (4, 32). Bonicel and coworkers have shown (33) that irradiation of adenine in DNA leads to saturation and fragmentation of the imidazole ring, forming 4,6-diamino-5-formamidopyrimidine. This compound is similar to 7-methylguanine whose imidazole ring has been opened by alkaline hydrolysis (34). Five years ago Chetsanga and Lindahl discovered a DNA glycosylase in E. coli which excises this compound from alkylated DNA (35). A similar enzyme exists in mammalian cells (30, 36). Recently, Boiteux and Laval (37) reported that the ring opened form of 7-methylguanine blocks chain elongation by E. coli DNA polymerase I in vitro, indicating that such altered purines may be regarded as cell-killing lesions. Consequently, I was curious to see whether the adenine derived formamidopyrimidine was excised from DNA (38).

A radioactively labelled poly(dA) polymer was synthesized using terminal transferase. It was irradiated in neutral potassium phosphate buffer with a dose of 200 Gy under nitrogen, ethanol precipitated, redisolved and dialyzed. 0.16% of the adenine was converted into 4,6-diamino-5-formamidopyrimidine (38). The polymer was made double stranded by the addition of an equimolar amount of poly(dT) and then incubated with crude cell extracts and partially purified enzyme fractions of E. coli. Free 4,6-diamino-5-formamidopyrimidine was enzymatically released (38). This DNA glycosylase is different from the one which excises oxidized thymine residues from DNA. It has been purified 4,500-fold by phosphocellulose and DNA-cellulose chromatography followed by AcA54 gel-filtration (38). The final fraction showed a major band at M_r = 29,000 on SDS-polyacrylamide gel electrophoresis and was judged to be 90% pure. The activities on 4,6-diamino-5-formamidopyrimidine and on the ring-opened form of 7-methylguanine copurified at a constant ratio throughout the purification steps and are consequently most likely to be functions of one single enzyme.

In summary, I believe that these two enzymes are active in the repair of base lesions caused by ionizing radiation and oxidation. Their physiological significance should now be evaluated by genetic methods.

REFERENCES

1. W. O. Fenn, R. Gerschman, D. L. Gilbert, and F. V. Tothran, Proc. Natl. Acad. Sci. (USA) 43:1027-1032 (1957).

2. W. J. Bruynickx, H. S. Mason, and S. A. Morse, Nature 274:606-607 (1978).

3. I. Fridovich, Science 201:875-880 (1978).

4. G. Scholes, in: "Photochemistry and Photobiology of Nucleic Acids, Vol. I," S. Y. Wang, ed., Academic Press, New York (1976), pp. 521-577.

5. R. Teoule and J. Cadet, in: "Effect of Ionizing Radiation on DNA, Chapter 2," A. J. Bertinchamps, J. Hutterman, W. Kohnlein, and R. Teoule, eds., Springer Verlag, Berlin (1978), pp. 171-203.

6. J. E. Repine, O. W. Pfenninger, D. W. Talmage, E. M. Berger, and D. E. Pettijohn, Proc. Natl. Acad. Sci. (USA) 78:1001-1003 (1981).

7. B. N. Ames, Science 221:1256-1264 (1983).

8. J. R. Totter, Proc. Natl. Acad. Sci. (USA) 77:1763-1767 (1980).

9. D. Harman, Proc. Natl. Acad. Sci. (USA) 78:7124-7128 (1981).

10. R. Cathcart, E. Schwiers, R. L. Saul, and B. N. Ames, Proc. Natl. Acad. Sci. (USA) 81:5633-5637 (1984).

11. P. A. Cerutti, in: "Photochemistry and Photobiology of Nucleic Acids, Vol. II," S. Y. Wang, ed., Academic Press, New York (1976), pp. 375-401.

12. D. E. Levin, M. Hollstein, M. F. Christman, E. A. Schwiers, and B. N. Ames, Proc. Natl. Acad. Sci. (USA) 79:7445-7449 (1982).

13. L. H. Breimer and T. Lindahl, Nucleic Acids Res. 8:6199-6211 (1980).

14. G. K. Darby, A. S. Jones, J. R. Tittensor, and R. T. Walker, Nature 216:793-794 (1967).

15. S. Iida and H. Hayatsu, Biochim. Biophys. Acta 240:370-375 (1971).

16. M. H. Benn, B. Chatamra, and A. S. Jones, J. Chem. Soc. 1014-1020 (1960).

17. A. S. Jones, G. W. Ross, S. Takemura, T. W. Thompson, and R. T. Walker, J. Chem. Soc. 373-378 (1964).

18. S. Iida and H. Hayatsu, Biochim. Biophys. Acta 213:1-13 (1970).

19. S. Iida and H. Hayatsu, Biochim. Biophys. Acta 228:1-8 (1971).

20. B. Doumas and H. G. Biggs, J. Biol. Chem. 237:2306-2310 (1962).

21. K. Burton and W. T. Riley, Biochem. J. 98:70-77 (1966).

22. M. Beer, S. Stern, D. Carmalt, and R. H. Mohleurich, Biochemistry 5:2283-2288 (1966).

23. T. Lindahl, Ann. Rev. Biochem. 51:61-87 (1982).

24. L. H. Breimer and T. Lindahl, J.Biol. Chem. 259:5543-5548 (1984).

25. M. Radman, J. Biol. Chem. 251:1438-1445 (1976).

26. F. T. Gates, III and S. Linn, J. Biol. Chem. 252:2802-2807 (1977).

27. H. R. Warner, B. F. Demple, W. A. Duetsch, C. M. Kane, and S. Linn, Proc. Natl. Acad. Sci. (USA) 77:4602-4606 (1980).

28. B. F. Demple and S. Linn, Nature 287:203-208 (1980).

29. H. L. Katcher and S. S. Wallace, Biochemistry 22:4071-4082 (1983).

30. L. H. Breimer, Biochemistry 22:4192-4197 (1983).

31. M. C. Hollstein, P. Brooks, S. Linn, and B. N. Ames, Proc. Natl. Acad. Sci. (USA) 81:4003-4007 (1984).

32. J. J. van Hemmen and J. F. Bleichrodt, Radiat. Res. 46:444-456 (1971).

33. A. Bonicel, N. Mariaggi, E. Hughes, and R. Teoule, Radiat. Res. 83:19-26 (1980).

34. J. A. Haines, C. B. Reese, and Lord Todd, J. Chem. Soc. 5281-5288 (1962).

35. C. J. Chetsanga and T. Lindahl, Nucleic Acids Res. 6:3673-3684 (1979).

36. G. P. Margison and A. E. Pegg, <u>Proc. Natl. Acad. Sci. (USA)</u> 78:861-865 (1981).

37. S. Boiteux and J. Laval, <u>Biochem. Biophys. Res. Commun.</u> 110:552-558 (1983).

38. L. H. Breimer, <u>Nucleic Acids Res.</u> 12:6359-6367 (1984).

AGE AND SPECIES SPECIFIC VARIATION IN DNA EXCISION REPAIR IN CULTURED SKIN FIBROBLASTS

J. Vijg, E. Mullaart, P. H. M. Lohman* and D. L. Knook

TNO Institute for Experimental Gerontology
P.O. Box 5815
2280 HV Rijswijk
The Netherlands
*TNO Medical Biological Laboratory
 P.O. Box 45
 2280 AA Rijswijk, The Netherlands

INTRODUCTION

The suggestion that "DNA repair" may be a determinant of life span frequently appears in the literature on fundamental aging research (1). This idea is mainly based on the correlation found by Hart and Setlow between the life span of a species and the activity of the excision repair pathway in its UV-irradiated fibroblasts (2). In this vision, rodent cells as compared with human cells would age more rapidly in vivo (maximum life spans of about 4 and 110 years, respectively) and in vitro (about 20 and 60 population doublings, respectively) because of their relatively deficient DNA repair. Following this line of reasoning, it can be hypothesized that the low level of DNA excision repair in rodent cells in comparison with human cells is causally related to the relative instability of the former cell type with respect to immortalization and neoplastic transformation in vitro. In this context it is of interest that (genetically unstable) transformed or tumor-derived mammalian cells are less capable of repairing DNA damage than are their normal counterparts (3, 4, 5). These findings led to the speculation that repair deficiencies may promote genetic alterations characteristic for transformed cells. Viewed in this way, the process of cellular senescence itself may be associated with changes in DNA repair activities leading to neoplastic transformation. This hypothesis is supported by the fact that certain types of cancer, the incidence of which increases greatly with age, have been shown to be associated with deficiencies in certain DNA repair pathways (6, 7). Moreover, decreases in the activities of DNA repair pathways during in vitro and in vivo aging have been frequently reported (8). In this paper we discuss the relevance of one form of DNA repair, excision repair, to the aging process on the basis of the state of the excision repair pathway in rat fibroblasts during in vitro and in vivo aging and the differences in the excision process between normal human and rat fibroblasts.

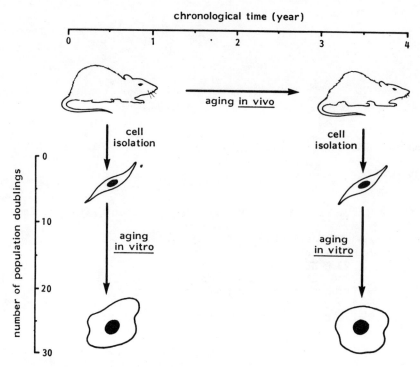

Fig. 1. Schematic representation of the longitudinal study of fibroblasts during aging in vitro and in vivo.

AGING CELLS FROM AGING RATS

When studying the occurrence of age-related changes, it is generally not sufficient to perform cross-sectional studies in which groups of young subjects are compared with groups of old ones. In this type of approach, each group has its own unique characteristics based on both individual and generational differences. A better way of determining whether certain factors change with age is to perform a longitudinal study in which the same population is followed over certain periods of time. However, longitudinal studies in humans are complicated because of the length of the human life span. Therefore, it is generally more appropriate to work with relatively short-lived mammals such as rats or mice having a maximum life span of about 4 years. In addition, diversity due to genetic and environmental variables can be excluded to a great extent by the use of inbred rodents kept under well-defined conditions (9). On the basis of these considerations, we have chosen a longitudinal approach to investigate some aspects of the DNA excision repair process in aging cells from individual animals of an inbred strain of Wistar rats (WAG/Rij ♀). The cell under study is the fibroblast, cultures of which can be established from skin biopsies taken from an individual animal at different times during its life span. The use of this cell type allows us to study DNA repair pathways simultaneously as a function of the chronological age of the donor and in vitro passaging of the established cell samples (in vitro age). This strategy, schematically depicted in Figure 1, was earlier applied in aging studies on humans (10).

Fibroblasts can be grown out of skin biopsies within several days (primary fibroblasts) and, when confluency is reached, further propagated by dividing them over 2 or more dishes after trypsinization. Each trypsinization cycle is termed a passage and if the population is each time

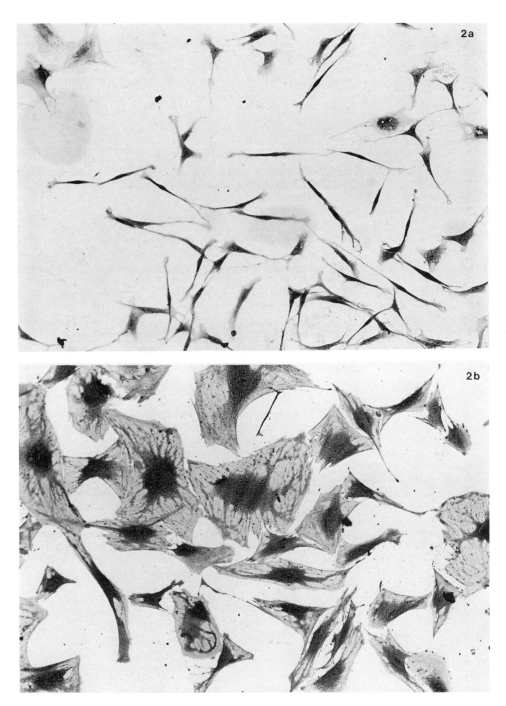

Fig. 2A and B.

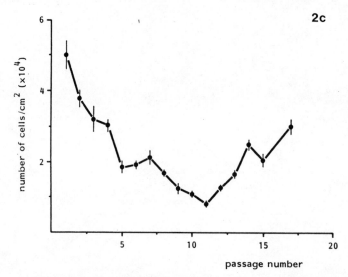

Fig. 2C. Morphological switch of fibroblasts after being placed in culture. (A) Primary cells (passage 0) among which some large cells (about 1% of the total population) can already be observed. (B) Secondary cells of passage 8. In this particular strain, senescence was not observed. In those strains that became senescent, however, the picture did not appear to be much different, although in a population that was kept senescent for about a month the cells were generally less densely packed and appeared to be extremely large and pleimorphic. (C) The effect of passaging on the cell surface area is indicated by a decrease in the number of cells per cm^2 at confluency. After about 11 passages, there appears to again be an increase, eventually leading to cell populations devoid of density dependent inhibition. This increase was observed for all cell strains which we isolated and cultured, except for those that became sensescent. Therefore, the dip in the curve may indicate the time when immortal cells become predominant at the cost of those cells predetermined for senescence.

divided into two parts one speaks of a population doubling as soon as the two daughter populations have again grown confluent. A striking observation that can be made during in vitro passaging of rat fibroblasts is the marked increase in cell surface area. This change from mostly small spindle shaped cells (Figure 2A) to large pleimorphic ones (Figure 2B) is clearly illustrated by an about 5-fold decrease in the number of cells per cm^2 at confluency between passage 1 and 11 (Figure 2C). The morphological switch of rat fibroblasts during in vitro passaging was first extensively described by Kontermann and Bayreuther (11), who considered its phenomenon essentially as a differentiation process. In some cell strains, the morphological shift was found to be accompanied by a decrease in the percentage of S-phase cells finally resulting in a senescent population in which the number of dying cells equalled or exceeded the number of newly emerging cells. In such a senescent population (consisting of vital cells that can be trypsinized and reseeded), we incidentally observed the emergence of "new' cell clones. Having a growth advantage, these newly emerging cells, eventually restored the proliferative capacity of the population. The same phenomenon has been described much earlier by Todaro and Green for mouse cells (12). However, in the majority of the fibroblast strains we followed, no significant decrease in proliferative capacity was observed and a senescent stage was never reached. The fact that initially

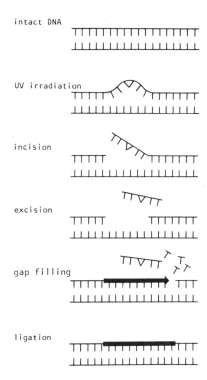

intact DNA

UV irradiation

incision

excision

gap filling

ligation

Fig. 3. Schematic representation of the steps
involved in excision repair of DNA
damaged by ultraviolet (UV) irradiation.

the same morphological shift was observed in these strains as in the cell
strains that became senescent suggests that there is no relationship
between the increase in cell surface area and the process that leads to
senescence. In some of the cell strains that were further monitored,
spontaneous transformation occurred, as indicated by the loss of density
dependent growth regulation.

Thus, rat skin fibroblasts in tissue culture have two options: to
become senescent after several passages or to become immortalized either
after passing through a senescent stage or "unnoticed" during the first
passages.

Finally, the changes observed in fibroblasts during passaging in vitro
did not appear to occur during the in vivo aging process. No apparent
differences were observed between fibroblasts from old and young rats when
placed in culture. However, it should be mentioned that Schneider and
Mitsui who systematically studied fibroblast cultures from old and young
human donors reported statistically significant differences in replicative
capacity as well as in cell surface area (13).

EXCISION REPAIR IN AGING CELLS

Cells are generally able to remove or tolerate lesions induced in
their DNA by mutagens and carcinogens in a variety of ways (14). One
mechanism of DNA repair is excision repair. This form of DNA repair is
induced by ultraviolet light (UV) and certain chemicals such as polycyclic
aromatic hydrocarbons. Its classical mode is schematically shown in

Figure 3. The relative importance of excision repair is difficult to estimate because no complete picture of the large variety of complex DNA repair systems in terms of their influence on cell survival and the induction of genetic variation has as yet been obtained. It is assumed that the excision repair pathway functions as the main channel via which a large variety of lesions frequently induced in cellular DNA can be repaired (15). For this purpose, there are various specific enzymes (e.g., endonucleases and DNA glycosylases) that recognize certain types of damage of which the repair is subsequently discharged into the excision pathway.

There are a few means for determining the activity of excision repair. A frequently applied method is to quantify the DNA synthesis step in the pathway by means of autoradiography. In this assay, cells attached to glass cover slips are exposed to a genotoxic agent (for instance UV) and allowed to repair the damage in the presence of radioactively labelled thymidine. The amount of incorporated radioactivity over a certain time interval which is a measure for the amount of unscheduled DNA synthesis (UDS) or DNA repair synthesis, can be quantified after autoradiography by counting the silver grains above the nuclei. S-phase cells can be easily distinguished from repairing cells on the basis of their much higher (about 100 times) number of grains above their nuclei.

With this system, UV induced excision repair activity was determined in early passage fibroblasts form rats varying in age between 6 and 44 months. Figure 4 shows the first results of this study. Both the initial rate (UDS over the first 3 h) and the end level (UDS over 24 h) were determined at two time points with an interval of nine months. The animals that died from old age during this time interval were replaced by young ones. According to this strategy, young animals can be compared with old ones while at the same time the young ones can be followed during their complete life span (time sequential cross-sectional study). Figure 4 shows that in the second cross-sectional study (performed at 9 months after the first) the overall UDS level was slightly lower than in the first. This illustrates the fact that UDS determinations are not very well reproducible when they are performed at different times (16). When all determinations are performed together as was done in each cross-sectional study, the errors generally do not exceed 5% of the mean. Consequently, UDS values for individual animals should be interpreted in terms of their relative position among data obtained from other animals assayed at the same time rather than that conclusions should be drawn from any observed variation in time.

It can be concluded from the results shown in Figure 4 that there is only a very small variation in UDS values among the individual animals. In addition, a slight but statistically significant age-related decrease in the initial rate of UDS was observed in both cross-sectional studies (P < 0.01 in both cases), whereas the end level of UDS at 24 h after irradiation remained constant. This suggests that possible differences in DNA repair synthesis between "old" and "young" cells are not absolute but merely reflect the rate at which the repair process is being carried out. In our opinion, however, the observed decrease in the initial rate of UDS is too small to have any dramatic biological significance; i.e., it might be a consequence but not a cause of aging. Furthermore, the lack of pronounced interindividual differences in UDS makes it unlikely that DNA excision repair is an important determinant of individual longevity in inbred rats of the same strain and sex.

When UV induced UDS was determined during in vitro aging of cultured fibroblasts, it appeared that UDS levels became significantly reduced in those cell strains where senescence occurred. Between passages 5 and 8, a reduction in initial rate and end level of UDS of about 50 and 20%,

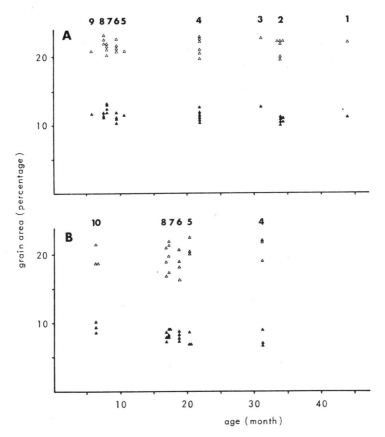

Fig. 4. Two cross-sectional studies of UV induced UDS in
fibroblasts from rats varying in age from 6 to 44
months. The second study (B) was performed at 9 months
after the first (A). Each point represents the mean
value of a triplicate determination in one rat. Each
group of points on a vertical line represents a
different cohort, indicated by a number. A cohort is
defined as the rats of a particular strain born during
the same week. Animals belonging to cohorts 4 to 8 were
included in both studies. Cohort 10 was newly
introduced into the second study. The animals belonging
to cohorts 1 to 3 died during the interval between the
first and the second study. Closed symbols, UDS over
the first 3 h after irradiation; open symbols, UDS over
24 h after irradiation. Data are from ref. 30.

respectively, was observed (Figure 5). As mentioned earlier, we consider a
fibroblast population as senescent solely on the basis of its greatly
reduced proliferative capacity. The senescent cells on which the UDS
determinations were carried out could be kept viable for months, during
which period they could be trypsinized, replated and assayed again for UDS,
yielding about the same low value as obtained one passage earlier. In
contrast to findings of other authors (17), we also found that almost all
cells in a UV-irradiated senescent population were, like actively dividing
early passage cells, able to perform UDS. These observations are not
consistent with the explanation of the decrease in UDS associated with
senescence in terms of a general deterioration of cellular functioning. On
the basis of our findings, the possiblity that the observed reduction in

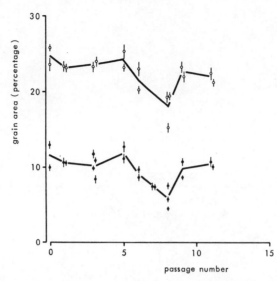

Fig. 5. UV induced UDS in rat fibroblasts over periods of 3
(closed symbols) and 24 h (open symbols) after
irradiation (10.3 J/m^2 during passaging in vitro.
Initially, the time required for 1 population doubling
(corresponding to about 1 passage in our splitting
scheme) was about 3 days. Between p 6 and p 7, the
culture stopped growing and was kept senescent for about
one month, after which the cells were transferred and
UDS was determined (p 7). After another period of about
1 month during which UDS was determined again (p 8),
newly growing cells appeared and the culture could be
transferred and split again. The phenomenon has been
reproduced in two other cell strains. In those strains
that did not become senescent, for instance, the one
from Fig. 2, UDS remained constant.

UDS is part of a programmed event should be taken into account. In this
context, it has been suggested that senescence in vitro might be terminal
differentiation rather than biological aging (18). This would be in accord
with the concept that the differentiated state is associated with reduced
DNA repair (19). However, the suggestion that the pronounced reduction in
UDS might be causally related to immortalization or neoplastic
transformation is an unlikely one, since in those senescent populations
that underwent immortalization UDS was restored to its old level (Figure
5). Finally, before drawing any definite conclusions with respect to DNA
excision repair from UDS determinations, it is necessary to confirm the
results obtained by use of other techniques. Studies for this purpose are
presently in progress.

EXCISION REPAIR IN TWO SPECIES AGING AT DIFFERENT RATES

Thus far, there has been no indication that nucleotide excision repair
may be a determinant of cellular aging. Therefore, the question of whether
the concept which relates cellular DNA excision repair to life span is
valid arises. According to this concept, DNA excision repair is one of
several so-called longevity assurance mechanisms which determine the
maximum life span of an organism (20). This assumption is based on
determinations of UV induced DNA repair synthesis in fibroblasts and later

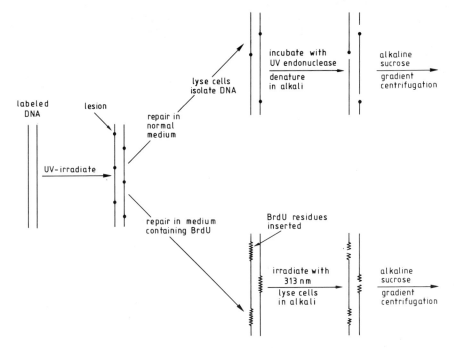

Fig. 6. Scheme of the assays for pyrimidine dimer sites and BrdU filled "repair patches." For a detailed description of how the techniques were employed, see ref. 27.

also in lymphocytes (21) taken from representatives of a number of species varying in their maximum life span (2). These and also other data (22, 23) leave little doubt about the generally higher UDS values in longer lived species, such as humans as compared with shorter lived ones such as rodents. Only few attempts have been made to investigate these interspecies differences in some more detail. Lohman et al. (24) showed that it can be dangerous to draw conclusions from interspecies differences in DNA repair synthesis by demonstrating that UV irradiated established hamster cell lines failed to remove pyrimidine dimers, the main UV photoproduct, although they were able to perform DNA repair synthesis. It was, therefore, suggested by these authors that any differences in excision repair between rodent and human cells might be due to mechanistic factors or the utilization of various DNA repair pathways instead of being a reflection of a different inherent capacity to restore DNA integrity. To investigate these possibilities in some more detail, it is necessary to compare the excision repair process in normal (untransformed) rodent and human cells by means of different techniques. For this purpose, in addition to UDS, we have applied the BrdU photolysis assay for determining DNA repair synthesis (25) and the UV endonuclease method for monitoring the removal of pyrimidine dimers (26) to analyze the kinetics of UV induced DNA excison repair in early passage rat and human skin fibroblasts (27). With the BrdU photolysis assay, the number and size of repaired sites per unit time can be determined. Together, these values should reflect the amount of UDS over a certain time interval. The number of removed pyrimidine dimers can be determined by the UV endonuclease method. Thus, the combined application of these techniques offers insight into all but the initial steps of the excision repair process in the two cell types (Figure 6). The results of our experiments essentially confirm those of Lohman et al. (24) and provide more detailed information on two normal untransformed mammalian cell types. Table 1 summarizes the results obtained by applying the three

Table 1. Comparison of UDS, UV-endo and BrdU photolysis over 3 and 24 h periods after irradiation with 4.6 J/m^2 of 254 nm UV

Cell type	Postirradiation time	UDS[a] grain area (%)	UV-endo[b] number of removed dimers per 10^9 mw DNA	BrdU photolysis number of repaired sites per 10^9 mw DNA	number of nucleotides per repair region
Human fibroblasts	3	13.1 ± 0.4	50 ± 10	83 ± 10	73 ± 10
	24	24.1 ± 0.5	121 ± 7	90 ± 10	63 ± 10
Rat fibroblasts	3	4.8 ± 0.1	0 ± 7	24 ± 10	66 ± 10
	24	14.9 ± 0.3	26 ± 7	52 ± 10	59 ± 10
Ratio rat/human	3	0.37 ± 0.01	–	0.3 ± 0.1	0.9 ± 0.2
	24	0.62 ± 0.02	0.21 ± 0.06	0.6 ± 0.1	0.9 ± 0.2

All determinations on rat and human cells were performed together in the same experiment. The errors in UDS and UV-endo were estimated from at least 4 experiments. The errors in BrdU photolysis were estimated from the photolysis curves of two experiments.
[a] UDS was determined noncumulatively, that is, over the complete time periods. These values are slightly lower than the ones presented earlier (ref. 27) which were based on cumulatively obtained data. This does not influence any of the conclusions since these are totally based on the ratios rat/human.
[b] The authenticity of the removed dimers was confirmed by their photoreactivability by a photolyase (ref. 27).

techniques to the two cell types. Determinations were made over 3 h (initial rate) and 24 h (end level) after irradiation.

Several conclusions can be drawn from the data presented in Table 1. Firstly, the mean repair patch size remains fairly constant over the 24 h repair period, and it does not significantly differ between the two species. Secondly, over both 3 and 24 h after irradiation, the ratio rat to human in UDS is the same as that in the number of created repair patches. This confirms the validity of UDS as a good measure for DNA repair synthesis. However, the ratio rat to human in dimer removal is significantly smaller than that in DNA repair synthesis. This finding underlines the discrepancy between dimer removal and DNA repair synthesis in rat cells.

Thirdly, dimer removal seems to proceed considerably more slowly than DNA repair synthesis in both species. This is, of course, especially obvious in rat cells, in which at 3 h after irradiation no significant dimer removal was observed, although 24 repair patches per 10^9 molecular weight of DNA were created over the same period. However, also in human cells, the number of repaired sites at 3 h after irradiation exceeded the number of removed dimers, in contrast to the situation at 24 h after irradiation. That in the latter case the number of removed dimers is somewhat greater than the number of created repair patches is most likely due to the fact that incorporation of BrdU becomes less efficient over such long periods. It should also be noted that, although it is tempting to directly compare the two assays, the conclusions we draw are based solely on the ratios rat to human. Determinations using one technique on the two cell types were always done together at the same time as part of one experiment.

In view of these findings, we suggest that in rat cells excision repair takes place primarily according to a mechanism in which DNA repair synthesis precedes dimer removal. A speculative model of how this might be

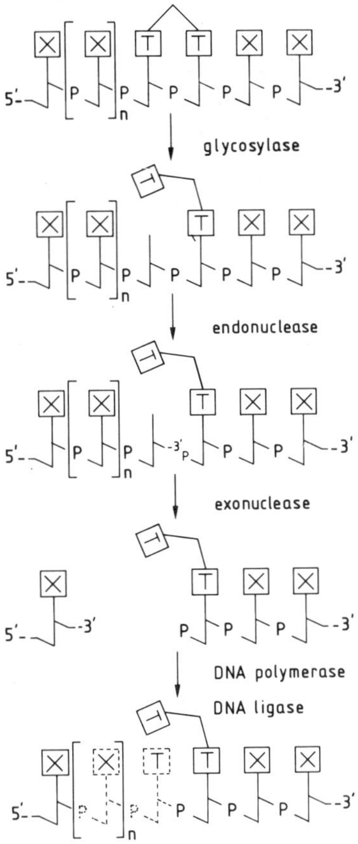

Fig. 7. Hypothetical model showing an alternative
pathway for excision repair of UV induced
pyrimidine dimers (described in the text).

realized is shown in Figure 7. It is based on the initial action of a
dimer specific glycosylase and an AP endonuclease as described by Haseltine
and Gordon (28) and the earlier suggestion of one of us (P.H.M.L.) that
pyrimidine dimers may remain hanging down in the DNA after repair synthesis
has been completed. In the model presented in Figure 7, it is assumed that
patching occurs only from 3' to 5' in order to remove the AP site and is
immediately followed by ligation. This would result in a semidetached
dimer still recognized by M. luteus UV endonuclease. In view of its
relatively small size as compared, for instance, with bulky adducts, this
structure may still be able to base pair and, therefore, not form a block
during replication. Eventually, the semidetached dimer may or may not be
removed via a pathway independent of DNA repair synthesis, which would
explain the occurrence of repair synthesis in rat cells while hardly any
dimers are removed. The model may also explain the discrepancy when dimer
removal is determined with antibodies and with M. luteus extract. It has
been shown that in Chinese hamster ovary cells dimer removal as determined
with antibodies proceeds even more rapidly than DNA repair synthesis (29).
This may be explained by assuming that, in contrast to the M. luteus
extract, the antibodies are able to select between genuine dimers and
semidetached ones. Removal of antibody binding sites would then rather be
a measure for glycosylase action than for dimer removal.

It is tempting to speculate that human cells may also partially remove pyrimidine dimers according to the mechanism proposed above. The balance between the classical mode of excision repair and the one suggested here would then differ for the two species; that is, rat cells would rely more heavily on the latter mode.

Although the model presented in Figure 7 is a speculative one, the data on which it is based illustrate the uncertainties one is dealing with when studying interspecies differences in DNA repair pathways. In our opinion, it is not wise to draw any conclusions with respect to a possible relationship between the level of activity of only one step in a DNA repair pathway and the capacity of a cell to maintain the integrity of its information content. The possibility of a correlation between "DNA repair" and species life span, however, is not invalidated by the findings discussed here; however, to obtain insight into the true nature of such an hypothetical relationship, a comparative analysis of the induction of DNA damage, its subsequent processing by DNA repair systems and the consequences for the aging cell in terms of survival and the emergence of genetic variations is required.

SUMMARY AND CONCLUSION

The possibility of whether variations in DNA excision repair may be involved in the predetermined in vivo and in vitro life span of cells is discussed in this paper. Data that indicate that the rate of excision repair in UV irradiated skin fibroblasts from old rats is slightly reduced as compared with that in cells derived from young rats are presented. There is, however, no indication for a dramatic age-related decrease in excision repair activities nor of extensive interindividual differences which could have corresponded with the great interindividual differences in life span in normal (inbred or outbred) populations. In view of the stability in the rate and extent of DNA excision repair, it is concluded that variations in these factors are not likely to determine in vivo variations in cellular life span among individuals of the same species.

During in vitro passaging of rat fibroblasts, a pronounced reduction in DNA repair synthesis occurs upon reaching the senescent phase (in vitro aging). In view of the characteristics of the senescent population, we suggest that this is more likely to be due to terminal differentiation than to a deterioration process. In addition, the reduced level of excision repair in senescent populations appears not to be causal to the spontaneous immortalization events frequently occurring in rodent cells in culture. This is indicated by the finding that the original level of excision repair was restored upon immortalization of some cells present in the senescent population.

A third aspect of cell aging, the high level of DNA repair synthesis in cells from long-lived species (such as man) in comparison with cells from short-lived species (such as rodents), was discussed in terms of the differences in UV induced excision repair between normal rat and human fibroblasts demonstrated after analysis by means of three different assays: UDS, UV-endo and BrdU-photolysis. The data provided indicate that in rat and human cells the excision repair process (partly?) takes place in a sequence in which DNA repair synthesis precedes dimer removal. A speculative model of this postulated new DNA excision repair pathway is presented. It is concluded that interspecies differences in the level of DNA repair synthesis do not necessarily reflect differences in excision repair capacity but may indicate a different mechanism or the utilization of alternative pathways. In this context, it should be taken into consideration that differences in characteristics or balance of activities of the many different DNA repair processes are involved in interspecies differences with respect to developmental processes, tumorigenesis and aging.

ACKNOWLEDGEMENTS

We thank Dr. F. Berends for helpful commentary on the manuscript. We are also grateful to Miss M. Roggenkamp for her help in typing the manuscript, Mr. E. J. van der Reijden and Mr. M. J. M. Boermans for preparing the figures and Dr. A. C. Ford for editing the English text.

REFERENCES

1. G. A. Sacher, Evolutionary theory in gerontology, Perspect. Biol. Med. 25:393-353 (1982).

2. R. W. Hart and R. B. Setlow, Correlation between deoxyribonucleic acid excision-repair and life span in a number of mammalian species, Proc. Natl. Acad. Sci. (USA) 71:2169-2173 (1974).

3. K. K. Sanford and V. J. Evans, A quest for the mechanism of "spontaneous" malignant transformation in culture with associated advances in culture technology, JNCI 68:895-913 (1982).

4. R. Parshad, R. Gantt, K. K. Sanford, G. M. Jones, and R. E. Tarone, Repair of chromosome damage induced by x-irradiation during G2 phase in a line of normal human fibroblasts and its malignant derivative, JNCI 69:409-414 (1982).

5. G. C. Elliot and R. T. Johnson, DNA repair in mouse embryo fibroblasts II. Responses of nontransformed, preneoplastic, and tumorigenic cells to ultraviolet irradiation, Mutat. Res. 145:185-194 (1985).

6. R. B. Setlow, Repair-deficient human disorders and cancer, Nature 271:713-717 (1978).

7. M. C. Paterson, Heritable cancer-prone disorders featuring carcinogen hypersensitivity and DNA repair deficiency, in: "Host Factors in Human Carcinogenesis," H. Bartsch and B. Armstrong, eds., IARC Scientific Publication No. 39 (1982), pp. 57-86.

8. J. R. Williams and K. L. Dearfield, DNA damage and repair in aging mammals, in: "Handbook of Biochemistry in Aging, J. R. Florini, ed., Boca Raton, Florida (1981), pp. 25-48.

9. C. F. Hollander, Current experience using the laboratory rat in aging studies, Lab. Anim. Sci. 26:320-328 (1976).

10. E. L. Schneider and J. R. Smith, The relationship of in vitro studies to in vivo human aging, Internatl. Rev. Cytology 69:261-270 (1981).

11. K. Kontermann and K. Bayreuther, The cellular aging of rat fibroblasts in vitro is a differentiation process, Gerontology 25:261-274 (1979).

12. G. J. Todaro and H. Green, Quantitative studies of the growth of mouse embryo cells in culture and their development into established lines, J. Cell Biol. 17:229-313 (1963).

13. E. L. Schneider and Y. Mitsui, The relationship between in vitro cellular aging and in vivo human age, Proc. Natl. Acad. Sci. (USA) 73:3584-3588 (1976).

14. A. R. Lehmann and B. Karran, DNA repair, Internatl. Rev. Cytology 72:101-146 (1981).

15. G. W. Teebor and K. Frenkel, The initiation of DNA excision-repair, in: "Advances in Cancer Research, Vol. 38," G. Klein and S. Weinhouse, eds., Academic Press, New York (1983), pp. 23-59.

16. J. E. Cleaver and G. H. Thomas, Measurement of unscheduled synthesis by autoradiography, in: A Laboratory Manual of Research Procedures, Vol. 1, Pt. B.," E. Friedberg and P. Hanawalt, eds., Dekker, New York (1981), pp. 277-287.

17. R. W. Hart and R. B. Setlow, DNA repair in late-passage human cells, Mech. Ageing Dev. 5:67-77 (1976).

18. E. Bell, L. Marek, S. Sher, C. Merrill, D. Levinstone, and I. Young, Do diploid fibroblasts in culture age? Internatl. Rev. Cytology Supplement 10:1-9 (1979).

19. C. Kidson, DNA repair in differentiation, in: "DNA repair mechanisms, ICN-UCLA Symposia on Molecular and Cellular Biology, Vol. IX," E. C. Friedberg and C. F. Fox, eds. (1978), pp. 761-768.

20. R. W. Hart and F. B. Daniel, Genetic stability in vitro and in vivo, in: "Aging, Cancer and Cell Membranes, Advances in Pathobiology," C. Borek, C. M. Fenoglio, and D. West King, eds., Georg Thieme, Verlag (1980), pp. 123-141.

21. K. Y. Hall, R. W. Hart, A. Kurt Benirischke, and R. L. Walford, Correlation between ultraviolet-induced DNA repair in primate lymphocytes and fibroblasts and species maximum achievable life span, Mech. Ageing Dev. 24:163-173 (1984).

22. H. Kato, M. Harada, K. Tsuchiya, and K. Moriwaki, Absence of correlation between DNA repair in ultraviolet irradiated mammalian cells and life span of the donor species, Jpn. J. Genet. 55:99-108 (1980).

23. A. A. Francis, W. H. Lee, and J. D. Regan, The relationship of DNA excision repair of ultraviolet induced lesions to the maximum life span of mammals, Mech. Ageing Dev. 16:181-189 (1981).

24. P. H. M. Lohman, M. C. Paterson, B. Zelle, and R. J. Reynolds, DNA repair in Chinese hamster cells after irradiation with ultraviolet light, Mutat. Res. 46:138-139 (1976).

25. J. E. Regan and R. B. Setlow, Two forms of repair in the DNA of human cells damaged by chemical carcinogens and mutagens, Cancer Res. 34:3318-3325 (1974).

26. B. Zelle and P. H. M. Lohman, Repair of UV-endonuclease-susceptible sites in the 7 complementation groups of xeroderma pigmentosum A through G, Mutat. Res. 62:363-368 (1979).

27. J. Vijg, E. Mullaart, G. P. van der Schans, P. H. M. Lohman, and D. L. Knook, Kinetics of ultraviolet induced DNA excision repair in rat and human fibroblasts, Mutat. Res. 132:129-138 (1984).

28. W. A. Haseltine and L. K. Gordon, A three-step incision model for early steps of excision repair of cyclobutane pyrimidine dimers, in: "Mechanisms of Chemical Carcinogenesis, UCLA Symposia on Molecular and Cellular Biology, New Series, Vol. 2," C. C. Harris and P. A. Cerutti, eds., Liss, New York (1982), pp. 449-456.

29. J. M. Clarkson, D. L. Mitchell, and G. M. Adair, The use of an immunological probe to measure the kinetics of DNA repair in normal and UV-sensitive mammalian cell lines, Mutat. Res. 112:187-199 (1983).

30. Y. Vijg, E. Mullard, P. H. M. Lohman and D. L. Knook, UV-induced unscheduled DNA synthesis in fibroblasts of aging inbred rats, Mutat. Res. 146:197-204 (1985).

NON-STOCHASTIC EFFECTS: COMPATIBILITY WITH PRESENT ICRP RECOMMENDATIONS

S. B. Field

MRC Cyclotron Unit
Hammersmith Hospital
London W12 OHS
England

The ICRP (International Commission on Radiological Protection has distinguished between "stochastic" and "non-stochastic effects" of ionizing radiation (1). In a recent report of the ICRP (2) the compatibility of present recommendations with non-stochastic effects has been considered. The present paper is a summary of the ICRP findings and is strongly based on ICRP 41 (2).

DEFINITIONS

The term stochastic has, in the present context, come to mean an event which is governed by the laws of probability. Stochastic effects are those for which the <u>probability</u> of occurrence is a function of dose, whereas the severity of the effect is dose independent. The principal stochastic effects of irradiation are thought to be cancer induction and heritable effects which are generally thought to arise from injury to one or a small number of cells. The probability of occurrence of such an effect increases with the number of cells at risk and with the nature and severity of the response. Its nature will depend on the particular change that has occurred. Because it is assumed that only a single cell need be affected, there is a finite probability of it occurring however small the dose and it follows that there will be an absence of threshold.

Non-stochastic effects, in contrast, are considered to be types of damage resulting from collective injury to substantial numbers or proportions of cells. For any given non-stochastic effect, a given number or proportion of cells will have to affects, so there will be a threshold dose below which the number of proportion of cells affected will be insufficient for the non-stochastic injury to occur. Any increase in dose above the threshold will result in an increasing level of injury. However, the threshold will depend on the choice of level of injury or the sensitivity of the apparatus used for its detection. For example, damage to mitochondria in rat intestinal cells has been demonstrated by electron microscopy after a fraction of gray, but 5-10 Gy are required for gross changes.

Non-stochastic effects may also occur which are "all or none" such as the probability of death. The relationship between the severity of an effect and the probability of occurrence of some level of injury is as illustrated in Figure 1.

Examples of non-stochastic effects include bone marrow damage, gonadal injury leading to impairment of fertility, lung damage leading to impaired function and fibrosis, etc. In each case, the injury is thought to originate from damage to individual cells resulting primarily in a loss of their reproductive capacity. It was pointed out by Hulse and Mole (3) that is is the nature of the damage to a cell that determines whether the final injury is in the category stochastic or non-stochastic, since the injurious event to any individual cell occurs at random. For example, neither malignant disease or hereditary effects can result if the cell is killed. These authors, therefore, propose that the terms stochastic and non-stochastic be replaced by haplocytic and polycytic.

RADIOBIOLOGICAL CONSIDERATIONS

Non-stochastic effects result primarily from the loss of reproductive integrity of individual cells, although other mechanisms may also be involved. For the vast majority of cell types radiation damage becomes manifest at the time of attempted cell division (lymphocytes and oocytes being principal exceptions). Thus, the responses of tissues _in vivo_

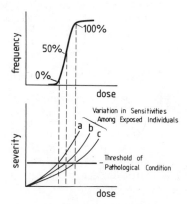

Fig. 1. Non-stochastic effects vary in severity as well as frequency with the dose. Since the mechanisms of nonstochastic effects include cell killing and other stochastic effects which may in themselves be observable at incipient stages, delineation of the dose-response relation for any given type of nonstochastic effect depends on the stage and severity at which the effect is scored. The upper and lower figures illustrate how the frequency and severity of a nonstochastic effect, defined as a pathologic condition, increases as a function of dose in a population of individuals of varying susceptibilities. The severity of the effect increases most steeply in those of the greatest susceptibility (lower figure), reaching the threshold of clinical detectability as a pathological condition at a lower dose in this subgroup than in less susceptible subgroups (curves b and c). The range of doses over which the different subgroups cross the same threshold of severity is reflected in the upper curve, which shows the frequency of the pathologic condition in the entire population, and which reaches 100 percent only at that dose which is sufficient to exceed the defined threshold of severity in all members of the population (from ICRP 41 (2)).

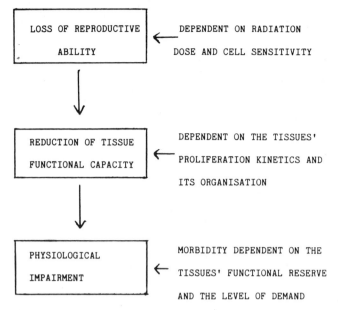

Fig. 2.   Factors affecting the expression of radiation
           damage as impairment of tissue specific function
           in proliferating normal tissues (from Wheldon, et
           al. (5)).

depend on the characteristics of cell survival and also substantially on
both the postirradiation cell proliferation kinetics and organization of
the particular tissue. Rapidly dividing tissues will characteristically
show a response soon after irradiation, the time depending on the turnover
rate of the constituent cells. The pathomechanism of late effects is more
controversial. One view is that radiation leads first to an increase in
vascular permeability resulting in leakage of plasma proteins into
interstitial spaces responsible for deposition of collagen and, ultimately,
atrophy of the parenchymal cells. Collapse of the radiation-damaged
capillary network might also be responsible for degenerative and atrophic
changes accompanied by progressive reduction in overall functional
capacity. An alternative view ascribes the delayed consequences of
irradiation to a loss of reproductive capacity by the parenchymal cells with
the rate of expression of damage determined by the physiological rate of
cell turnover. A gradual depopulation then leads to replacement fibrosis.
However none of these hypotheses fully accounts for radiation effects in
slowly proliferating tissues and organs. A summary of the factors
affecting the expression of non-stochastic injury is indicated in Figure 2.

Tissue Kinetics and Organization

        The rate at which the cells of a tissue are replaced and their dynamics
of production, differentiation, aging and loss determine the time course of
the radiation response. These considerations and most of the factors
summarized in Figure 2 have been well documented in detail in the
literature but less has been written of differences due to the
proliferative organization. The majority of the more rapidly proliferating
tissues are thought to be composed of a population of stem cells with the
property of indefinite proliferation. These produce mature, post mitotic
cells by differentiation through a transit compartment in which a limited
umber of divisions may occur, amplifying the mature cell input (Figure 3).
Mature cells are lost naturally. Radiation sterilizes the proliferative
cells, stopping the input into the mature compartment. The rate of

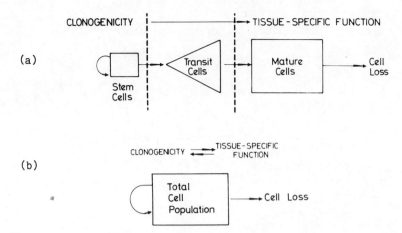

Fig. 3. Two types of proliferative organization. (a) In "hierarchical" (type H Proliferative Organization) tissues (e.g. haemopoietic tissues) a small minority of cells (stem cells) are clonogenic. Functional but non-clonogenic cells are derived from stem cells via the transit compartment which may incorporate a limited number of obligatory developmental divisions, so amplifying stem cell input. (b) In "flexible" (type F Proliferative Organization) tissues (e.g. liver parenchyma) all cells are equally capable of clonogenic (or at least, extensive proliferation or function. In both cases, proliferation normally takes place to balance physiological cell loss (from Wheldon et al., (5)).

functional cell depletion and thus the time course of the morbidity depend on the normal loss of the mature cells, i.e., on the normal steady state kinetics of renewal. This type of tissue organization is termed "hierachical" and examples include epidermis, intestinal mucosa, haemopoietic system.

However, the above scheme may not be universal and some tissues appear to have the ability to react to irradiation by a massive proliferative response of previously quiescent cells (Figure 3). The liver parenchyma is probably a good example. Michalowski and his colleagues (4, 5) have used the term "flexible" or F-type to describe this type of tissue response. An important difference between the radiation responses of these two types of tissue is that the time course of injury is relatively dose independent in H-type, but damage occurs earlier with increasing dose in F-type. F-type tissues possibly also include endothelium, mesothelium, kidney parenchyma. All are tissues with a slow turnover. By modelling the response of F-type tissues Michalowski and his colleagues have drawn attention to several important differences in their response from that of H-type tissues. Some of these are summarized in Table 1.

Protraction of Irradiation

When a dose of radiation is divided into two or more dose fractions, its effectiveness is reduced. This is due to two main factors, repair of intracellular damage and replacement of cells by repopulation or migration. These two components of "repair" are illustrated in Figure 4. A cell survival curve for a single acute exposure is characterized by an initial shoulder region relating to repair of sublethal injury. As the dose is given in more fractions or increasingly protracted, there is a increasing

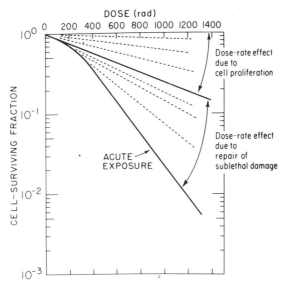

Fig. 4. Illustration of the dose-rate effect due to (a) repair
of sublethal radiation damage, and (b) cell
proliferation. The usual dose-response curve for low
LET radiation (lower solid line) has a broad initial
shoulder. As the dose rate is reduced, the slope of
the survival curve becomes shallower and the
extrapolation number tends towards unity, reflecting
repair of sublethal damage taking place during the
exposure. A limiting slope is reached (upper solid
line), corresponding to complete repair of such damage.
If the dose rate is reduced below a critical value,
which varies with the cell cycle of the population
exposed, cell proliferation may occur during
irradiation and there will be an additional dose-rate
effect as the exposure is further protracted (from Hall
(6)).

proportion of the total injury inflicted in the form of sublethal damage,
but repaired so that it is not expressed. As a result, an increasing
proportion of the lethal injury results from non-repairable types of
damage. The net result will be a tendency of the curve to become shallower
with decreasing dose rate or increasing number of dose fractions, finally
becoming exponential with a slope equal to the initial slope of the curve
derived from a single acute exposure. Such a situation will be reached
when the dose rate is reduced to the order of 0.1 Gy per hour (6).

    If the dose rate is further reduced, the slope of the curve may become
even shallower due to cellular repopulation, the extent depending on the
characteristics of cell turnover and organization of the exposed population.
For example, the stem cells in the small intestine of the rat, which have a
high capacity for proliferation, enable the tissue to tolerate continuous
irradiation at 4 Gy per day in contrast with the slowly proliferating testis
of the dog for which the critical dose rate is approximately 1000 times
less than that for intestine (2).

    In the vast majority of cases these factors are not known, especially
for man. They must be estimated by extrapolation from available data. For
example, the known responses to radiotherapy will give information on
human tissue responses for conventional dose fractionation regimes.

Table 1. Consequences of Proliferative Organization

	type H (three-compartmental)	type F (one-compartmental)
Rate of depopulation after irradiation	constant and dose-independent	accelerating for any given dose ("avalanche") and increasing with dose
Time to reach a fixed level of depopulation	predicatble from normal (steady-state) kinetics	shorter than calculated from steady-state kinetics
Limited (sub-clonogenic) proliferation of radiation-sterilised cells	usually of minor consequence	invariably critically protective
Highly sensitive hemeo-static regulation of population size	beneficial (earlier recovery following less severe impairment of function)	deleterious (earlier and more severe functional deficit)
Deliberate stimulation of cell proliferation after irradiation	assists repopulation	precipitates the avalanche ("recall" reactions)

from Dr. A. Michalowski (personal communication)

However, to obtain information relative to occupational exposure involves extrapolating from the known effects of a treatment divided into many small dose fractions to the unknown effects of much smaller dose fractions or continuous irradiation. In terms of cell survival curves, this requires a knowledge of the shape of the initial region of the curve.

For decades radiotherapists have devised methods to equate treatments given in different numbers of fractions and overall treatment time. A widely used empirical formula is that from Ellis (7),

$$\text{i.e., Total Dose} = (\text{NSD}) \; N^{0.24} T^{0.11}$$

where N = number of fractions, T = overall treatment time and NSD is a constant. This formula has been greatly used and has often been modified for more convenient application.

However, the Ellis formula has been shown to have limited application. The exponent of N is known to vary with the tissue, e.g., 0.4 for paralysis after irradiated of the CNS. With increasing protraction of irradiation to large values of N (dose fractions less than approximately 1 Gy), the formula will overestimate the sparing resulting from sublethal damage. It is extremely difficult in the present state of knowledge to estimate the sparing by repopulation but $T^{0.11}$ is unlikely to give a reasonable estimate for all tissues.

An alternative approach to the problem of extrapolating to small dose fractions and one which is currently much favoured is based on the linear quadratic model of the cell survival curve, applied to tissue endpoints,

$$\text{i.e., } E = \alpha D + \beta D^2$$

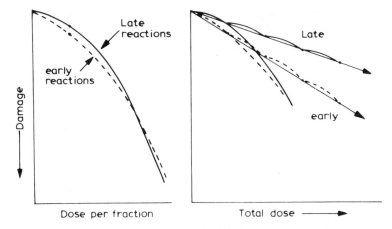

Fig. 5.   Cell survival curves of different shapes for early
          reactions (high values of α/β) and late reactions (low
          values of α/β) with fractionated irradiation. These
          differences in shape correspond to greater sparing for
          late effects as shown (from Fowler (11)).

where E is a given effect of a dose D. This formulation ignores the
effects of repopulation which must be accounted for separately. However,
the formula has been found to provide a good fit for variety of endpoints
over a wide range of doses per fraction. At very low doses and dose rates
the response is determined by α, which unfortunately is difficult to
measure <u>in vivo</u>. However, it is not difficult to establish the ratio α/β
from experimental studies. This parameter represents the dose at which the
αD and βD^2 components contribute equally to the damage and is therefore an
indication of the shape of the relevant dose response curve. In general,
values of α/β range from 1-15 Gy. Low values imply a large repair
capacity and are typical of the slowly proliferating, late responding
tissues. High values imply less repair and are typical for the rapidly
turning over tissues which show damage soon after irradiation. These
differences are illustrated in Figure 5.

The dose equal to 0.1 α/β indicates that dose up to which the
response curve is effectively linear, i.e., negligible sparing due to
fractionation will occur as the dose per fraction is reduced below 0.1 α/β.
The subject has been reviewed recently (8, 9, 10).

With caution, the linear quadratic formula may be used to extrapolate
from conventional radiotherapy exposures, i.e., 20-30 fractions given in 4-
7 weeks duration to very low doses per fraction given in the same overall
treatment time. This results in a further decrease in effectiveness per Gy
by a factor of the order of 1.2 for the more rapidly turning over tissues
which generally have high values of α/β and by a factor of about 1.5-2 for
the more slowly turning over tissues which have low values of α/β. The
effect of repopulation over long periods is even more difficult to assess.
In general, the tissues with high values of α/β (moderate repair capacity)
are those with high rates of turnover and hence a great capability for
repair by repopulation. Tissues with low values of α/β (high capacity for
repair of sublethal injury) are those with low turnover and probably
limited capacity for repair by repopulation. However, the proliferation
kinetics of such tissues is complex and not fully understood as discussed
above.

Table 2. Summary of factors relevant to extrapolation from radio-
          therapy experience to occupational exposure.

	Rapidly Proliferating	Slowly Proliferating
Timing of Response	early	late
Repair by proliferation	considerable	probably only moderate
Repair of sublethal damage	moderate	considerable
Ratio α/β	high ($\sim$ 10)	low ($\sim$ 2)
Extrapolation factor (excluding repopulation)	1.2	1.5 – 2.0

A summary of these conclusions regarding the influence of repair and
repopulation in extrapolating from radiotherapy to occupational exposures
is given in Table 2.

High LET Radiation

With increasing LET both the initial and final slopes of the dose-
survival curves become steeper. A maximum of effectiveness is reached, and
with further increase in LET the sensitivity then decreases. As a result
of the reduced capacity for repair of intracellular injury at high LET, the
RBE increases as the dose or dose per fraction is decreased (Figure 6).
With decreasing dose or dose rate, the RBE will reach a constant value at
sufficiently low doses or dose rates when only single-hit events become
effective. In terms of the linear quadratic equation, α/β for high LET
radiation is very large. β is though not to vary greatly but becomes less
important as the dose rate is decreased.

RBE values at low doses and dose rates are highly uncertain, but for
fast neutrons are known for many tissues in the range used for
radiotherapy. It is reasonable for the purposes of radiation protection to
assume that extrapolation from high LET radiotherapy to occupational
exposure should not contain a factor to allow for further increase in dose
due to repair of sublethal damage. However, repopulation is thought not to
vary with radiation quality.

Table 3. Organs and Tissues Considered in ICRP 41

SKIN	REPRODUCTIVE SYSTEM

DIGESTIVE SYSTEM
    including liver
        salivary glands
        pancreas
	URINARY TRACT
	    including kidneys
	        ureters
	        bladder

HAEMOPOIETIC SYSTEM	RESPIRATORY SYSTEM
CARDIOVASCULAR SYSTEM	MUSCLOSKELETAL SYSTEM

EYE	ENDOCRINE SYSTEM
	    including thyroid
	        pituitary
	        adrenals

NERVOUS SYSTEM	

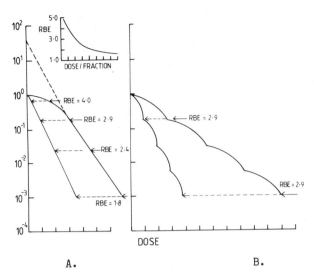

Fig. 6.   Typical survival curves for mammalian cells exposed to
          X-rays or fast neutrons. A. Single Doses. With X-rays
          the survival curve has a large initial shoiulder; with
          fast neutrons the initial shoulder is smaller and the
          final slope steeper. As a result of the differences in
          shapes the RBE is large for small doses, decreasing
          with increasing dose, as illustrated in the inset
          diagram. B. Fractionated Doses. The effect of giving
          4 equal fractions of X-rays or fast neutrons each of
          which would give rise to an RBE of 2.9 (as illustrated
          in Panel A) is shown. Providing sufficient time is
          allowed for full recovery of sublethal injury the
          shoulder of each survival curve is expressed with each
          fractionated treatment and the RBE for 4 fractions is
          the same as for single treatment of the same dose per
          fraction. Thus the curve relating RBE against dose, as
          shown in inset in Panel A, applies either to single
          doses or, in the case of fractionated treatments, to
          dose per fractioon (from ICRP 41 (2)).

RESPONSES OF DIFFERENT TISSUES AND ORGANS

     Table 3 shows the tissues and organs considered by ICRP (2).   The
following discussion will compare estimates of threshold doses for
detrimental effects with the present ICRP recommended dose limits, much of
the information on normal tissue injury having been derived from UNSCEAR
REPORT 1982 (12).

     The starting point for assessment of threshold doses in man is largely
dependent on accepted values in radiotherapy. There is, of course, some
uncertainty in this procedure since the responses of radiotherapy patients
are not necessarily typical of the normal working population. In addition,
there is not uniform agreement amongst radiotherapists on the question of
normal tissue sensitivity. However, for the purposes of radiation
protection it was considered by ICRP adequate to rely mainly on the
published summary of Rubin and Casarett (Table 4) (13). These authors give
the dose required, in their opinion, to cause a particular effect in 1-5%
of individuals exposed to conventional radiotherapy, i.e., 20-30 fractions
given in an overall time of 3-7 weeks. Since the dose response curves are

Table 4. Estimates of approximate threshold doses for clinically detrimental non-stochastic effects in various tissues, based on responses of patients to conventionally fractionated therapeutic X- or -irradiation

Organ	Injury at 5 years	Dose Causing Effect in 1-5% of Patients (Gy)	Dose Causing Effect in 25-50% of Patients (Gy)	Irradiation Field (Area)
Skin	Ulcer, severe fibrosis	55	70	100cm^2
Oral mucosa	Ulcer, severe fibrosis	60	75	50cm^2
Oesophagus	Ulcer, stricture	60	75	75cm^2
Stomach	Ulcer, perforation	45	50	100cm^2
Intestine	Ulcer, stricture	45	65	100cm^2
Colon	Ulcer, stricture	45	65	100cm^2
Rectum	Ulcer, stricture	55	80	100cm^2
Salivary glands	Xerostomia	50	70	50cm^2
Liver	Liver failure, ascites	35	45	whole
Kidney	Nephrosclerosis	23	28	whole
Urinary bladder	Ulcer, contracture	60	80	whole
Ureters	Stricture, obstruction	75	100	5-10cm
Testes	Permanent sterilization	5-15	20	whole
Ovary	Permanent sterilization	2-3	6-12	whole
Uterus	Necrosis, perforation	> 100	> 200	whole
Vagina	Ulcer, fistula	90	> 100	5cm
Breast, child	No development	10	15	5cm^2
Breast, adult	Atrophy and necrosis	> 50	100	whole
Lung	Pneumonitis, fibrosis	40	60	lobe
Capillaries	Telangiectasia, sclerosis	50-60	70-100	--
Heart	Pericarditis, pancarditis	40	> 100	whole
Bone, child	Arrested growth	20	30	100cm^2
Bone, adult	Necrosis, fracture	60	150	100cm^2
Cartilage, child	Arrested growth	10	30	whole
Cartilage, adult	Necrosis	60	100	whole
CNS (brain)	Necrosis	50	> 60	whole
Spinal cord	Necrosis, transection	50	> 60	5cm^2
Eye	Panophthalmitis, haemorrhage	55	100	whole
Cornea	Keratitis	50	> 60	whole
Lens	Cataract	5	12	whole
Ear (inner)	Deafness	> 60		whole
Vestibulum auris	Meniere's syndrome		60	100whole
Thyroid	Hypothyroidism	45	150	whole
Adrenal	Hypoadrenalism	> 60		whole
Pituitary	Hypopituitarism	45	200-300	whole
Muscle, child	Hypoplasia	20-30	40-50	whole
Muscle, adult	Atrophy	> 100		whole
Bone marrow	Hypoplasia	2	5.5	whole
Bone marrow	Hypoplasia	20	40-50	localized
Lymph nodes	Atrophy	35-40	> 70	--
Lymphatics	Sclerosis	50	> 80	--
Fetus	Death	2	4.5	whole

From Rubin and Casarett (13).

rather steep (as illustrated in Figure 1 for the probability of causing an effect), the above dose is likely to be close to the threshold dose.

It should be noted that the recommended limit for non-stochastic effects to any organ is 0.5 Sv per year for all tissues, i.e., a total accumulated lifetimes' occupational exposure of 25 Sv during 50 years. The recommended limit for the lens is an exception, being 0.15 Sv per the year, i.e., 7.5 SV total accumulated exposure. However, in many cases recommended limit will be much lower on the basis fo stochastic effects.

The following brief review of incidental tissues and organs should be seen in the light of these recommendations.

Skin   Irradiation of the skin produced a transient erythema within hours, resulting from capillary dilatation. After 2-4 weeks there may be waves of erythema followed by epilation, dry desquamation, moist desquamation and necrosis. Long-term effects, occurring after several months or years, include changes in pigmentation, atrophy of the epidermis, sweat glands, sebaceous glands and hair follicles, fibrosis and increased susceptibility to subsequent trauma. The severity is dependent on dose, irradiated area and site.

In man the threshold dose in skin, in a radiotherapy treatment regime is in the order of 50 Gy (Table 4). For occupational exposure this figure would be increased considerably, mainly by repopulation, and is therefore well in excess of the recommended limit. However, occupational exposures of 10-30 Gy accumulated during 8-25 years have revealed subclinical microscopic changes in skin.

Digestive System   Amongst the organs of the digestive tract the liver is though to have the lowest threshold. Impairment of hepatic function follows 20-25 Gy of radiotherapy of the whole organ, although partial liver irradiation results in much greater tolerance.

The mucosa of the gastrointestinal tract, with comparable structure to skin in some respects, responds rapidly to irradiation, resulting in denudation and ulceration. A single acute exposure of the order of 10 Gy to a large volume may result in a rapidly fetal dysentery-like syndrome. Late effects of radiation in the gastrointestinal tract include fibrosis, stricture, perforation, and fistula formation. The salivary glands and pancreas are more resistant, the threshold for conventional radiotherapy being in the region of 50 Gy, compared with 45 Gy for intestine.

Haemopoietic System   The haemopoietic system is one of the most sensitive elements in the body. Within minutes of whole body irradiation of 1 Gy or more cytological changes in bone marrow and lymphoid follicles can be seen. Also changes in peripheral blood occur through killing of haematopoietic stem cells and circulating lymphocytes, the latter dying rapidly in interphase. The threshold for cell depletion after a single acute exposure is approximately 0.5 Gy whilst the LD/50 within 60 days is in the range 2.5-5 Gy.

On fractionation or protraction of irradiation, tolerance is markedly increased by repopulation and to a lesser extent by repair of sublethal injury. Available data imply that the threshold for detectable depression of haemopoiesis is probably greater than 0.4 Sv per year and for fatal aplasia is greater than 1 Sv per year.

These data are summarized in Table 5, in comparison with the presently rcommended animal dose limits. In the case of whole body irradiation, the stochastic dose limit of 0.05 Sv/year will apply. For irradiation, the stochastic dose limit of 0.05 Sv/year will apply. For irradiation of the bone marrow alone, e.g., by internal radionuclide contamination, the limit is 0.4 Sv/year but it is likely that bone will also be irradiated thus reducing the recommended limit to 0.33 Sv/year. If non-skeletal tissues are also irradiated then the recommended limits will be lower still.

Hence, detrimental stochastic effects in the bone marrow are likely to be totally excluded by the present limits for stochastic effects, but the margin is small.

Table 5. Estimates of the thresholds for nonstochastic effects in the adult human testes, ovaries, lens, and bone marrow

Tissue and Effect	Threshold			Presently recommended annual dose equivalent limit (Sv)[a]	
	Total dose equivalent received in a single brief exposure (Sv)	Total dose equivalent received in highly fractionated or protracted exposures (Sv)	Annual dose rate if received yearly in highly fractionated or protracted exposures for many years (Sv yr^{-1})	(if irradiated alone)	(if irradiated with the whole body)
Testes					
Temporary Sterility	0.15	NA[b]	0.4	0.2	0.05
Permanent Sterility	3.5	NA	2.0	0.2	0.05
Ovaries					
Sterility	2.5–6.0	6.0	> 0.2	0.2	0.05
Lens					
Detectable Opacities	0.5–2.0	5.0	> 0.1	(0.15)	0.05
Visual Impairment (cataract)	5.0	> 3.0	> 0.15	(0.15)	0.05
Bone marrow					
Depression of Hematopoeisis	0.5	NA	> 0.4	0.4	0.05
Fatal Aplasia	1.5	NA	> 1.0	0.4	0.05

a Values listed, except those in parentheses, denote annual dose-equivalent limits for stochastic effect, these values being limiting for the tissues in question.

b NA denotes Not Applicable, since threshold dependent on dose rate rather than on total dose.

From ICRP 41 (2).

Cardiovascular System   A degree of myocardial degeneration is likely to result from 40 Gy conventional radiotherapy to the whole heart or from higher doses if only a part of the organ is irradiated. Higher doses cause pericardial effusion or constrictive pericarditis. The basic cause of such an inflammatory reaction is not known for certain but is thought to result from damage to blood vessels.

The present recommended levels would exclude any detrimental non-stochastic effects in the cardiovascular system.

Eye   The relevant sensitivities of the various parts of the eye are given in Table 6 from which it is seen that the lens is the most sensitive. Irradiation causes damage to the slowly dividing cells in the anterior epithelium. The damaged cells and products of cell breakdown migrate posteriorly and accumulate beneath the capsule at the posterior pole of the lens, causing displacement of the lens bow. Sufficient damage results in dots of opacity which at this stage do not impair vision. The lesion may or may not progress to cataract, depending on the radiation dose, when it may involve the anterior cortex and nucleus of the lens and severely impair vision. It appears that the ability for recovery, or the sparing of injury due to protraction of exposure is less in the lens than in other organs.

The threshold dose of X-rays for induction of minimally detectable lens opacities is estimated as 2 Gy in a single exposure and 5.5 Gy in a fractionated exposure over 3-13 weeks. The lowest dose to cause a progressive cataract is thought to be 5 Gy, which might be extrapolated to a threshold of 8 Gy necessary to produce such a lesion under the conditions of occupational exposure.

These threshold values are summarized in Table 5 in comparison with the recommended dose limits for the lens. It is seen that for irradiation of the eye alone, at the maximum recommended limit of 0.15 Sv/year, it is unlikely that any impairment of vision would result, but the threshold for opacities which are detectable ophthalmologically might be reached.

Nervous System   It has long been known that relatively small doses to the brain can cause transitory electrophysiological responses (14). Larger doses are required to result in morphological lesions and functional impairment.

Irradiation of the spinal cord primarily results in demyelination and delayed necrosis in the white matter and damage to the fine vasculature. It characertistically takes 6 months to two years to develop. The symptoms include numbness, tingling, anaesthesia, paraesthesia, weakness and paralysis. The threshold for such damage is in the region of 10 Gy in a single acute exposure of 40 Gy in conventional radiotherapy.

Both the spinal cord and brain show considerable capacity for repair of sublethal damage, i.e., a large reduction in effectiveness per Gy as the dose per fraction is decreased, and a small degree of repair by repopulation.

Table 6. Estimated radiotherapy threshold doses for certain non-stochastic effects of radiation on tissues of thge human eye

Tissue	Effect	Single Dose	Fractionated
Lid skin	Early erythema	4-6	6 x days$^{0.33}$
Lachrymal gland	Atrophy	20	50-60 (6 weeks)
Conjunctiva	Late telangiectasia		30-50 (3-5 weeks)
Cornea	Early oedema and keratitis	10	30-50
Sclera	Late atrophy		200-300
Retina	Early oedema		30-35
	Late degeneration		30-50
Lens	Cataract	2-10	4 x days$^{0.17}$

(from Merriam, et al. (15)).

Damage to the brain, i.e., white matter necrosis and vascular injury has a high threshold, in the order of 55 Gy in conventional radiotherapy. However, single acute doses of 1-6 Gy have been shown to produce morphological and physiological changes in children (Ron et al. 1982).

Peripheral nerves normally require 60 Gy or more before damage is expressed.

Thus, the recommended dose limits are sufficient to ensure that no detrimental effects occur in the central nervous system.

Testis   The germ cells of the testis are by far the most sensitive in the male reproductive system and their death results in imparied fertility, the degree of which is dose dependent. The most sensitive period of sperm development is during the early stage of development of spermatogonia. After irradiation the sperm count will start to decline as the more mature germ cells are eliminated from the reproductive tract, which takes several weeks. Fertility will be restored if enough "stem" cells survive to repopulate the seminiferous tubules, although this may take several years. After a dose of 3-5 Gy few stem cells will survive so that sterility may be effectively permanent. The threshold single acute dose for impaired fertility is in the order of 0.15 Gy because of the high sensitivity at the one particular stage of sperm development (Table 7).

Table 7. Radiotherapy threshold doses to the testes reported to cause temporary or permanent sterility in some men.

	Dose (Gy)[b]	Ref.
Temporary Sterility	0.15-3 (single)	Heller, 1967
		Hahn, et al., 1976
	2.5 (single)	Glucksmann, 1947
	4 (single)	Oakes and Lushbaugh, 1952
	0.1-1 (fractionated)	Sandeman, 1966
	1-2 (fractionated)	Speiser, et al., 1973
Permanent Sterility	0.5 (single)	Hahn, et al., 1976
	6 (single)	Heller and Rowley (Personal Communication)
	5-6 (single)	Glucksmann, 1947
	4.5-6 (fractionated)	Lushbaugh and Ricks, 1972
	2-3 (fractionated)	Sandeman, 1966

[b] Therapeutic irradiation received in a single brief exposure or in multiple exposures fractionated over a period of days.

From UNSCEAR, 1982 (12).

It is important to note that the threshold dose for sterility is relatively independent of dose rate of fractionation. From data derived from man and dogs it is is inferred that the threshold for impairment of fertility is approximately 0.4 Sv per year of occupational exposure. This is compared with the recommended dose limit of 0.05 Sv/year for whole body irradiation or 0.2 Sv/year for irradiation of the testes alone (which is most unlikely to occur) (Table 5). However, it is theoretically possible that the limits allow sufficient exposure in a single acute dose to both testes alone to give rise to a temporary sterility.

Ovary   The oocyte is at its most radiosensitive when mature. The threshold for permanent sterility decreases with age, which must be partly due to the age dependent natural depletion of oocytes, since the ovary contains no proliferating oogonial stem cell pool. From the data given in Table 8, the threshold dose in a single acute exposure is in the region of 1 Gy for temporary impairment of fertility and 2.5 Gy for permanent sterility. There is a considerable sparing effect of fractionation or protraction so that the threshold for permanent sterility is considered to be in the order of 6 Gy for a protracted exposure. Table 5 compares these values with the recommended dose limits. Since the ovaries are unlikely to be irradiated selectively, the whole body stochastic limit of 0.05 Sv per year is applicable. Only if the ovaries were selectively irradiated at the recommended maximum level continuously for 30 years could the threshold for sterility theoretically be reached.

Urinary Tract   The kidney appears to be more sensitive than the bladder which is more sensitive than the ureters. Clinical signs and symptoms of radiation nephropathy may occur months or years after fractionated radiotherapy with total doses exceeding approximately 20 Gy, including polyuria, sodium wasting, proteinuria, azotaemia, and anaemia with some patients developing arterial hypertension. Progressive renal ischaemia occurs resulting from damage to glomerular arterioles and/or interstitial capillaries, but some investigators view tubular depopulation as the primary event. In advanced cases, the affected kidneys are characterized microscopically by hyalinized glomeruli, atrophic tubules, interstitial fibrosis and arteriosclerosis. In line with other late responding normal organs, the degree of interfraction sparing of radiation damage to the kidney is greater than in early responding tissues although repopulation is

Effect	Tolerance Dose (Gy)[b]		Ref.
Temporary Sterility	1.7	(single)	Glucksmann, 1947
or	4	(single)	Paterson, 1963
Reduced Fertility	0.65	(single)	Hahn, et al., 1982
	1.5	(fractionated)[c]	Thomas, et al., 1976
	12	(fractionated)	Ray, 1970
		(3/day)	Paterson, 1963
	17.4	(in 3 series/ 2.5 years)	Gans, et al., 1963
Permanent Sterility	3.2	(single)	Glucksmann, 1947
	4	(single)	Paterson, 1963
	6.25	(single)	Peck, et al., 1940)
	8-10	(single)	Lacassagne, et al., 1940
	2.5-5	(fractionated)	Ray, 1970
	6.25-12	(fractionated) (30F/6 weeks)	Rubin and Casarett, 1972
	6-20	(fractionated) (30F/6 weeks)	Lushbaugh and Ricks, 1972
	3.6-7.2	(fractionated) (2-4F)	Doll and Smith, 1968
	2	(in 3 series/2 years)	Jacox, 1939

[b] Therapeutic irradiation received in a single brief exposure or in multiple exposures fractionated over a period of days.

[c] No effect in women aged < 40 years

From UNSCEAR, 1982 (12).

probably limited. Hence, at the recommended dose limits no non-stochastic renal or other urinary tract damage is likely to occur, the safety margin being moderate.

Respiratory System   Irradiation of the lungs results in pneumonitis followed by pulmonary fibrosis. The pneumonitic phase occurs within 2-6 months and is thought to result from damage to type II penumoncytes which are the cells responsible for production of alveolar surfactant. It is less clear which cells are primarily responsible for the later fibrosis, the pneumonocytes or capillary endothelial cells being the most likely targets.

The threshold dose for pneumonitis and fibrosis in fractionated radiotherapy is 20-30 Gy, but the capacity to repair both sublethal damage and the existence of a slow repair mechanism in lung is considerable, so that the threshold for occupational exposure will be much greater. This is compared with the recommended limit for selective irradiation of the lung of 0.4 Sv per year, i.e., 20 Sv over 50 years. The tissues of the upper respiratory tract appear to be less sensitive than lung.

Musculoskeletal System   Mature bone and muscle are relatively resistant to irradiation. However, in the proliferative state, as in children or during healing, these tissues are far more sensitive. For example, 1 Gy in children may result in retardation of growth, depending on age at exposure.

Nevertheless, occupational exposure (irrelevant for children) at the maximum recommended limits is extremely unlikely to exceed the threshold to cause non-stochastic injury to muscle or bone.

Endocrine System   Effective irradiation of the thyroid is rather age dependent. Hypothyroidism and retardation of growth has resulted from exposure of young children to radioactive fall out. Older children have experiences overt hypothyroidism or subclinical evidence of a reduction in thyroid reserve, i.e., increased levels of thyroid stimulating hormone (TSH) or increased TSH response to thyrotropic-releasing hormone. In adults excess fractionated irradiation may result in myxoedema. The threshold for functional change in the adult thyroid, when totally irradiated in conventional radiotherapy, is in the region of 25 Gy which is similar to the non-stochastic limit for 50 years occupational exposure selectively to the thyroid. The adult adrenal and pituitary glands are more resistant.

The childhood female breast is particularly sensitive. Doses of 10 Gy in fractionated radiotherapy given before adolescence may impair normal development. Hence, the endocrine organs are not expected to suffer detrimental non-stochastic effects for occupational exposure below the recommended dose limits.

SUMMARY AND CONCLUSIONS

In 1977 the ICRP recommended that the aim in radiation protection should be to avoid totally any detrimental non-stochastic effects. Few non-stochastic effects are fatal and hence cannot be strictly compared either with cancer induction or a disabling genetic disorder. However, the dose effect curves for non-stochastic injury are relatively steep so that the difference in dose between the threshold for a detrimental effect and that to cause a severe injury is relatively small, justifying the ICRP recommendation.

Although there are many data on dose effect relationships for acutely responding tissues, quantitative data on late effects are relatively fragmentary. Much of our knowledge is based on radiotherapy experience so that the estimated thresholds are frequently derived by extrapolations from 20-35 exposures given in 4-7 weeks to the conditions of occupational exposure. For many slowly dividing tissues this will result in an increase in dose to reach the threshold by a factor of approximately 1.5-2, on account of repair of sublethal damage and an additional factor due to repopulation. The increase for rapidly dividing, early responding tissues will be less, i.e., only about 1.2 due to repair of sublethal damage, but there will be a very large factor resulting from repopulation.

Most radiotherapeutic observations are on elderly patients whose response may not be typical of the working population. However, for most tissues the threshold for a detrimental effect is likely to be well above the 25 Sv applicable to all tissues, so that the presently recommended dose limits provide a substantial margin of safety. For thyroid, liver and lung, the margin of safety is rather less and for lens of the eye, haemopoietic tissues and reproductive organs, it is possible to conceive theoretically of ways in which either the margin of safety is very small relative to the present recommended dose limits or even that the threshold for a non-stochastic effect may be exceeded. However, in reality, it is highly improbable that the threshold for any non-stochastic effect could be exceeded in any worker even if individual tissues received the annual dose limit continually, year after year.

For members of the public, the recommended dose equivalent limits are 10 times lower than for radiation workers and are, therefore, completely adequate to ensure the prevention of non-stochastic effects.

For members of the public, the recommended dose equivalent limits are 10 times lower than for radiation workers and are, therefore, completely adequate to ensure the prevention of non-stochastic effects.

The data on high LET radiation are fragmentary, but there is no evidence that the value of Q need be revised upwards to prevent non-stochastic effects.

REFERENCES

1. International Commission on Radiological Protection, in: "Recommendations of the International Commission on Radiological Protection," ICRP Publication 26, Annals of the ICRP, Vol. 1, No. 3, Pergamon Press, Oxford (1977).

2. International Commission on Radiological Protection, in: "Nonstochastic Effects of Ionizing Radiation: A Report of a Task Group of Committee 1 of the International Commission on Radiological Protection," ICRP Publication 41, Annals of the ICRP, in press.

3. E. V. Hulse and R. H. Mole, Reflections on the terms stochastic and non-stochastic, Br. J. Radiol. 55:321-324 (1982).

4. A. Michalowski, Effects of radiation on normal tissues: hypothetical mechanisms and limitations of in situ assay of clonogenicity, Radiat. Environ. Biophys. 19:157-172 (1981).

5. T. E. Wheldon, A. S. Michalowski, and J. Kirk, The effect of irradiation on function in self-renewing normal tissues with differing proliferative organization, Br. J. Radiol. 55:759-766 (1982).

6. E. J. Hall, "Radiobiology for the Radiologist, 2nd Edition," Harper and Row, New York, New York (1978).

7. F. Ellis, The relationship of biological effects to dose-time fractionation factors in radiotherapy, in: "Current Topics in Radiation Research, Vol. IV" (Ebert and Howard, eds.) 1968, pp. 357-397.

8. H. D. Thames, H. R. Withers, L. J. Peters, and G. H. Fletcher, Changes in early and late radiation responses with altered dose fractionation: Implications for dose-survival relationships, Int. J. Rad. Oncol. Biol. Phys. 8:219-226 (1982).

9. J. F. Fowler, Review: Total doses in fractionated radiotherapy - implications of new radiobiological data, Int. J. Radiat. Biol. 40:103-120 (1984).

10. G. W. Barendsen, Dose fractionation, dose rate, and iso-effect relationships for normal tissue responses, Int. J. Radiat. Oncol. Biol. Phys. 8:1982-1998 (1982).

11. J. F. Fowler, Fractionation and therapeutic gain, in: "The Biological Basis of Radiotherapy" (Steel, Adams, and Peckham, eds.) Elsevier (1983), pp. 181-194.

12. United Nations, "Ionizing Radiation: Sources and Biological Effects," United Nations Scientific Committee on the Effects of Atomic Radiation, Report to the General Assembly with Annexes, United Nations, New York, New York (1982).

13. P. Rubin and G. W. Casarett, "Clinical Radiation Pathology, Vol. 1 and 2," W. B. Saunders, Philadelphia, PA (1968).

14. United Nations, "Report of the United Nations Scientific Committee on the Effects of Atomic Radiation," General Assembly Official Records, 24th Session, Supplement No. 13 (A/7613), United Nations, New York, New York (1969).

15. G. R. Merriam, A. Schechter, and E. F. Focht, The effects of ionizing radiation on the eye, Front. Radiat. Ther. Oncol. 6:346-385 (1972).

CARCINOGENIC POTENTIAL OF INCINERATED LOW-LEVEL RADIOACTIVE WASTE:

CYTOPATHOLOGIC EVALUATION

I. V. Brown and J. M. Browne

Department of Biology
Cytopathology and Cell Biology Laboratories
Atlanta University
Atlanta, Georgia 30314

ABSTRACT

Fundulus sp., a ubiquitous estuarine fish, was used in cytopathologic
evaluations of the carcinogenic potential of incinerated ash from low-level
radioactive waste, currently, disposed in the marine environment. We
correlated the increased biosynthesis of Epoxide Hydrolase of liver
microsomes with ultrastructural changes in livers of Fundulus sp.,
following exposure to non-radioactive and radioactive ash (7 ppm,
radioisotope = S^{35}, specific activity: 1410 Ci/mmol/kg ash). Fish were
exposed to incinerated ash suspended in filtered artificial sea water in
closed aerated/temperaturecontrolled marine tank systems. Macroscopic
observation of animals exposed to radioactive ash revealed enlargement of
the belly at the level of or just behind the pectoral fins. Livers from
these animals had a yellowish brown appearance and were enlarged.
Microscopic examination of some liver specimens revealed diffuse
hyperplasia, hypertrophy, and fatty degeneration of hepatocytes.
Ultrastructurally, there was an increased number of residual bodies
containing undigested lipid, a proliferation of both rough and smooth
endoplasmic reticula, and dilation of endoplasmic reticulum vesicles. The
endomembrane changes correlated with observed epoxide hydrolase induction
above control levels. The data obtained in these studies will be used to
ascertain the safety and efficiency of incinerated low-level radioactive
waste disposal in the marine environment.

INTRODUCTION

The marine environment is, currently, the receptacle for the disposal
of, putatively, nonhazardous refuse such as incinerated ash from low-level
radioactive waste. However, the possible carcinogenic potential of this
practice has not been evaluated.

Polycyclic aromatic hydrocarbons and other carcinogens are capable of
inducing the liver microsomal enzyme, epoxide hydrolase, which is associated
with detoxification/toxification efforts in mammals and fish (1, 2).
Morphologic changes in liver cells following exposure to these xenobiotics

have, also, been reported (3-5). The early carcinogen-induced changes included proliferation and dilation of the endoplasmic reticulum, fatty degeneration, hyperplasia, loss of glycogen, pigment deposition and necrosis (4-5).

Fish have been shown to have a high sensitivity to carcinogens (4). Further, _Fundulus_ sp., a fish which traverses both fresh, estuarine and marine waters, is an excellent model for assessing the carcinogenic potential of incinerated ash from radioactive waste disposed in the marine environment.

In these initial studies we correlated two early assay points, the increased biosynthesis of epoxide hydrolase of liver microsomes previously reported by Browne and Jideama, 1984 (6) with morphologic changes in livers of _Fundulus_ _grandis_, following exposure to non-radioactive and radioactive ash in long-term studies involving biochemical and cytopathologic evaluations of the carcinogenic potential of incinerated ash from low-level radioactive waste.

MATERIALS AND METHODS

Fish

Adult male _Fundulus_ _grandis_ were obtained from Gulf Specimen Co., Panacea, Florida and kept in closed aerated/temperaturecontrolled marine tank systems containing filtered artificial sea water.

Ash Exposure

Fish were exposed for 18-24 hours to non-radioactive and radioactive ash (7 ppm, radioisotope - S^{35}, specific activity: 1410 Ci/mmol/kg ash) suspended in the sea water.

Light and Electron Microscopy

The animals were killed by immersion in the fixative, 3% glutaraldehyde in 0.2 M sodium cacodylate buffer (pH 7.4 at 4°C). Livers were excised, minced and fixed in the glutaraldehyde fixative overnight. The specimens were post-fixed in 2% osmium tetroxide, dehydrated through graded ethanols, rinsed in two changes of propylene oxide, and embedded in Poly/Bed 812 (Poly-Sciences, Inc., Warrington, PA). One micron sections, stained with toluidine blue, were examined with a light microscope. Selected areas were then sectioned with an LKB Ultratome, stained with lead citrate, and examined with an RCA EMU-4A transmission electron microscope. At least three specimens from different regions of each liver were examined.

RESULTS

Summarily, in early cytopathologic evaluations, we found: (1) endomembrane changes which correlated with the observed epoxide hydrolase induction (6); and (2) exacerbated liver changes in specimens exposed to radioactive ash which included some diffuse hyperplasia, hypertrophy, fatty degeneration, and an increased number of residual bodies containing partially digested lipid.

Macroscopic observation of fish exposed to radioactive ash revealed enlargement of the belly at the level of or just behind the pectoral fins. Livers from these animals had a yellowish brown appearance and were

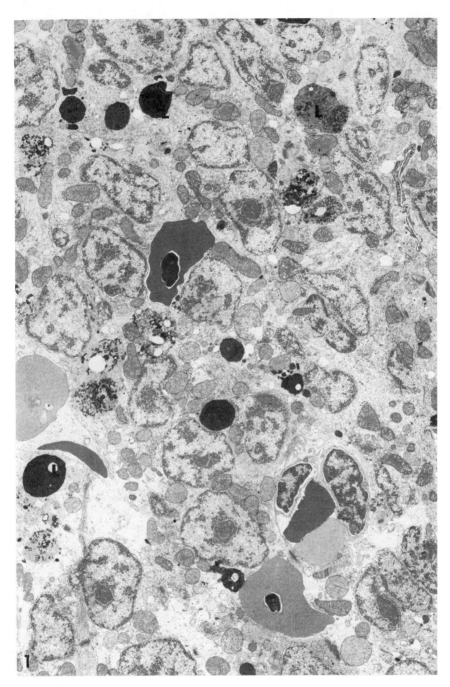

Fig. 1.   Non-radioactive ash exposed liver. Cells show moderate
          cytoplasm, normal nuclei and mitochondria, as well as,
          regular continuity. Large residual bodies (L)
          containing undigested lipids are seen in some cells.
          Note the intact nucleated red blood cells.
          Glutaraldehyde and OsO_4. Lead citrate. X 4,500.

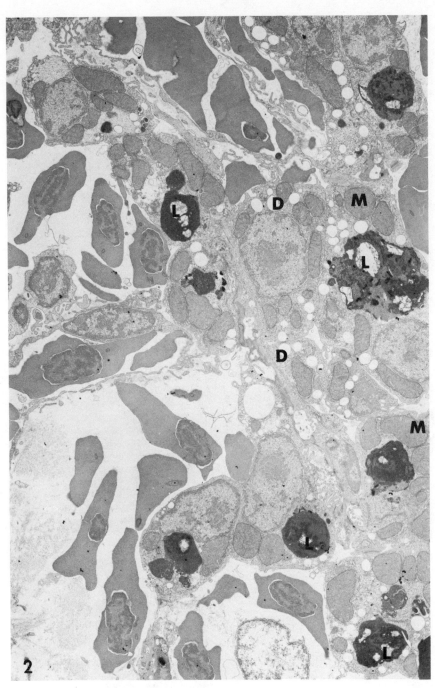

Fig. 2.   Radioactive ash exposed liver. Almost all cells
          contain enlarged   residual bodies (L) and mitochondria
          (M). Accumulation of non- membranebound lipid droplets
          (D) is seen. (Much of the lipid was lost during
          preparation for electron microscopy.) Note the
          intercellular edema and absence of obvious nuclear
          changes. Blood sinuses contain intact nucleated red
          blood cells. Glutaraldehdye and O_sO_4. Lead citrate.
          X 4,500.

enlarged. Microscopic examination of some liver specimens revealed some diffuse hyperplasia, hypertrophy, and fatty degeneration of hepatocytes. These changes were confirmed, ultrastructurally.

Ultrastructurally, liver specimens from fish exposed to non-radioactive ash revealed cells with moderate cytoplasm, normal nuclei and mitochondria, regular continuity and intact nucleated red blood cells

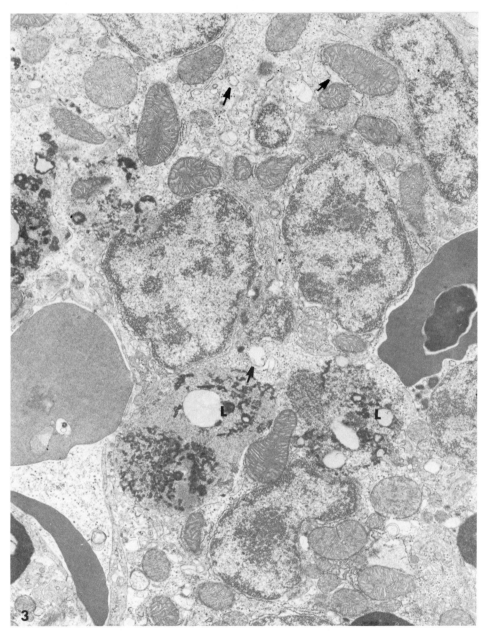

Fig. 3. Non-radioactive ash exposed liver. The cells are unremarkable in appearance with the exception of residual bodies of multidensities (L) and dilation of endoplasmic reticula (smooth and rough) (arrows). Glutaraldehyde and O_sO_4. Lead citrate. X 13,200.

(Figure 1). Large residual bodies were found in some liver cells (Figure 1). This change may be correlated with the presence of xenobiotics,

benzo(a)pyrene and dimethylbenz(a)-anthracene, found in incinerated ash (both non-radioactive and radioactive (7). Alternately, it could reflect stress or a cellular response to injury. However, almost all of the cells in liver specimens from fish exposed to radioactive ash contained residual bodies (Figure 2). In addition, these cells showed an accumulation of non-membranebound lipid droplets, intercellular edema, and enlarged mitochondria. There were no obvious nuclear changes.

Higher magnification of non-radioactive ash exposed specimens showed that the cells were unremarkable in appearance with the exceptions of residual bodies of multidensities and dilation of the endoplasmic reticula (smooth and rough) (Figure 3).

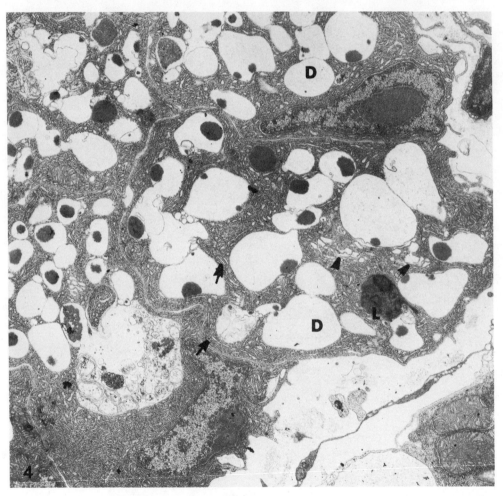

Fig. 4.   Radioactive ash exposed liver. The cells show an exacerbation of the changes seen in non-radioactive ash exposed specimens. Note the dense residual bodies (L) and accumulation of lipid droplets (D). Proliferation of smooth rough (arrowheads) and (arrows) endoplasmic reticula is conspicuous. Glutaraldehyde and O_sO_4. Lead citrate. X 6,000.

Higher magnifications of radioactive ash exposed specimens showed an exacerbation of these changes (Figures 4 and 5). Proliferation of both rough and smooth endoplasmic reticula, as well as, dilation of endoplasmic reticulum vesicles were conspicuous (Figure 5).

DISCUSSION

The results obtained in these initial studies do not demonstrate an obvious carcinogenic potential of incinerated ash from low-level radioactive waste. We have, however, shown an early morphologic response to radioactive ash in excess of that seen to non-radioactive ash (containing the xenobiotics benzo(a)pyrene and dimethylbenz(a)anthracene only). To our knowledge, there is no literature on liver changes in fish exposed to radioactive ash. Some of the observed early liver changes are consistent with those reported for this tissue following exposure to polycyclic aromatic hydrocarbons and other carcinogens (4-5). Since it has

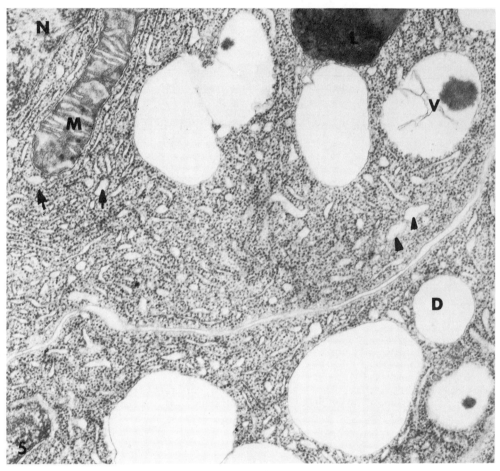

Fig. 5.   Radioactive ash exposed liver. A higher magnification of Figure 4 shows dilation of endoplasmic reticulum vesicles (smooth = arrowheads; rough = arrows; mitochondria = M; residual body = L; lipid droplets = (D); nucleus = N). Some membrane-bound vacuoles (V), with and without, their containing dense material are seen. G lutoaraldehyde and O_sO_4. Lead citrate. X 28,800.

been shown that hepatocarcinogenesis develops in fish as in mammals gradually through various stages (4, 8) time course studies may yield information on the possible progression of carcinogenesis in _Fundulus grandis_ following exposure to radioactive ash. Morphological and biochemical studies of liver specimens from the ubiquitous estaurine fish, _Fundulus_ sp., may be useful in assessing the carcinogenic potential of incinerated ash from radioactive waste disposed in the marine environment.

ACKNOWLEDGEMENT

This study was supported by grants from the Department of Energy (Grant: R10-001) and the National Science Foundation (RIMI Grant: RII 8405927), Washington, D. C., USA.

REFERENCES

1. J. Seidegard and J. W. DePierre, Microsomal epoxide hydrolase propertiesregulation and function, _Biochimica et Biophysica Acta_ 695:251 (1983).

2. M. J. Griffin, and N. Ganqozian, Epoxide hydrolase: A marker for experimental hepatocarcinogenesis, _Ann. Clin. Lab. Sci._ 14:27 (1984).

3. E. A. Smucker and M. Arcasoy, Structural and functional changes of the endoplasmic reticulum of hepatic parenchymal cells, _Rev. Exper. Path._ 1:305 (1969).

4. G. B. Pliss and V. V. Khudoley, Tumor induction by carcinogenic agents in aquarium fish, _JNCI_ 55:129 (1975).

5. W. P. Schoor and J. A. Couch, Correlation of mixed function oxidase activity with ultrastructural changes in the liver of a marine fish, _Cancer Biochem. Biophys._ 4:95 (1979).

6. J. M. Browne and N. Jideama, Carcinogenic potential of incinerated low-level radioactive waste: Electrophoretic resolution. (Paper presented at the NATO Advanced Study Institute on "Radiation Carcinogenesis and DNA Alterations," Corfu, Greece, October, 1984.)

7. J. M. Browne, _in:_ "DOE/AMF-R10-002 Interim Report: Test system for detecting mutagenic and/or carcinogenic potential in low-level radio-waste," (1981), pp. 1-17.

8. S. R. Wellings, Neoplasia and primitive vertebrates phylogeny, Echinoderms, prevertebrates and fishes, _Natl. Cancer Inst. Monogr._ 31:59 (1969).

CARCINOGENIC POTENTIAL OF INCINERATED LOW-LEVEL RADIOACTIVE WASTE:

ELECTROPHORETIC RESOLUTION

J. M. Browne and N. Jideama

Cell Biology Laboratory
Biology Department
Atlanta University
Atlanta, Georgia 30314

ABSTRACT

The presumed causal connection between the presence of radiowastes and carcinogenic potential are currently speculative. Xenbiotics are extended to include those accumulated in laboratory wastes from experimentation involving the use of radioisotopes. The presence of heightened biosynthesis of putative detoxifying enzymes (mixed-function oxidases and Epoxide Hydrolase) in the liver of vertebrates exposed to xenobiotics suggests a toxic and possible carcinogenic risk environment. We have exploited such an environment, (incinerated low-level radioactive waste), to assay for biochemical indicators of potential cancer risks. In the aquatic environment the estuarine fish, Fundulus sp. has been subjected to 7 ppm incinerated radiowaste ash (specific activity = 1410 Ci/mmol/kg ash). Microsomal fractions from fish liver were isolated and Epoxide Hydrolase(s) purified and resolved in SDS-Polyacrylaminde slab gels. An induced three-fold increase in epoxide hydrolase was observed in fish exposed to both incinerated non-radioactive and radioactive ash. The presence of these enzymes indicate a carcinogenic risk in aquatic and land animals exposed to incinerated ash, however, whether the potential is increased by the presence of radiowaste as a source of ash was not resolved.

INTRODUCTION

Epoxide hydrolase (EC3.3.2.3), a detoxifier of a variety of epoxides has been detected in a number of animal species (1, 5, 7, 8, 10, 11). Evidence of the existence of multiple forms of this enzyme in some animals has been stated most basically on their substrate specificities (4) and the slight differences in their C-terminal amino-acid sequences (6). We are now reporting experimental results, visualized electrophoretically, of two microsomal forms of epoxide hydrolase from non-radioactive and radioactive incinerated ash from laboratory waste. The molecular weights of these two forms were also determined.

MATERIALS AND METHODS

Induction of Epoxide Hydrolase

Two plexiglass marine aquaria, each containing 12.0 gallons of artificial sea water and six fish (Gulf Specimen Company, Inc., Panacea, Florida) were allowed to equilibrate overnight. In one of the aquaria, 120.0 grams of ash obtained from incinerated radioactive laboratory waste (radioactive paper filter discs and laboratory bench coverings), 7 ppm (specific activity = 1410 Ci/mmol/kg ash) were added and the fish exposed for 18 hours. Control fish were housed in marine tanks containing 7 ppm ash from non-radioactive waste in aerated, filtered artificial sea water.

Purification of Epoxide Hydrolase

The liver from exposed fish and controls was harvested and homogenized in 0.25 M sucrose TKM (50 mM KCl, 50 mM triethanolamine, 5 mM $MgCl_2$) buffer. The homogenate was centrifuged at 6,000 and 10,000 rpms for five and ten minutes, respectively. The acquired post mitochondrial supernatant was further centrifuged for 1 hour at 40,000 rpm.

The microsomal pellets were solubilized in 5.0 mM K_2PO_4 containing 0.05% lubrol at pH 7.4. The solubilized microsomes were dialyzed overnight in 4 liters of the same buffer. Dialyzed fractions were passed through previously equilibrated DE52 cellulose columns and eluted with 5 mM K_2PO_4 buffer at pH 7.4, Oesch, et al. (7). The eluates were washed overnight with the same buffer but at pH 6.5 and passed through CM52 cellulose columns previously equilibrated with the same buffer. The purified epoxide hydrolase was quantitated using the Bio-Rad protein assay methods (2).

Epoxide Hydrolase Activity

Enzyme activity was determined, spectrophotometrically, by assaying for the concentration of the excess, unconverted substrate. The incubation mixture, composed of 28 1 0.03 mM styrene oxide as the substrate, buffered by 1.0 ml 0.5M Tris at pH 9.0, 0.1% lubrol ad 3 ml distilled water interacted with 0.02 ml of epoxide hydrolase solution. The incubation period was 5 minutes at room temperature (20°C). The action of the enzyme was stopped by adding 4 ml of petroleum ether and shaking gently.

Extraction of the excess styrene oxide from the incubation mixture was by the method of Oesch and Daly (9). The optical densities of the extracted styrene oxide were read at 245 nm using a Gilford Spectrophotometer model 249.

SDS Polyacrylamide Gel Electrophoresis

The purified epoxide hydrolase from hepatic cells of Fundulus grandis was alkylated and loaded onto a 10% SDS polyacrylamide gel and electrophoresed for 17 hours at 15 mA using an ISCO power source.

RESULTS

Incinerated (both radioactive and non-radioactive) ash are efficient inducers of increased epoxide hydrolase synthesis in Fundulus grandis (Table 1). In the three separate experiments shown, the induction of epoxide hydrolase is approximately three fold. The enzyme assay has shown that the purified epoxide hydrolase catalyzed the hydration of styrene oxide (Table 2). Our electrophoretic profiles shows two protein bands

Table 1. Concentration of epoxide hydrolase per gram weight of fish liver in mg

EXPERIMENT	CONTROL	NON-RADIOWASTE ASH-TREATED	RADIOWASTE ASH TREATED
1	3.20	11.08	10.84
2	3.47	11.43	11.49
3	3.64	12.52	13.07

Table 2. Recovered styrene oxide from epoxide hydrolase enzyme assay mixture*

EXPERIMENT	OD_{254} CONTROL (ENZYME ABSENT)	OD_{254} UNTREATED**	OD_{254}ASH-TREATED*	OD_{254} - RADIO-ASH-TREATED*
1	0.0200	-----	0.0040	0.0042
2	0.0190	0.0046	0.0028	0.0030
3	0.0187	0.0045	0.0036	0.0033
4	0.0210	0.0035	0.0025	0.0028

----NOT DETERMINED
*PURIFIED FROM LIVER MICROSOMES
**RESULTING FROM STYRENE OXIDE ADDITION TO ASSAY MEDIUM CONTAINING MICROSOMES FROM ANIMALS WHICH WERE NOT PRETREATED.

indicating that there are two forms of the purified microsomal enzymes (Figure 1).

DISCUSSION

This study has revealed that there are, putatively, two microsomal forms of fish liver microsomal epoxide hydrolase induced to increased levels by both non-radioactive and radioactive incinerated laboratory waste. Our results raise the question as to whether inclusive radioisotopes at the concentration used have any causal role in observed increases in epoxide hydrolase biosynthesis. Our postulation in addressing this question is that the incinerated ash in both instances used in this investigation contained among other compounds, benzo(a)pyrene and dimethylbenzanthracene (13, 14), well known polycyclic aromatic hydrocarbons, generally characterized as xenobiotics. It is, therefore, probable that each xenobiotic found in the processed ash is capable of inducing increased synthesis of substrate specific forms of epoxide hydrolase.

The rationale for this postulation is that each epoxide resulting from xenobiotic conversion pathways has a different structural configuration. This, putatively, allows for a specific epoxide hydrolase requirement. It is not, therefore, surprising when previous investigations have reported that epoxide hydrolase is substrate specific.

In conclusion, we have determined that the liver microsomes of one vertebrate the estuarine fish, _Fundulus grandis_ contains multiple forms of epoxide hydrolase. The biochemical assay and electrophoretic resolution of

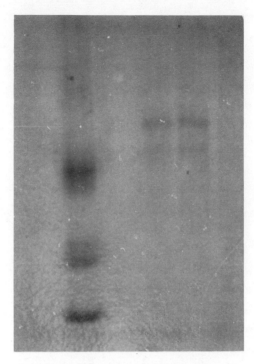

Fig. 1. The electrophoretic resolution of microsomal
forms of epoxide hydrolase isolated from non-
radioactive incinerated laboratory waste.

this enzyme from induced increased biosynthesis in both radioactive and
non-radioactive ash show summarily that the presence of radioactive
isotopes, at least 35-sulfur, does not resolve any differences in forms
utilized in converting produced epoxides.

ACKNOWLEDGEMENTS

We thank Mrs. Joyce Lockhart for her excellent proofing and typing of
this manuscript. This reported work was partially supported by DOE-AMAF
Contract No. R10-002 and NSF Grant No. RII-8405927.

REFERENCES

1. S. K. Bhat and G. Padmanaban, Biochem. Biophys. Res. Commun. 84:1-6
   (1978).

2. "Bio-Rad Protein Assay Methodology Bulletin," (1979), pp. 1-17.

3. E. M. Gozukara, Molec. Pharmacol. 19:152-161 (1980).

4. T. Guenthner and F. Oesch, in: "Polycyclic Hydrocarbons and Cancer,
   Vol. 3," Academic Press, New York (1981), pp. 183-212.

5. D. M. Jerina, J. W. Daly, and B. Witkop, Arch. Biochem. Biophys.
   128:176-183 (1968).

6. J. Siedegard and J. DePierre, <u>Biochim. Biophys. Acta</u> 695:251-270 (1983).

7. R. G. Knowles and B. Brain, <u>Biochem. J.</u> 163:181-183 (1977).

8. D. W. Nebert and H. V. Gelboin, <u>J. Biol. Chem.</u> 243:6242-6249 (1968).

9. F. Oesch, D. M. Jerina, and J. Daly, <u>Biochim. Biophys. Acta</u> 227:685-691 (1971).

10. K. Pyykko, <u>Acta Pharmacol. Toxicol.</u> 52:39-46 (1983).

11. S. G. Sarject, <u>Biochem. Biophys, Res. Commun.</u> 112:763-769 (1983).

12. J. Seidegard, <u>Biochem. Biophys. Res. Commun.</u> 112:763-769 (1978).

13. J. S. Smith, <u>Science</u> 211:180-183 (1981).

14. J. Stegman, <u>in</u>: "Polycyclic Hydrocarbons and Cancer, Vol. 3," Academic Press, New York (1981), pp. 1-59.

X-RAYS LOW DOSE RELATIONSHIPS WITHIN THE G_2 PHASE OF CHINESE HAMSTER CELLS

Geza Mindek

Radiobiological Institute of the University of Zurich
August Forel-Str. 7
8029 Zurich
Switzerland

SUMMARY

Heterogeneous chromosomal radiosensitivity was found in the G_2 phase of a newly established cell line (line 19/1) of Chinese hamster (Cricetulus griseus, 2 n = 22) during the first five-hour testing period after 100 cGy x-irradiation. Metaphases showed maximal aberration frequencies when they were fixed in the first or fourth hour after irradiation. Dose effect correlations for the first hour colchicine collection time show between 5-100 cGy irradiations significantly more aberrations than non-irradiated control cells within the lowest radiation dose of 5 cGy too.

INTRODUCTION

The most sensitive stage of the cell cycle for radiation induced visible structural changes in chromosomes of mammalian cells is in the G_2 phase (3, 15). The general use of this phase for the study of dose effect correlations is doubtful because of its heterogenous radiation sensitivity (14) and the lack of stage specific markers. On the other hand, it is well known that a partial synchronization can be induced by irradiation with low doses up to 4.5 rad X-rays (13). Cells which remain in G_2 phase 45-60 minutes before metaphase at the time of irradiation, will be blocked depending on the dose. Cells which are between this "G_2 blockade" (7) and metaphase continue their cycle irrespective of irradiation towards metaphase.

If a mitotic collection will begin immediately after irradiation, only such cells, including those in prophase, will reach methaphase first which are between G_2 blockade and mitosis. But, if the collection begins later after prophase reach ana- or telophase (5), only G_2 cells from a very narrow and distinct part of this phase will be collected during a short colchicine treatment period.

The objective of the present study is to try to use this part of the G_2 phase as a test system for dose effect correlations in low dose ranges of x-irradiation. It could be an useful experimental contribution in regard to the increasing interest on the biological effects of low dose irradiations (1).

MATERIALS AND METHODS

Cell Culture

In order to work with a simple and unchanged karyotype, we made use of a newly established cell line from Chinese hamster. This line was developed from a 16-19 day old female embryo. An ordinary cell suspension resulted after trypsinization of back and flank skin which multiplied quickly in early passages a a fibroblast-like monolayer (line 19/1). A part of this was preserved in liquid nitrogen as a reserve. Young passage numbers (22-75) were made use of for experiments. A slight aneuploidy was frequently evident in the form of trisomy in the chromosome groups 6-8 or 9-11. The cells were cultured in Pyrex Milk Dilution bottles (corning) at 37°C with a 5% CO_2 atmosphere in a medium consisting of Basal Medium Eagle (BME, Gibco G-13), 16% fetal calf serum (Microbiological Assoc. 14-414), Na-Bicarbonate, Phenol red and antibiotic-antimycotic mixture (Gibco 5214). The cultures were subcultivated (Difco, TC-Bacto Trypsin) 2-3 times weekly. Cells were preserved in liquid nitrogen in a 1:9 DMSO:Medium mixture.

Radioactive Labelling and Autoradiography

Thymidine (methyl-^{3}H-thymidine, spec. act. 6.7 Ci/mM, NEN NET-027) with a final concentration of 0.5 µCi/ml medium was applied in order to label the S phase. The 20 minute pulse labelling tie ended immediately prior to irradiation. After pulse labelling the cells were washed twice in PBS (Phosphate Buffer Solution, Gibco 420) at 37°C. They were dyed with

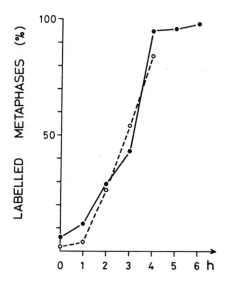

Fig. 1.   Percentage of labelled metaphases as a function of the incubation time (h) after 20 minutes pulse labelling with 0.5 Ci/mi ^{3}HTdR.Cell line 19/1 on 2nd day after trypsinisation.   o,●: two independent experiments.

Orcein and exposed for 7 days following routine autoradiography procedures
(11).

Irradiation Procedures

A Picker X-ray apparatus (200 kV, 12 mA, 1 mm A1 + 0.25 mm Cu,
HVL:0.70 mm Cu, 46 cGy/min) was used to irradiate the cells 24 hours after
trypsinization. Cells were irradiated in T 30 bottles (Falcon Plastics)
with 10 ml previously warmed PBS, and the irradiation was carried out at
room temperature. Dose measurements were done with a Victoreen chamber in
a plexiglas phantom under 6 mm water. For the 5 cGy experiment with short
exposure times a dose output of 23 cGy/min and 6 mA was used.

Preparation

The PBS in which the cells were irradiated was replaced shortly after
irradiation with a warmed mixture of medium and conditioned medium (CM),
from the same line, in a 1:1 ratio, in a 37°C walk-in room. Colchicine
(0.006 mg/ml final concentration) was added 30 minutes after irradiation.
Sixty minutes after irradiation a series of trypsinization, at a
predetermined intervals (between 0.0-5.0 hours), was started. The general
method of Moorhead et al. (1960) was used for the preparation of
metaphases. The hypotonic treatment was carried out with 0.17% NaCl at
room temperature for 20 minutes. Cells were then fixed twice in
methanol:acetic acid (3:1) 10 min. each and allowed to stand for a further
few hours, or overnight at 4°C in the second fixative. Cells were dropped
onto cold wet slides and dried over flame.

The Length of the G_2 Phase

The fraction of labelled mitoses (FLM method of Quastle and Sherman,
1959) was used to determine the average duration of the G_2 + 1/2 M
(mitosis). Cells cultured on Thermanox (Lux) sheets in Petri dishes
(Sterilin HP 3) were treated on the second day with ^{3}HTdR for 20 minutes
and fixed at hourly intervals. Five hundred metaphases per fixing time
were counted.

Determination of the Most Sensitive Section of the G_2 Phase

Two sampling regimes were used:

(1) Two days after trypsinization of the culture the cells were pulse
labelled, irradiated with 100 cGy, treated with colchicine and fixed after
0, 0.5, 1.0, 2.0, 2.5, 4.0, and 5.0 hours, respectively. The addition of
colchicine followed half an hour after irradiation. During this half hour,
the irradiated prophases and metaphases reached (5) and, therefore, were
not evaluated.

The increasing durations of colchicine treatments in the remaining
samples lead to progressive accumulation of G_2 cells covering a wide range
of cells in each successive sample.

(2) In two further samples, colchicine was added at either 0.5 h or
4.5 h following irradiation, and fixation of both was at 5.0 h. The 1/2 h
accumulation from 4.5-5.0 h contains predominately early G_2 cells.

Dose Effect Curve for the First Hour Sampling Time

Cells were pulse labelled with ^{3}HTdR as below on the second day after
trypsinization. After washing cells were irradiated in PBS at room
temperature with doses of 5,12, 15, 50 or 100 cGy. Cells were reincubated

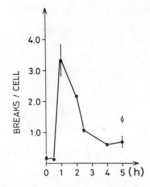

Fig. 2.   Frequency of breaks in the G_2 cells
           irradiated with 100 cGy as a function of
           incubation time in hours (h) after
           irradiation. a: aberrant metaphases
           (%), b: average number of breaks per
           cell ($S_x = s/ n$)√●: start of colchicine
           treatment 0.5 hour after irradiation,○:
           fixation immediately after irradiation,△:
           without colchicine (see Table 1).

within 5 minutes in a prewarmed mixture of EBM and conditioned medium
(1:1). Cells were fixed in the 60th minute following irradiation after
colchicine treatment during the last 30 min.

Evaluation of Metaphases

    Whenever possible, 100 unlabelled metaphases (20-24 centromeres) per
experiment were evaluated in order to determine the aberration frequency
(1000x magnification, WILD microscope). Single and isochromatid breaks,
acentric fragments, interchanges and dicentric chromosomes were taken into
consideration for the evaluation. We considered single chromatid breaks as
one break. With regard to the irradiated post synthetic stage, at least in
the case of radiation quality used, isochromatid breaks, acentri fragments
and exchanges were regarded as two breaks. Gaps were not counted as
breaks. Breaks and gaps were differentiated as by Schmid and Stiager (12);
break is defined as a complete discontinuity that is wider than the
diameter of the single chromatid. This criterion is presently used in
routine cytogenetic investigations on rodents as well as for humans (10).

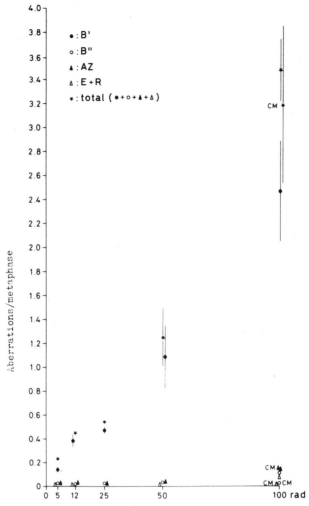

Fig. 3.   Dose effect curve for the G_2 phase of the cell
line 19/1. Ordinate: aberrations per metaphase,
abscissae: dose in cGy.Aberration types (average
values, see Table 1); ●: single chromatid breaks
(B'), ○: isochromatid breaks (E+R), ▲: acentric
fragments (AZ),△ : exchanges and rings (E+R), *:
total number of aberrations. Single chromatid
breaks were considered as one break and all other
types as two. Symbols with CM: irradiated in
conditioned medium.

RESULTS AND DISCUSSION

Heterogenous Sensitivity and Dose Effect Relationship

The average length of the G_2 + 1/2 M in the cell line 19/1 is 2.5-3.5
h (Figure 1) and the maximum depression of mitotic yield is 0.1% in the
first hour after 100 cGy irradiation (data not shown). The maximum
aberration yield was observed in the first hour after irradiation, i.e., in
the G_2 part before blockade with 3.4 breaks per cell. Higher doses induced
so many breaks that it was not possible to count them. The results

Table 1. Aberration frequency in the 5-100 cGy irradiated G_2 cells 1 h after irradiation. D: dose in cGy. N_1 number of evaluated metaphases. N_2: metaphases with aberrations (%). B': number of single chromatid breaks. i: number of isochromatid breaks. Azc : number of acentric fragments. E: number of exchanges. Dic: number of dicentric chromosomes. SR: number of sister reunions. R: number of ring chromosomes. Total: sum of aberrations. Br/C: number of breaks per cell. B' is considered as one break and all others as two breaks. S_X: average and distribution, using formula $S_X = s/n$ a: control. b: irradiated. *: labelled metaphases. *: irradiated in conditioned medium CM. The average values of 0 cGy and 5 cGy are different (t-test, p<2%). The average values of 100 cGy in PBS and 100 cGy in CM do not differ (t-test, p>20%).

D_0	N_1	N_2	B'	i	Az	E	Dic	SR	R	Total	Br/C	S_X a	S_X b
0	100	4	4	--	1	--	--	--	--	5	0.06		
5	92	18	19	--	3	--	--	--	--	22	0.27		
5	100	14	13	--	--	--	--	--	--	13	0.13		
5	100	21	19	3	1	--	--	--	--	23	0.27		
0	100	6	4	2	--	1	--	--	--	7	0.10	0.08±0.02	0.23±0.02
5	100	11	8	4	2	--	--	--	--	14	0.20		
5	100	15	10	4	4	--	--	--	--	18	0.26		
5	100	15	11	2	3	1	1	--	--	18	0.25		
0	100	7	2	2	4	--	--	--	--	8	0.14		
12	100	24	28	2	--	--	--	--	--	30	0.32		
0	100	6	2	--	3	1	--	--	--	6	0.10		
12	100	29	34	--	1	--	--	--	--	35	0.36		
0	100	8	5	--	4	--	--	--	--	9	0.13	0.11±0.02	0.45±0.08
12	100	31	32	--	5	--	--	--	--	37	0.42		
0	50	4	1	--	1	--	--	--	--	2	0.06		
12	100	43	56	--	5	1	--	--	--	62	0.68		
0	100	5	2	--	3	--	--	--	--	5	0.08		
25	100	33	47	--	3	--	--	--	--	50	0.53		
0	50	6	3	--	--	--	--	--	--	3	0.06	0.07±0.01	0.54±0.01
25	100	32	42	4	--	2	--	--	--	48	0.54		
25	99	30	46	1	3	--	--	--	--	50	0.55		

Table 1. Continued

D_0	N1	N2	B'	i	Az	E	Dic	SR	R	Total	Br/C	$S_{\bar{X}}$ a	$S_{\bar{X}}$ b
0	100	4	3	—	2	—	—	—	—	5	0.07		
50	100	51	150	—	4	1	—	—	—	155	1.60		
0	50	6	1	1	1	—	—	—	—	3	0.10		
50	83	67	96	4	3	1	—	—	—	104	1.35	0.06±0.02	1.25±0.24
0	50	2	1	—	—	—	—	—	—	1	0.02		
50	100	49	62	3	4	1	—	1	—	71	0.80		
0	100	8	9	3	3	—	—	—	—	15	0.21		
100	50	84	158	—	9	5	—	1	—	173	3.76		
100	96	91	354	—	12	7	—	—	—	373	4.08		
0	55	9	4	—	1	—	—	—	1	6	0.15	0.19±0.02	3.49±0.26
100	98	84	202	9	22	13	—	—	1	247	2.98		
0	50	14	7	—	2	—	—	—	—	9	0.22		
100	100	92	271	13	6	2	—	—	—	292	3.13		
0	100	7	2	2	4	2	—	—	—	10	0.18		
100*	100	7	2	2	4	2	—	—	—	220	2.51		
100*	100	93	391	13	13	2	—	—	—	419	4.47		3.87±0.68
100*	50	94	188	—	22	—	—	—	—	210	4.64		

correspond qualitatively with those of Hsu et al. (3). However, we found the same aberration frequency with 100 cGy as they did with 250 cGy. We suggest that the reason for this difference is dependent on the experimental set-up; the inserting of the 0.5 h waiting time between irradiation and colchicine treatment in contrast to Hsu et al. (3) does not allow the inclusion of the relatively "radioresistant" irradiated metaphases in the analysis. There is a significant difference between the averages of the 1 and 5 h sampling times. THis means that with regard to radiation-induced chromatid breaks, the G_2 phase of the cell line 19/1 shows a non-uniform radiosensitivity during the 5 h sampling time after irradiation. These findings agree with the experiment on Vicia faba (14), which was due to shorter and non-overlapping colchicine treatments.

The higher frequency in the 1/2 h sampling time between 4.5-5.0 h as compared to the 41/2 h accumulation may represent a "dilution" phenomenon, since the latter period contains a much wider range of G_2 cells than the former.

For a dose effect correlation in low dose ranges, we have irradiated cells with 5, 12, 25, 50, and 100 cGy in the most sensitive part (first hour collecting time). It is significant to note that even with doses as low as 5 cGy, irradiation induced a significantly higher rate of breaks than in the unirradiated controls (t-test, t = 3.63; p 0.02%, Table 1, Figure 3). We observed a slight plateau in the dose effect curve between effect curve between 12 and 25 cGy, similar to the one found by Luchnik and Sevankaev (4) and Takahashi (16).

The non-uniform radiosensitivity of different sections of the G_2 phase may depends on various factors. Different sensitivities could signify different chromosome condensations or different physiological conditions at the time of irradiation. Rao's finding (8) may thus be interesting. He found that at least nine specific proteins are synthesized in the G_2 phase, these being necessary for the transition of G_2/mitosis or for chromosome condensation. Cells irradiated in specific conditions (2h, 3h, Figure 2) become less sensitive than other stages (1h, 4h, Figure 2). The reason for low sensitivity in classical terms is that these cells become either less defective or they are characterized by a higher repair capacity than others.

In the one hour experiments, the irradiated cell population comes from a very narrow range of the latest G_2 phase. Thus, the irradiated metaphase and prophase would pass the mitosis during the 0.5 h incubation time after irradiation (5). In this way, G_2 cells will be captured close to the prophase. Cells which stay in G_2 45-60 min before metaphase (13, 2) will be blocked at the time of irradiation. Therefore, our reference cell population represents in the first h sampling time a very distinct part of the population, namely between prophase and G_2 blockade. If a perturbation (9) is induced after irradiation, this will barely affect our reference cells, and this uncertainty can be neglected within the 30 min colchicine collecting time.

A possible perturbation may arise after irradiation with lower doses by this collection time. The lowest documented dose of 4.5 cGy X-rays caused a drop of the mitotic yield of the CHO line to about 80% of the control value for the next 80-90 min (13). The mitotic rate of the line 19/1 falls to 0.1% in the first hour after 100 cGy X-rays irradiation (5) and by the CHO line to 0 after 150 cGy X-rays (13). It is, therefore, possible that the dose-dependent radiosensitivity of the lower range does not reflect the response of identical cell populations, but their average sensitivity is high enough to react to 5 cGy irradiation. To obtain information concerning the radiation sensitivity of a cell from a narrow segment of the cell cycle has disadvantages and advantages. A disadvantage is that this segment gives only information from a short period of the whole cycle. Otherwise, a specific part could let us detect specific sensitivities. The advantage of this system is that the first h collection time is a well defined stage in the postreplicative phase. The long time repair is missing within the same cycle so the probability of a G_2 cell to the transmission of chromosomal damage to daughter cells is higher than that of an S cell or the former "earlier" G_2 cell. It is a suitable stage for further investigations in combination with sensitizers and radioprotective agents.

REFERENCES

1. BEIR III, National Academy Press, National Academy of Sciences, New York (1980).

2. Y. Doida and S. Okada, Radiat. Res. 38:513 (1969).

3. T. C. Hsu, W. C. Dewey, and R. M. Humphrey, Expl. Cell Res. 27:441 (1962).

4. N. V. Luchnik and A. V. Sevankaev, Mutat. Res. 36:363 (1976).

5. G. Mindek, Rev. Suisse Zool. 83:858 (1976).

6. P. S. Moorhead, P. C. Nowell, W. J. Mellman, D. M. Battips, and D. A. Hungerford, Expl. Cell Res. 20:613 (1960).

7. H. Quastler and F. G. Sherman, Expl. Cell Res. 17:420 (1959).

8. P. N. Rao, Molecular Cellular Biochem. 29:47 (1980).

9. J. R. K. Savage and D. G. Papworth, J. Theoret. Biol. 38:17 (1973).

10. A. Schinzel and W. Schmid, Mutat. Res. 40:139 (1976).

11. W. Schmid, in: "Human Chromosome Methodology," J. J. Yunis, ed., Academic Press, New York/London (1965), p. 91.

12. W. Schmid and G. R. Staiger, Mutat. Res. 7:99 (1969).

13. M. H. Schneiderman, L. A. Braby, and W. C. Roesch, Radiat. Res. 70:130 (1977).

14. D. Scott and H. J. Evans, Mutat. Res. 4:579 (1967).

15. W. K. Sinclair, in: "Proceedings of the Third International Congress of Radiation Research Cortina d'Ampezzo," G. Silini, ed., North-Holland Publishing Co., Amsterdam (1967), p. 607.

16. E. Takahashi, in: "Seventh International Chromosome Conference, Oxford," (1980), p. 99, Abst.

THE DEPENDENCE OF DOSE-EFFECT RELATIONS FOR VARIOUS RESPONSES IN MAMMALIAN

CELLS ON RADIATION QUALITY, IMPLICATIONS FOR MECHANISMS OF CARCINOGENESIS

G. W. Barendsen

Radiobiological Institute TNO
Rijswijk
Laboratory for Radiobiology
Amsterdam, The Netherlands

INTRODUCTION

The induction and expression of malignant properties of cells, initiated by radiation or by other agents, involves a complex sequence of events. Some of the early processes can be studied with cells in culture which can be transformed by various treatments. The transformed characteristics are expressed as irregular growth, loss of contact inhibition and anchorage independence. Other processes required for the development of tumours, e.g., angiogenesis, and modification of tumour growth by immunological, hormonal or other factors, can only be studied in intact animals or in man. The analysis and interpretation of dose-effect relationships for radiation carcinogenesis must take into account physical, chemical, cellular and tissue factors which determine responses to this agent. In this cont ribution I want to discuss in particular some of the characteristic parameters of dose-response relationships which depend on energy deposition characteristics of ionizing radiations. These parameters have been determined for effects in cells, but they are in various aspects relevant for dose-effect relations for the development of tumours observed after irradiation.

Chromosomes as Critical Structures in Radiation Carcinogenesis

The fundamental change required for initiation of the development of a tumour is a hereditary cellular alteration which can result in changes of variety of metabolic and proliferative properties. This alteration is a cytogenetic change which is transferred to all descendants of the transformed cells. Because genes are located in the chromosomes, it is logical to expect that the radiation induced changes conferring malignant properties to cells are associated with chromosomal alterations. These alterations can be very subtle and difficult to detect as changes in karyotype, but in other cases they may involve large parts of chromosomes.

During the past few years, evidence has been obtained that specific types of tumours are associated with specific types of translocations of genes from one chromosome to another chromosome (1). For instance the aberrant chromosome characteristic of chronic myelocytic leukemia, is a shortened chromosome number 22, whereby in many cases the deleted region is translocated to the long arm of chromosome number 9. Recent results on transforming genes inducing morphologic changes of cells in culture, indicate that oncogenes are genes which are normally present in mammalian cells and are possibly only active during embryonal development, but which can be activated as a result of repositioning. However, the discovery that specific non-random cytogenetic abnormalities are associated with a given type of tumour is not sufficient to demonstrate that this translocation is the first initiating step in the induction of the cancer studied. In particular, the induction of cancer by ionizing radiation is likely to involve a series of changes, only some of which may consist of chromosomal rearrangements characteristic of specific tumours. It is possible that radiation causes as a primary effect non-specific chromosomal aberrations which, for instance due to instability, only predispose cells to further changes. The later secondary changes could be specific and finally cause fully malignant characteristics through a multi-stage process involving a number of chromosomal aberrations. A series of progressive chromosome changes has been observed in the spontaneous neoplastic evolution of Chinese hamster cells in culture, which was shown by analysis of subsequent karyograms over a long period to be a multi-step process (2). Support for the idea that the primary change is non-specific can be derived from various observations. It is known that in certain rare conditions in man, e.g., Fanconi's anemia, there is an increased spontaneous rate of chromosomal breakage, rearrangement, and recombination, which is also associated with an increased risk of the development of certain tumours. It is also often observed that tumour progression in patients is associated with an increasing complexity of chromosomal aberrations, indicating the influence of an underlying instability.

All these new insights lead to the conclusion that radiation carcinogenesis, even at the cellular level, involves a complex series of changes and insufficient insight is presently available to predict the shapes of dose effect relationships on the basis of knowledge about fundamental mechanisms. Consequently, it is important to derive information on characteristics of dose-effect relations for radiation carcinogenesis on the basis of other considerations. In particular, a comparison of dose-effect relations for various cellular endpoints can provide significant insights. Ionizing radiations can induce a variety of changes in cultured mammalian cells, many of which are initiated by damage to the chromosomes. Important examples are cell reproductive death, chromosome structural changes, morphological transformation and specific gene mutations.

Several types of primary lesions have been demonstrated in the DNA of irradiated cells: single strand breaks, double strand breaks, base damage and cross linking of DNA to DNA or to other macromolecules. All of these changes might cause observable cellular effects, but the effectiveness per unit dose is likely to depend on the type of lesion assessed and the region of DNA involved. If the primary mechanisms of damage at the molecular level are similar, it can be expected that dose-effect relationships for the different cellular responses should exhibit common characteristics, e.g., with respect to the influence of dose-rate, dose-fractionation and linear energy transfer of the ionizing particles. If the primary mechanisms differ, this might be expected to be expressed in differences in the dependence of the effectiveness on dose, radiation quality and on modifying factors.

Biophysical Aspects of Radiation Effectiveness

Ionizing radiation, in contrast to UV-light and chemical agents, has a special characteristic: with respect to energy deposition it does not discriminate between different types of chemical constituents of cells, because individual energy transfers are large enough to break all kinds of chemical bounds. Thus, damage can be induced in principle at all sites on all chromosomes and in all genes. This initial damage produced by ionizations can result in chromosomal aberrations observable at mitosis, in cell reproductive death, in mutations and, as mentioned earlier, in induction of malignant characteristics of cells. It is of interest to compare some characteristic parameters which can be obtained from the dose-effect relations for different types of effects and to consider their dependence on the linear energy transfer (LET), because the differences observed may provide insight in some of the early changes involved in the induction of these various cellular responses. An analysis of cellular effects can be based on a few general assumptions concerning biophysical mechanisms:

a. Notwithstanding the complex nature of the induction of cellular damage by ionizing radiation, the local energy transfers involved in traversals of primary and secondary charged particles through critical structures of cells, are large enough to cause observable biological effects as a result of energy deposited by a single track. Although only a fraction of the changes induced in a given track may be effective, it must be concluded that at sufficiently low doses, where the probability of two independent tracks striking a cell nucleus is small, the dose-effect relationship for responses of isolated single cells must be linear. This applies to low LET radiations and with a higher effectiveness over a wider dose range to high LET radiation.

b. In addition to damage with a linear dependence of the frequency of effective lesions on the dose, cellular effects may also be caused by interaction of sublesions or accumulation of subeffective damage from independent tracks, i.e., from different particles passing through the same cell. This latter contribution to the total number of cells showing a given response, is generally observed to become more important with increasing dose. This is consistent with the general feature that the frequency of many types of cellular effects can be described to a first approximation by

$$F(D) = - (a_1 D + a_2 D^2) \qquad (1)$$

in which a_1 and a_2 are constants with values depending on the effect studied, on the cell type investigated and on the conditions of exposure to a dose D (3).

Dose-effect relationships which can be described by formula 1 have been measured for various types of effect, e.g., for dicentric chromosome aberrations and specific mutations. A few examples of such relations are presented in Figure 1. This figure illustrates that the slopes and shapes of these curves depend on the type of radiation applied (4). For different cell lines, values of a_1, a_2, the ratio of a_1/a_2 and of the RBE for high LET radiations vary widely (3).

c. For the induction of cell reproductive death, the endpoint assessed in an experiment is not the number of cells which show a given response, but the number of cells which fail to respond, i.e., which retain the capacity for unlimited proliferation. It can be shown that for random

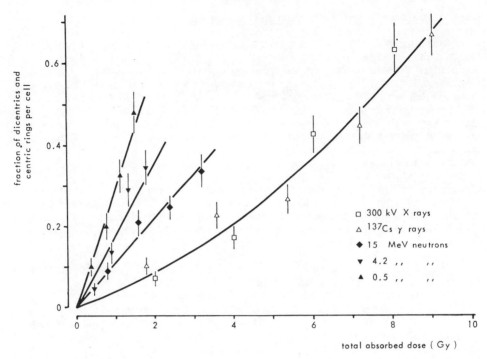

Fig. 1. Induction of dicentrics and centric rings per cell in V-79 cells
by various types of radiation as a function of total absorbed
dose. (4)

distributions of lethal lesions among cells, the number of cells
without one or more of these lesions can be described by

$$S(0)/S(D) = \exp - F(D) = \exp - (a_1D + a_2D^2) \qquad (2)$$

This formula describes the well known cell survival curves whereby the
fraction of cells in which no lethal lesions have occurred is generally
presented on a logarithmic scale as a function of the dose on a linear
scale (3).

Analysis of Experimental Data

In Figure 2 results are presented from an analysis of published dose-
effect relations for the induction of reproductive death, chromosome
aberrations, malignant transformation and specific mutations in cultured
cells treated with low LET and high LET radiation (5).

Comparison of the different values of the parameters for lethal
lesions shows that various types of cells have different sensitivities to
low LET as well as to high LET radiation. Values of a_1 for cell
reproductive death have been shown to range from about 10^{-1} to 1 Gy^{-1} in
the case of photons and between about 1 and 3 Gy^{-1} in the case of the most
effective fast neutrons with a mean energy of 0.4 to 1.0 MeV (3). Values
of a_2 for low LET radiation also vary considerably over a range of about
10^{-2} to 10^{-1} Gy^{-2}. The a_1/a_2 values (for both types of radiation) vary
somewhat less, with a range of 2 to 10 Gy (6). RBE values of fast neutrons

586

with a mean LET of about 50 keV/μm derived as ratio's a_{1x}/a_{1n} vary between 3 and 15.

Results of many types of experiments suggest that reproductive death induced by ionizing radiation is due mainly to structural chromosome abnormalities, although not all of these aberrations are readily detectable (3).

Relative to the incidence of reproductive death, the commonly scored chromosome aberrations, dicentrics and centric rings, are induced with a frequency which is lower by a factor ranging from 2 to about 10. It is evident that dicentrics and centric rings constitute only a proportion of all aberration types. Deletions are also potentially lethal, but the minimal size of the lost or translocated chromosome portion needed for lethality, is not known. RBE values of fast neutrons range up to values of about 20 (4).

Data on morphological transformation of cells in culture by different radiations are relatively scarce and have been measured for only two cell types. The values for a_1 show that this effect is much less frequently induced than reproductive death or chromosome structural abnormalities, i.e., by a factor of about 50 less for hamster embryo cells and by one of about 10^3 less for C3H 10T1/2 cells.

The results on mutations shown in Figure 2, although limited for high LET radiations, show a_1 values which are a factor of 10^4 to 10^5 smaller than for reproductive death. In the UNSCEAR 1982 report, an average value of 4×10^{-5} mutations per lethal event is mentioned, which is similar to that which can be deduced from the data in Figure 2 (7). It can be concluded that with ionizing radiations, specific mutations are less frequently induced than morphological cell transformation by a factor of 30 to 1000.

With respect to the ratio a_1/a_2, which represents the dose at which the quadratic term contributes equally to the total frequency as does the linear term, no general differences can be deduced between the dose-effect relations for the different types of effect.

A Hypothesis about Radiation Induced Cellular Transformation

The observation that various cellular effects are induced with different frequencies per unit dose but with a similar dependence on LET, can be used to obtain some insights with respect to the mechanisms involved. Cell reproductive death and chromosome aberrations can presumably be induced as a result of damage in any one of the chromosomes. As noted earlier, ionizing radiation is an a-specific agent. Although with low LET radiation, the interpretation of relations between effectiveness per unit dose and the size of the volume or structure associated with a given effect involves various uncertainties, equivalent data on fast neutrons of different energies eliminate part of these problems and provide significant information on the relative size of the structures involved. Chromosome breaks leading to various types of effects may occur at many sites. The probability of breaks may not be uniform along chromosomes, but this is difficult to establish because not all aberrations are observable with the presently available techniques. Compared to lethal events and visible chromosome abnormalities, specific gene mutations, for which changes at a specific site on a given chromosome are required, are less frequently induced by radiation by a factor of 10^4 to 10^5. This lower frequency can be attributed to the requirement that for a specific mutation a given chromosome must be damaged at a specific site containing the gene responsible for the mutation assessed.

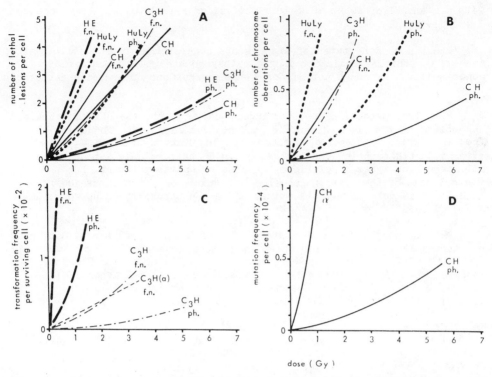

Fig. 2. Curves showing relations between the frequency of induction of
various types of changes in cultured cells as a function of the
radiation dose.

A: Cell lethality, curves derived from survival curves.
B: Chromosome aberrations.
C: Cell morphological transformation.
D: Cell mutation, resistance to 6 thioguanine.
H.E.:   Hamster embryo.
HuLy: Human Lymphocytes.
CH: Chinese Hamster V-79 line.
C3H: Mouse C3H 10T1/2 line.
f.n.:   Fission neutrons, neutrons with mean energies between 0.5
        and 1 MeV.
ph: Photons, X-rays or -rays
α: α-particles of 5-10 MeV energy.

    Because cell transformation is more frequently (30 to 1000 times)
induced by ionizing radiations than specific gene mutations, it may be
inferred that the critical sites for transformation are larger and/or are
present in larger numbers. This indicates that many, if not all,
chromosomes may contain one or more sites with genes which, if damaged,
deleted, or transposed to another site, may cause morphological malignant
transformation. It is unlikely, however, that so many sites on chromosomes
contain specific transformation genes.

    A hypothesis which can account for many features of the induction and
development of malignant tumours may be based on the assumption that the
primary chromosomal changes induced by radiation do not affect transforming
genes (oncogenes) directly, but that the primary changes can occur at many

other sites, presumably located on many or all chromosomes. These primary changes could be thought to be associated with functions or genes which are necessarily present on all chromosomes. A notable candidate representative of such a function is the replication process of chromosomes during DNA synthesis, which is presumably under control of several genes present on each chromosome. If one of these genes is damaged or changed in its expression, then during subsequent cell cycles an instability or fragility of chromosomes could develop, which may result in enhancement of the probability of gene transposition. These secondary steps, in turn, could lead to the derepression or activation of oncogenes. In addition, the development of further mutations in later stages may also be facilitated by the primary instability or fragility of the chromosomes induced as a primary change by radiation. This hypothesis might also provide an explanation for the observation that the expression of cell transformation can be modified during subsequent cell generations. Transformation is not necessarily the uniquely determined consequence of the primary induced chromosome fragility, but may be thought of as the consequence of a series of secondary changes, promoted by the initial induction of chromosomal fragility by radiation. An important consequence of the suggestion that the primary effect of radiation in the sequence of events of the induction of tumours constitutes a relatively frequently occurring type of chromosome damage which is characterized by a_1/a_2 values and RBE values similar to the values obtained for other aberrations and mutations, is that interpretation of dose-effect relations for tumour induction from 1 Gy down to very low doses can be based on the relatively simple formula (3) as explained in the next section.

The Relationship Between Tumour Development and Cell Reproductive Integrity

In addition to the evaluation of differences and similarities between dose-effect relations for the induction of cell lethality and transformation and their implications for mechanisms of tumour induction, it is of interest to discuss characteristics of cell-survival curves with respect to their influence on the probability of tumour development. It is evident that if a cell which is transformed by radiation is to develop into a tumour, it must have retained the capacity for unlimited proliferation. The frequency of tumours which after irradiation actually develop as a result of the transformation of normal cells, depends, therefore, on the probability of cell survival. As a consequence, the tumour yield as a function of the dose can be represented to a first approximation by:

$$y = (p_0 + p_1D + p_2D^2) \times \exp - (a_1D + a_2D^2) \qquad (3)$$

in which p_0 is the incidence without radiation, p_1D and p_2D^2 are the linear and quadratic terms for the malignant transformation processes, while a_1D and a_2D^2 are the linear and quadratic terms which determine the induction of cell reproductive death. From this formula, it can be deduced that the yield of tumours as a function of the dose has a complex shape with general features illustrated in Figure 3. At low doses of low LET radiation, where the influence of cell death is small, the yield increases linearly with the dose, while at somewhat larger doses the quadratic term may start to contribute significantly. The dose at which the term p_2D contributes a number of transformations equal to p_1D is given by $D = p_1/p_2$. The available data, illustrated in Figure 2, indicate that for low LET radiation values of p_1/p_2 may vary over a range of 0.5 to 2 Gy. This value of p_1/p_2 depends on the radiation quality, mainly because of the increase of p_1 with LET (8, 9). The influence of cell reproductive death generally becomes significant only at doses in excess of a few Gy of low-LET radiation. At a dose which depends on the actual values of a_1 and a_2 for induction of cell reproductive death, the yield of tumours will reach a maximum, as illustrated in Figure 3 and subsequently a decrease of the

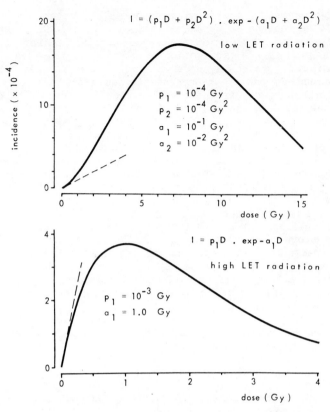

$$I = (p_1 D + p_2 D^2) \cdot \exp - (a_1 D + a_2 D^2)$$

low LET radiation

$$p_1 = 10^{-4} \text{ Gy}$$
$$p_2 = 10^{-4} \text{ Gy}^2$$
$$a_1 = 10^{-1} \text{ Gy}$$
$$a_2 = 10^{-2} \text{ Gy}^2$$

$$I = p_1 D \cdot \exp - a_1 D$$

high LET radiation

$$p_1 = 10^{-3} \text{ Gy}$$
$$a_1 = 1.0 \text{ Gy}$$

Fig. 3. Examples of incidence versus dose relationships for tumours induced by low LET radiation and high LET radiation. Parameters have been chosen to demonstrate the importance of linear and quadratic terms in the induction of transformation and cell lethality. The broken lines represent initial slopes determined by the parameter p_1.

yield will be observed as cell killing becomes a dominant factor. For high-LET radiations only the parameters p_1 and a_1 are important and the shape of the yield versus dose curve is less complicated as illustrated in Figure 3. This general shape of the yield versus dose curve has first been suggested by Gray (10) and this analysis has subsequently been applied by other investigators (11). The yield of tumours as well as the values of dose at which the maximum yield is obtained, depends on parameters of the cell survival curves.

REFERENCES

1. J. J. Yunis, The chromosomal basis of human neoplasia, Science 221:227-236 (1983).

2. P. M. Kraemer, G. L. Travis, F. A. Ray, and L. S. Cram, Spontaneous
    Neoplastic Evolution of Chinese hamster cells in culture:
    Multistep progression of phenotype, Cancer Res. 43:4822-4827
    (1983).

3. G. W. Barendsen, Influence of radiation quality on the effectiveness
    of small doses for induction of reproductive death and chromosome
    aberrations in mammalian cells.Int. J. Radiat. Biol. 36, no. 1,
    49-63 (1979).

4. J. Zoetelief and G. W. Barendsen, Dose-effect relationships for
    induction of cell inactivation and asymmetrical chromosome
    exchanges in three cell lines by photons and neutrons of different
    energy. Int. J. Radiat. Biol., 43, 349-362 (1983).

5. G. W. Barendsen, Comparison of the effectiveness of different
    radiations for the induction of reproductive death, chromosome
    aberrations, morphological transformation and specific mutations in
    cultured mammalian cells, in: "Proc. 7th Int. Congr. Radiation
    Research, Section C: Somatic and Genetic Effects, C5-02," J. J.
    Broerse, G. W. Barendsen, H. B. Kal, and A. J. Van der Kogel, eds.,
    Martinus Nijhoff Publishers, The Hague (1983).

6. G. W. Barendsen, Dose fractionation, dose rate and iso-effect
    relationships for normal tissue responses, Int. J. Radiat. Biol.
    Phys. 8:1981-1997 (1982).

7. United Nations Scientific Committee on the Effects of Atomic
    Radiation, "Ionizing Radiation: Sources and Biological Effects. Annex
    Genetic Effects of Radiation," (1982), pp. 425-570.

8. C. K. Hill, F. M. Bounoguro, C. P. Myers, A. Han, and M. M. Elkind,
    Fission-spectrum neutrons at reduced dose rates enhance neoplastic
    transformation, Nature 298:67-69 (1982).

9. A. Han and M. M. Elkind, Transformation of mouse C3H/101/2 cells by
    single and fractionate doses of X-rays and fission spectrum
    neutrons, Cancer Research 39:123-103 (1979).

10. L. H. Gray, Radiation biology and cancer, in: "Cellular Radiation
    Biology," Proc. 18th Ann. Symp. Found. Ca. Res. 7-25, M. D.
    Anderson Inst., The Williams and Wilkins Co., Baltimore (1965).

11. G. W. Barendsen, Fundamental aspects of cancer induction in relation
    to the effectiveness of small doses of radiation, in: "Late
    Biological Effects of Ionizing Radiation, Vol. 2," International
    Atomic Energy Agency, Vienna (1978), pp. 263-275.

THE PHYSICS OF ABSORBED DOSE AND LINEAR ENERGY TRANSFER

J. J. Broerse and G. W. Barendsen

Radiobiological Institute TNO
Rijswijk, The Netherlands

ABSTRACT

The objectives of dosimetry and dose specification concern the description of the temporal and spatial distribution of the energy deposition at a macroscopic and microscopic level.

The incident radiation field is defined when the type of particles and their initial energy spectrum are specified. Knowledge of interaction coefficients is required to convert the particle fluence to energy imparted to biological tissue. The absorbed dose is defined as the differential quotient of mean energy imparted and mass. It is pointed out that the energy deposition is a stochastic process, and this becomes important if small doses and small volumes of tissue are considered.

The quality of the radiation can be related to the linear energy transfer spectra or the lineal energy spectra. Lineal energy spectra for different types of radiation are described and the expectation values: frequency mean lineal energy and dose mean lineal energy for neutrons of different energies are compared.

To explain the differences in biological effectiveness of different types of radiation, the energy deposition processes have to be correlated with the sizes of the biological structures involved. Some of the biophysical approaches to understand the biological effects of ionizing radiation are summarized.

INTRODUCTION

For the evaluation of biological effects of ionizing radiation, the energy deposition processes have to be described in a quantitative and qualitative way. Ionizing radiation consists of charged particles (e.g., positive or negative electrons, protons, alpha particles, and heavier ions) which cause ionization by primary processes (directly ionizing radiation) and/or uncharged particles (e.g., photons or neutrons) which can only ionize by secondary processes (indirectly ionizing radiation). The most elementary description of a radiation field is one in terms of the type, energy, direction, and number of particles. The radiation quantities associated with the radiation itself have been defined by the ICRU (1) under the category radiometry. A second category of quantities entitled interaction coefficients deals with the interaction of radiation and biological material. In the third category dosimetric quantities are devised to provide a physical measure to be correlated with actual or potential effects. In essence, these dosimetric quantities are products of the quantities mentioned in the first two categories. A number of definitions recommended by the ICRU (1) are summarized.

Investigations in radiobiology and radiotherapy have demonstrated that differences of 10 percent in absorbed dose will produce observable quantitative variations in biological response. It has, therefore, been suggested that an accuracy of better than about 5 percent and a precision of within 2 percent is required for the determination of absorbed dose in biomedical applications.

The energy deposition processes are subject to random fluctuations which become significant if the mass of interest is small or the fluence of charged particles is small. Quantities subject to statistical fluctuations are termed stochastic while their means are non-stochastic quantities. Examples will be provided of the differences between stochastic and non-stochastic quantities as introduced by the ICRU (1).

Equal absorbed doses of various types of ionizing radiation do not necessarily produce the same frequency or incidence of biological effects. This implies that specification of absorbed dose alone is inadequate to predict the quantitative effects of radiation on biological specimens. Information should, therefore, be provided on the microscopic distribution of energy dissipation, i.e., radiation quality. Attempts to account for radiation quality led first to the concept of linear energy transfer (LET) and its distributions and later to the stochastic quantity lineal energy (y) and its distributions. Lineal energy spectra for various fast neutron beams will be shown and the adequacy of mean values of y distributions will be discussed. The possibilities for experimental determination of meaningful y spectra are directly connected with the dimensions of the critical biological structures. Biophysical evidence accrues that the relevant biological effects are determined by stochastic interactions in target molecules with diameters in the nanometer range.

SPECIFICATION OF RADIATION FIELDS

Radiometric quantities have been introduced to specify radiation fields in terms of type, energy, direction, and number of particles. These quantities deal primarily with either particle number or energy and this is denoted in their names, e.g., particle fluence or energy fluence. The word particle can be replaced by the more specific term for the considered entity, e.g., neutron fluence or electron fluence. The ICRU (1) recommends that the quantities are expressed in SI units, a coherent system of units in which all derived units can be obtained from a selected set of base units without the introduction of any numerical factors.

The (particle) fluence, Φ, is the quotient of dN by da, where dN is the number of particles incident on a sphere of cross sectional area da:

$$\Phi = \frac{dN}{da} \text{ (SI unit: } m^{-2})$$

The area da must be perpendicular to each radiation's direction. A sphere arranges this in the simplest manner.

The (particle) fluence rate, ϕ, is the quotient of Φ by dt, where dΦ is the increment of particle fluence in the time interval dt:

$$\phi = \frac{d\Phi}{dt} \quad \frac{d^2N}{da\ dt} \qquad \text{(SI unit: } m^{-2}.s^{-1})$$

The term particle flux density is also used as the name for this quantity. As the word density has several connotations, the term particle fluence rate is preferable.

Definitions of other quantities, such as energy fluence and energy fluence rate, used to describe the radiation field, can be found elsewhere (1). For photon irradiation, the ionization in air has been used extensively in the past for field specification.

The exposure, X, is the quotient of dQ by dm where the value of dQ is the absolute value of the total charge of the ions of one sign produced in air when all the electrons (negatrons and positrons) liberated by photons in air of mass dm are completely stopped in air:

$$X = \frac{dQ}{dm} \qquad \text{(SI unit: } C.kg^{-1})$$

The special unit of exposure, rontgen (R), may be used temporarily but will be abandoned after 1985, $1R = 2.58 \times 10^{-4}$ Ckg^{-1}. With present techniques, it is difficult to measure exposure when the photon energies involved lie above a few MeV or below a few keV. Difficulties associated with the introduction of SI units for exposure will most likely lead in the future to the adoption by the standardization laboratories of the quantity kerma in air to characterize the photon field. It has to be stressed that the quantity exposure is not directly applicable for biomedical applications. Specifications of the exposure at the positions where the experimental animal will be irradiated are of very limited value. The actual irradiation conditions have to be investigated with phantoms which simulate the biological specimen with respect to size, shape, density, and atomic composition (2). Measurement of the exposure in a small quantity of air inside the phantom can be used to derive the absorbed dose in the biological material applying conversion factors as given in Table 1 for monoenergetic photons. These conversion factors are slightly different from those recommended earlier by the ICRU (3), since new values have been used for W and the mass energy transfer coefficients (2, 4). Mean factors for conversion of exposure to absorbed dose for various X-ray spectra have also been re-evaluated (2).

MACROSCOPIC ASPECTS OF ENERGY DEPOSITION

Radiobiological effects are the consequence of energy deposition by ionizing radiations in tissue. This energy transfer occurs in discrete events, i.e., interactions of fast charged particles with atoms and molecules in the irradiated material which give rise to ionizations and excitations. The following dosimetric quantities are of special relevance:

The kerma, K, defined as the quotient of dE_{tr} by dm, where dE_{tr} is the sum of the initial kinetic energies of all the charged ionizing particles liberated by uncharged ionizing particles in a material of mass dm:

$$K = \frac{dE_{tr}}{dm} \qquad \text{(SI unit: } J.kg^{-1})$$

The special name for the unit of kerma is gray (Gy). The special unit of kerma, rad, will be abandoned in the near future, $1 \text{ rad} = 10^{-2} \text{ J.kg}^{-1}$.

Table 1. Factor f relating absorbed dose to exposure for
monoenergetic photons with energies from 10 keV to 2
MeV under conditions of secondary charged-particle
equilibrium

Photon Energy (keV)	Water (mGy/R)	Muscle (mGy/R)	Bone (mGy/R)
10	9.11	9.21	34.6
15	9.00	9.21	38.5
20	8.92	9.19	40.7
30	8.84	9.18	42.4
40	8.87	9.22	40.3
50	9.00	9.29	35.2
60	9.16	9.37	29.0
80	9.42	9.49	19.4
100	9.56	9.56	14.5
150	9.67	9.60	10.6
200	9.69	9.61	9.78
300	9.70	9.62	9.41
400	9.71	9.62	9.33
600	9.71	9.62	9.28
1000	9.71	9.62	9.27
2000	9.71	9.62	9.27

After ICRU report 30, revised[2,4].

The energy imparted, ε, by ionizing radiation to the matter in a volume
is defined as:

$$\varepsilon = R_{in} - R_{out} + \Sigma Q \quad (\text{SI unit:} \quad J)$$

where

R_{in} = the radiant energy incident on the volume, i.e., the sum of the
energies (excluding rest energies) of all those charged and
uncharged ionizing particles which enter the volume,

R_{out} = the radiant energy emerging from the volume, i.e., the sum of the
energies (excluding rest energies) of all those charged and
uncharged ionizing particles which leave the volume,

and ΣQ = the sum of all changes (decreases: positive sign, increases:
negative sign) of the rest mass energy of nuclei and elementary
particles in any nuclear transformations which occur in the
volume.

The energy imparted, ε, is a stochastic quantity. The expectation value of
ε, termed the mean energy imparted, $\bar{\varepsilon}$, is a non-stochastic quantity.

The absorbed dose, D, defined as the quotient of d by dm, where d is the mean energy imparted by ionizing radiation to matter of mass dm:

$$\frac{d\bar{\varepsilon}}{dm} \quad \text{(SI unit:} \quad J \cdot kg^{-1})$$

The special name for the unit of absorbed dose is gray (Gy). The special unit of absorbed dose, rad, will be abandoned in the near future, 1 rad = 10^{-2} J.kg^{-1}. Absorbed dose is defined for both charged and uncharged particles, in contrast to kerma which is only defined for indirectly ionizing radiations. For biomedical purposes absorbed dose is usually specified in ICRU muscle tissue (3) or water. Equality of absorbed dose and kerma is approached to the degree that charged particle equilibrium is achieved and bremsstrahlung production is negligible. The absorbed dose rate and the kerma rate are defined as the increment of absorbed dose and kerma, respectively, in the time interval dt.

When the amount of mass is reduced, the stochastic aspects of the energy deposition process will become evident. This has led to the introduction of stochastic dosimetric quantities such as:

The specific energy (imparted), z, defined as the quotient of ε by m, where ε is the energy imparted by ionizing radiation to matter of mass m:

$$z = \frac{\varepsilon}{m} \quad \text{(SI unit:} \quad J \cdot kg^{-1})$$

The special name for the unit of specific energy is gray (Gy). The specific energy, z, is a stochastic quantity. It is, therefore, useful to consider also the probability distribution of z. Definitions of the probability density, f(z), and the distribution function can be found elsewhere (1).

The specific energy may be due to one or more energy deposition events, i.e., traversals of charged particles through a volume element considered. The statistical fluctuations will be less apparent when the mass of the irradiated material is increased (5, 6) as shown in Figure 1. The solid line covers the region in which the absorbed dose can be established in a single measurement. At large masses the energy density is reduced due to attenuation of the indirectly ionizing particles. The shaded portion represents the range where statistical fluctuations are important.

The mean specific energy,

$$\bar{z} = \int_{0}^{\infty} z f(z) dz$$

is a non-stochastic quantity that can be used for an alternative definition for D.

$$D = \lim_{m \to 0} z$$

This formula indicates the relation between D and z. The absorbed dose, D, is equal to the limit of z as the mass, m, approaches zero. The mean absorbed dose in a volume is equal to the mean specific energy, $\bar{z}$, in that volume.

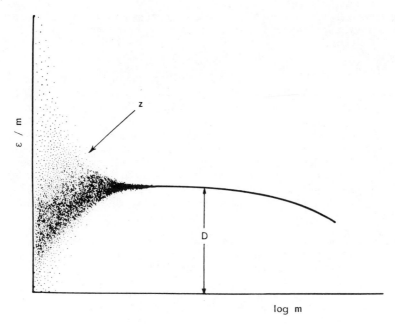

Fig. 1. Energy density as a function of mass showing the
statistical fluctuations which become apparent at
small masses (5).

The mean absorbed dose can be derived from the particle fluence and
the energy losses of the charged particles along their tracks. This is
schematically shown in Figure 2 for various groups of cells with individual
diameters of 10 µm irradiated with secondary electrons with an average LET
of 0.6 keV µm^{-1} such as produced by 1 MeV gamma radiation. It can be
concluded that an average passage of one electron through the cell and its
nucleus is equivalent to a mean absorbed dose of 1 mGy. For an irradiation
with 5 MeV α-particles (LET 94 keV µm^{-1}), the passage of one α-particle
per cell would result in an absorbed dose of 0.15 Gy. In view of the
random spatial distribution of the tracks and the stochastic nature of the
energy deposition processes along the tracks, the above calculations are a
simplified approach. At the higher dose levels, the energy imparted will
be due to multiple tracks in the same cell.

The biological effects of low doses of ionizing radiation attract at
the moment appreciable attention, especially with regard to the risk of
radiation carcinogenesis. For isolated single cells, the dose-effect
relations are expected to be linear in the range of sufficiently low doses
when there is a negligible probability of a cell being traversed by two
independent charged particle tracks. Goodhead (7) calculated the maximum
dose limits at which the role of two-track effects can be ignored with a
confidence of 90% for cells with diameters of 4-32 m irradiated with
gamma-rays, alpha particles and monoenergetic neutrons (see Figure 3). For
typical mammalian cells with a diameter of 12 µm, these maximum dose limits
are 0.1 mGy for 1 MeV gamma-rays, 0.4 mGy for 250 kV X-rays, 8 mGy for
monoenergetic 1 MeV neutrons and 20 mGy for 5 MeV alpha particles.

MICROSCOPIC ASPECTS OF ENERGY DEPOSITION

On the microscopic level the energy dissipation patterns of various
types of radiation are considerably different as shown schematically in

598

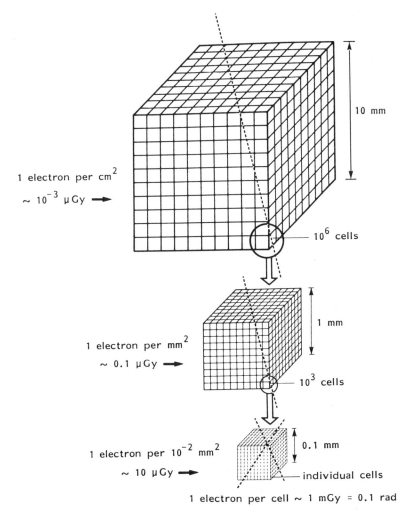

1 electron per cm^2

$\sim 10^{-3}$ μGy ➡

10 mm

10^6 cells

1 electron per mm^2

~ 0.1 μGy ➡

1 mm

10^3 cells

1 electron per 10^{-2} mm^2

~ 10 μGy ➡

0.1 mm

individual cells

1 electron per cell $\sim$ 1 mGy = 0.1 rad

Fig. 2.   Mean absorbed dose as a function of electron-fluence
            with an average LET of 0.6 keV μm^{-1} for various groups
            of cells.

Figure 4 for sparsely ionizing electrons produced by X-rays and a densely
ionizing alpha-particle. The differences in biological effects produced by
equal doses of different radiations have to be attributed to these
differences in the spatial distribution of the energy deposition.   To
quantify the local energy transfer, the following quantities have been
introduced:

     The linear energy transfer or restricted linear collision stopping
power L , of a material for charged particles is defined as the quotient of
dE by dl, where dE is the energy lost by a charged particle in traversing a
distance dl due to those collisions with electrons in which the energy loss
is less than :

$$L \;=\; \left(\frac{dE}{dl}\right)_{\!\triangle} \qquad (\text{SI unit:} \quad J.m^{-1})$$

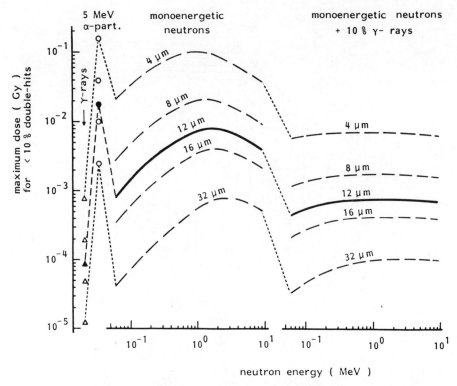

Fig. 3. Maximum dose limits for which it can be assumed that cells or nuclei are hit by one, rather than two, radiation tracks with a confidence of 80%. Cells or nuclei are assumed to be spherical with diameters of 4 to 32 μm (7).

The energy may also be expressed in eV (1 eV = 1.6×10^{-19} J) and hence, L may be expressed in eV m^{-1} or some convenient submultiple or multiple, such as keV m^{-1} (1 keV m^{-1} = 1.6×10^{-10} Jm^{-1}). In order to simplify the notation, may be expressed in eV. Thus, L_{100} is understood to be the linear energy transfer for an energy cut off of 100 eV.

As a measure of differences in effectiveness of various radiations, the term relative biological effectiveness (RBE) has been introduced (3), which is defined as the ratio of the absorbed dose of a reference radiation to the absorbed dose of a test radiation required to produce the same level of biological effect, other conditions being equal. When two radiations produce an effect that is not of the same extent and/or nature, an RBE cannot be specified.

For any given type of radiation, environmental factors such as the oxygen concentration can modify the radiation response. In this connection, the term oxygen enhancement ratio has been introduced, which is defined as the ratio of the absorbed dose required under conditions of hypoxia to that under conditions in air to produce the same level of effect.

Experiments with cultured cells irradiated with charged particles of well-defined LET, as those performed by Barendsen (8, 9), have shown that the RBE and OER are clearly dependent on LET (see Figure 5). Irradiation with charged particles with LET values in excess of 30 keV μm^{-1} of tissue

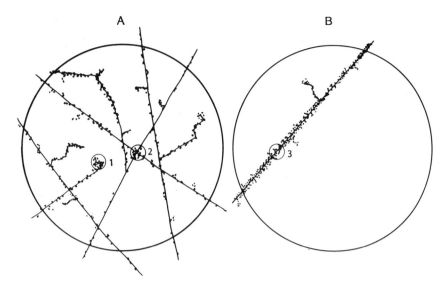

Fig. 4. Schematic representation of energy dissipation patterns in
small volumes in cells irradiated with equal doses of X-rays
(A) or high-LET α-particles (B). High concentrations of
energy events occur for both types of radiation (small circles
1, 2 and 3), but they are per unit dose much less frequent for
low-LET radiation.

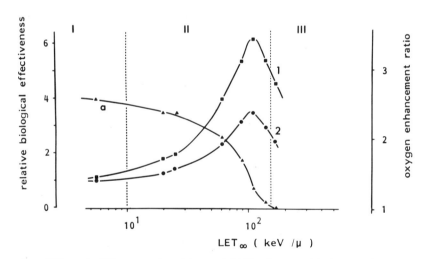

Fig. 5. RBE and OER as a function of LET of α-particles and deuterons,
measured for damage to the reproductive capacity of cultured
cells of human origin. Curve A represents the OER, the RBE
Curves 1 and 2 correspond 50 percent and 1 percent survival,
respectively. In the LET region I, cell reproductive death is
produced predominantly through accumulation of damage,
corresponding to survival curves with a pronounced shoulder.
In region III cell reproductive death can be produced by
single traversals of particles, resulting in exponential
survival curves (Barendsen (9)).

result in exponential survival curves which implies that the biological effect is due to single events:

$$S(D) = e^{-D/D_0} = e^{-\sigma_{eff} \cdot \Phi}$$

where $1/D_0$ is the slope of the exponential survival curve, σ_{eff} is the effective cross section and Φ the particle fluence. The effective cross section can be derived from the D_0 and the LET since

$$\sigma_{eff} = \frac{L}{\rho D_0}$$

Examples of the dependence of σ_{eff} on LET are shown in Figure 6 for cultured mammalian cells and bacterial spores.

The quantity linear energy transfer, mostly in terms of L_∞, has been useful to estimate the biological effectiveness of various types of radiation and their risks in radiation protection applications, however, the LET concept has some inherent limitations. For a given type of particle with a given kinetic energy, LET is a mean value and does not

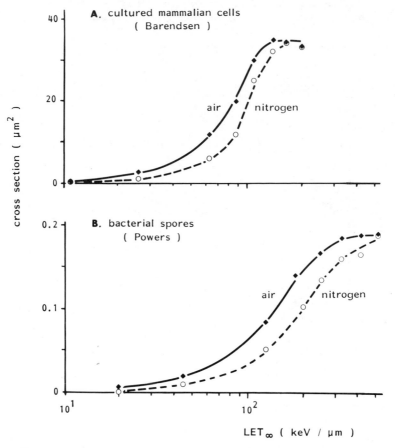

Fig. 6.   Effective cross sections for impairment of the reproductive capacity of cultured mammalian cells (Barendsen 8)) and spores of Bacillus megaterium (Powers (10)) as a function of linear energy transfer.

explicitly describe the discrete nature of the energy loss events. Energy loss-straggling, radial extension of the tracks, and the finite range of the recoil nuclei account for the fact that it is not possible to obtain accurate distributions of LET from energy deposition patterns measured with spherical proportional counters. Such considerations have led to the introduction of microdosimetric quantities which are stochastich such as:

The lineal energy, y, defined as the quotient of ε by $\bar{\ell}$, where ε is the energy imparted to the matter in a volume of interest by an energy deposition event and $\bar{\ell}$ is the mean chord length in that volume.

$$y = \frac{\varepsilon}{\bar{\ell}} \quad (\text{SI unit:} \quad J.m^{-1})$$

The unit most commonly used for this quantity is keV.μm^{-1}. The mean chord length in a volume is the mean length of randomly oriented chords in that volume. For a convex body: $\bar{\ell}$ equals 4V/a, were V is the volume and a is the surface area of this body. In the special case of a sphere, $\bar{\ell}$ equals 2d/3 where d is the diameter of the sphere.

The lineal energy is similar to the linear energy transfer since both quantities are defined as quotient of energy by length. However, while linear energy transfer is a non-stochastic quantity subject to an energy cut off, lineal energy in a stochastic quantity subject to a geometric cut off. Another difference is that linear energy transfer applies to a differential track element and must be determined over distances that are short compared with the range of the directly ionizing particle, while lineal energy is defined without reference to track structure and is, therefore, applicable even if the range is less than $\bar{\ell}$.

Lineal energy spectra can be measured with tissue equivalent proportional counters, with spherical or cylindrical volumes simulating biological structures. A description of the technical features of these instruments can be found elsewhere (6). Generally, the proportional counters are filled with tissue equivalent gas. The dimension of the gas cavity can be converted to those of the simulated regions by a factor which is equal to the density ratio between tissue and counter gas. The lineal energy spectra for sparsely ionizing radiation and two different neutron energies for a 1 μm sphere of tissue (11) are shown in Figure 7. There is

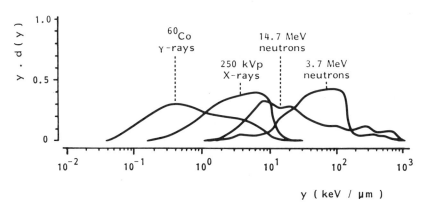

Fig. 7. Lineal energy spectra for sparsely ionizing radiation and two different neutron energies. The spectra refer to a 1 μm sphere of tissue (Kellerer and Rossi 11)).

a wide range of lineal energies involved for the photons as well as for the neutrons, and a shift of the distributions with energy.

To compare the radiation quality of different particle beams, it is useful to derive a mean y value from the differential distributions of the frequency of events in y, f(y), or from the differential distribution of absorbed dose in y, d(y). The corresponding expectation values are the frequency-mean lineal energy

$$\overline{y_F} = \int_0^\infty y\ f(y)dy$$

and the dose-mean lineal energy

$$\overline{y_D} = \int_0^\infty y\ d(y)\ dy,$$

which are both non-stochastic quantities.

An algorithm developed by Kellerer (12) to derive LET spectra from energy deposition distributions demonstrated a linear relationship between $\overline{y_F}$ and the track average LET and between $\overline{y_D}$ and the dose average LET. Studies by Broerse et al. (13) have shown that the track average LET values for neutrons are considerably lower than those of directly ionizing particles, which would have an identical relative biological effectiveness (RBE) for cell reproductive death. For homogeneous spheres with a 1 m diameter, $\overline{y_D}$ and $\overline{y_F}$ have been calculated as a function of neutron energy (see Figure 8). The dose average lineal energy values are unsatisfactory in that the $\overline{y_D}$ for neutron energies above 10 MeV is higher than that for neutron energies below 10 MeV; this is incompatible with the findings of higher RBE values for the lower energy neutrons. It should be realized that a given y event becomes less effective in producing a biological effect per unit dose when y becomes too high, since some of the energy in such a track of very dense ionization is wasted. To correct for this phenomenon, Kellerer and Rossi (11) introduced the saturation-corrected dose-averaged lineal energy y*. However, irradiation experiments for different biological endpoints show different RBE values, whereas y* is constant (16).

The evaluation and interpretation of the biological effectiveness of different radiations should be based on the nature of the biological lesions produced in the DNA, protein or membrane of the cells, the local energy requirements and the sizes of the critical structures involved. The exposure of a biological system will result in a vast background of biologically irrelevant atomic damage (17) which is unlikely to lead to biological damage, e.g., cell reproductive death. This is schematically illustrated in Figure 9. Only above a certain threshold (T) the lesions will become lethal, with a small transit zone in which the damage is potentially lethal (level P) but in appropriate conditions can still be repaired. Another important aspect is the correlation of the complex spatial structure of radiation tracks and the likely biological target molecules such as DNA and chromatin. The organization of DNA in mammalian cells is summarized in Table 2. Goodhead and colleagues (18) applied Monte Carlo methods to calculate frequency distributions of energy deposition by protons and α-particles in cyclindrical volumes. The results of their

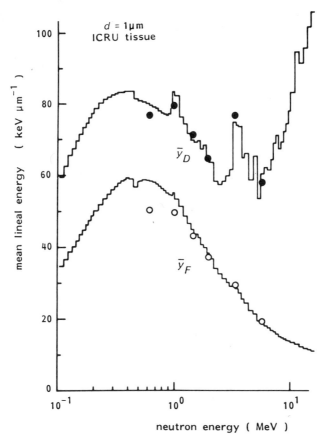

Fig. 8. Calculated volumes of $\overline{y}_D$ and $\overline{y}_F$ of fast neutrons
for homogeneous spheres of tissue of 1 m diameter
as a function of neutron energy. The solid and
open circles have been derived from Monte Carlo
calculations (14) and the solid lines from bin-
averaged analytical calculations (15).

calculations on local energy deposition have been compared with the
biological effectiveness of these particles. An illustration of their
approach is given in Figure 10. All data are normalized to unity for 4 MeV α
-particles. The solid points show experimental data of numbers of lethal
lesions per cGy in human cells derived from survival curves. The lines
show frequencies of deposition of selected threshold energies in target
cylinders of various sizes. For each size the threshold energy was
selected to best fit the experimental data on lethal lesions. The shape of
the curve of RBE of α-particles of varying LET can be fitted by the
appropriate assumptions of threshold energies at approximate dimensions of
5 to 10 nm. Acceptable fits do not seem possible at all for smaller
targets of approximately 2 nm (DNA diameter) or larger diameters of
approximately 25 nm (elementary fibre). Thus, a "window" of possible
target sizes and threshold energies seems to exist in which local energy
deposition by α-particles correlated well with biological effectiveness.
Goodhead and colleagues (18) conclude that good agreement is possible for a
threshold energy deposition of 340 eV in a target cylinder of diameter 10
nm and length 5 nm. These are approximately equal to the dimensions of
nucleosomes which are the basic DNA plus protein repeat units of mammalian
cell genetic material.

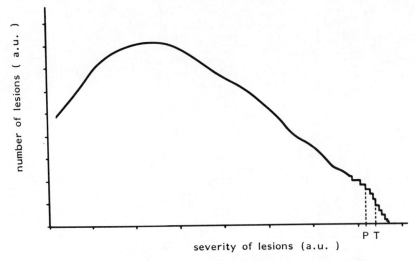

Fig. 9.   Hypothetical spectrum of lesions in a group of
1000 cells irradiated with 2 Gy X-rays.
T indicates the threshold beyond which lesions
cause cell reproductive death. P indicates the
threshold for damage which is only lethal in
specific conditions, e.g., when repair is
diminished (Barendsen 17)).

Table 2. Organization of DNA in mammalian cells (Goodhead et al. (18))

Structure	Diameter	Comment
DNA	~2 nm	Total length ~2 metres
Nucleosome	~10 nm	~5 nm 'disc' holding ~50 nm DNA
Elementary fibre	~25 nm	'Solenoid' of nucleosomes
Coiled fibre	~300 nm	
Condensed chromosome	~1 μm	Human cell nucleus contains
Cell nucleus	~10 μm	46 chromosomes

The results of the Monte Carlo track structure calculations confirm
the earlier conclusion of Barendsen (8), derived on the basis of cell
reproductive death induced by α-particles and deuterons of various LET that
an energy deposition event of about 200 to 300 eV within a distance of
about 10 nm is required to initiate the damage by single ionizing particles
which causes the initial slope of a survival curve. Experimental
determination of lineal energy distribution at these small simulated
diameters cannot be performed with proportional counters presently
available.

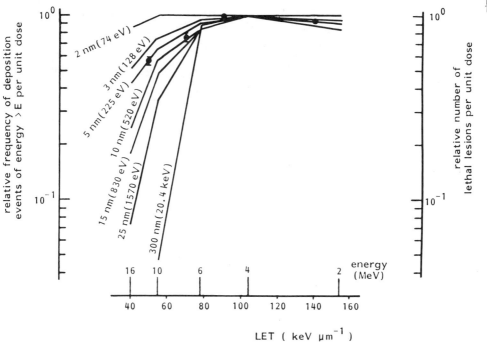

Fig. 10. Frequencies of local energy depositions by α-particles in small targets compared with their observed lethal effectiveness in human cells (18).

CONCLUSIONS

The concepts and dosimetric quantities discussed provide the physical basis for a prediction and better understanding of detrimental effects which may occur after exposure to ionizing radiation. A number of definitions have been summarized according to the recommendations formulated by the ICRU. The following aspects of the dosimetry of ionizing radiation need specific attention:

1. For biomedical applications the absorbed dose should be assessed with an accuracy of better than about 5 percent and precision of within 2 percent.

2. Specification of exposure at the position, where the biological specimen will be irradiated, has limited practical value.

3. The absorbed dose should be determined for the actual exposure arrangement. This can be accomplished by using phantoms which simulate the biological specimen.

4. The stochastic aspects of the energy deposition processes become evident if the amount of mass and/or the particle fluence are reduced.

5. On the average the passage of one electron (LET 0.6 keV μm^{-1}) or an α-particle (LET 94 keV μm^{-1}) through a cell will be equivalent to mean absorbed doses of 1 mGy and 150 mGy, respectively.

6. The relative biological effectiveness of various types of ionizing radiation are dependent on the linear energy transfer, L, and the lineal energy, y.

7. The dose average lineal energy $\overline{y_D}$ shows some inadequacies in relation to the dependence of RBE on neutron energy.

8. Lineal energy spectra can be measured with proportional counters generally for 1 μm spheres and minimally for a 0.25 m tissue sphere.

9. There is increasing evidence that relevant biological effects are determined by stochastic interactions in target molecules with dimensions of approximately 10 nm.

REFERENCES

1. ICRU Report 33, "Radiation Quantities and Units," International Commission on Radiation Units and Measurements, ICRU, Washington, D.C. (1980).

2. J. Zoetelief, R. W. Davies, G. Scarpa, G. H. Hofmeester, A. Dixon-Brown, A. J. van der Kogel, and J. J. Broerse, Protocol for X-ray dosimetry and exposure arrangements employed in studies of late somatic effects in mammals, Int. J. Radiat. Biol. 47:81-102 (1985).

3. ICRU Report 30, "Quantitative Concepts and Dosimetry in Radiobiology," International Commission on Radiation Units and Measurements, ICRU, Washington, D.C. (1979).

4. H. O. Wijckoff, Corrected f factors for photons from 10 keV to 2 MeV, Medical Physics 10:715-716 (1983).

5. H. H. Rossi, Microscopic energy distribution in irradiated matter, in: "Radiation Dosimetry," F. H. Attix and W. C. Roesch, eds., Academic Press, New York (1968), pp. 43-92.

6. ICRU Report 36, "Microdosimetry," International Commission on Radiation Units and Measurement, ICRU, Washington, D.C. (1983).

7. D. T. Goodhead, Deductions from cellular studies of inactivation, mutagenesis and transformation, in: "Radiation Carcinogenesis: Epidemiology ad Biological Significance," J. D. Boice, Jr. and J. F. Fraumeni, Jr., eds., Raven Press, New York (1984), pp. 369-385.

8. G. W. Barendsen, Impairment of the proliferative capacity of human cells in culture by α-particles with differing linear-energy transfer, Int. J. Radiat. Biol. 8:453-466 (1964).

9. G. W. Barendsen, Responses of cultured cells, tumours and normal tissues to radiations of different linear energy transfer, in: "Current Topics in Radiation Research, Vol. 4," M. Ebert and A. Howard, eds., North-Holland Publishing Company (1968).

10. E. L. Powers, Some physiochemical bases of radiation sensitivity in cells, in: "Cellular Radiation Biology, Proceedings Eighteenth Annual Symposium on Fundamental Cancer Research," The Williams and Wilkins Company, Baltimore (1965), pp. 286-304.

11. A. M. Kellerer and H. H. Rossi, The theory of dual radiation action, in: "Current Topics in Radiation Research Quarterly" Vol. 8, North-Holland Publishing Company (1972), pp. 85-158.

12. A. M. Kellerer, An algorithm for LET-analysis, Phys. Med. Biol. 17:232-240 (1972).

13. J. J. Broerse, G. W. Barendsen, and G. R. van Kersen, Survival of cultured human cells after irradiation with fast neutrons of different energies in hypoxic and oxygenated conditions, Int. J. Radiat. Biol. 13:559-572 (1968).

14. J. Booz, U. Oldenburg, and M. Coppola, Das Problem der Gewebeaquivalenz fur schnelle Neutronen in der Mikrodosimetrie, in: Proceedings of the First Symposium on Neutron Dosimetry in Biology and Medicine," EUR 4896, G. Burger, H. Schraube and H. G. Ebert, eds., Commission of the European Communities, Luxembourg (1972), pp. 117-136.

15. J. J. Coyne and R. S. Caswell, Microdosimetric energy deposition spectra and their averages for bin-averaged and energy-distributed neutron spectra, in: "Proceedings of the Seventh Symposium on Microdosimetry, EUR 7147," J. Booz, H. G. Ebert, and H. D. Hartfield, eds., Harwood Academic Publishers, London (1980), pp. 689-696.

16. J. Booz, Neutron dosimetry, radiation quality and biological dosimetry, in: "High LET Radiations in Clinical Radiotherapy," G. W. Barendsen, J. J. Broerse, and K. Breur, eds., Pergamon Press, New York (1979), pp. 147-150.

17. G. W. Barendsen, Linear and quadratic terms in dose-effect relationships for cellular responses and implications for normal tissue tolerance at small doses per fraction and low dose rates, in: "Proceedings of the Eighth Symposium on Microdosimetry," EUR 8395, J. Booz and H. G. Ebert, eds., Commission of the European Communities, Luxembourg (1983), pp. 811-821.

18. D. T. Goodhead, D. E. Charlton, W. E. Wilson, and H. G. Paretzke, Current biophysical approaches to the understanding of biological effects of radiation in terms of local energy deposition, in: "Proceedings of the Fifth Symposium on Neutron Dosimetry," EUR 9762 Commission of the European Communities Luxembourg (1985), pp. 57.68.

AUTHOR INDEX